Fitness Professional's Handbook

SIXTH EDITION

Edward T. Howley, PhD

Dixie L. Thompson, PhD

University of Tennessee at Knoxville

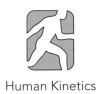

Human Kinetics

Library of Congress Cataloging-in-Publication Data

Howley, Edward T., 1943-
 Fitness professional's handbook / Edward T. Howley and Dixie L. Thompson. -- 6th ed.
  p. ; cm.
 Includes bibliographical references and index.
 ISBN 978-1-4504-1117-2 (print) -- ISBN 1-4504-1117-7 (print)
 I. Thompson, Dixie L., 1960- II. Title.
 [DNLM: 1. Exercise--physiology. 2. Physical Fitness--physiology. 3. Health Behavior. 4. Nutritional Physiological Phenomena. QT 255]

 613.7--dc23

2011043137

ISBN-10: 1-4504-1117-7
ISBN-13: 978-1-4504-1117-2

The web addresses cited in this text were current as of August 2011, unless otherwise noted.

Acquisitions Editor: Amy N. Tocco; **Developmental Editor:** Melissa J. Zavala; **Assistant Editor:** Kali Cox; **Copyeditor:** Alisha Jeddeloh; **Indexer:** Nancy Ball; **Permissions Manager:** Dalene Reeder; **Graphic Designer:** Nancy Rasmus; **Graphic Artist:** Dawn Sills; **Cover Designer:** Keith Blomberg; **Photographer (cover):** © Human Kinetics; **Photographer (interior):** © Human Kinetics, unless otherwise noted; **Photo Asset Manager:** Laura Fitch; **Visual Production Assistant:** Joyce Brumfield; **Photo Production Manager:** Jason Allen; **Art Manager:** Kelly Hendren; **Associate Art Manager:** Alan L. Wilborn; **Printer:** Courier Companies, Inc.

Printed in the United States of America   10   9   8   7   6   5

The paper in this book was manufactured using responsible forestry methods.

Human Kinetics
Website: www.HumanKinetics.com

United States: Human Kinetics
P.O. Box 5076
Champaign, IL 61825-5076
800-747-4457
e-mail: humank@hkusa.com

Canada: Human Kinetics
475 Devonshire Road Unit 100
Windsor, ON N8Y 2L5
800-465-7301 (in Canada only)
e-mail: info@hkcanada.com

Europe: Human Kinetics
107 Bradford Road
Stanningley
Leeds LS28 6AT, United Kingdom
+44 (0) 113 255 5665
e-mail: hk@hkeurope.com

Australia: Human Kinetics
57A Price Avenue
Lower Mitcham, South Australia 5062
08 8372 0999
e-mail: info@hkaustralia.com

New Zealand: Human Kinetics
P.O. Box 80
Torrens Park, South Australia 5062
0800 222 062
e-mail: info@hknewzealand.com

E5468

To Ann, for her love and support.
Ed Howley

To my parents, Jean and Felton Thompson. Thank you for your unwavering love and support. To Penny. Thank you for helping make the journey one full of adventure.
Dixie Thompson

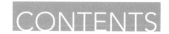CONTENTS

PART III Fitness Assessment

PART IV Exercise Prescription for Health and Fitness

PART VI Exercise Programming

You are different from most people. In all likelihood you are physically active, exercise each week, and are concerned about your fitness. In contrast, more than 60% of American adults do not engage in the recommended amounts of physical activity and are overweight. Further, the epidemic of obesity reaches right into the elementary classroom.

Your timing is perfect if you are interested in helping children, adults, or older citizens become more active and improve fitness, health, and quality of life. Support is growing in the government and private sector to do something about the problems of inactivity and obesity, and success stories already exist. This text will help you get on your way. You will learn how to screen participants for exercise programs, evaluate the various fitness components, and prescribe exercise to improve each fitness component. In addition, you will learn how to help people with chronic disease (e.g., hypertension) or specific conditions (e.g., pregnancy). Recent advances in how to approach these issues demanded a revision of the text, and we hope you enjoy the result.

Updates to the Sixth Edition

In 2008, the U.S. government published its first ever Physical Activity Guidelines for Americans. These guidelines were the result of a systematic review of research published in the area of physical activity, fitness, and health, and they provide physical activity recommendations for people of all ages, those with chronic disease, those who are pregnant, and so on. We have used that document, as well as others published by major national organizations and societies, to update the information in this edition of the text.

Given the aging of the population and the chronic diseases that accompanies it, the development of the Exercise is Medicine program by the American College of Sports Medicine (ACSM) will be of interest to many readers, be they interested in a career in fitness, allied health, or medicine. The career goals of our undergraduates at the University of Tennessee reflect this diversity of interests, with the majority choosing careers in physical therapy. The Exercise is Medicine program emphasizes the importance of communication between professionals in medicine and allied health with those in the fitness arena (and vice versa) when patients are discharged. This textbook will help that conversation along by giving you a sound foundation on which to prescribe exercise and deliver physical activity and fitness programs for various populations.

In this edition of the text, every chapter has been updated based on the latest standards, guidelines, and research, be they related to special populations or low-back pain and injury prevention. As you might expect, some chapters have required more updates than others. The chapters that received the most significant updates are the following:

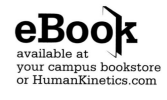

- Chapter 1, Health, Fitness, and Performance, links physical activity to health, fitness, and performance as a logical continuum of outcomes. It clarifies the distinction between moderate and vigorous physical activity in terms of health outcomes, and it deals with the importance of fitness versus fatness relative to health risk.

- Chapter 2, Health Appraisal, adds a flow chart to assist with risk stratification and determination of the need for physician consent prior to fitness testing and beginning an exercise program. A table to assist in the identification of cardiovascular, metabolic, and pulmonary diseases is also included.

- Chapter 3, Functional Anatomy and Biomechanics, has been extensively revised, with new figures, new concepts, and more focused objectives included.

- Chapter 5, Nutrition, has been updated based on the latest *Dietary Guidelines for Americans* as well as the current standards for nutritional intake, including recommended diets (e.g., MyPlate, DASH diet). A special section has been added to discuss scope of practice issues for fitness professionals.

- Chapter 6, Energy Costs of Physical Activity, has a new section on measuring physical activity and shows how to calculate exercise volume in MET-minutes.

- Chapter 8, Assessment of Body Composition, provides a comparison of the various techniques for measuring body composition and adds new photos of skinfold sites.

- Chapter 11, Exercise Prescription for Cardiorespiratory Fitness, provides details related to Exercise is Medicine, and it emphasizes progression and the use of both moderate-intensity and vigorous-intensity physical activity to realize health and fitness goals. The use of pedometers and exercise diaries is addressed as a means to increase physical activity.

- Chapter 13, Exercise Prescription for Muscular Fitness, has been updated with special attention to the most recent and relevant position stands for children, seniors, and pregnant women.

- Chapter 14, Exercise Prescription for Flexibility and Low-Back Function, provides a new emphasis on the coordination aspect of muscle function related to muscular strength and endurance.

- Chapter 15, Exercise and Children and Youth, updates the acute and chronic effects of exercise on children, adds current guidelines for children under age 5, expands the discussion of clinical exercise testing, and discusses the use of criterion-referenced fitness standards.

- Chapter 16, Exercise and Older Adults, emphasizes the use of progression in all programs for seniors, expands the discussion of balance and strength in preventing falls, and describes the role of physical activity in psychological health and well-being.

- Chapter 17, Exercise and Women's Health, provides updates on pregnancy, osteoporosis, and the female athlete triad.

- Chapter 18, Exercise and Heart Disease, shows new ways to reach patients who cannot attend traditional cardiac rehabilitation programs.

- Chapter 19, Exercise and Obesity, provides new information on medications and the treatment of obesity, the cost of obesity, and the role of physical activity.

- Chapter 20, Exercise and Diabetes, provides the latest criteria for diagnosing diabetes, common medications used by those with diabetes, and the latest exercise testing and prescription guidelines.

- Chapter 23, Behavior Change, expands the discussion of self-determination theory and describes ways to enhance exercise self-efficacy and goal setting to support changes in physical activity.

- Chapter 24, Mindful Exercise for Fitness Professionals, provides new research that supports mindful exercise as part of a regular physical activity program, expands information on the use of yoga, and describes the difficulty of evaluating the impact of such programs using conventional fitness tests.

- Chapter 27, Legal Considerations, is a completely new addition to the text. Dr. JoAnn Eickhoff-Shemek, a recognized expert on legal issues related to the fitness industry, provides an up-to-date and easy-to-read discussion of these issues.

Although many updates have been made, former users of the text will be comfortable with this new edition. The text continues to use *ACSM's Guidelines for Exercise Testing and Prescription* as a primary source of standards and expectations for fitness professionals. This has been and remains the standard-setting reference for professionals delivering fitness programs in any setting, whether club or hospital-based. Consequently, the text is helpful to those interested in taking appropriate ACSM certification exams as well as those offered by other organizations.

In addition, we have included study questions at the end of each chapter to help students review for regular examinations. This edition also includes many reproducible forms, interesting sidebars, useful key points, case study questions and answers, key terms and a glossary, and extensive references, making it a useful textbook for students as well as a valuable reference for practitioners.

Intended Audience

This text continues to be written for the upper-level undergraduate or beginning graduate student with a general background in anatomy and physiology. The purpose of the text to is enable people with limited knowledge of fitness testing and prescription to screen participants, carry out standardized fitness tests to evaluate the major components of fitness, and write appropriate fitness prescriptions. Many academic programs incorporate laboratory experiences to drive the mastery of skills needed to accomplish these tasks. In that way, the class is not simply an academic experience, but one that allows a person to move into practicum or internship experiences with the requisite skills and abilities. This text will work seamlessly with most laboratory experiences associated with fitness assessment because of its attention to detail regarding the most common fitness tests, from pretest concerns to posttest evaluation of results.

Text Organization

Part I, Activity, Health, and Fitness, contains two chapters that provide an overview of the connections among health, fitness, and performance; general information to set up the remainder of the text; and a step-by-step approach on how to screen potential participants for fitness programs.

Part II, Scientific Foundations, covers basic anatomy and biomechanics and exercise physiology, useful for a quick review. In addition, chapters are provided on nutrition assessment and how to evaluate the energy cost of activity, both of which are central to energy balance.

Part III, Fitness Assessment, provides extensive detail on how to assess cardiorespiratory fitness, body composition, flexibility, and muscular strength and endurance.

Part IV, Exercise Prescription for Health and Fitness, provides a separate chapter on how to deal with the test results for each of the fitness components assessed in part III, and it describes how to formulate an exercise prescription consistent with a client's goals and abilities.

Part V, Special Considerations, provides chapters on exercise testing and prescription for the following: children and youth, older adults, women, and people with heart disease, obesity, diabetes, or pulmonary disease.

Part VI, Exercise Programming, leads off with a chapter on general principles related to exercise programming. In addition, separate chapters are provided on successful behavioral science approaches to changing behavior, mind–body exercise programs and their benefits, exercise electrocardiograms (ECGs) and medications, injury prevention and rehabilitation, and legal considerations.

Instructor Resources

In addition to the thoroughly updated content, this edition also has several instructor resources available to aid in teaching a class with this textbook: a new instructor guide and a revised test package and presentation package.

- The new instructor guide includes a syllabus; course outlines that detail lecture topics and lab and classroom activities; initial and final practical exams, including checklists for easy grading; and a laboratory notebook that students can use to track their completion of 12 fitness assessment and programming activities.

- The test package includes more than 700 questions, including true or false, multiple choice, and short answer and essay questions.

- The Microsoft PowerPoint presentation package contains 593 slides that present the textbook material in a lecture-friendly format, including art, photos, and tables pulled from the text.

- The image bank contains all of the art, tables, content photos, and reproducible forms from the text. Instructors may print the reproducible forms and use the art, tables, and photos to create class presentations.

We hope that this book is helpful to you, whether you are using it as a textbook or a resource to help you stay up to date.

ACKNOWLEDGMENT

To Don Franks

The current emphasis on being physically active and fit is not new. Over 40 years ago Don Franks, the principal architect of this text, was immersed in research on the physiology of fitness in adults and children. He did his graduate work at the University of Illinois with T.K. Cureton, an internationally recognized 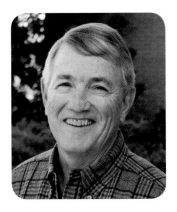 leader in fitness. Don was an active and productive scholar throughout a career that resulted in 12 books and chapters and 75 research publications. He focused his efforts on the translation of research into the improvement of exercise testing, prescription, and programming for both healthy people and those with chronic disease. His commitment to research was shown in the quality of the departments in which he served as chair (at the University of Tennessee, Louisiana State University, and the University of Maryland), in the professional organizations he served as president of (the AAHPERD Research Consortium and the American Academy of Kinesiology and Physical Education), and in his long-term work with the President's Council on Physical Fitness and Sports (PCPFS). He received the prestigious Honor Award from both the AAHPERD and the PCPFS in recognition of his contributions. Throughout his career, Don's commitment to gender and racial equality was made manifest in his hiring of faculty, recruitment and training of graduate students, and mentoring of young professionals. This commitment influenced the communities, universities, and professional societies in which he lived and worked and has had a lasting impact.

We want to add a special thank-you to Don for his leadership and dedication to making this text a reality and making sure it maintained its quality over multiple editions. We will miss his thoughtful input and support.

I also want to add a personal thank-you to Don for his friendship and support over my career. Although Don will no longer be involved with the text, I will continue to play golf and paddleball with him and listen to his funny stories.

Ed Howley

Activity, Health, and Fitness

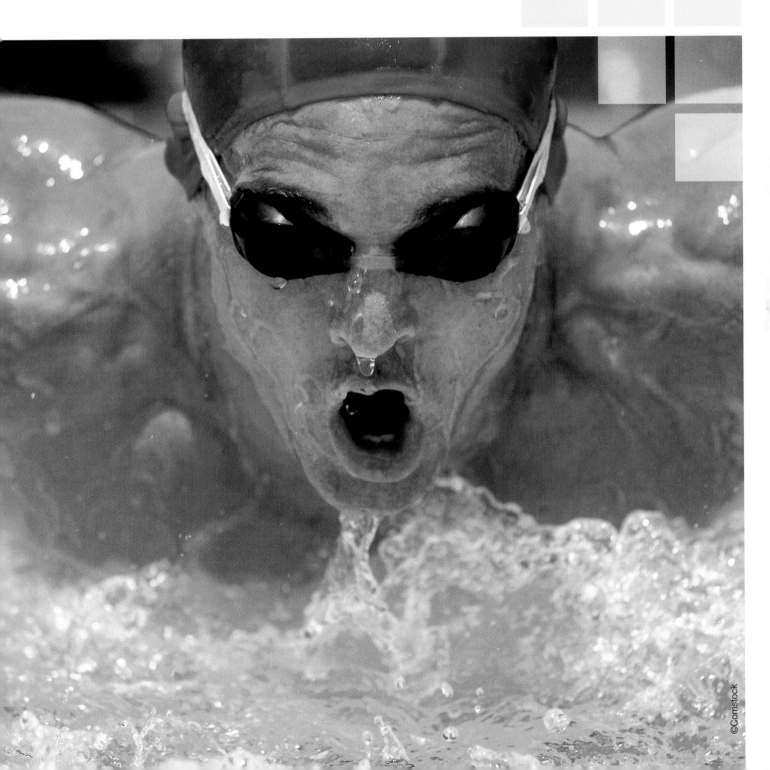

PART I

Physical activity is an essential element in health and well-being. With that in mind, we wrote this book for current and future fitness professionals who help individuals, communities, and groups gain the benefits of regular physical activity in a positive and safe environment.

The chapters of part I provide the background underlying the study of physical activity and its relevance to fitness. In chapter 1, we summarize the current evidence regarding physical activity and health, and we provide insights into the connections among health, fitness, and performance. In chapter 2 we provide a process for screening potential fitness participants and recommend criteria for medical referrals and the development of supervised and unsupervised programs.

Health, Fitness, and Performance

OBJECTIVES

The reader will be able to do the following:

1. Contrast the physical activity requirements for achieving health benefits, fitness, and performance.

2. Contrast the top three leading causes of death with the top three actual causes of death.

3. Describe the difference between absolute and relative intensity for physical activity recommendations.

4. Explain the difference between moderate-intensity and vigorous-intensity physical activity as well as how volume of physical activity is calculated.

5. List the health-related benefits gained through regular participation in physical activity.

6. Contrast the changes in physical activity guidelines over the past 40 years in terms of exercise volume, intensity, and outcomes.

7. Describe the *2008 Physical Activity Guidelines for Americans* recommendations for moderate-intensity and vigorous-intensity physical activity for realizing substantial health benefits.

8. Describe the physical activity guidelines for increasing or maintaining strength.

9. Define *adverse events*, and explain how the potential for such events affects the intensity of physical activity recommended for those who have been sedentary.

10. Describe the progression in physical activity for someone who is sedentary or someone who wishes to move from a moderate-intensity to a vigorous-intensity physical activity program.

11. Contrast fitness versus fatness as they relate to chronic disease.

12. Contrast health-related fitness components with performance-related fitness components.

13. Describe the continuum of physical activity recommendations for realizing health, fitness, and performance goals.

One of the main questions we address throughout this text is "How much exercise is enough?" In order to answer that question, we must first address another: "Enough for what?" In other words, what is the goal of the exercise program? Is it fitness, **performance**, or avoidance of disease? As figure 1.1 shows, the amount and intensity of physical activity needed to realize each goal is quite different, representing a continuum from low to high volume and from moderate to vigorous (hard) intensity. On the left side of the figure, we see that avoidance of disease (e.g., lowering the risk of heart disease, type 2 diabetes, and so on) can be achieved with moderate-intensity activity done 30 min · day^{-1}, 5 days · wk^{-1}. To achieve **cardiorespiratory fitness (CRF)**, as well as the health benefits associated with moderate-intensity physical activity, vigorous-intensity exercise is done 3 to 4 days · wk^{-1}, 30 to 45 min · day^{-1}, which is equivalent to jogging or running about 3 mi (4.8 km) 3 to 4 days · wk^{-1}. What about those who want to be elite marathon runners? In contrast to the previous two examples, those interested in being elite marathon runners must work at the extreme end of the intensity scale (very hard) for hours every day. Few elite marathoners run less than 100 mi (170 km) per week (11), which is about 10 times what is needed to achieve a reasonable level of CRF.

We begin with this example because this text focuses on the amount of physical activity and exercise needed for health and fitness rather than on the performance of elite athletes. That said, the information on nutrition, CRF, body composition, strength, and flexibility forms the foundation for those wanting to achieve performance-related goals. In this chapter we discuss how physical activity is connected to health, fitness, and performance. Later chapters provide more extensive detail about how to help sedentary individuals become active and realize the many benefits of a physically active lifestyle.

Health and Avoidance of Disease

What does being healthy mean? For some it is the simple avoidance of disease, but it is also more than that. **Health** has been defined as a human condition possessing social, psychological, and physical dimensions. **Positive health** is associated with a capacity to enjoy life and withstand challenges. **Negative health** is associated with morbidity (incidence of disease) and premature mortality (34). The highest quality of life includes mental alertness and curiosity, positive emotional feelings, meaningful relationships with others, awareness and involvement in societal strivings, recognition of the broader forces of life, and the physical capacity to accomplish personal goals with vigor. These aspects of positive health are interrelated; a high level of accomplishment in one area enhances the other areas, and, conversely, a low level of function in any area restricts the accomplishments possible in other areas. Although physical activity plays a major role in the physical dimension, it also contributes to learning, relationships, and a sense of human limitations within the broader perspective. An optimal quality of life requires individuals to strive, grow, and develop, though they may never achieve the highest level of positive health. What are the risks or challenges to our health and well being?

Factors Affecting Health and Disease

The five leading causes of death in the United States in 2007 were cardiovascular diseases (CVD) (31.0%), cancers (23.2%), chronic lower-respiratory diseases (5.3%), accidents (5.1%), and Alzheimer's disease (3.1%) (35). Although infectious diseases are not in the top five, we are warned each year to make sure that our flu shots and other vaccinations are up to date in order to prevent a problem

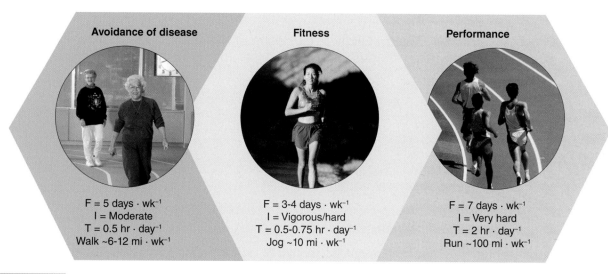

Avoidance of disease

F = 5 days · wk^{-1}
I = Moderate
T = 0.5 hr · day^{-1}
Walk ~6-12 mi · wk^{-1}

Fitness

F = 3-4 days · wk^{-1}
I = Vigorous/hard
T = 0.5-0.75 hr · day^{-1}
Jog ~10 mi · wk^{-1}

Performance

F = 7 days · wk^{-1}
I = Very hard
T = 2 hr · day^{-1}
Run ~100 mi · wk^{-1}

FIGURE 1.1 How much physical activity is enough?

Photos 2 and 3: © Photodisc/Getty Images

from occurring. Most of the top five leading causes of death are chronic degenerative diseases whose onset can be delayed or prevented. Risk factors associated with chronic diseases can be divided into three categories (see figure 1.2) (38).

Inherited or Biological Factors

These factors include the following:

- Age—older adults have more chronic diseases than younger people.
- Gender—men develop CVD at an earlier age than women, but women experience more strokes than men (6).
- Race—African Americans develop about 30% more heart disease than non-Hispanic white Americans (36).
- Susceptibility to disease—several diseases have a genetic component that increases the potential for having them.

People can achieve health and fitness goals up to their genetic potential, but it is not possible to establish the relative portion of a person's health that is determined by heredity. Although heredity influences physical activity, fitness, and health (27), most people can lead healthy or unhealthy lives regardless of their genetic makeup. Thus, genetic background neither dooms a person to poor health nor guarantees good health.

Environment

We are born not only with fixed genetic potentials but also into environments that affect our development. An environment includes physical factors (e.g., climate, water, altitude, pollution), socioeconomic factors (e.g., income, housing, education, workplace characteristics), and family (e.g., parental values, divorce, extended family, friends) that affect our opportunities to be active, level of fitness, and health status. Some elements, such as our nutrition or the air we breathe and water we drink, affect us directly. Other elements, such as the values and behaviors of people we admire, influence our lifestyles indirectly. We can control certain aspects of our environments; for instance, we choose many of the mental and physical activities we undertake. However, our past and current environments affect us in various ways. For example, some children have inadequate food because of their environment and cannot think about other aspects of health until that basic need is fulfilled.

Behaviors

We have discussed the leading causes of death, but what are the *actual causes* of death? The list of behaviors in figure 1.2 helps answer that question. That smoking is at the top of the list should be no surprise given its connection to both lung cancer and CVD. In fact, it is the number one actual cause of death, accounting for 18% of all deaths (23, 24). The existence of smoking-cessation programs and laws to restrict areas in which one can smoke speak to the seriousness with which our society takes that risk to health. The number two actual cause of death is poor diet and physical inactivity (15.2%), with alcohol consumption coming in at number three (3.5%). The emphasis on healthy eating at work and school and the creation of new parks and bike trails to enhance opportunities to be physically active are examples of responses to these actual causes of death. Figure 1.3 shows that healthy eating and physical activity affect a large number of factors that influence health and disease. Clearly, your ability to help establish and reinforce the behaviors of healthy eating and physical activity in the people you serve during your professional life will do much to improve their health and well-being. (See chapter 5 for information on nutrition and chapter 23 for steps to help clients change their behaviors.) This chapter introduces the role that physical activity and fitness play in a healthy lifestyle. However, before we begin, we need to review a few terms that will be important in the following sections of this chapter.

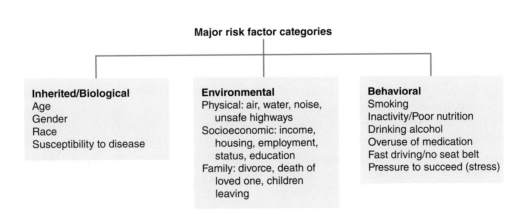

FIGURE 1.2 Major categories of risk factors with examples of each.

Reprinted from Healthy People, 1979, *The Surgeon General's report on health promotion and disease prevention.*

HE	Health benefits	PA
✓	Lowers risk for heart disease	✓
✓	Reduces risk for certain cancers	✓
✓	Lowers blood pressure	✓
✓	Improves lipid profile	✓
✓	Prevents obesity	✓
✓	Prevents diabetes	✓
✓	Builds healthy bones	✓
✓	Enhances immune function	✓
?	Relieves stress, improves mood, promotes self-esteem	✓
X	Increases functional health	✓

FIGURE 1.3 Effect of healthy eating (HE) and physical activity (PA) on health benefits.
Reprinted, by permission, from R.A. Carpenter.

Important Definitions

We will introduce you to key terms as we move through the chapters of the text; however, we need to begin here in order to facilitate your understanding of the various parts of an exercise prescription or physical activity recommendation (9, 33, 34).

- **Physical activity** is defined as any bodily movement produced by skeletal muscle that results in energy expenditure (e.g., it is associated with occupation, leisure time, household chores, and sport).

- **Exercise** is a subset of physical activity that is planned, structured, and repetitive and has the objective of improving or maintaining physical fitness.

- **Physical fitness** refers to a set of health- or skill-related attributes that can be measured by specific tests.

- **Health-related fitness** refers to muscular strength and endurance, CRF, flexibility, and body composition (relative leanness).

- **Skill-related (performance-related) fitness** refers to agility, balance, coordination, speed, power, and reaction time that are linked to games, sport, dance, and so on.

- Exercise **intensity** describes the rate of work (i.e., how much energy is being expended per minute)

and the degree of effort required to carry out the task. The rate of work is the **absolute intensity** and can be expressed in a number of ways: kilocalories (kcal) of energy produced per min (kcal · min^{-1}), milliliters of oxygen consumed per kilogram of body weight per minute (ml · kg^{-1} · min^{-1}), or metabolic equivalents (METs), where one MET is taken as resting metabolic rate and is equal to 3.5 ml · kg^{-1} · min^{-1}. Walking at 3 mi · hr^{-1} (4.8 km · hr^{-1}) requires 3.3 METs (11.5 ml · kg^{-1} · min^{-1}), and jogging at 6 mi · hr^{-1} (9.7 km · hr^{-1}) requires 10 METs (35 ml · kg^{-1} · min^{-1}). You will see more on this in chapter 6.

- **Relative intensity** describes the degree of effort required to expend that energy and is influenced by maximal aerobic power or cardiovascular fitness ($\dot{V}O_2$max). Relative intensity can be expressed as a percentage of $\dot{V}O_2$max or a percentage of maximal heart rate (HRmax). You will see more on this in chapter 11.

- **Moderate intensity** refers to an absolute intensity of 3 to 5.9 METs and a relative intensity of 40% to 59% $\dot{V}O_2$max or 64% to 76% HRmax.

- **Vigorous intensity** refers to an absolute intensity of 6 or more METs and a relative intensity of 60% to 84% $\dot{V}O_2$max or 77% to 93% HRmax.

- **Frequency** refers to the number of days per week physical activity is done.

- **Duration** refers to the amount of time a physical activity is done.
- **Volume** refers to the total amount of energy expended or work accomplished in an activity, and it is equal to the product of the absolute intensity, frequency, and time. For example, a person expending 5 kcal · min⁻¹ for 20 min on 3 days · wk⁻¹ will have an exercise volume of 300 kcal · wk⁻¹ (5 kcal · min⁻¹ × 20 min · day⁻¹ × 3 days · wk⁻¹). The volume can also be expressed using the MET scale: A 10 MET activity done 3 days · wk⁻¹ for 20 min · day⁻¹ generates a volume of 600 MET-min · wk⁻¹ (10 METs × 3 days · wk⁻¹ × 20 min · day⁻¹).

Physical Activity and Health

From the beginning of recorded history, philosophers and health professionals have observed that regular physical activity is an essential part of a healthy life. Hippocrates wrote the following in *On Regimen in Acute Diseases,* about 400 BC:

> Eating alone will not keep a man [woman] well; he [she] must also take exercise. For food and exercise, while possessing opposite qualities, yet work together to produce health. . . . And it is necessary, as it appears, to discern the power of various exercises, both natural exercises and artificial, to know which of them tends to increase flesh and which to lessen it; and not only this, but also to proportion exercise to bulk of food, to the constitution of the patient, to the age of the individual . . . (21)

Over the past four decades, thousands of studies have examined the relationship between physical activity and the risk of various diseases and death. The overwhelming conclusion is that regular participation in physical activity results in a reduced risk of numerous diseases and death from all causes. As shown in figure 1.4, regular participation in physical activity reduces the risk of death from all causes by about 40% (relative risk decreased from 1.0 to 0.6). Doing physical activity on a regular basis also has been shown to have a similar impact on the following (33):

- Cardiorespiratory health: Physical activity reduces the risk of heart disease and stroke, lowers blood pressure (BP), improves the blood lipid profile, and increases CRF.
- Metabolic health: Physical activity reduces the risk of developing type 2 diabetes and helps to control blood glucose in those who already have type 2 diabetes.
- Musculoskeletal health: Physical activity slows the loss of bone density that occurs with aging, and it lowers the risk of hip fractures. In addition, it improves pain management in people with arthritis. Finally, progressive

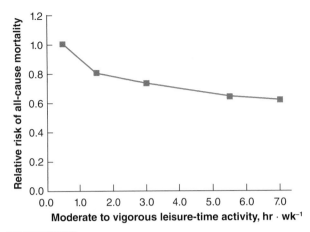

FIGURE 1.4 Dose–response of physical activity related to all-cause mortality.

Reprinted from U.S. Department of Health and Human Services, 2008, *Physical activity guidelines advisory report.*

muscle-strengthening activities increase or preserve muscle mass, strength, and power.

- Cancer: Physically active people have a significantly lower risk of colon cancer and breast cancer. In addition, there is some evidence that physical activity reduces the risk of endometrial cancer and lung cancer.
- Mental health: Physical activity lowers the risk of depression and age-related cognitive decline, and it improves the quality of sleep.
- Functional ability and fall prevention: Physical activity reduces the risk of functional limitations (e.g., ability to do activities of daily living), and for those older adults at risk of falling, physical activity is safe and reduces this risk.

Physical Activity Guidelines

Given the large number of benefits derived from participation in physical activity, it should be no surprise that professional societies such as the American College of Sports Medicine (ACSM), the American Heart Association (AHA), and various governmental agencies (e.g., Centers for Disease Control and Prevention [CDC]) have developed physical activity guidelines for the general public. The following paragraphs provide a brief overview showing how the focus of these guidelines shifted from fitness to public health outcomes and finally to obesity over the past 40 years.

Vigorous Exercise, Fitness, and Health

In the early and mid-1970s, three major organizations published guidelines or recommendations for improving fitness and health:

1. In 1972, the AHA published *Exercise Testing and Training of Apparently Healthy Individuals: A Handbook for Physicians* (5). The exercise prescription was to begin at 75% HRmax for 15 to 20 min, 3 days · wk⁻¹.

2. In 1973, the YMCA published it first edition of *The Y's Way to Physical Fitness* (16). The exercise prescription was to exercise at 80% $\dot{V}O_2$max for 40 to 45 min, 3 days · wk⁻¹.

3. In 1975, ACSM published the first edition of *ACSM's Guidelines for Exercise Testing and Prescription* (1). The exercise prescription was to exercise at ~70% to 90% $\dot{V}O_2$max for 20 to 45 min, 3 to 5 days · wk⁻¹.

In each case the focus was on higher-intensity exercise, with both CRF and health outcomes being important.

Volume of Physical Activity and Health Outcomes

In 1978, ACSM published its first position stand (2): "The Recommended Quantity and Quality of Exercise for Developing and Maintaining Fitness in Healthy Adults." The focus was on improving CRF as well as achieving health outcomes. The emphasis was again on higher-intensity exercise to achieve these goals. However, in that same year, a now classic study on Harvard alumni by Paffenbarger, Wing, and Hyde (25) showed a 36% lower risk of developing a heart attack in those who accumulated 2,000 kilocalories or more of leisure-time physical activity per week (that did not have to be done at a high intensity). This study and many that followed shifted the focus to three variables associated with physical activity guidelines:

- Activity volume (e.g., kilocalories expended) rather than intensity

- Health outcomes (e.g., reduced risk of heart attack) rather than CRF

- Leisure activity rather than structured exercise programs

Throughout the 1980s there was a growing body of research showing a strong relationship between regular participation in physical activity and a lower risk of chronic disease. It became clear that we needed to rethink our understanding of how physical activity and exercise were linked to a reduced risk of chronic disease (7-9). Dr. William Haskell took a leadership role in helping us to understand the potential links among physical activity, fitness, and health (17, 18). Figure 1.5 shows the following:

- In our earliest understanding, we thought that physical activity improved fitness, which, in turn, was linked to improved health outcomes (number 1).

- However, it was just as likely that physical activity could improve health and fitness separately and by different mechanisms (number 2).

- Lastly, some physical activity programs could improve fitness and not health outcomes, and vice versa (numbers 3 and 4).

These distinctions helped shape our understanding of how physical activity is connected to fitness and health outcomes, that is, physical activity could achieve health outcomes independent of fitness.

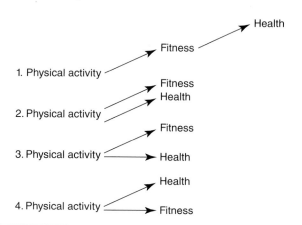

FIGURE 1.5 Possible causal relations among physical activity, physical fitness, and health.

Reprinted, by permission, from W.L. Haskell, 1994, Dose-response issues from a biological perspective. In *Physical activity, fitness, and health: International proceedings and concensus statement*, edited by C. Bouchard, R. J. Shephard, and T. Stevens (Champaign, IL: Human Kinetics) 1031; Adapted from *American Journal of Cardiology*, Vol. 55, W. Haskell, pg. 5D, "Physical activity and health: The need to define the required stimulus," Copyright 1984, with permission of Elsevier.

One of the most important decisions that accelerated the drive to promote physical activity in a public health context occurred in 1992, when the AHA made physical inactivity a major risk factor for CVD, the same as smoking, high BP, and high serum cholesterol (15). Following up on that important decision, in 1995 the ACSM and CDC published their public health physical activity recommendation to reduce the risk of chronic disease (26): Every U.S. adult should accumulate 30 min or more of moderate-intensity physical activity on most, preferably all, days of the week. The shift in focus was clearly spelled out, with exercise volume (total kilocalories expended) being crucial and somewhat independent of intensity (as long as it was equal to or higher than moderate intensity). It is important to remember that this was a minimum recommendation (*at least* 30 min, 5 times a week) for realizing health benefits. In the following year, the Surgeon General's *Report on Physical Activity and Health* was published (32). This document supported the 1995 ACSM and CDC statement and brought even more attention to the need for Americans to become physically active. The emphasis on physical activity from a public health perspective also was incorporated into *ACSM's Guidelines for Exercise Testing and Prescription*, which is revised every 5 years.

Physical Activity and Obesity

The United States and many other industrialized countries have seen an incredible increase in the prevalence of overweight and obesity over the last 20 years. In the United States, 32.3% of men and 35.5% of women are obese, with combined overweight and obesity prevalence being 68% and 72.3%, respectively (14). The increase in obesity during the 1990s prompted the Institute of Medicine (IOM) to evaluate the research on how much physical activity was needed to prevent weight gain (20). The IOM recommended 60 min of moderate-intensity activity to prevent weight gain and achieve the full health benefits of physical activity, twice the amount that ACSM and the CDC recommended for reducing the risk of chronic diseases. This was supported by recommendations from the International Association for the Study of Obesity (IASO) to do 45 to 60 min of physical activity to prevent weight gain (29) and the International Obesity Task Force (IOTF) recommendation of 60 to 90 min of activity to prevent weight regain in those who have lost a great deal of weight (12). In 2005, the *Dietary Guidelines for Americans* endorsed the ACSM and CDC recommendation of 30 min of physical activity to reduce the risk of chronic diseases, the IOM recommendation of 60 min to prevent weight gain, and the IOTF recommendation of 60 to 90 min to sustain weight loss (37).

Current Physical Activity Guidelines

As you can imagine, there was confusion among both fitness professionals and the general public about how much activity was enough. Which was it—30, 60, or 90 min? Was moderate-intensity activity the only way to achieve these various goals? In 2007, ACSM and the AHA published an updated position stand on physical activity and health that addressed some of these questions (19):

- Moderate or vigorous: The position stand supported the 1995 minimum recommendation of 30 min of moderate-intensity activity 5 days a week for reducing the risk of chronic disease. However, one could do 20 min of vigorous-intensity activity 3 days a week to achieve the same goal or do some combination of both.

- More is better: Doing more than the minimum (e.g., doing 60 min of moderate-intensity activity 5 days a week) increases health benefits.

This brief historical tour through physical activity recommendations shows how guidelines change as we learn more about the effects of physical activity. The review also provides a jumping-off point for the most recent and comprehensive series of recommendations that affects much of what is presented in this text. The U.S. Department of Health and Human Services published *Physical Activity Guidelines for Americans* in 2008—the first set of national physical activity recommendations related to health and fitness (33). This document was based on an extensive review of the literature that was carried out by an advisory committee (34). These guidelines provide physical activity recommendations for children and adolescents, adults, older adults (65 yr and older), women during and following pregnancy, people with disabilities, and people with chronic medical conditions. You will read more about the specific guidelines for each of these populations as you move through the textbook; however, the following findings from the advisory committee's report are provided to help prepare you for what is ahead (34):

- Substantial health-related benefits occur at a volume of activity in the range of 500 to 1,000 MET-min $\cdot$ wk^{-1}. If you did a brisk walk at a moderate intensity of 3.5 METs for 150 min, you would meet the low end of that range (3.5 METs $\cdot$ 150 min $\cdot$ wk^{-1} = 525 MET-min$\cdot$ wk^{-1}). Another person could do vigorous activity at 7 METs for half that time and accomplish the same volume of activity.

   One min of vigorous-intensity physical activity is equal to 2 min at a moderate intensity. This is important because moderate-intensity activity accommodates the fitness levels of most individuals, and a fit person who can do vigorous-intensity activity can accomplish the recommended volume in a shorter time.

- Many health outcomes follow a dose–response relationship with physical activity, meaning that, in general, more is better (see the later section on adverse events).

- For those who cannot meet the lower end of the guideline, it is recommended that they be as active as they can; some activity is better than none.

- The health-related benefits of physical activity are independent of body weight, so overweight and obese adults should engage in a program of regular physical activity regardless of whether weight is being lost.

In spite of what we know about the effects of physical activity on health, we have not been very successful in helping individuals begin and maintain a physically active lifestyle. This is shown in figure 1.6, which reports physical activity done by adults in the United States between 1997 and 2006 (34). As you can see, only 30% to 35% of adults report doing regular moderate or vigorous physical activity that meets current recommendations. Forty percent of adults report doing no leisure-time physical activity, and only 10% to 20% report doing muscle-strengthening activities. Looking at the flatness of these lines over the years, it is clear that fitness professionals have had little success in getting more adults to become and remain physically active. Our work is cut out for us.

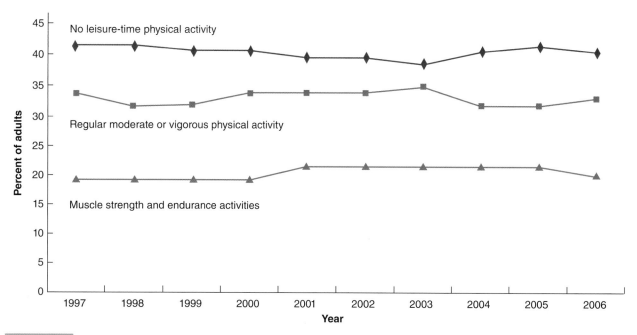

FIGURE 1.6 Reported physical activity by adults in the United States: 1997 to 2006.

Reprinted from U.S. Department of Health and Human Services, 2008, *Physical Activity Guidelines Advisory Committee report.*

Strength Training

In the previous discussion, little was said about muscular-strengthening activities because the vast majority of studies examining the relationship between physical activity and chronic disease have measured only aerobic activity. That said, ACSM has recommended exercises to enhance muscular strength and endurance since their 1990 position stand (3), and that has remained the case since then. As you might expect, the *2008 Physical Activity Guidelines for Americans* also provided guidelines for improving muscular strength and endurance. Recommendations include the following (19, 33):

- Do 8 to 10 exercises for the major muscle groups: legs, hips, back, chest, shoulders, and arms.

- To maximize strength development, use a resistance that allows 8 to 12 repetitions (number of times each lift is done in one set) of each exercise, at which point fatigue is experienced.

- One set of each exercise is sufficient, although more can be gained with 2 or 3 sets.

- Do resistance training on 2 or more nonconsecutive days each week.

There is no question that muscular strength and endurance activities provide benefits, including improvements in muscle mass, strength, and bone health (33). But there is also evidence that resistance training is associated with a lower risk of all-cause mortality, potentially linked to the role that increased muscle mass plays in glucose metabolism (19), as well as a lower risk of cancer mortality (28). Individuals need adequate muscular strength and endurance

to be able to carry out activities of daily living (ADLs), do leisure activities (e.g., gardening, mowing, sport), and realize performance goals. An increase in muscle mass has implications beyond sport performance, since muscle mass determines to a large extent the number of calories expended per day (see chapter 12). This is tied to energy balance and the ability to maintain body weight as we age. In addition, adequate endurance of the muscles in the trunk (core) is important to reduce the risk of low-back pain (see chapter 14). As strength declines with aging, the ability of older adults to maintain an independent lifestyle is compromised (see chapter 16). The evaluation of muscular strength and endurance is discussed in chapter 9, and the design of programs to improve muscular strength and endurance is presented in chapter 13.

Adverse Events

In contrast to the many benefits of participating in physical activity, there is also the potential for an adverse outcome: an injury or medical complication (e.g., heart attack). Figure 1.7 captures the potential for risk associated with exercise. The risk of musculoskeletal injuries increases with the amount of activity done (i.e., more risk for someone jogging 30 mi [48 km] a week compared with 10 mi [16 km] a week). In addition, participation in collision sports has a higher injury risk than participation in non-collision sports. Cardiac events such as a heart attack or sudden death are rare, but this risk is higher when someone becomes more active than usual, emphasizing the need for a progressive introduction to physical activity.

The risk of cardiovascular problems during exercise is directly related to the severity of preexisting heart disease. The risk of exercise testing is low, based on a mixed population of subjects, with about 6 cardiac events per 10,000 tests. The fact that most of these tests were symptom-limited tests indicates that the risk is lower when submaximal tests are used. As mentioned, the risk of death is higher during vigorous activity (about 1 per year for every 15,000 to 18,000 people) and for sedentary individuals who perform unaccustomed or infrequent exercise (4). The good news, as shown in figure 1.7, is that healthy people have a low risk of adverse events when participating in moderate-intensity physical activity such as brisk walking (33). To reduce the risks associated with exercise testing and participation in physical activity programs, you will learn how to

- screen individuals using health-risk questionnaires (chapter 2),
- measure important physiological variables at rest before taking exercise tests (chapters 7, 8, 10), and
- gradually progress a sedentary individual through a physical activity program (chapters 11, 13, 14, 22).

KEY POINT

Current physical activity guidelines recommend both moderate-intensity and vigorous-intensity aerobic physical activity to realize substantial health benefits and strengthening exercises to help maintain muscle mass and bone health. These recommendations have evolved as a result of a growing research base that shows beyond any doubt the substantial health benefits that can be realized through regular physical activity.

Fitness

Figure 1.1 presented health (avoidance of disease), fitness, and performance as three distinct goals, with a physical activity recommendation tied to each. It should be clear at this point, however, that health and fitness goals are not so much distinct as connected. They are two sides of the same coin—a coin that represents an investment in achieving health outcomes through regular participation in physical activity. As previously stated, health outcomes are realized by doing a minimum of

- 150 min · wk^{-1} of moderate-intensity physical activity, or
- 75 min · wk^{-1} of vigorous-intensity physical activity.

The vigorous-intensity recommendation is the traditional exercise prescription for increasing or maintaining CRF. Are there any benefits to doing vigorous- versus moderate-intensity physical activity?

Moderate- Versus Vigorous-Intensity Activity

Swain and Franklin (31) addressed this question in a systematic review of the literature examining the relationship of physical activity to the incidence of **coronary heart disease (CHD)** and risk factors for CHD. In their review, it was important to control for the total energy expenditure associated with the physical activity in order to accurately compare the difference between moderate-intensity and vigorous-intensity activity (since for any duration of vigorous activity, more energy would be expended compared with moderate-intensity activity). Their findings follow.

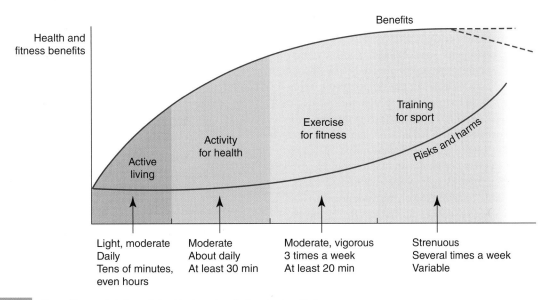

FIGURE 1.7 Benefits and risks related to levels of physical activity.

From van Sluijs, Verhagen, van der Beek, van Poppel, van Mechelen, 2003, Risks of physical activity. In *Perspectives on health and exercise*, edited by J. McKenna and C. Riddoch (United Kingdom: Palgrave Macmillan), 112. Reproduced with permission from Palgrave MacMillan.

- The vast majority of epidemiological studies found a greater reduction in the risk of CVD with vigorous-intensity (≥6 METs) than with moderate-intensity (3-5.9 METs) physical activity. In addition, more favorable risk-factor profiles were observed for individuals engaged in vigorous- as opposed to moderate-intensity activity.

- Clinical intervention studies generally showed greater improvement in diastolic blood pressure (DBP), glucose control, and CRF after vigorous-intensity physical activity versus moderate-intensity activity. However, there was no intensity effect on improvements in systolic blood pressure (SBP), blood lipid profile, or body-fat loss.

Thus, although moderate-intensity physical activity was good, vigorous-intensity activity was better. In addition, one can obtain faster and larger gains in CRF with vigorous-intensity exercise programs (see chapter 11). However, as mentioned, fitness professionals must use good judgment when working with individual clients, recognizing that vigorous-intensity exercise is associated with more adverse events and that some clients may simply wish to stay with a successful moderate-intensity program that meets their needs than progress to a vigorous-intensity exercise program.

Fitness or Fatness: Which Is More Important?

Some investigators, notably Dr. Steven Blair and associates with the Aerobics Research Institute in Dallas, have used CRF as an index of physical activity, reasoning that more active individuals would have higher levels of CRF. Many of the classic studies linking physical activity to various health outcomes have used this approach and have both confirmed and expanded on what we know from research that uses questionnaires or objective measures of physical activity (e.g., pedometers or accelerometers) to obtain information on the activity levels of individuals. The advantage of using CRF as a measure of physical activity is that it can be objectively determined using treadmill or cycle ergometer tests (see chapter 7), and it is easily tracked over time. Having information on CRF as a measure of physical activity also allows us to ask another question: Which is more important in terms of health status, having a higher level of physical activity or having a lower body fatness?

This is no small question given our attention to the obesity epidemic. As we will see in chapters 8, 12, and 19, obesity is linked to a variety of chronic diseases. However, from a health-promotion perspective, should we focus more on getting people to be physically active or on achieving a normal body weight? Figure 1.8 is an example of the kind of data that allow one to separate the impact of fitness from fatness (10). In this study, investigators measured

the CRF and body fatness of individuals with diabetes and then followed them over time to determine how many died from CVD. Those who had a high fitness score and were at a normal body weight were used as the reference group to compare with the others; this group was assigned a risk value of 1.0. As you can see, for the normal-weight group, those who had low fitness levels had about a four-fold greater risk of dying from CVD compared with those who had high fitness levels, indicating the importance of being fit. This was also true for the other weight classes. In contrast, as you look across the figure, moving from normal weight to overweight and then to obese has little impact on the risk of dying from CVD in this group of subjects. Similar observations have been made for a wide variety of health outcomes (13, 22, 30). In addition, recent work shows that a change in fitness, not fatness, is the best predictor of future health outcomes.

The message is clear: Being physically active provides substantial health benefits independent of body weight. This is consistent with a central theme of the Physical Activity Guidelines for Americans: Health-related benefits of physical activity occur in people of all body weights and whether one is gaining or losing weight. The primary focus, then, should be on getting people physically active so they can realize the health benefits and then deal with body-weight concerns as the physical activity program is being established. This is a powerful message to current and future fitness professionals.

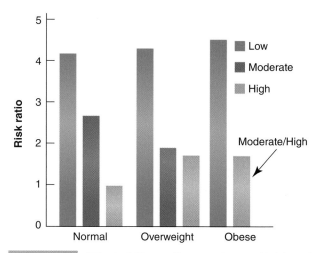

FIGURE 1.8 Effect of fitness (low, moderate, high) and fatness on the risk of death from CVD in men with diabetes.
Based on Church et al. 2005.

Performance

The term *performance* means different things to different people. At its most basic level, it means being able to complete daily tasks efficiently; at a higher level, it speaks to an ability to engage successfully in sport-related performance.

Completing Daily Tasks

To get through the day efficiently, we must have fundamental motor skills that allow us to accomplish various tasks. We must be able to move from place to place and push, pull, pick up, carry, and perform other tasks requiring the hands and arms. Moderate levels of **muscular strength** and **endurance**, **flexibility**, **body composition** or **relative leanness**, and CRF are essential for these routine tasks. In addition, we need special abilities to perform the unique activities related to work or home. The term *functional fitness* has entered our vocabulary to describe fitness programming that uses a variety of exercises to simulate tasks individuals do routinely, rather than using traditional aerobic or resistance training exercises.

Achieving Desired Sport Performance

Some clients may want to engage in selected games, sports, and high-level physical performances. In addition to requiring good physical fitness, these activities require specific motor abilities (such as agility, balance, coordination, power, and speed) as well as the particular skills of the sport. Given that it is beyond the scope of this textbook to discuss sport performance, we direct the interested reader to the Human Kinetics website (www.humankinetics.com) for information on publications dealing with the performance of virtually all sports.

Performance Components

Appropriate CRF, body composition, muscular strength and endurance, and flexibility allow people to achieve performance goals. First, modest levels of these fitness components increase the efficiency with which we can perform daily tasks around the home, in the yard, and at work. Although successful daily living is important at all ages, it is a top priority for the elderly because it allows them to live independently.

Second, higher levels of these fitness components also support successful participation in sport and performance activities. Although an individual can attain health and fitness goals through other activities, sports and games are enjoyable health and fitness supplements. In addition to requiring basic fitness, each sport places unique demands on energy, body composition, strength, endurance, and flexibility, and each requires specific skills. Many sports demand **agility**, **balance**, **coordination**, **power**, and **speed**.

Because most of this book deals with health and fitness, the following example illustrates the differing needs for meeting the two performance goals. As discussed, the first goal is to complete daily tasks efficiently. Most people move around during the day, bending, lifting, carrying, pushing, and pulling, all of which require appropriate CRF, muscular strength and endurance, flexibility, and

body leanness. In addition, a person's lifestyle adds other needs. Contrast, for example, a computer programmer, a firefighter, and a parent staying at home with an infant. The computer programmer needs stretching and relaxation activities to prevent low-back and postural problems and can benefit from short activity breaks. The firefighter is sedentary for most of the time but must be able to respond quickly with near-maximal levels of anaerobic energy and muscular strength and endurance, all within an adverse environment with heavy equipment. Thus, this person must engage in regular vigorous aerobic, anaerobic, and resistance exercise to maintain the conditioning necessary to respond to emergencies. The parent needs flexibility, strength, and endurance to lift and carry the infant and other items through an obstacle course of toys, clothes, and so on, in addition to learning to perform under sleep deprivation.

The second performance goal is to achieve desired levels in selected sports, games, and competitions. Although high fitness levels are desirable as an athletic base, individuals also have specific needs in this area. Compare, for example, 10K runners, basketball players, and golfers. The runners rely on aerobic power that comes from lots of distance running, with careful stretching before and after. Basketball players depend on aerobic and anaerobic energy, coordination, and specific passing, shooting, and defensive skills. Golfers require a moderate cardiorespiratory base, some muscular power, and coordination of a complex skill used in a variety of settings (e.g., fairway, bunker, woods).

KEY POINT

Being physically fit (achieving appropriate levels of CRF, body composition, strength, and flexibility) is linked to a low risk of health problems and an improved ability to engage in daily tasks with adequate energy. A higher level of these fitness components is associated with sport performance, along with attention to the unique skills related to each sport or game.

Pulling It All Together

We end this chapter where we began, with the question of how much exercise is enough (see figure 1.9). At this point you know that the goals of health, fitness, and performance represent a continuum of outcomes that result from regular participation in physical activity and exercise. It is clear that participation in both moderate- and vigorous-intensity physical activity is associated with numerous substantial health benefits and improvement in the various fitness components of CRF, body fatness, flexibility, and strength. Achieving a level of fitness is a first step in the quest to realizing performance-related goals. The progression from moderate-intensity physical activity to structured vigorous

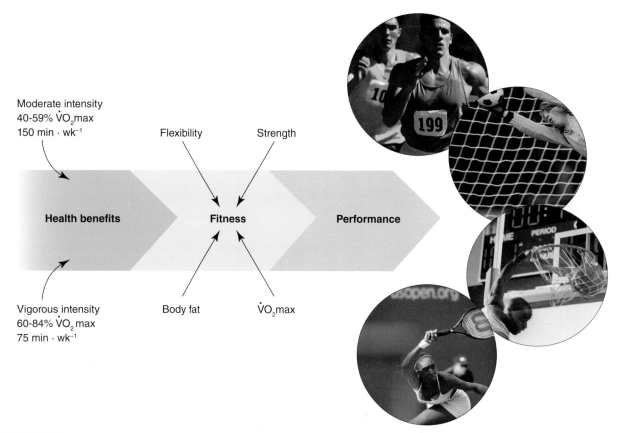

FIGURE 1.9 The continuum of health, fitness, and performance outcomes linked to physical activity.
Photos 1, 2, and 3: © Comstock

exercise programs and then sports and games reflects a logical and appropriate pathway that minimizes risk and maximizes the chance of success along the way.

One of the most frustrating yet exciting aspects of dealing with health problems is that individuals can modify their health status and control major health risks. The frustrating side is that many people find it difficult to change an unhealthy lifestyle. The exciting element is that they can gain control of their health. Fitness professionals are at the cutting edge of health in much the same way the scientists discovering vaccines for major diseases were at the turn of the 20th century. The opportunity to help people alter their unhealthy lifestyles carries the responsibility of making recommendations based on the best scientific evidence available. This text will lead you through the steps

KEY POINT

Fitness professionals live in an exciting time because of the increasing evidence and recognition that regular physical activity is essential to a good life. It is a worthwhile challenge to motivate people to begin and continue an active lifestyle, especially when there is so much competition for everyone's time.

to evaluate health-related risk factors and behaviors, test the various fitness components, and prescribe exercise to improve each.

STUDY QUESTIONS

1. What is the difference in the physical activity requirements for achieving health benefits, fitness, and performance?
2. List the top three leading causes of death and compare them with the behaviors linked to the top three actual causes of death.
3. What is the difference between absolute and relative intensity?
4. What is moderate-intensity and vigorous-intensity physical activity in terms of METs?
5. Calculate the volume of physical activity done per week for someone exercising at 5 METs for 40 min · day^{-1}, 3 days · wk^{-1}.

6. How does regular participation in physical activity affect the top two leading causes of death?

7. What are the *2008 Physical Activity Guidelines for Americans* moderate-intensity and vigorous-intensity physical activity recommendations for realizing substantial health benefits?

8. Describe the physical activity guidelines for increasing or maintaining strength.

9. What are adverse events, and how can they be minimized?

10. What does progression mean for someone wishing to move from a moderate-intensity to a vigorous-intensity physical activity program?

11. What impact does fitness versus fatness have on the risk of chronic disease?

12. What performance-related fitness components are linked to sport?

13. Describe the continuum of physical activity recommendations for realizing health, fitness, and performance goals.

CASE STUDIES

You can check your answers by referring to appendix A.

1. A client complains that she has been deceived by all the physical activity recommendations you have given her over the past several years. She just read a government report indicating that a person has to only do moderate-intensity physical activity (walking) to achieve health benefits. She wants to know if she should continue her vigorous exercise program in which she exercises at her target heart rate (THR) for 30 min 3 to 4 times each week or whether she should switch to a walking program. How do you respond?

2. You have just presented a speech on physical fitness to a local service club. One of the members says that he knows of two men who died in incidents related to exercise during the past few years and that he has read of other exercise-related deaths. He has decided that it will be safer to lead a quiet life and not take the risk of exercising. How do you respond?

3. You are working with an obese client who has been sedentary for several years. He indicates that he would like to lose weight before beginning a physical activity program. What information might you provide to encourage him to begin a moderate-intensity physical activity program as plans are developed to accomplish weight-loss goals?

REFERENCES

1. American College of Sports Medicine (ACSM). 1975. *Guidelines for graded exercise testing and exercise prescription*. Philadelphia: Lea & Febiger.

2. American College of Sports Medicine (ACSM). 1978. The recommended quality and quantity of exercise for developing and maintaining fitness in healthy adults. *Medicine and Science in Sports and Exercise* 10:vii-x.

3. American College of Sports Medicine (ACSM). 1990. Position stand: The recommended quantity and quality of exercise for developing and maintaining cardiorespiratory and muscular fitness in healthy adults. *Medicine and Science in Sports and Exercise* 22:265-274.

4. American College of Sports Medicine (ACSM). 2010. *ACSM's guidelines for exercise testing and prescription*. Philadelphia: Lippincott Williams & Wilkins.

5. American Heart Association (AHA). 1972. *Exercise testing and training of apparently healthy individuals: A handbook for physicians*. New York: Author.

6. American Heart Association (AHA). 2011. Women and cardiovascular diseases—statistics. www.heart.org/idc/groups/heart-public/@wcm/@sop/@smd/documents/downloadable/ucm_319576.pdf

7. Bouchard, C., R.J. Shephard, and T. Stephens. 1994. *Physical activity, fitness, and health*. Champaign, IL: Human Kinetics.

8. Bouchard, C., R.J. Shephard, T. Stephens, J.R. Sutton, and B.D. McPherson. 1990. *Exercise, fitness, and health*. Champaign, IL: Human Kinetics.

9. Caspersen, C.J., K.E. Powell, and G.M. Christenson. 1985. Physical activity, exercise, and physical fitness: Definitions and distinctions for health-related research. *Public Health Reports* 100:126-131.

10. Church, T.S., M.J. LaMonte, C.E. Barlow, and S.N. Blair. 2005. Cardiorespiratory fitness and body mass index as predictors of cardiovascular disease mortality among men with diabetes. *Archieves of Internal Medicine* 165:2114-2120.

11. Daniels, J.T. 2002. Personal communication.

12. Erlichman, J., A.L. Kerbey, and W.P.T. James. 2002. Physical activity and its impact on health outcomes. Paper 2: Prevention of unhealthy weight gain and obesity by physical activity: an analysis of the evidence. *Obesity Reviews* 3:273-287.

13. Farrell, S.W., L. Braun, C.E. Barlow, Y.J. Cheng, and S.N. Blair. 2002. The relation of body mass index, cardiorespiratory fitness, and all-cause mortality in women. *Obesity Research* 10:417-423.

14. Flegal, K.M., M.D. Carroll, C.L. Ogden, and L.R. Curtin. 2010. Prevalence and trends in obesity among U.S. adults,

1999-2008. *Journal of the American Medical Association* 303:235-241.

15. Fletcher, G.F., B.S. N., J. Blumenthal, C.J. Caspersen, B. Chaitman, S. Epstein, H. Falls, E.S. Sivarajan Froelicher, V.F. Froelicher, and I.L. Pina. 1992. American Heart Association statement on exercise. *Circulation* 86:340-344.

16. Golding, L.A., C.R. Myers, and W.E. Sinning. 1973. *The Y's Way to Physical Fitness.* Emmaus, PA: Rodale Press.

17. Haskell, W.L. 1985. Physical activity and health: Need to define the required stimulus. *American Journal of Cardiology* 55:4D-9D.

18. Haskell, W.L. 1994. Dose–response issues from a biological perspective. In *Physical activity, fitness and health*, ed. C. Bouchard, R.J. Shephard, and T. Stephens, 1030-1039. Champaign, IL: Human Kinetics.

19. Haskell, W.L., I.M. Lee, R.R. Pate, K.E. Powell, S.N. Blair, B.A. Franklin, C.A. Macera, G.W. Heath, and P.D. Thompson. 2007. Physical activity and public health: Updated recommendation for adults from the American College of Sports Medicine and the American Heart Association. *Medicine and Science in Sports and Exercise* 39:1423-1434.

20. Institute of Medicine. 2002. *Dietary reference intakes for energy, carbohydrates, fiber, fat, fatty acids, cholesterol, proteins, and amino acids.* Washington, D.C: National Academy of Sciences.

21. Jones, W.H.S. *Regimen (Hippocrates).* 1953. Cambridge, MA: Harvard University Press.

22. Lee, C.D., S.N. Blair, and A.S. Jackson. 1999. Cardiorespiratory fitness, body composition, and all-cause and cardiovascular disease mortality in men. *American Journal of Clinical Nutrition* 69:373-380.

23. Mokdad, A.H., J.S. Marks, D.F. Stroup, and J.L. Gerberding. 2004. Actual causes of death in the United States, 2000. *Journal of the American Medical Association* 291:1238-1245.

24. Mokdad, A.H., J.S. Marks, D.F. Stroup, and J.L. Gerberding. 2005. Correction: Actual causes of death in the United States, 2000. *Journal of the American Medical Association* 293:293-294.

25. Paffenbarger, R.S.J., A.L. Wing, and R.T. Hyde. 1978. Physical activity as an index of heart attack risk in college alumni. *American Journal of Epidemiology* 108:161-175.

26. Pate, R.R., M. Pratt, S.N. Blair, W.L. Haskell, C.A. Marcera, and C. Bouchard. 1995. Physical activity and public health: A recommendation from the Centers for Disease Control and Prevention and the American College of Sports Medicine. *Journal of the American Medical Association* 273:402-407.

27. Rankinen, T., and C. Bouchard. 2007. Genetic differences in the relationships among physical activity, fitness, and health. In *Physical activity and health*, ed. C. Bouchard, S.N. Blair, and W.L. Haskell. Champaign, IL: Human Kinetics.

28. Ruiz, J.R., X. Sui, F. Lobelo, S. Lee, J.R. Morrow, A.W. Jackson, J.R. Hébert, C.E. Matthews, M. Sjöström, and S.N. Blair. 2009. Muscular strength and adiposity as predictors of adulthood cancer mortality in men. *Cancer Epidemiology Biomarkers Prevention* 18:1468-1476.

29. Saris, W.H.M., S.N. Blair, M.A. Van Baak, S.B. Eaton, P.S. Davies, L. DiPietro, M. Fogelholm, A. Rissanen, D. Schoeller, B. Swinburn, A. Tremblay, K.R. Westerterp, and H. Wyatt. 2003. How much physical activity is enough to prevent unhealthy weight gain? Outcomes of the IASO 1st Stock Conference and consensus statement. *Obesity Reviews* 4:101-114.

30. Sui, X., M.J. LaMonte, J.N. Laditka, J.W. Hardin, N. Chase, S.P. Hooker, and S.N. Blair. 2007. Cardiorespiratory fitness and adiposity as mortality predictors in older adults. *Journal of the American Medical Association* 298:2507-2516.

31. Swain, D.P., and B.A. Franklin. 2006. Comparison of cardioprotective benefits of vigorous versus moderate intensity aerobic exercise. *American Journal of Cardiology* 97:141-147.

32. U.S. Department of Health and Human Services (HHS). 1996. *Surgeon General's report on physical activity and health.* Washington, DC: Author.

33. U.S. Department of Health and Human Services (HHS). 2008. *2008 Physical Activity Guidelines for Americans.* www.health.gov/paguidelines/guidelines/default.aspx.

34. U.S. Department of Health and Human Services (HHS). 2008. Physical Activity Guidelines Advisory Committee report 2008. www.health.gov/paguidelines/committeereport.aspx.

35. U.S. Department of Health and Human Services (HHS). 2010. Deaths: Final data for 2007. *National Vital Statistics Reports* 58:1-136.

36. U.S. Department of Health and Human Services (HHS). 2010. Heart disease and African Americans. http://minorityhealth.hhs.gov/templates/content.aspx?ID=3018.

37. U.S. Department of Health and Human Services (HHS) and U.S. Department of Agriculture (USDA). 2005. *Dietary guidelines for Americans.* Washington, DC: U.S. GPO.

38. U.S. Department of Health, Education, and Welfare. 1979. *Healthy people: The Surgeon General's report on health promotion and disease prevention.* Washington, DC: U.S. GPO.

Health Appraisal

Michael Shipe

OBJECTIVES

The reader will be able to do the following:

1. Understand the purpose of evaluating the health status of potential participants in fitness programs and identify appropriate instruments for preactivity appraisal.

2. Identify the presence of cardiovascular, pulmonary, or metabolic disease, including signs and symptoms.

3. Identify primary risk factors for heart disease and understand how they are used in risk stratification.

4. Describe the categories of participants who should receive physician consent before undergoing exercise testing or participation.

5. Understand how to classify fitness test results relative to the participant's age and gender.

6. Recommend an appropriate fitness program for participants based on their preactivity screening and fitness test results.

Fitness professionals in both clinical and commercial settings will encounter individuals with low cardiovascular fitness (CRF) and an array of health and medical conditions. The fitness professional is responsible for properly screening prospective exercise participants to determine their current health status and whether physician consent is warranted prior to undergoing fitness testing or beginning regular physical activity. To properly screen an exercise participant, the fitness professional should begin with a preactivity screening questionnaire, such as the Physical Activity Readiness Questionnaire (PAR-Q) or the Health Status Questionnaire (HSQ). The choice of questionnaire should be linked to the target population with whom the fitness professional will be working. (These two questionnaires are discussed in detail later in this chapter.)

In some instances, physician consent or referral of the participant to a clinic-based supervised exercise program may be necessary before starting an unsupervised exercise program. Unfortunately, there are no universal guidelines for determining when physician consent is necessary before exercise participation or when supervised exercise in a clinical setting is warranted. To help the fitness professional make these decisions, this chapter provides the recommendations of the AHA and ACSM for both situations. When in doubt, the fitness professional should rely on the participant's primary care physician and the fitness director of the facility to make the final decision regarding the approval for exercise participation.

Initially, the participant's preactivity screening questionnaire should be evaluated for the presence of chronic diseases or symptoms that increase the risk of cardiovascular events during exercise. If they are present, physician consent is necessary *before* fitness testing or exercise participation (1-3). The participant's primary risk factors and desired level of activity should be determined to estimate the risk for CVD (i.e., low, moderate, or high). Next, the participant undergoes a fitness test and the results are evaluated relative to age and gender norms. The fitness professional now has the necessary information to develop an appropriate exercise prescription for improving the participant's health and fitness in relation to present health status and personal exercise goals. To update records of the participant's health status, the preactivity screening questionnaire and fitness tests should be readministered periodically.

Evaluating Health Status

The AHA and ACSM recommend that exercise facilities provide their adult members with a preactivity health screening that is consistent with the exercise programs they plan to pursue (1-4). Although an exercise facility may not have an expressed legal responsibility to conduct a preactivity screening, this screening is in the best interest of exercise participants. Further, the results of the preactivity screening should be interpreted and documented by qualified staff (1-3).

Preactivity Screening

A well-designed preactivity screening questionnaire identifies symptoms or chronic diseases that increase the risk of cardiovascular events during exercise participation (5). It is the first step in the fitness professional's health appraisal of exercise participants, and it includes the following categories:

- **M**edical history review
- **R**isk-factor assessment and stratification
- **P**rescribed medications
- **L**evel of physical activity
- **E**stablishment of the necessity of physician consent
- **A**dministration of fitness tests and evaluation of results
- **S**etup of exercise prescription
- **E**valuation of progress with follow-up tests

It may help the fitness professional to remember the recommended health appraisal categories and the order in which they are performed by using the acronym *MR. PLEASE*, which could represent the participant asking, "Mister, may I please exercise?" This protocol expands on previous recommendations for working with new clients in fitness settings (11).

Two standard preactivity screening questionnaires commonly used in the fitness industry are the PAR-Q and HSQ. Each level of MR. PLEASE is discussed in detail following the descriptions of the PAR-Q and HSQ, and additional categories of screening are discussed after that.

Physical Activity Readiness Questionnaire

The Physical Activity Readiness Questionnaire (PAR-Q; see form 2.1) is a simple and effective preactivity screening tool for identifying people at high risk for cardiovascular complications during light to moderate exercise (e.g., 20%-60% $\dot{V}O_2R$) (4). Therefore, when participants want to pursue only moderate-intensity physical activity, the PAR-Q might be an appropriate screening tool.

If participants answer *yes* to any of the seven questions in this self-administered questionnaire, they are directed to contact a physician before undergoing a fitness test or pursuing regular physical activity. The PAR-Q produces

FORM 2.1

Physical Activity Readiness
Questionnaire - PAR-Q
(revised 2002)

PAR-Q & YOU

(A Questionnaire for People Aged 15 to 69)

Regular physical activity is fun and healthy, and increasingly more people are starting to become more active every day. Being more active is very safe for most people. However, some people should check with their doctor before they start becoming much more physically active.

If you are planning to become much more physically active than you are now, start by answering the seven questions in the box below. If you are between the ages of 15 and 69, the PAR-Q will tell you if you should check with your doctor before you start. If you are over 69 years of age, and you are not used to being very active, check with your doctor.

Common sense is your best guide when you answer these questions. Please read the questions carefully and answer each one honestly: check YES or NO.

YES	NO		
☐	☐	1.	**Has your doctor ever said that you have a heart condition <u>and</u> that you should only do physical activity recommended by a doctor?**
☐	☐	2.	**Do you feel pain in your chest when you do physical activity?**
☐	☐	3.	**In the past month, have you had chest pain when you were not doing physical activity?**
☐	☐	4.	**Do you lose your balance because of dizziness or do you ever lose consciousness?**
☐	☐	5.	**Do you have a bone or joint problem (for example, back, knee or hip) that could be made worse by a change in your physical activity?**
☐	☐	6.	**Is your doctor currently prescribing drugs (for example, water pills) for your blood pressure or heart condition?**
☐	☐	7.	**Do you know of <u>any other reason</u> why you should not do physical activity?**

If you answered

YES to one or more questions

Talk with your doctor by phone or in person BEFORE you start becoming much more physically active or BEFORE you have a fitness appraisal. Tell your doctor about the PAR-Q and which questions you answered YES.

- You may be able to do any activity you want — as long as you start slowly and build up gradually. Or, you may need to restrict your activities to those which are safe for you. Talk with your doctor about the kinds of activities you wish to participate in and follow his/her advice.
- Find out which community programs are safe and helpful for you.

NO to all questions

If you answered NO honestly to <u>all</u> PAR-Q questions, you can be reasonably sure that you can:
- start becoming much more physically active — begin slowly and build up gradually. This is the safest and easiest way to go.
- take part in a fitness appraisal — this is an excellent way to determine your basic fitness so that you can plan the best way for you to live actively. It is also highly recommended that you have your blood pressure evaluated. If your reading is over 144/94, talk with your doctor before you start becoming much more physically active.

DELAY BECOMING MUCH MORE ACTIVE:
- if you are not feeling well because of a temporary illness such as a cold or a fever — wait until you feel better; or
- if you are or may be pregnant — talk to your doctor before you start becoming more active.

PLEASE NOTE: If your health changes so that you then answer YES to any of the above questions, tell your fitness or health professional. Ask whether you should change your physical activity plan.

<u>Informed Use of the PAR-Q</u>: The Canadian Society for Exercise Physiology, Health Canada, and their agents assume no liability for persons who undertake physical activity, and if in doubt after completing this questionnaire, consult your doctor prior to physical activity.

No changes permitted. You are encouraged to photocopy the PAR-Q but only if you use the entire form.

NOTE: If the PAR-Q is being given to a person before he or she participates in a physical activity program or a fitness appraisal, this section may be used for legal or administrative purposes.

"I have read, understood and completed this questionnaire. Any questions I had were answered to my full satisfaction."

NAME _____

SIGNATURE _____   DATE_____

SIGNATURE OF PARENT _____   WITNESS _____
or GUARDIAN (for participants under the age of majority)

Note: This physical activity clearance is valid for a maximum of 12 months from the date it is completed and becomes invalid if your condition changes so that you would answer YES to any of the seven questions.

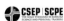 **CSEP | SCPE**
THE GOLD STANDARD IN EXERCISE
SCIENCE AND PERSONAL TRAINING

© Canadian Society for Exercise Physiology www.csep.ca/forms

(continued)

...continued from other side

PAR-Q & YOU

Physical Activity Readiness
Questionnaire - PAR-Q
(revised 2002)

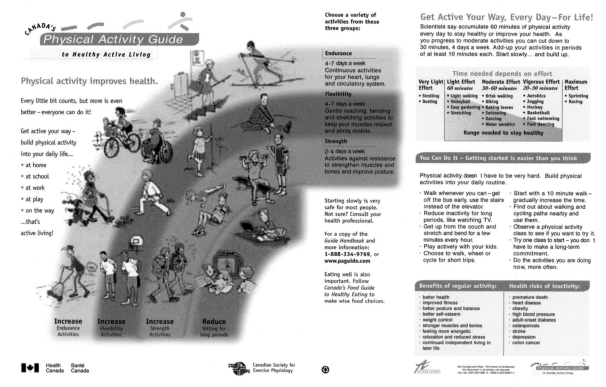

Source: Canada's Physical Activity Guide to Healthy Active Living, Health Canada, 1998 http://www.hc-sc.gc.ca/hppb/paguide/pdf/guideEng.pdf
© Reproduced with permission from the Minister of Public Works and Government Services Canada, 2002.

FITNESS AND HEALTH PROFESSIONALS MAY BE INTERESTED IN THE INFORMATION BELOW:

The following companion forms are available for doctors' use by contacting the Canadian Society for Exercise Physiology (address below):

The **Physical Activity Readiness Medical Examination (PARmed-X)** – to be used by doctors with people who answer YES to one or more questions on the PAR-Q.

The **Physical Activity Readiness Medical Examination for Pregnancy (PARmed-X for Pregnancy)** – to be used by doctors with pregnant patients who wish to become more active.

References:
Arraix, G.A., Wigle, D.T., Mao, Y. (1992). Risk Assessment of Physical Activity and Physical Fitness in the Canada Health Survey
Follow-Up Study. **J. Clin. Epidemiol.** 45:4 419-428.
Mottola, M., Wolfe, L.A. (1994). Active Living and Pregnancy, In: A. Quinney, L. Gauvin, T. Wall (eds.), **Toward Active Living: Proceedings of the International Conference on Physical Activity, Fitness and Health**. Champaign, IL: Human Kinetics.
PAR-Q Validation Report, British Columbia Ministry of Health, 1978.
Thomas, S., Reading, J., Shephard, R.J. (1992). Revision of the Physical Activity Readiness Questionnaire (PAR-Q). **Can. J. Spt. Sci.** 17:4 338-345.

For more information, please contact the:

Canadian Society for Exercise Physiology
202-185 Somerset Street West
Ottawa, ON K2P 0J2
Tel. 1-877-651-3755 • FAX (613) 234-3565
Online: www.csep.ca

The original PAR-Q was developed by the British Columbia Ministry of Health. It has been revised by an Expert Advisory Committee of the Canadian Society for Exercise Physiology chaired by Dr. N. Gledhill (2002).

Disponible en français sous le titre «Questionnaire sur l'aptitude à l'activité physique - Q-AAP (revisé 2002)».

 © Canadian Society for Exercise Physiology   Supported by: Health Canada   Santé Canada

---

From E.T. Howley and D.L. Thompson, 2012, *Fitness professional's handbook, 6th ed.* (Champaign, IL: Human Kinetics). Source: Physical Activity Readiness Questionnaire (PAR-Q) © 2002. Reproduced with permission from the Canadian Society for Exercise Physiology. www.csep.ca/forms.asp.

an inordinate number of false-positives with older adults (e.g., 60 yr and older), especially those with orthopedic problems (7). The fitness professional should ask additional questions to those individuals who check *yes* to a given question to determine whether they have legitimate medical reasons to seek physician consent before exercising. Given that most facilities offer unsupervised vigorous-intensity exercise, the remainder of this chapter addresses how to screen participants for this level of activity.

Health Screening Questionnaire

A more thorough preactivity screening tool, the Health Screening Questionnaire (HSQ; see form 2.2), provides the fitness professional with enough information to quickly and accurately identify the presence of cardiovascular, pulmonary, or metabolic disease by recognizing their major signs and symptoms, **risk factors** for CHD, and lifestyle behaviors that may affect the ability to begin exercising safely. The HSQ provided in this text has been expanded from the AHA and ACSM health and fitness facility preactivity screening questionnaire to include specific physical activity patterns, current medications, and a patient information release form (1). This information should be evaluated *before* conducting any fitness testing or recommending exercise prescriptions.

A completed HSQ will contain a significant amount of personal health information, which is protected under the Health Insurance Portability and Accountability Act of 1996 (HIPAA) (15). Thus, a completed HSQ should be kept in a secure location and be accessible only by designated staff. A participant's medical history and fitness test results constitute personal health information. This information should be shared only with other health care professionals who will be working with the participant and should only be discussed in a private setting in which fellow staff or participants cannot overhear. For instance, a violation of HIPAA regulations would occur if a participant's body composition results were discussed with another participant or staff member when other individuals could listen in on the conversation. Additional legal concerns that may be involved in the exercise testing and prescription process are addressed in chapter 27.

Fitness professionals should note the patient information release form at the end of the HSQ. Participants must provide their signature in this section so that their physicians may release their pertinent medical information to the fitness professional, if warranted, in accordance with HIPAA regulations (15).

Aside from legal rights that protect personal health information, the fitness professional should consider that many participants may feel uncomfortable sharing their detailed medical history with a person they have just met.

Using a conversational style to ask questions about medical diagnoses may help to alleviate the discomfort that clients may feel. For instance, when a participant has checked the box for having a heart attack, relevant questions providing further insight into this medical history would include the following: "Are your heart symptoms present? If so, are they stable?" "Has your heart attack affected your activities of daily life?" "Have you been able to return to the activities you were doing before the event?" "Did you participate in cardiac rehabilitation?" "Were you given any restrictions?" The participant's responses should be documented on the HSQ. Reviewing the HSQ conversationally allows the fitness professional to learn more about the participant's health status and to convey **empathy**, making participants more likely to consider the fitness professional as being genuinely concerned with helping them improve their health.

No questionnaire can address all possible medical conditions that might warrant physician consent. Thus, the fitness professional is encouraged to ask additional questions relevant to the participant's medical history while reviewing the HSQ. The line of questioning should be directed by any condition that is checked as being present. By doing so, all probable medical diagnoses or symptoms that may possibly place the participant at additional cardiovascular risk during exercise are more likely to be addressed. A fitness facility may want to make minor alterations to the HSQ so that it is more applicable to their participant population.

If prospective exercise participants refuse to complete an HSQ, then they cannot be properly screened according to the standards of care for fitness facilities advocated by the AHA and ACSM. In this case, the participant should be informed that the HSQ is a safety-oriented screening tool and the information will be shared only with the appropriate health care professionals. If the prospective participant still refuses, the ACSM recommends that they be permitted to sign a release or waiver before exercising. The release or waiver should entail the following: acknowledgment that a preactivity screening was provided, that the participant has been informed of the inherent risks of exercise participation, that the participant has chosen not to be screened, and that the participant agrees not to file any claims or suits arising from exercise participation (3).

MR. PLEASE: Medical History Review

The first step in evaluating health status—the medical history review—is addressed in section 2 of the HSQ. The AHA and ACSM recommend that individuals who mark any of the statements in this section should consult a physician or appropriate health care provider before pursuing a regular exercise program because they may need to exercise

FORM 2.2 Health Screening Questionnaire

This questionnaire identifies adults for whom physical activity might be inappropriate or adults who should consult a physician before beginning a regular physical activity program.

SECTION 1   PERSONAL AND EMERGENCY CONTACT INFORMATION

Name:_____ Date of birth:_____

Address: _____ Phone: _____

Physician's name: _____

Height: _____ Weight: _____

Person to contact in case of emergency

Name: _____ Phone:_____

SECTION 2   GENERAL MEDICAL HISTORY

Please check the following conditions you have experienced.

Heart History

_____Heart attack   _____Cardiac rhythm disturbance

_____Heart surgery   _____Heart valve disease

_____Cardiac catheterization   _____Heart failure

_____Coronary angioplasty (PTCA)   _____Heart transplantation

_____Cardiac pacemaker/implantable cardiac defibrillator   _____Congenital heart disease

Symptoms

_____You experience chest discomfort with exertion.

_____You experience unreasonable shortness of breath at any time.

_____You experience dizziness, fainting, or blackouts.

_____You take heart medications.

Additional Health Issues

_____You have diabetes (type 1 or type 2).

_____You have asthma or other lung disease (e.g., emphysema).

_____You have burning or cramping sensations in your lower legs with minimal physical activity.

_____You have joint problems (e.g., arthritis) that limit your physical activity.

_____You have concerns about the safety of exercise.

_____You take prescription medications.

_____You are pregnant.

SECTION 3 RISK-FACTOR ASSESSMENT

Risk Factors for Coronary Heart Disease

_____You are a man ≥45 yr.

_____You are a woman ≥55 yr.

_____You smoke or you quit smoking within the previous 6 mo.

_____Your blood pressure is ≥140 or ≥90 mmHg.

_____Your total cholesterol is ≥200 mg · dl⁻¹, or low-density lipoprotein (LDL-C) is ≥130 mg · dl⁻¹, or high-density lipoprotein (HDL-C) is <40 mg · dl⁻¹.

_____You have prediabetes.

_____You have a close male blood relative (father or brother) who had a heart attack or heart surgery before the age of 55 or a close female blood relative (mother or sister) who had a heart attack or heart surgery before the age of 65.

_____You are physically inactive (you do not participate in at least 30 min of moderate intensity (40%-60% $\dot{V}O_2R$) physical activity at least 3 days · wk⁻¹).

_____Your body mass index (BMI) is ≥30 kg · m⁻² or your waist circumference is >40 in. (102 cm) for men or >35 in. (89 cm) for women.

SECTION 4 MEDICATIONS

Are you currently taking any medication?   ○ Yes   ○ No

If yes, please list all of your prescribed medications and how often you take them, whether daily (D) or as needed (PRN).

_____

_____

Of the medications you have listed, are there any you do not take as prescribed?

SECTION 5 PHYSICAL ACTIVITY PATTERNS AND OBJECTIVES

List the type, frequency, intensity (e.g., light, moderate, vigorous), and duration of your weekly exercise. Note the intensity at which you plan to exercise and list the specific goals for your exercise program.

Please inform the fitness professional immediately of any changes that occur in your health status.

Patient Information Release Form

If you have answered *yes* to questions indicating that you have significant cardiac, pulmonary, metabolic, or orthopedic problems that may be exacerbated with exercise, you agree it is permissible for us to contact your physician regarding your health status in compliance with the Health Information Portability and Accountability Act of 1996 (HIPAA).

Signature: _____   Date: _____

Fitness staff signature: _____   Date:_____

To be completed by fitness professional (circle one):

AHA and ACSM risk stratification: ○ Low   ○ Moderate   ○ High

Physician consent: ○ Yes   ○ No

From E.T. Howley and D.L. Thompson, 2012, *Fitness professional's handbook,* 6th ed. (Champaign, IL: Human Kinetics). Adapted from American College of Sports Medicine 2010.

in a facility with medically qualified staff(1-3). The main objective of this section is to identify the presence of the following three common chronic diseases.

- Cardiovascular disease (CVD): coronary heart disease (CHD), peripheral artery disease (PAD), and cerebrovascular disease
- Pulmonary disease: chronic obstructive pulmonary disease (COPD), asthma, interstitial lung disease, and cystic fibrosis
- Metabolic disease: diabetes mellitus (type 1 or 2 diabetes), thyroid disorders, and renal or liver disorders

People who have one of these three diseases (i.e., the big three) are considered at *high risk* for CHD and require physician consent before any fitness testing or exercise participation (1-3).

KEY POINT

Evaluation of a preactivity screening questionnaire helps the fitness professional determine a participant's current health status and whether it is appropriate for the participant to undergo fitness testing or begin regular physical activity. In addition, fitness professionals can assess the presence of relevant medical conditions, risk factors for CHD, lifestyle behaviors, and medications that will assist in determining the necessity of a physician's consent before beginning an exercise program. This information is protected by HIPAA.

When analyzing the HSQ, it is imperative to acknowledge that the risk status of individuals both with and without CHD varies significantly. Regular physical activity reduces cardiovascular morbidity and mortality for people with established CHD (9). Yet, the incidence of a coronary event during exercise for these individuals is estimated to be 10 times greater than that of healthy adults (10). In addition, some factors dramatically increase a person's risk for a cardiac event. For example, a diagnosis of diabetes is considered a CHD equivalent. A person who has diabetes but has not been diagnosed with CHD is as likely to have a coronary event as is a person who has CHD (8). These facts underline the need for fitness professionals to understand a participant's medical history before administering fitness tests or designing exercise prescriptions.

After determining the presence or absence of the big three chronic diseases (cardiovascular, pulmonary, or metabolic diseases), the fitness professional should further evaluate section 2 of the HSQ to ascertain if the participant has major signs or symptoms suggestive of these diseases

(see table 2.1). Note that just because participants have one of these signs or symptoms, it does not mean that they have cardiovascular, pulmonary, or metabolic disease. For instance, a participant may present with a resting heart rate (RHR) greater than 100 beats · min^{-1} but have no other symptoms suggestive of CVD. Upon further inquiry, the fitness professional finds that the participant has rushed to make the appointment and recently consumed a large dose of caffeine. Thus, the elevated heart rate (HR) may be the result of these recent events as opposed to an indication of possible CVD. This scenario demonstrates the importance of the fitness professional asking additional questions to help ensure the HSQ is interpreted properly.

Another designation that is often checked is the use of heart medications. Many prospective exercisers may have high BP that requires daily medication. Yet if this is the only sign or symptom checked, it does not warrant physician consent. These situations highlight the importance of fitness professionals using their knowledge and professional experience when evaluating a participant's medical history. In the event that the fitness professional is still uncertain whether a medical history requires physician consent before performing a fitness test, administrative personnel should be consulted.

Finally, section 2 of the HSQ addresses additional concerns the fitness professional should consider, such as pregnancy and orthopedic issues. Pregnant women always require physician consent before exercise testing or participation (1-3). Additionally, an area that sometimes causes confusion is a diagnosis of arthritis. For example, it is unlikely that people who have arthritis in the shoulders will have limitations related to walking or cycling; thus, they may not need additional physician consent to begin those types of exercise programs. One's professional judgment must be used in these circumstances.

MR. PLEASE: Risk-Factor Assessment and Stratification

Risk-factor assessment and stratification involve reviewing section 3 of the HSQ, which contains specific information concerning risk factors for CHD. For the remainder of this chapter, the term *risk factor* refers to a primary risk factor for CHD. The AHA and ACSM recommend obtaining consent from a physician or an appropriate health care provider before exercise participation if two or more statements are marked in section 3 and the participant wants to pursue vigorous-intensity exercise (1-3).

The fitness professional should establish and quantify the participant's specific CHD risk factors using the thresholds listed in table 2.2. The scope of this table is not exhaustive, because emerging risk factors such as elevated triglycerides, which have been highly correlated with the progression of CHD, are not included (1). The conditions

TABLE 2.1 Major Signs or Symptoms of Cardiovascular, Pulmonary, and Metabolic Disease

Sign or symptom	Clarification and significance
Angina (i.e., heart pain) may present in the chest, neck, jaw, or arms. Women may also present with unusual nausea.	Angina is a hallmark of heart disease, especially CHD, and indicates the blood supply to the heart is insufficient. Key features of angina include a constricting or heavy feeling in the middle of the chest, shoulders, or arms. These sensations may be provoked by exercise or exertion and other forms of stress.
Palpitations or tachycardia (i.e., RHR >100 beats · min^{-1})	A palpitation is the unpleasant awareness of a forceful or rapid heartbeat, which may indicate an irregular heartbeat. The fitness professional may be able to sense the palpitation by taking the HR manually at the carotid or radial artery. Palpitations can originate from unusual stress, fever, anemia, or a high cardiac output. Tachycardia is a common palpitation, and it can be due to recent actions (e.g., caffeine ingestion) or a sign of other cardiovascular problems.
Shortness of breath at rest or with mild exertion	Dyspnea is an abnormally uncomfortable awareness of breathing and is a principal symptom of cardiac and pulmonary disease. It occurs naturally during heavy exertion in individuals with high CRF and during mild exertion in untrained individuals. Dyspnea may be considered abnormal when it occurs at an atypical (e.g., low-intensity) level of exertion.
Dizziness or syncope	Syncope is the loss of consciousness and occurs most often due to lack of blood flow to the brain. Dizziness and especially syncope during exercise can be the product of cardiac disorders that prevent the normal increase or decrease in cardiac output. These cardiac output disorders are potentially life threatening. Dizziness or syncope can occur in healthy individuals after completing an exercise bout and should be addressed. These symptoms may occur because of reduced blood flow to the heart.
Ankle edema	Ankle edema is an unnatural accumulation of fluid surrounding the ankles and is characteristic of CHF, a common CVD. Individuals with CHF may exhibit generalized edema, whereas swelling in one limb may result from a venous thrombosis or blockage in the lymphatic system.
Intermittent claudication	Intermittent claudication is a burning or cramping pain (typically in the gluteal region) that is exacerbated by exertion. It occurs in a muscle with inadequate blood supply secondary to localized atherosclerosis. The pain should be consistent at a given exertion level and should resolve within 1-2 min after exercise cessation. Intermittent claudication is more prevalent in individuals with CHD and type 1 or 2 diabetes.

Based on American College of Sports Medicine 2010.

and values listed in the table were chosen to help fitness professionals identify individuals who likely have CHD but have not been clinically diagnosed.

Fitness professionals are encouraged to be conservative when identifying CHD risk factors. When a specific risk factor is unknown or unavailable, aside from prediabetes, it is designated as a risk factor (see table 2.2 for prediabetes defining criteria). If glucose levels are not known, prediabetes should be counted as a risk factor if the participant is >45 years, especially if BMI is >25 kg/m^2. Regarding younger individuals, prediabetes should be counted as a risk factor if BMI > 25 kg/m^2 and additional CHD risk

factors (e.g., physical inactivity, hypertension, hyperlipidemia) are present. Another good indicator of prediabetes for younger individuals is if they have a first-degree relative diagnosed with diabetes (1).

Section 3 also requires the fitness professional to properly interpret the ACSM and AHA guidelines for seeking physician consent. For instance, let's consider a woman older than 55 yr who has blood cholesterol levels greater than 200 mg · dl^{-1}, is physically active, and wants to participate in vigorous-intensity exercise. According to the ACSM and AHA guidelines, physician consent is recommended because she checked two statements

TABLE 2.2   Atherosclerotic Cardiovascular Disease Risk-Factor Thresholds for Risk Stratification

Positive risk factors	Defining criteria
Age	Men ≥45 yr; women ≥55 yr
Family history	Myocardial infarction (MI), coronary revascularization, or sudden death before age 55 in father or other male first-degree relative or before age 65 in mother or other female first-degree relative
Cigarette smoking	Current cigarette smoker *or* quit within previous 6 mo *or* exposure to environmental tobacco smoke
Sedentary lifestyle	Not participating in at least 30 min of moderate intensity (40%-59% $\dot{V}O_2R$) aerobic physical activity on at least 3 days · wk^{-2} for at least 3 mo
Obesity*	BMI ≥30 kg · m^{-2}, *or* waist girth >40 in. (102 cm) for men and >35 in. (88 cm) for women
Hypertension	SBP ≥140 mmHg or DBP >90 mmHg confirmed by resting measurements on at least two separate occasions, *or* on antihypertensive medications
Dyslipidemia	LDL-C ≥130 mg · dl^{-1} (3.37 mmol · L^{-1}), HDL-C <40 mg · dl^{-1} (1.04 mmol · L^{-1}), *or* total serum cholesterol (if only measurement available) ≥200 mg · dl^{-1} (5.18 mmol · L^{-1}), *or* on lipid-lowering medication
Prediabetes	Impaired fasting glucose (IFG) = fasting plasma glucose ≥ 100 mg · dl^{-1} (5.50 mmol · L^{-1}) but < 126 mg · dl^{-1} (6.93 mmol · L^{-1}), *or* impaired glucose tolerance (IGT) = 2 hr values in oral glucose tolerance test (OGTT) > 140 mg · dl^{-1} (7.70 mmol · L^{-1}) *but* < 200 mg · dl^{-1} (11.00 mmol · L^{-1}) confirmed by measurements on at least two separate occasions

Negative risk factor	Defining criteria
High serum HDL-C**	≥60 mg · dl^{-1} (1.55 mmol · L^{-1})

*Professional opinions vary regarding the most appropriate thresholds for obesity; thus, allied health professionals should use clinical judgment when evaluating this risk factor.

**It is common to sum risk factors in making clinical judgments. If HDL-C is high, subtract one risk factor from the sum of positive risk factors, since high HDL-C decreases CVD risk.

Adapted, by permission, from American College of Sports Medicine, 2010, *ACSM's guidelines for exercise testing and prescription,* 8th ed. (Philadelphia, PA: Lippincott, Williams & Wilkins), 28.

and wants to exercise vigorously. Yet the prudent fitness professional knows that blood cholesterol can be elevated either by high bad cholesterol (i.e., LDL-C or VLDL) or high good cholesterol (i.e., HDL-C). After asking the participant if she knows her HDL-C level and finding that it is 65 mg · dl^{-1}, physician consent is no longer necessary. Why? Because high HDL-C levels (i.e., ≥60 mg · dl^{-1}) are considered a negative risk factor (see the bottom of table 2.2). This negates a positive risk factor, and thus she only has a net of one risk factor. Therefore, the sum of risk factors should be properly established before determining a participant's risk stratification. If information on her HDL-C level is not available, then the fitness professional must use the total cholesterol value to determine if she has high cholesterol. Further, if total cholesterol level is missing or unknown, the risk factor should be counted as being present. This conservative approach to risk stratification

protects individuals who may actually be at a higher, but unknown, level of risk (1).

Fitness professionals should inform participants about their risk factors for CHD and the significance of those factors. Initially, they should explain the meaning of a risk factor (i.e., a clinical diagnosis or lifestyle behavior that increases the chances of developing heart disease). Some fitness professionals may want to quantify the severity of a participant's individual risk factors and overall relative risk for developing CHD by using the Framingham algorithm (13). Instructions for using this tool can be found in an article written by Wilson et al. (16).

The fitness professional should then address which risk factors can be modified, which include all of the factors except family history and age. The participant should be informed that regular physical activity can positively influence most risk factors for CHD and decrease the risk of developing new ones (1, 2, 5). The fact that regular physical activity may help manage and prevent these risk factors can serve as powerful motivation for long-term exercise adherence.

At this juncture, the fitness professional should consider the medical history, symptoms, and risk factors and classify the participant into one of the following three risk strata (adapted from table 2.1 in *ACSM's Guidelines for Exercise Testing and Prescription* [1]).

- Low risk. Asymptomatic men and women who have ≤1 risk factor from table 2.2.

- Moderate risk. Asymptomatic men and women who have ≥2 risk factors from table 2.2.

- High risk. Men and women who have known cardiovascular, pulmonary, or metabolic disease or who show signs or symptoms suggestive of these diseases (see table 2.1 and table 2.2). Major signs and symptoms are angina, shortness of breath at rest or with mild exertion, dizziness, loss of consciousness, ankle swelling, palpitations, tachycardia, heart murmurs, and intermittent claudication.

To ensure that each participant is stratified, the last notation of the HSQ prompts the fitness professional to document whether the participant is considered low, moderate, or high risk. Proper stratification is combined with the participant's desired activity level to determine whether physician consent is warranted before beginning fitness testing or regular exercise participation.

MR. PLEASE: Prescribed Medications

The next section of the HSQ requires the participant to document prescribed medications. The fitness professional should study appendix D of this book to be aware of common medications and their effects. Information on medication provides additional insight into the medical history and diagnosed risk factors. For example, a participant may indicate that she does not have high cholesterol in section 3 but lists Lipitor as one of her medications in section 4. Reviewing table D.1 in the appendix, the fitness professional can deduce that Lipitor is a class of drug known as a statin and is prescribed to treat high cholesterol. Some participants may indicate that they don't have a given medical condition because they are taking medication to treat it. However, taking a prescription medication to manage a chronic disease doesn't mean that the condition is absent, just that it is more likely to be effectively controlled. Thus, the participant still has the risk factor of high cholesterol and the fitness professional should note this accordingly.

In addition, the fitness professional should be able to determine whether a prescribed medication will alter the typical physiological responses to physical activity. For example, if a participant is taking a medication from the class of drugs known as beta-blockers, the fitness professional should be aware that the participant's HR will be substantially reduced (e.g., may not exceed 120 beats · min^{-1}) even though the participant is exercising strenuously. This response should not be considered abnormal; instead, it indicates the efficacy of the medication and necessitates the use of a perceived exertion scale (see chapter 7) to monitor exercise intensity.

KEY POINT

Analyzing the first three sections of the HSQ allows the fitness professional to identify the presence of cardiovascular, pulmonary, or metabolic disease; symptoms suggestive of these diseases; and primary risk factors for CHD. This information should be evaluated to categorize the participant's health risks (i.e., low, moderate, or high). This information coupled with the participant's desired activity level determines whether a participant requires physician consent to begin exercising.

As mentioned previously, section 2 of the HSQ asks whether the participant takes any prescribed medications. Checking these questions should prompt the fitness professional to review the participant's medication list to determine whether she takes medications commonly prescribed for chronic diseases such as high BP, elevated cholesterol, or diabetes. In this manner, risk factors can be more readily identified, which expedites the participant's risk stratification and the determination of whether physician consent is warranted. This point underlines the importance of evaluating the overall HSQ rather than simply relying on one section to determine whether physician consent is necessary.

MR. PLEASE: Level of Physical Activity

This section indicates present level and intensity of physical activity. It is important to identify whether the participant is physically inactive since heart attacks and sudden death are more common in people who are inactive (5). As indicated in table 2.2, if someone has not been accumulating 30 min of moderate-intensity (40%-59% $\dot{V}O_2R$) physical activity on at least 3 days · wk^{-1} for 3 mo, then that person has the risk factor of physical inactivity (1, 14). This section asks participants to note the intensity of exercise they perform as light, moderate, or vigorous. Because exercise intensity is subjective, the fitness professional should discuss examples of these intensity designations (e.g., slow walking as light intensity, brisk walking as moderate intensity, and jogging as high intensity). Thus, the fitness professional will have greater insight regarding the participant's actual physical activity level, which can be useful in guiding the exercise prescription. Further, the fitness professional should ask if exercising causes any physiological responses the participant considers unusual (e.g., exceptional shortness of breath, significant joint or muscle pain or soreness). If so, the participant's remarks should be documented and taken into consideration when determining whether or not physician consent is warranted.

MR. PLEASE: Establishment of the Necessity of Physician Consent

The fitness professional can now compile the information obtained in the previous sections of the HSQ to determine if the participant needs physician consent before starting a moderate- or vigorous-intensity exercise program. At this point the fitness professional should know if the participant has cardiovascular, pulmonary, or metabolic disease or related symptoms; the number of risk factors; and the intensity of activity to be pursued.

Individuals in the low-risk category do not need physician consent before undergoing exercise testing or participation in vigorous exercise (1-3). For instance, a 43-yr-old female with hypertension who walks for 30 min 5 times · wk^{-1} is considered a low-risk participant since she has only one risk factor. Further, ACSM does not recommend physician consent for individuals in the moderate-risk category if they plan to engage in no greater than moderate-intensity exercise (e.g., $<60\% \dot{V}O_2R$) (1). Therefore, a person who has two or more risk factors for CHD (see table 2.2) can safely initiate a walking program without physician consent. Fitness professionals should provide participants in this category with specific examples of recommended exercise (e.g., walking briskly at 3-4 mi · hr^{-1}, or 4.8-6.4 km · hr^{-1}) as well as adequate supervision to ensure they are exercising in the correct intensity range.

Most health or fitness facilities offer vigorous-intensity physical activity, and the staff at the facilities cannot closely supervise each moderate-risk participant during each visit. Thus, facilities might consider developing a standard protocol in which anyone classified as moderate risk or greater must receive physician consent before pursuing a vigorous-intensity exercise program (12). This protocol helps ensure the greatest safety for exercise participants.

Individuals classified as moderate or high risk should obtain physician consent before they begin a vigorous-intensity exercise program (e.g., $>60\% \dot{V}O_2R$) (1, 2, 12). For example, a 48-yr-old physically inactive male with high cholesterol and hypertension who wants to pursue a jogging program, which is high intensity, has four risk factors (age, sedentary lifestyle, high BP, elevated cholesterol). He would be classified as being at moderate risk, and thus physician consent is required before he can participate in the program. The fitness professional should be aware that participants with diabetes (type 1 or type 2) are classified as high risk regardless of additional risk factors for CHD and need physician consent before exercising (1, 2, 12).

Although the AHA and ACSM offer specific recommendations regarding medical clearance before exercise participation, it is in the best interest of fitness facilities for the director to determine the preactivity screening policy based on personnel qualifications, emergency preparedness, and target population (1-4). Remember, individuals classified as low risk never need physician consent before exercise testing or participation, whereas individuals at high risk always do. Individuals who are at moderate risk only need physician consent before maximal exercise testing or participation at high intensities. Figure 2.1 provides an overview of the protocol for medical history, risk stratification, and physician consent.

MR. PLEASE: Administration of Fitness Tests and Evaluation of Results

The next step of the health appraisal involves administering and evaluating fitness tests. When combined with the HSQ, the test results provide greater insight into an individual's current level of physical fitness. Common measurements obtained before fitness testing are RHR and BP, percent body fat, waist circumference, and low-back flexibility. Next, a submaximal graded exercise test is conducted to determine how the participant's HR, BP, and rating of perceived exertion (RPE) respond to gradually increasing exercise workloads. Additional fitness tests may determine muscular strength and endurance. Fitness testing procedures are included in chapters 7, 8, 9, and 10. If symptoms suggestive of cardiovascular or pulmonary disease occur during fitness testing, the fitness professional should determine if the participant warrants physician referral. Possible indications of these diseases that require a physician referral include the participant complaining of chest pain, experiencing a failure of SBP to rise appropriately with increases in exercise intensity, or indicating a pronounced shortness of breath at low exercise intensities.

KEY POINT

The last two sections of the HSQ enable the fitness professional to learn what medications participants are taking and their specific level of physical activity. These results should be considered along with participants' risk factors so that they can be readily risk stratified and the fitness professional can determine whether physician consent is necessary before undergoing fitness testing. In addition, if symptoms suggestive of cardiovascular, pulmonary, or metabolic disease occur during fitness testing, physician referral may be necessary.

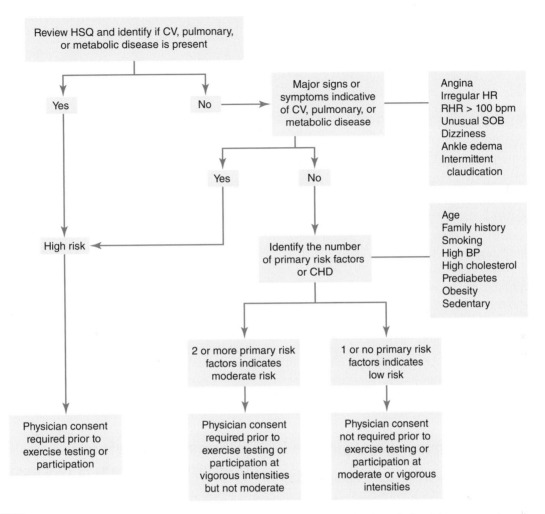

FIGURE 2.1 Flow chart for medical history, risk stratification, and determination of physician consent.

Based on American College of Sports Medicine 2010.

The results of the fitness tests should be compared with normative data based on the participant's age and gender (1). The classification of the fitness test values, combined with the participant's medical history, risk stratification, and exercise goals, should serve as the framework for the exercise prescription.

MR. PLEASE: Setup of Exercise Prescription

At this point, the fitness professional should be prepared to address the next step in the health appraisal process: setting up the exercise prescription by following current guidelines (1-3). An appropriate exercise prescription considers a person's health status, risk stratification, personal goals, and fitness test results. Chapters 11 through 14 address exercise prescriptions for aerobic fitness, weight management, muscular strength and endurance, flexibility, and low-back function for generally healthy adults. In addition, chapters 15 through 21 provide information on prescribing exercise for special populations.

MR. PLEASE: Evaluation of Progress With Follow-Up Tests

The participant's exercise goals and health status are certain to change over time, which necessitates the last step in the health appraisal: evaluating progress with follow-up tests. Fitness tests should be periodically repeated and an HSQ readministered. Follow-ups involving fitness tests and updates to the participant's health status serve several purposes: documenting the participant's health and fitness progress, identifying any changes in health status or response to activity, and indicating whether changes in the exercise prescription or level of supervision are necessary. A follow-up fitness test may be conducted 3 mo after the participant has been exercising regularly, with biannual testing thereafter.

Health Appraisal Overview

*M*edical history review. Use a preactivity screening questionnaire to determine if any symptoms of the big three chronic diseases (i.e., cardiovascular, pulmonary, metabolic) are present, indicating that physician consent is necessary before undergoing exercise testing or participation.

*R*isk-factor assessment and risk stratification. Identify risk factors and stratify participants (e.g., low, moderate, high) based on their sum of risk factors for CHD.

*P*rescribed medications. Identify medications that will alter the typical physiological responses to exercise and document that medications are being taken as prescribed.

*L*evel of physical activity. Determine if the participant is physically inactive. If the person already exercises, assess the frequency, intensity, duration, and type of exercise performed.

*E*stablishing the need for physician consent. The participant's medical history should be evaluated for the presence of the big three chronic diseases, risk stratification, and current level of physical activity. This information should be used to determine if physician consent is necessary prior to fitness test administration and regular physical activity participation according to the AHA and ACSM standards of practice.

*A*dministration of fitness tests and evaluation of results. Determine what fitness tests are appropriate given the participant's health status and compare the results with normative values based on age and gender.

*S*etup of exercise prescription. Consider the participant's medical history, past physical activity patterns, fitness results, and personal goals to prescribe an appropriate exercise program.

*E*valuation of progress with follow-up tests. Determine if the participant's fitness level and risk stratification have changed.

Fitness Program Decisions

This chapter has addressed the guidelines supported by the AHA and ACSM concerning when physician consent is necessary before a participant undergoes fitness testing or begins an exercise program. The following section discusses additional criteria to consider as the fitness professional decides which of the following actions to pursue:

- Immediate referral for physician consent or proper medical consultation
- Admission to one of the following fitness programs:
  - Clinic-based supervised exercise program
  - Appropriately prescribed exercise under the supervision of a fitness professional
  - Vigorous-intensity exercise
  - Any unsupervised physical activity
- Educational information, seminars, or referral to other health professionals

Fitness professionals will encounter individuals who are on the verge of meeting the criteria for moderate or high risk but are not quite there. Do they require physician consent? Should they exercise in a supervised program? The following section helps resolve these dilemmas.

Determining If Referral to a Supervised Program Is Necessary

The fitness professional should consider the participant's health status and desired activity level to determine whether referral to a supervised exercise program is necessary. A supervised program, sometimes referred to as a *phase III program*, entails professionally qualified staff who have academic training in and clinical knowledge of monitoring special populations classified as high risk (e.g., individuals diagnosed with cardiovascular, pulmonary, or metabolic disease) (1-3). These types of programs are also better suited for individuals with special conditions (e.g., emphysema, chronic bronchitis, cancer, epilepsy) that warrant additional supervision by medically qualified personnel (e.g., nurses or registered clinical exercise physiologists) who have experience with special populations.

Section 2 of the HSQ helps identify health conditions that require constant supervision. For example, the HSQ of a prospective participant reveals he has chronic bronchitis and typically requires supplemental oxygen when exercising. The participant has been walking regularly and independently but never monitors his blood oxygen levels (i.e., O_2 saturation levels). In this case, the pulmonary condition dictates that the participant's oxygen levels should be monitored before, during, and after exercise participation to ensure that O_2 saturation levels are maintained. This individual would benefit by initially exercising in a clinic-based supervised exercise program, such as a supervised pulmonary rehabilitation or cardiac rehabilitation program (e.g., phase III). As with physician consent, there are no universal guidelines for referring an individual to supervised programs. Each exercise facility should have standards regarding the health conditions it considers itself qualified to supervise, and these standards should be based on the qualifications of its fitness professionals, the availability of medical equipment (e.g., supplemental O_2, automatic external defibrillator [AED]), and its emergency preparedness (4). As always, fitness professionals should use their personal experience, as well as consultation with a supervisor or physician, to determine whether referral to a supervised program is necessary.

KEY POINT

The fitness professional should consider the participant's health status, risk stratification, desired activity level, and fitness test results, in addition to the facility's preactivity screening standards and emergency preparedness, to determine whether referral to a supervised exercise program is necessary.

Obtaining Physician Consent

After determining that a person requires physician consent, the fitness professional should promptly inform the participant of this requirement. The appropriate medical personnel, typically the participant's primary care physician, should provide the consent. A sample physician form is presented in form 2.3 (4). The form provides the physician with the option to refer the patient to a clinic-based supervised exercise facility. When a physician makes this recommendation, the fitness professional should contact the participant promptly and place him in contact with the nearest supervised exercise facility. In accordance with HIPAA regulations, the request for physician consent must be accompanied by a notation indicating that the participant understands that personal health information will be shared with appropriate allied health professionals. This permission is granted with the participant's signature in the medical release section of the HSQ (15).

Physician consent can be sought in one of two ways. First, the participant can be given the paperwork to be signed by a physician. After consulting with a physician, the participant can return the paperwork to the fitness professional for verification. Second, fitness professionals can contact the appropriate physician directly (e.g., fax the consent form to the physician's administrative office). Taking the initiative to contact a physician has both ben-

efits and challenges. The following are benefits of taking the initiative:

- Demonstrates recognition of conditions requiring physician consent.
- Permits a relatively prompt reply from the physician.
- Acquires additional medical information so that the participant receives appropriate exercise testing and prescription.
- Builds rapport with local physicians conducive to obtaining future exercise referrals from them.

The workload of primary care physicians does not allow them to quickly respond to each medical request they receive. Thus, it is recommended to wait 3 business days before sending a second physician consent request. Thereafter, participants should be encouraged to contact the physician personally to expedite the return of the consent form. Participants requiring physician consent should be informed of the facility's protocol for contacting physicians so that they understand that their clearance to begin exercising may take time. Although they may have to wait to exercise, participants should be assured that the steps taken in accordance with established protocols are serving their best health interests.

KEY POINT

The participant's physician or appropriate medical personnel should be contacted immediately when physician consent is required for exercise participation.

To prevent the delay of fitness tests for individuals requiring physician clearance, the HSQ should be completed and furnished to the appropriate fitness professional for review 2 to 3 business days before a fitness test is scheduled. This will provide time to secure physician clearance and ensure that the appropriate paperwork is completed before the fitness test, allowing the participant to begin an exercise program shortly thereafter.

Education

All participants with documented primary risk factors or borderline clinical values for CHD should be provided with information about their increased risk for CHD, such as calculating their 10 yr CHD risk using the Framingham algorithm (16). In addition, the fitness professional should discuss sensible lifestyle changes that participants can pursue to more readily control their risk factors. However, information alone is unlikely to lead participants to make significant changes. Chapter 23 provides several

FORM 2.3   Sample Physician Consent Form*

Dear Dr.:_____

Your patient would like to begin an exercise program at _____ (name of health or fitness facility). After reviewing _____ (patient's name)'s responses to our health status questionnaire, we would appreciate your medical opinion and recommendations concerning participation in regular exercise. Please provide the following information and return this form to the following:

Name: _____

Address: _____

Phone/fax: _____

1. Are there specific concerns or conditions our staff should be aware of before this individual engages in regular exercise at our facility? Yes/No. If yes, please specify.

   _____

2. If this individual has completed a graded exercise test, please provide the following:

   a. Date of test _____

   b. A copy of the final exercise test report and interpretation

   c. Your specific recommendations for exercise training, including HR limits during exercise:

   _____

3. Please provide the following information so that we may contact you if we have any further questions:

   _____ I AGREE to the participation of this individual in regular exercise activity at your fitness facility.

   _____ I DO NOT AGREE that this individual is a candidate for exercise at your fitness facility, and this individual should be referred to a supervised exercise facility because _____.

Physician's signature _____

Physician's name _____

Address _____

Thank you for your consideration.

(Signature of fitness staff member) _____

*Must be accompanied by a medical release form in accordance with HIPAA regulations.

From E.T. Howley and D.L. Thompson, 2012, *Fitness professional's handbook, 6th ed.* (Champaign, IL: Human Kinetics). Adapted, by permission, from American College of Sports Medicine and American Heart Association, 1998, "Recommendations for cardiovascular screening, staffing, and emergency policies at health/fitness facilities," *Medicine and Science in Sports and Exercise* 30: 1009-1018.

approaches to changing behavior that fitness professionals can use to help the participant. In addition, the fitness professional can inform the participant of support groups, upcoming educational seminars, and other health professionals (e.g., dietitians) who can assist with healthy lifestyle choices.

Changing Health or Fitness Status

People who regularly participate in physical activity are likely to experience positive changes in their fitness and in their risk factors for CHD, such as greater CRF and lower resting BP. These changes can be readily observed by an increase in participants' exercise duration or intensity and when resting BP measurements are taken. Changes such as these improve quality of life and reduce the risk for chronic disease (see chapter 1).

However, new medical conditions may develop and not be readily apparent after a participant completes preactivity screening and fitness tests. Unless specifically asked about new conditions, participants may not reveal this information. For instance, a participant may begin to experience chest pain during exercise but may keep this information private. The HSQ directs participants to contact the fitness director when they experience significant changes in their health status, but not all clients may understand the importance of this communication. Although some people will notify staff members when health changes occur, many will not. Therefore, periodic fitness retesting and readministration of the HSQ are advisable to determine whether participants experiencing changes in health status should seek physician consent or be assigned to a clinic-based supervised program.

If participants develop symptoms such as significant chest pain during exercise, they should be referred to a physician. In addition, participants initially classified as low to moderate risk who develop a medical condition that reclassifies them as high risk should be referred to a physician (1-3). Additional situations in which moderate- and vigorous-intensity exercise should be discontinued are musculoskeletal problems exacerbated with activity and severe psychological, medical, or drug or alcohol problems that are not responding to therapy (2). In addition, exercise should be deferred with major changes in resting BP (1). It is the responsibility of the fitness professional to determine the length of time between follow-up fitness tests or HSQ administrations to ensure participants are properly risk stratified and pursuing an appropriate exercise program.

KEY POINT

Fitness professionals should be aware of temporary or chronic conditions that alter a participant's health status and warrant medical clearance, additional supervision, or changes in exercise recommendations. These conditions can be identified with periodic readministration of the HSQ and follow-up fitness tests.

STUDY QUESTIONS

1. What is the first step in the preactivity screening process, and what is its main objective?

2. When is it appropriate to use the PAR-Q versus the HSQ?

3. The categories of health appraisal can be recalled using the acronym *MR. PLEASE*. Provide a brief example of what each letter represents.

4. If a prospective exercise participant chooses not to complete a PAR-Q or HSQ, what is the next course of action?

5. Explain a sign or symptom that may indicate a participant has cardiac, pulmonary, or metabolic disease.

6. Section 3 of the HSQ addresses the identification of primary risk factors for CHD. Explain what a primary risk is and provide three examples, including the threshold for each.

7. Consider a 35-yr-old female who is 5 ft 6 in. (168 cm) and weighs 160 lb (72.6 kg), smokes occasionally on the weekends, and walks 3 days · wk^{-1} for 35 min. Her HSQ indicates that she does not have high BP or cholesterol or type 2 diabetes. Her resting BP is 118/60 mmHg and her RHR is 85 beats · min^{-1}. What are her primary risk factors, and why did you designate them as such?

8. Why is it important to consider participants' HDL-C levels when determining the number of risk factors?

9. What is an example of a chronic disease that puts an individual at high risk for cardiovascular complications during exercise participation?

10. Provide an example of an individual who would be at moderate risk for cardiovascular complications during exercise participation. When does this risk stratification require physician consent prior to exercise testing or participation?

11. Why is it important to review participants' medications?

12. Why is it important to determine if a prospective exercise participant is physically active or not?

13. After obtaining fitness test results, what standards should the fitness professional compare them with?

14. Explain two scenarios in which a participant may be referred to a clinic-based supervised exercise program.

CASE STUDIES

You can check your answers by referring to appendix A.

1. Barbara is a 48-yr-old female who has recently joined your fitness facility. She appears to be somewhat apprehensive as she taps her foot while you review her HSQ. After reviewing her medical history and determining her risk stratification, you conclude she can engage in unsupervised exercise. Next, you assess her resting measurements. Her resting HR is 112 beats · min^{-1} and BP is 158/94 mmHg. What do you do?

2. You are the instructor for a chair-based arthritis class that involves moderate-intensity aerobic exercise, stretching, and weightlifting and is open to the public. Everyone in the class completes a PAR-Q and answers *no* to all of the questions on the checklist. One of the participants is a woman of normal weight who mentions that she is 67 yr old when you speak with her. Upon further questioning, you find out she does not have any additional risk factors, and she walks 5 days · wk^{-1} for 35 min at a brisk pace. She saw her physician recently for her annual physical and was given a clean bill of health. She recently read that resistance training would be good for her and therefore wants to attend your class. What are her primary risk factors? Do you permit her to participate in the class? Why or why not? What advice do you give her?

3. Tom, a 47-yr-old marketing agent who has been physically inactive for several years, visits your fitness facility to begin his fitness assessment. He has seen his physician recently and brings his lab results with him. Reviewing his HSQ, you note that he does not have a family history of heart disease. He is 5 ft 9 in. (1.75 m), weighs 185 lb (83.9 kg), and has a 38 in. (99.1 cm) waist. His resting BP is 124/82 mmHg and his resting pulse rate is 76 beats · min^{-1}. His blood chemistry values include a total cholesterol of 195 mg · dl^{-1}, an LDL-C of 134 mg · dl^{-1}, and an HDL-C of 40 mg · dl^{-1}. (Consult table 2.2 for the defining criteria for CHD risk factors.). However, his HSQ states that he is taking medication for high BP and high cholesterol. His fasting blood glucose is 88 mg· dl^{-1}, and he wants to pursue vigorous-intensity exercise.

   a. Identify Tom's risk factors for CHD and list the clinical threshold for each one.

   b. Does he warrant physician consent before exercise testing and participation? Why or why not?

REFERENCES

1. American College of Sports Medicine (ACSM). 2010. *ACSM's guidelines for exercise testing and prescription.* 8th ed. Philadelphia: Lippincott Williams & Wilkins.

2. American College of Sports Medicine (ACSM). 2006. *ACSM's resource manual for guidelines for exercise testing and prescription.* 5th ed. Philadelphia: Lippincott Williams & Wilkins.

3. American College of Sports Medicine (ACSM). 2007. *ACSM's health/fitness facility standards and guidelines.* 3rd ed. Champaign, IL: Lippincott Williams & Wilkins.

4. American College of Sports Medicine (ACSM) and American Heart Association (AHA). 1998. ACSM/AHA joint position statement: Recommendations for cardiovascular screening, staffing, and emergency policies at health/fitness facilities. *Medicine and Science in Sports and Exercise* 30:1009-1018.

5. American College of Sports Medicine (ACSM) and American Heart Association (AHA). 2007. Exercise and acute cardiovascular events: Placing the risks into perspective. *Medicine and Science in Sports and Exercise* 39:886-897.

6. Canadian Society for Exercise Physiology (CSEP). 2005. Canadian fitness safety standards and recommended guidelines. www.csep.ca/forms.asp.

7. Cardinal B., J. Esters, and M. Cardinal. 1996. Evaluation of the revised physical activity readiness questionnaire in older adults. *Medicine and Science in Sports and Exercise* 28:468-472.

8. Expert Panel on Detection, Evaluation, and Treatment of High Blood Cholesterol in Adults. 2001. Executive summary of the third report of the National Cholesterol Education Program (NCEP) (Adult Treatment Panel III). *Journal of the American Medical Association* 285:2486-2497.

9. Fletcher, G., G. Balady, S. Blair, J. Blumenthal, C. Caspersen, B. Chaitman, S. Epstein, E. Froelicher, V. Froelicher, I . Pina, and M. Pollock. 1996. Statement on exercise: Benefits and recommendations for physical activity programs for all Americans. *Circulation* 94:857-862.

10. Fletcher, G., G. Balady, V. Froelicher, L. Hartley, W. Haskell, and M. Pollock. 1995. Exercise standards: A statement from the American Heart Association. *Circulation* 91:580-615.

11. Franke, W. 2005. Covering all bases: Working with new clients. *ACSM's Health and Fitness Journal* 9:13-17.

12. Gibbons, R., G. Balady, J. Bricker, B. Chaitman, G. Fletcher, V. Froelicher, D. Mark, et al. 2002. ACC/AHA 2002 guideline update to exercise testing: Summary article. A report of the American College of Cardiology/American Heart Association task force on practice guidelines (committee to update the 1997 exercise testing guidelines). *Journal of the American College of Cardiology* 40:1531-1540.

13. Grundy, S., R. Pasternak, P. Greenland, S. Smith Jr., and V. Fuster. 1999. Assessment of cardiovascular risk by use of multiple-risk-factor assessment equations: A statement for healthcare professionals from the American Heart Associa-tion and the American College of Cardiology. *Circulation* 100:1481-1492.

14. Haskell, W., I.M. Lee, R. Pate, K. Powell, S. Blair, et al. 2007. Physical activity and public health: Updated recommendation for adults from the American College of Sports Medicine and the American Heart Association. *Medicine and Science in Sports and Exercise* 39:1423-1434.

15. *Health Insurance Portability and Accountability Act (HIPAA), Subtitle F Section 1171 4(a).* August 21, 1996. Public law 104-191, 104th Cong.

16. Wilson, P., R. D'Agostino, D. Levy, A. Belanger, H. Silbershatz, and W. Kannel. 1998. Prediction of coronary heart disease using risk factor categories. *Circulation* 97:1837-1847.

Scientific Foundations

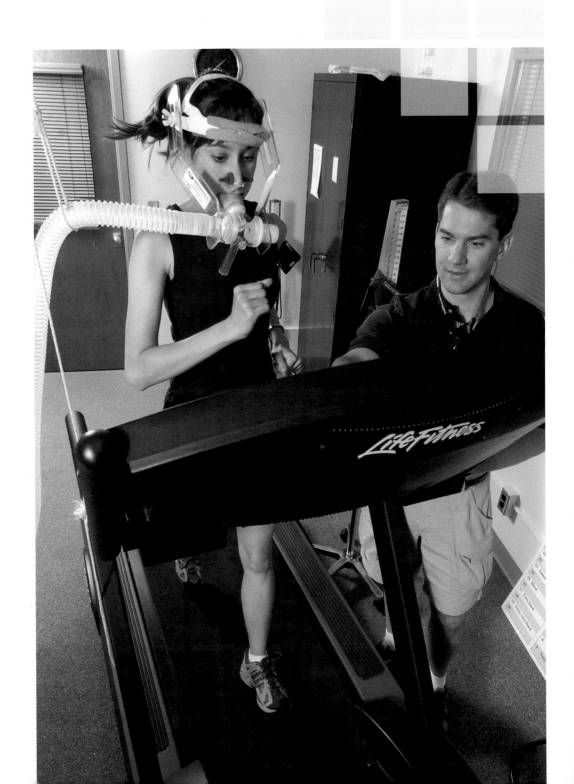

PART II

Part II provides the basic scientific foundation for understanding the structure and function of the human body, nutrition, and energy expenditure. In chapter 3, we review the bones, joints, and muscles of the body and their biomechanical functions during common physical activities. In chapter 4, we cover the basic concepts of energy, muscle function, and the physiological response to acute and chronic physical activity. Differences due to gender, type of exercise, and temperature are described. In chapter 5, we cover the basics of nutrition, and in chapter 6, we address the energy cost of physical activity.

Functional Anatomy and Biomechanics

Jean Lewis and Clare E. Milner

OBJECTIVES

The reader will be able to do the following:

1. Identify the major bones of the skeletal system and classify them by shape.

2. Name each synovial joint and demonstrate the movements possible.

3. Explain the differences among concentric, eccentric, and isometric muscle actions.

4. List the major muscles in each muscle group, and identify the major actions at the joints involved (shoulder girdle, shoulder joint, elbow joint, radioulnar joint, wrist joint, lumbo-sacral joint, spinal column, hip joint, knee joint, ankle joint, and subtalar joint).

5. Cite common exercises involving the major muscle groups and point out potential errors in their execution.

6. Describe the three factors that determine stability and describe the relationships among them during physical activity.

7. Explain how contracting muscles produce torque at a joint.

8. Describe how an exerciser can change positions of body segments to alter the resistance torque.

9. Define the mechanical principles of *rotational inertia* and *angular momentum* as applied to human movement.

10. Describe the key muscle groups involved in locomotion, throwing, cycling, jumping, swimming, and carrying objects.

11. Discuss common errors seen in locomotion, throwing, and striking.

The fitness professional must have knowledge of the bones, joints, and muscles; must understand muscle forces and other forces (e.g., gravity); and must be able to apply biomechanical principles to human movement. With this knowledge, the fitness professional is better equipped to direct safe physical activity for participants seeking the health-related benefits of exercise. This knowledge also helps earn the respect of clients, who will view the instructor as a professional in the field rather than a technician who may know what to do but not why. This chapter is merely a summary; for greater detail on anatomy and biomechanics, see the reference list (1-7).

Skeletal Anatomy

Most of the 200 distinct bones in the human skeleton are involved in movement. Their high mineral component gives them rigidity, while their protein component reduces their brittleness. The two types of bone tissue are cortical and trabecular bone. Cortical, or compact, bone is the dense, hard outer layer of a bone. Trabecular bone, also known as spongy or cancellous bone, has a lattice-like structure to provide greater internal strength along the lines of stress within a bone but with less overall weight than solid bone. Bones are living tissue and are constantly being remodeled in adaptation to the loading demands placed on them. Bones are divided into four classifications according to their shape: long, short, flat, and irregular.

Long Bones

The long bones, found in the limbs and digits, serve primarily as levers for movement. Each long bone has several distinct features. The **diaphysis**, or shaft, is made up of thick, compact bone surrounding the hollow medullary cavity. It is characteristic of long bones that the shaft is longer than it is wide. The **epiphyses**, or expanded ends, are composed of spongy bone with a thin outer layer of compact bone. The **articular cartilage** is a thin layer of hyaline cartilage covering the articulating surfaces (the surfaces of a bone that come into contact with another bone to form a joint) that provides a smooth, low-friction surface and helps absorb shock. The **periosteum** is a fibrous membrane covering the entire bone (except where the articular cartilage is present) to serve as an attachment site for muscles (see figure 3.1). Examples of long bones include the femur in the thigh, the ulna in the forearm, and the phalanges in the digits.

Short, Flat, and Irregular Bones

In addition to long bones, the skeleton is made up of short bones, flat bones, and irregularly shaped bones (see figure 3.2). The tarsals (in the ankle) and carpals (in the wrist) are the short bones, and they are approximately as wide as they are long. Their composition (internal trabecular bone

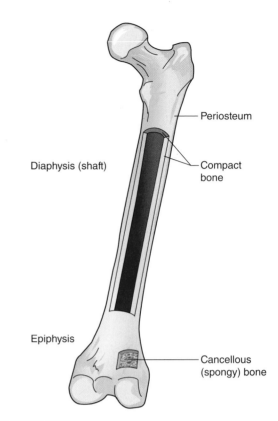

FIGURE 3.1 Structure of the femur, a long bone in the thigh.

covered with a thin outside layer of cortical bone) provides light weight and strength. Their roughly cubic shape decreases the potential for movement between adjacent bones. The flat bones, such as the ribs, ilia (wings of the pelvis), and scapulae (shoulder blades), serve primarily as broad sites for muscle attachments and, in the case of the ribs and ilia, to enclose cavities and protect internal organs. These bones have a broad, flattened structure. They are composed of trabecular bone covered with a thin layer of cortical bone. The ischium (inferior part of the pelvis), pubis (anterior part of the pelvis), and vertebrae are irregularly shaped bones that protect internal parts and support the body in addition to being sites for muscle attachments. An additional category of bone is reserved for those few bones in the body that are embedded within a tendon. The role of these bones is to modify the way a tendon crosses a joint. The patella (kneecap) is a sesamoid bone embedded in the quadriceps tendon at the knee.

KEY POINT

Bones are living tissues that are light in weight but strong and stiff. The combination of solid cortical bone on the outside and a lightweight scaffold of trabecular bone inside provides strength with less weight than solid bone.

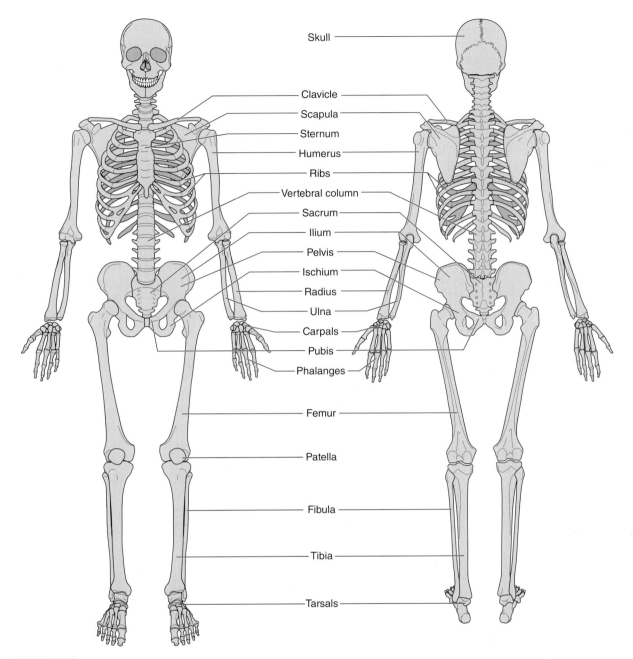

FIGURE 3.2 Anterior (front) and posterior (back) views of the human skeleton in the anatomical position.

Reprinted, by permission, from NSCA, 2000, The biomechanics of resistance training, by E. Harman. In *Essentials of strength training and conditioning*, 2nd ed., edited by T.R. Baechle and R.W. Earle (Champaign, IL: Human Kinetics), 27.

Ossification of Bones

The skeleton begins as a cartilaginous structure that is gradually replaced by bone during growth and maturation in a process known as **ossification**. This process begins at the diaphysis of long bones (in centers of ossification) and spreads toward the epiphyses. The **epiphyseal plates** between the diaphyses and epiphyses are the growth areas where the cartilage is replaced by bone; bone growth continues in length and width until the epiphyseal plates are completely ossified. During growth, additional cartilage is laid down to be replaced eventually by bone. When no further cartilage is produced and the cartilage present is replaced by bone, growth ceases. Secondary centers of ossification develop in the epiphyses and in some bony protuberances, such as the tibial tuberosity and the articular condyles of the humerus; however, short bones have one center of ossification. The age when growth plates close varies among individuals. Although bone fusion at some centers of ossification may occur by puberty or earlier, most of the long bones do not completely ossify until the late teens. Premature closing, which results in a shorter bone length, can be caused by trauma, abnormal stresses, malnutrition, and drugs.

Planes and Axes of Movement

Anatomical terminology enables the accurate description of position and movement of the human body. To describe joint movements, reference is made to rotation about one or more of three axes and to movement in one of three cardinal planes. These planes are perpendicular to each other and represent a side view (sagittal plane), front or back view (frontal or coronal plane), and top view, looking down from above (transverse plane). Movement observed in each plane is a rotation about an axis that is perpendicular to the plane. The reference position for describing movement is the anatomical position (standing erect, arms hanging at sides, palms facing forward, feet shoulder-width apart; see figure 3.3). The mediolateral axis is perpendicular to the sagittal plane, and joint rotations about this axis are flexion and extension. The anteroposterior axis is perpendicular to the frontal plane, and joint rotations about this axis are abduction and adduction. The longitudinal or vertical axis is perpendicular to the transverse plane, and rotations about this axis are **internal** and **external rotation**. Joint rotations are described according to how the distal segment (body

part just below the joint) moves relative to the proximal segment (body part just above the joint).

Structure and Function of Joints

Joints, which are the places where two or more bones meet, or articulate, are often classified according to the amount of movement that can take place at those sites. **Ligaments**, which are tough, fibrous bands of connective tissue, connect bones to each other across all joints. Joints are classified as synarthrodial, amphiarthrodial, or synovial based on how much they can move. **Synarthrodial joints** are immovable joints. The bones merge into each other and are bound together by fibrous tissue that is continuous with the periosteum. The sutures, or lines of junction, of the cranial (skull) bones are prime examples of this type of joint. **Amphiarthrodial joints**, or cartilaginous joints, allow only slight movement between bones. Usually a fibrocartilage disc separates the bones, and movement can occur only by deformation of the disc. Examples of these joints are the tibiofibular and sacroiliac joints and the joints between the bodies of the vertebrae in the spine.

Diarthrodial joints, more commonly known as synovial joints, are freely movable joints that allow greater movement direction and range; most of the joint movements during physical activity occur at these joints. The synovial joints are the most common type and include most joints of the extremities. Strong and inelastic ligaments, along with connective and muscle tissue crossing the joint, maintain their stability. Synovial joints have several distinguishing characteristics. The articulating surfaces of the bones are covered by articular cartilage, a type of hyaline cartilage that reduces friction and contributes to shock absorption between the bones. Each joint is completely enclosed by an **articular capsule**, whose thickness varies from thin and loose to thick and tight. The **synovial membrane** lines the inner surface of the capsule. It secretes synovial fluid into the **joint cavity**, the space enclosed by the articular capsule. Synovial fluid bathes the joint to nourish the articular cartilage and reduce friction when bones move. Normally, the joint cavity is small and, therefore, contains little synovial fluid, but an injury to the joint can increase the secretion of synovial fluid and cause swelling.

Some synovial joints, such as the sternoclavicular and knee joints, also have a partial or complete fibrocartilage disc between the bones to aid shock absorption and, in the case of the knee, to give greater stability to the joint. The partial, C-shaped discs between the femur and the tibia at the knee are called **menisci**. To reduce friction or rubbing as tendons move during muscle contraction, tendons often are surrounded by tendon sheaths—cylindrical, tunnel-like sacs lined with synovial membrane. For example, the two proximal tendons of the biceps brachii pass through these tunnels in the bicipital groove of the humerus. **Bursae**, or

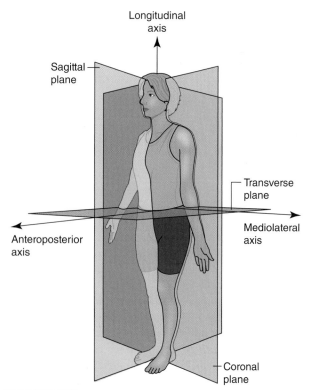

Longitudinal axis

Sagittal plane

Transverse plane

Mediolateral axis

Anteroposterior axis

Coronal plane

FIGURE 3.3 The anatomical position and the cardinal planes and axes of movement.

sacs of synovial fluid that lie between muscles, tendons, and bones, also reduce friction between the tissues and act as shock absorbers. Many bursae are found around the shoulder, elbow, hip, and knee. Bursitis, or the inflammation of a bursa, can result from repeated friction or mechanical irritation.

KEY POINT

The moveable joints in the body are diarthrodial (synovial) joints. The bony surfaces are covered in smooth articular cartilage and the joint cavity is filled with synovial fluid, which lubricates the joint.

Factors Determining Direction and Range of Motion

The primary movement at a joint is rotation about one or more axes. Some joints may exhibit a small amount of sliding (translation) between the bones. The limits to direction and the range of motion (ROM) at a joint are determined primarily by the shape of the bones at their articulating ends. Depending on the bone shape, joints may rotate about one, two, or three axes. Ball-and-socket joints, which are found at the hip and shoulder, allow a wide range of movement in all directions as the ball rotates within the socket. Hinge joints, such as the elbow and ankle joints, have only one axis of rotation due to the structure of the interlocking bones. Other types of joints include ellipsoidal joints, such as the wrist, and saddle joints, such as the sternoclavicular joint, whose shapes permit rotation about two axes. Pivot joints, such as the proximal radioulnar joint, permit rotation about one axis only, the longitudinal axis. Gliding joints, such as between the tarsal bones in the foot, have minimal sliding movement between the bones. The length of the ligaments and to a lesser extent their **elasticity**, or ability to stretch passively and return to their normal length, also limit ROM. For example, the iliofemoral ligament at the anterior hip joint is a strong but short ligament that prohibits much hip extension.

KEY POINT

The limits to range and direction of motion at a joint are determined by the shape of the articulating bones and the length of ligaments crossing the joint.

Specific Joint Movements

Specific terminology is used to describe the direction of movement at the various joints. This ensures that movements are described accurately and can be immediately understood. The anatomical position (see figure 3.3) serves as a point of reference. Terminology generally relates to movements within planes and about axes. **Flexion** and **extension** are movements in the sagittal plane about a mediolateral axis. Flexion is moving the distal segment forward and upward from the anatomical position to bring two body segments closer together. Extension is the return from flexion, moving the segment in the opposite direction. **Abduction** and **adduction** are movements in the frontal plane about an anteroposterior axis. Abduction is moving the distal segment out to the side and away from the body from the anatomical position, whereas adduction is the return toward the anatomical position from abduction, moving the segment in the opposite direction. Internal and external rotation are movements in the transverse plane about a longitudinal axis. **Internal rotation** is turning a segment toward the midline of the body from the anatomical position. **External rotation** is the return toward the anatomical position, turning the segment in the opposite direction. Exceptions to these general descriptions are noted in the following text where they occur for specific joints.

Shoulder Girdle

The primary articulation between the scapula (shoulder blade) and the thoracic cage (ribs) is not a traditional joint because there is no direct contact between the bones, which have several muscles between them. However, there is a large ROM of the scapula on the thoracic cage that has its own terminology. Vertical movements are *elevation* (upward movement) and *depression* (downward movement). Horizontal movements are *protraction* or *abduction* (out to the side) and *retraction* or *adduction* (in toward the spine). Rotational movements are *upward* and *downward rotation* (see figure 3.4). Movements of the shoulder girdle combine with movements of the shoulder joint to provide the large ROM found at the shoulder. The shoulder girdle also includes the sternoclavicular joint, between the sternum (breastbone) and clavicle (collarbone), and the acromioclavicular joint, between the scapula and clavicle. These joints move when the scapulothoracic joint moves.

Shoulder Joint

The glenohumeral joint is a ball-and-socket joint, so it can move in all directions—flexion, extension, abduction, adduction, internal and external rotation, and circumduction (tips of the fingers trace a circle in the sagittal plane). Horizontal adduction and horizontal abduction are additional movements of the upper limb toward and away from the midline when it is positioned in the transverse plane (parallel to the ground) (see figure 3.5).

The relationship between the scapulothoracic and shoulder joints is called *scapulohumeral rhythm*. The glenohumeral joint alone cannot reach the full ROM seen at the shoulder because it is restricted by the bone structure at the joint. However, the glenoid fossa that makes up part

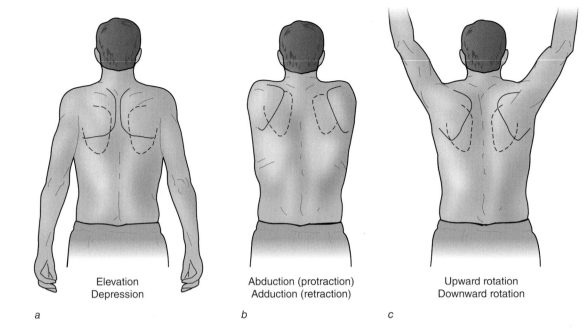

Elevation
Depression

a

Abduction (protraction)
Adduction (retraction)

b

Upward rotation
Downward rotation

c

FIGURE 3.4 Movements of the scapulae (scapulothoracic joint).

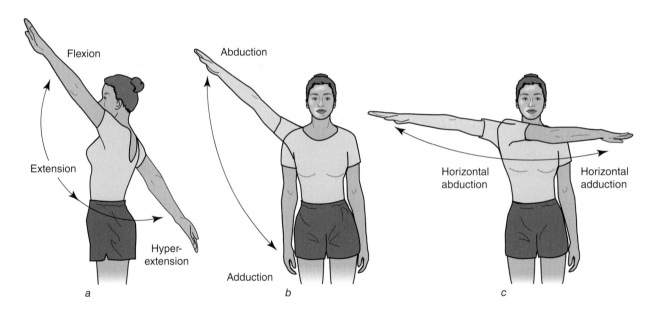

Flexion

Extension

Hyper-
extension

a

Abduction

Adduction

b

Horizontal
abduction

Horizontal
adduction

c

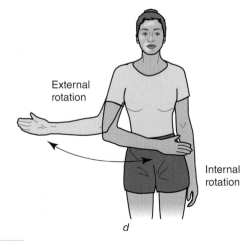

External
rotation

Internal
rotation

d

FIGURE 3.5 Movements of the shoulder (glenohumeral) joint.

of the glenohumeral joint is part of the scapula, so if the scapula also moves, greater ROM can occur.

Elbow Joint

The elbow joint is the articulation between the humerus and the two forearm bones, the radius and ulna. The ulnohumeral joint is the primary joint, and as a hinge joint, it limits movements to flexion and extension (see figure 3.6). The radiohumeral joint is also part of the elbow joint, but it does not provide much bony stability. The ability of some individuals to hyperextend the elbow joint is due to differences in the shape of their articulating surfaces.

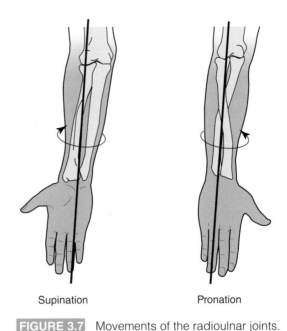

Supination   Pronation

FIGURE 3.7 Movements of the radioulnar joints.

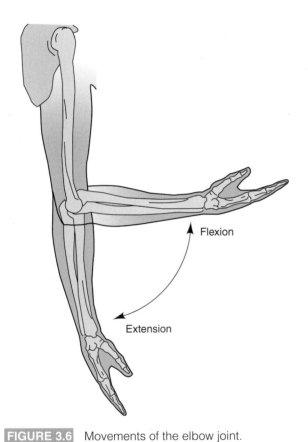

Flexion

Extension

FIGURE 3.6 Movements of the elbow joint.

Wrist Joint

The wrist joint consists of the radiocarpal and ulnocarpal articulations between the forearm bones and the carpal bones of the wrist. Movements at the wrist include joint flexion, extension, abduction (radial flexion), and adduction (ulnar flexion) (see figure 3.8).

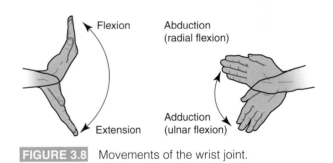

Flexion   Abduction (radial flexion)

Extension   Adduction (ulnar flexion)

FIGURE 3.8 Movements of the wrist joint.

Radioulnar Joints

The radius and ulna articulate with each other both proximally and distally in the forearm. The joint movements are pronation and supination (see figure 3.7). Although the wrist is not involved in these movements, the position of the radioulnar joints can be identified by the direction the palms face. When the arms hang down alongside the trunk, the palms face forward in the supinated position and toward the back in the pronated position. In the supinated position, the radius and ulna are parallel with each other; in the pronated position, the radius lies across and on top of the ulna.

Metacarpophalangeal and Interphalangeal Joints

The metacarpophalangeal joints are the knuckles of the hand. The second through the fifth joints move in flexion and extension as well as abduction and adduction of the fingers. The metacarpophalangeal joint of the thumb allows only flexion and extension. The ability of the opposable thumb to touch the tips of all the other digits comes from movement at the carpometacarpal joint. The interphalangeal joints of the fingers and thumb are hinge joints that flex and extend.

Vertebral Column

The vertebral column contains 24 individual vertebrae and the sacrum. Although movement between adjacent vertebrae is just a few degrees, when combined over the whole vertebral column, the ROM of the trunk is substantial. Movements of the trunk occur in all three planes: flexion and extension, lateral flexion to the left and right, and rotation to the left and right (see figure 3.9).

Lumbosacral Joint

The pelvis (see figure 3.10) tilts mainly at the joint formed by the fifth lumbar vertebra and the sacrum. A reference for the direction of pelvic tilt is a line between the anterior and posterior superior iliac spines in the sagittal plane. When the pelvis tilts anteriorly, the angle between the horizontal and the line between the iliac spines increases. With posterior pelvic tilt, the angle of the line between the iliac spines becomes closer to the horizontal. Anterior pelvic tilt is accompanied by extension of the lumbar spine, whereas a backward tilt results in a flattening out of the lumbar spine.

Hip Joint

The hip joint is a ball-and-socket joint similar to the shoulder (glenohumeral joint), but the bony socket at the hip is much deeper compared with the shoulder. The deep socket makes the hip more stable than the shoulder at the expense of total ROM (see figure 3.11). For example, extension is less at the hip than at the shoulder. Movements at the hip joint are flexion, extension, abduction, adduction, internal rotation, external rotation, and circumduction (a movement

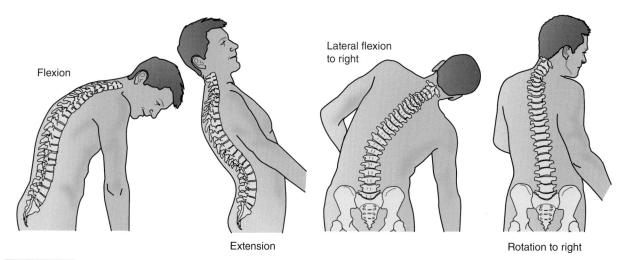

FIGURE 3.9 Movements of the vertebral column and trunk.

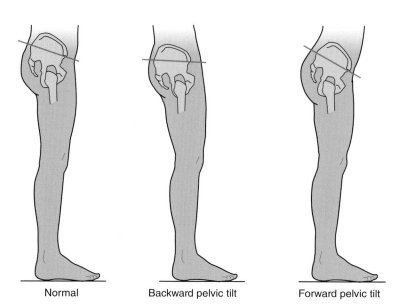

Normal   Backward pelvic tilt   Forward pelvic tilt

FIGURE 3.10 Movements of the lumbosacral joint and pelvis.

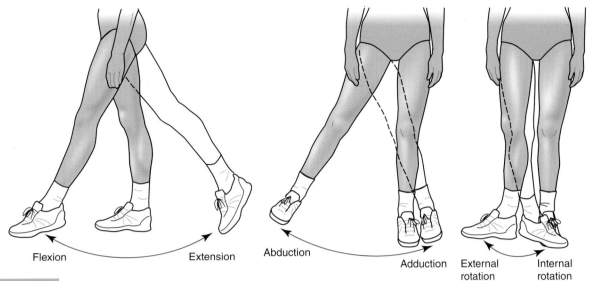

Flexion   Extension   Abduction   Adduction   External rotation   Internal rotation

FIGURE 3.11 Movements of the hip joint.

combining flexion, extension, abduction, and adduction that results in the foot moving in a circular motion).

Knee Joint

The tibiofemoral joint is the primary knee joint. The knee does not have good bony stability in flexion due to the flattened surface of the tibial plateau; therefore, it relies on ligaments to provide stability, making it vulnerable to injury. Flexion and extension are the major movements at the knee (see figure 3.12). When the knee is in a flexed position, limited rotation, abduction, and adduction are possible.

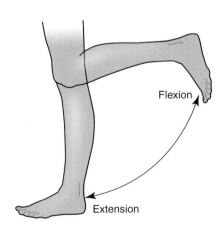

Flexion

Extension

FIGURE 3.12 Movements of the knee joint.

Ankle Joint

Also called the **talocrural joint**, the ankle joint is limited to movement in one plane only. Plantar flexion is pointing the foot downward and dorsiflexion is pulling the foot up toward the shin (see figure 3.13).

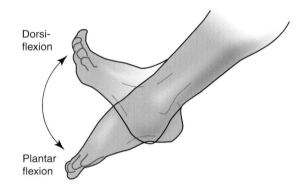

Dorsi-flexion

Plantar flexion

FIGURE 3.13 Movements of the ankle joint.

Subtalar Joint

The subtalar joint contributes to pronation and supination movements of the foot. In the frontal plane, these movements are eversion and inversion (see figure 3.14). In combination with other foot joints, the subtalar joint lowers the medial longitudinal arch (pronation) via a combination of eversion, dorsiflexion, and abduction. The

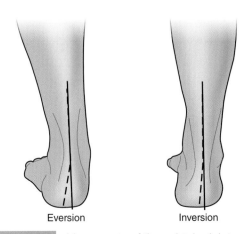

Eversion   Inversion

FIGURE 3.14 Movements of the subtalar joint.

Adapted, by permission, from J. Johnson, 2011, *Postural assessment* (Champaign, IL: Human Kinetics), 63.

opposite movement is supination, and it raises the arch via a combination of inversion, plantar flexion, and adduction.

Skeletal Muscle

Skeletal, or voluntary, muscles consist of thousands of muscle fibers (e.g., the brachioradialis has approximately 130,000 fibers; the gastrocnemius has more than 1 million) and connective tissue. Each fiber is enclosed by the endomysium, a type of connective tissue. The **fascicles**, or bundles of fibers grouped together, are surrounded by the **perimysium**, and the entire muscle is enclosed by the **epimysium**. The **tendon** is the passive part of the muscle and is made up of elastic connective tissue. Each muscle attaches to bone at the periosteum or alternatively to deep, thick fascial tissue via tendons and the perimysium and epimysium connective tissues. The size and shape of tendons depend on the functions and shape of the muscles. Some tendons can be easily seen and palpated just under the surface of the skin, such as the hamstring muscle tendons at the sides of the posterior aspect of the knee and the Achilles tendon inserting into the posterior heel. Other muscles, such as the supraspinatus and infraspinatus (muscles of the rotator cuff in the shoulder), are attached directly to the bone with no observable tendon. Broad and flat tendons, such as the proximal tendinous sheath of the latissimus dorsi, are **aponeuroses**. Refer to figure 3.15 for anterior and posterior views of surface muscles. Other muscles lie underneath the surface muscles.

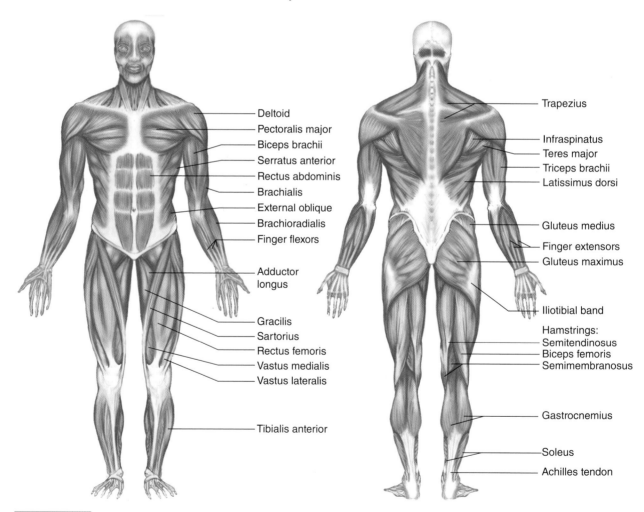

FIGURE 3.15 Anterior (front) and posterior (back) views of the human body in the anatomical position with surface muscles illustrated.

Reprinted, by permission, from NSCA, 2008, Biomechanics of resistance training, by E. Harman. In *Essentials of strength training and conditioning*, 3rd ed., edited by T.R. Baechle and R.W. Earle (Champaign, IL: Human Kinetics), 68.

TABLE 3.1 Movements at Main Synovial Joints

Joint	Movements
Shoulder girdle (scapulothoracic joint)	Elevation, depression; protraction (abduction), retraction (adduction); upward rotation, downward rotation
Shoulder joint (glenohumeral joint)	Flexion, extension; abduction, adduction; internal rotation, external rotation; horizontal adduction, horizontal abduction
Elbow joint	Flexion, extension
Radioulnar joint	Pronation, supination
Wrist joint	Flexion, extension; abduction (radial flexion), adduction (ulnar flexion)
Metatarsophalangeal joints	Flexion, extension; abduction, adduction
Vertebral column	Flexion, extension; lateral flexion; rotation
Lumbosacral joint	Anterior pelvic tilt, posterior pelvic tilt
Hip joint	Flexion, extension; abduction, adduction; internal rotation, external rotation
Knee joint	Flexion, extension
Ankle joint	Plantar flexion, dorsiflexion
Subtalar joint	Eversion, inversion

Forces That Cause Movement

Joint movement is caused primarily by either the shortening of a muscle or the action of gravity, although other forces, such as another person pushing or pulling on a body part, may cause joint movement. Whether a muscle contraction causes movement depends on the combined effect of the force developed and the amount of resistance from other forces.

Forces That Resist or Prevent Movement

The same forces that can cause movement may also resist or prevent movement. Joint movement caused by gravity can be resisted or decelerated by eccentric muscle action (which lengthens the muscle; see the section on eccentric action later in the chapter). Gravity always resists movement occurring in a direction away from the earth. Other forces that can resist movement include internal soft-tissue restriction by ligaments and tendons. Outside the body, exercise bands, hydraulic or air-pressure devices on resistance training equipment, and the drag provided by air and water against bodies moving through them can resist movement.

Muscle Action

Each muscle fiber is innervated, or receives stimuli, by a branch of a motor neuron. A **motor unit** consists of a single motor neuron, its branches, and all the muscle fibers that it innervates. With a sufficiently strong stimulus, each muscle fiber within that motor unit responds maximally; muscular tension increases as a result of the stimulation of more motor units (**recruitment**) or an increased rate of stimulation (**summation**). A muscle whose primary purpose is a strength or power movement (e.g., the gastrocnemius) rather than a delicate movement (e.g., the finger muscles) has a large number of muscle fibers and many muscle

fibers per motor unit. When a muscle develops tension, it tends to shorten toward the middle, pulling on all of its bony attachments. Whether the attached bones move as a result of that muscle action depends on the amount of muscle force and the resistance to that movement from other forces. The three major muscle actions are concentric, eccentric, and isometric.

Concentric Action

Concentric action occurs when a muscle shortens under tension. This shortening pulls the points of attachment on each bone closer to each other, causing movement at the joint. Figure 3.16 illustrates elbow flexion moving a dumbbell against gravity as a result of a concentric action. The muscles responsible for flexion act with sufficient force to shorten, which pulls the forearm toward the humerus. Although the pull is on all the bones of attachment, usually only the bone farthest from the trunk (i.e., more distal) moves during a concentric action. To stand up from a semisquat position, the body must extend at the hip joints and knee joints, but gravity resists that extension. The muscles must develop sufficient force to overcome the force of gravity as the muscle shortens in a concentric action, pulling on the bones to cause extension. Resistance training with free weights uses gravity as the resistance. The use of pulleys in resistance training machines changes the direction of the force needed to overcome gravity acting on the weight stack, offering resistance to movement in other directions. Water resists the movement of submerged body parts in all directions.

To exercise muscles by using gravity as the resisting force, the movements must be done in the direction opposite the pull of gravity (i.e., away from the Earth). Shoulder abduction from a standing position occurs opposite the pull of gravity, so a concentric action is required by the muscles that will pull the humerus into the abducted position. Movements such as shoulder horizontal abduction and adduction (see figure 3.5) executed from a standing position occur parallel to the ground and, therefore, are not resisted by gravity. During these movements, gravity is still trying to draw the upper limb toward the Earth (requiring concentric action of the shoulder abductors to overcome it). To perform horizontal abduction and adduction against the resistance of gravity, the performer must get into a position in which these movements are away from the pull of gravity. To horizontally abduct the shoulder against gravity, the performer can lie prone on a bench or stand with the trunk flexed 90° at the hip. Horizontal adduction against gravity can be done from a supine position on a bench.

A concentric action is also necessary for a rapid movement, regardless of the direction of other forces. When an external force could cause the desired movement without any muscular action but would be too slow, concentric actions produce the desired speed. An example of this is seen in the upper-limb movements during the second count of a jumping jack, when the arms adduct from their abducted position. Gravity would adduct the arms, but concentrically acting muscles speed up the adduction.

A muscle that is very effective in causing a certain joint movement is a prime mover, or **agonist**. Assistant movers are muscles that are not as effective for the same movement. For example, the peroneus longus and brevis are prime movers for eversion of the foot, but they assist plantar flexion of the ankle joint only a little. During a concentric action, muscles that act opposite to the muscles causing the concentric action, the **antagonist** muscles, are mostly passive and lengthen as the agonists shorten. For example, for the elbow to flex against gravity, the muscles responsible for elbow flexion act concentrically, while the antagonists, or the muscles responsible for elbow extension, relax and lengthen passively.

Eccentric Action

An **eccentric action** occurs when a muscle generates tension that is not great enough to cause movement but instead slows the speed of movement in the opposite direction caused by another force (see figure 3.16). The muscle exerts force, but its length increases while it is under tension. Shoulder abduction requires concentric action, but gravity will adduct the upper limb back to the side of the body. To adduct the upper limb more slowly than gravity does, the same muscles that acted concentrically to abduct the upper limb now act eccentrically to control the speed of upper limb. Eccentric actions may also occur when the maximum effort of a muscle is not great enough to overcome the opposing force. Movement due to the opposing force will still occur despite the maximally activated muscle, which is lengthening under tension. An example of this may occur when a person with the elbow joint flexed to 90° is handed a heavy weight. The exerciser tries to flex the elbow joint or even maintain the 90° position but lacks the strength to do so. The elbow joint extends despite the efforts to flex it. Muscles that are antagonists to the eccentrically acting muscles will passively shorten during the movement.

Ballistic Movements and Muscle Action

A **ballistic movement** is a fast movement that occurs when resistance is minimal, as in throwing a ball, and requires a burst of concentric action to initiate it. Once movement has begun, these initial muscles relax because any further action would slow the movement. Other muscles actively guide the movement in the appropriate direction. At the end of the movement, eccentric action of muscles that are antagonist to the initial muscles decelerates and stops the movement. For example, one of the most important movements in throwing is internal rotation of the shoulder joint. The muscles responsible for internal rotation act quickly and concentrically to begin the throwing motion. After the ball is released, the muscles responsible for external rotation act eccentrically to slow and stop the movement during the follow-through. The reverse is true for the windup, or preparation for the actual throw.

Jumping jacks require repeated ballistic movements in which opposing muscles come into play. The upper-limb movements require concentric action by the agonist muscles to initiate the rapid movement. Once the movement is initiated, these muscles relax. To stop the abduction movement and initiate the upper-limb movement in the opposite direction, muscles antagonistic to those that

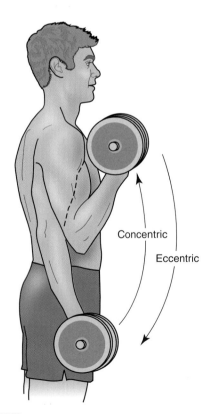

Concentric

Eccentric

FIGURE 3.16 Concentric and eccentric action of the elbow flexors during a biceps curl.

acted concentrically act eccentrically to decelerate the movement and then act concentrically to initiate the next movement (adduction).

Isometric Action

During an **isometric action**, or static action, the muscle exerts a force that is equal in magnitude to an opposing force. The muscle length does not change and the joint position is maintained: The contractile part of the muscle shortens, but the elastic connective tissue lengthens proportionately, so there is no overall change in the entire muscle length. Holding the upper limb in an abducted position or maintaining a semisquat position requires isometric action, producing just enough muscle force to counteract the pull of gravity and result in no movement. The effort involved in trying to move an immovable object (e.g., pushing against a wall) is another example of an isometric action; although the amount of muscular force can be maximal, the joint does not move (see figure 3.17).

The posterior pelvic tilt desired during some exercises is maintained by isometric action of the anterior trunk muscles after they have acted concentrically to tilt the pelvis backward. During all resistance exercises that involve the arms or legs, the trunk muscles should act isometrically to stabilize the trunk and help prevent injury.

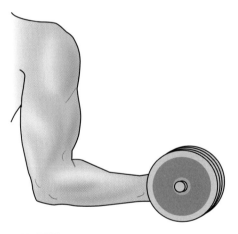

FIGURE 3.17 Isometric action of the elbow flexor muscles holding a dumbbell.

KEY POINT

During concentric muscle action, the muscle shortens and the joint moves in the direction the muscle is pulling. During eccentric muscle action, the muscle lengthens and the joint moves in the opposite direction than the muscle is pulling. During isometric muscle contraction there is no change in length and the joint does not move.

Role of Muscles

Skeletal muscles can act in several ways and have a variety of effects on joint movement. They can cause movement via concentric action or decelerate movement caused by another force via eccentric action. Muscles may also act isometrically to stabilize or prevent undesirable movement. For example, during a push-up, gravity tends to cause the lumbar spine to hyperextend. Isometric action of the trunk muscles prevents this sagging and stabilizes the lumbar region in a neutral position.

Another function of muscle is to counteract an undesirable action caused by the concentric action of another muscle. The concentric action of many muscles causes more than one movement at the same joint or causes movement at more than one joint. If only one of those movements is intended, another muscle must act to prevent the undesirable movement. For example, concentric action of fibers in the upper trapezius both elevates and adducts the scapula. If only adduction is desired, fibers in the lower trapezius, which cause depression and adduction, neutralize the undesirable scapula elevation. In this example, different fibers of the same large trapezius muscle neutralize the unwanted action. As another example, the biceps brachii causes both elbow flexion and radioulnar supination, so for only flexion to occur, the pronator teres counteracts the supination movement.

Muscles can also guide movements caused by other muscles. During activities against a great resistance, such as lifting free weights, additional muscles help maintain balance and proper direction of the movement. After the force of a prime mover has initiated a ballistic movement, other muscles guide the movement in the proper direction.

KEY POINT

The major roles of the muscles are to cause movement (concentric action) regardless of an opposing force, decelerate or control the speed of movement (eccentric action) caused by another force, and prevent movement (isometric action). Other muscle functions include counteracting an undesirable action caused by the concentric action of another muscle and guiding movements caused by another muscle.

Muscle Groups

A **muscle group** includes all of the muscles that cause the same movement at the same joint. The group is named for the joint where the movement takes place and for the movement commonly caused by the concentric action of those muscles. The elbow flexors, for example, are a muscle group composed of the muscles responsible for flexion at the elbow joint when the muscles act concentrically. Table

3.2 lists the prime and assistant movers at each joint. A movement being observed at a joint does not necessarily involve the muscle group for the movement that is occurring; the muscle group responsible for the opposite action may be acting eccentrically to control the movement. For example, the elbow flexor muscle group flexes the elbow joint during an elbow curl. To return to the starting position, the pull of gravity extends the joint to the original position, but the elbow flexor muscle group is still exerting force to eccentrically control the speed of that movement. Maintaining the elbow in a flexed position requires an isometric action by those same elbow flexors (see figure 3.17). Specific muscles that cause more than one action at a joint or cause movement at more than one joint belong to more than one muscle group. For example, the flexor carpi ulnaris belongs in both the wrist flexor and wrist adductor muscle groups, and the biceps brachii is part of the elbow flexor and radioulnar supinator muscle groups.

KEY POINT

A muscle group includes all the muscles that act concentrically to cause a specific movement at a given joint.

Tips for Exercising Muscle Groups and Common Exercise Mistakes

Many errors that occur during exercise and movement activities result from a lack of knowledge of musculoskeletal anatomy rather than a lack of muscular strength or coordination. Applying basic knowledge allows exercisers to perform better and more safely. This section offers tips for each major muscle group.

Shoulder Girdle and Shoulder Joint

Movement can be enhanced and more muscles involved if shoulder girdle movements are deliberately incorporated with shoulder joint movements. These muscles can be optimally involved in the following exercises and movements:

• Forward reaching. Glenohumeral joint flexion can be accompanied by scapular elevation and upward rotation if the exerciser reaches the fingertips as far forward as possible.

• Push-up. At the completion of a push-up, the scapulae can be protracted to raise the chest a bit more off the floor.

• Overhead reaching. Normally, some scapular elevation is involved when the upper limb is overhead. A conscious effort to reach as high as possible will involve the scapula elevators more. Conversely, a deliberate attempt to keep the shoulders down and the neck long requires concentric action by the scapula depressors.

• Sideward reaching. During horizontal abduction at the shoulder joint, the upper limb can be moved farther back with scapular retraction.

Elbow and Radioulnar Joints

Flexion against resistance requires concentric action of the flexor muscles at the elbow joint. The degree to which these muscles are strengthened, however, is affected by supination and pronation—a good point to remember when instructing participants on how to perform curls. The biceps brachii attaches to the radius, and this bone rotates when the forearm pronates, stretching out the biceps and reducing its contribution to elbow flexion. Thus elbow flexion with the radioulnar joint in a pronated position (a reverse curl) is a weaker movement than a traditional curl with the forearm in a supinated position. The brachialis muscle is not affected by the position of the radioulnar joint because it is attached to the ulna; therefore, its relationship to the humerus does not change with pronation and supination of the radius. Thus, a reverse curl puts more emphasis on the brachialis at the expense of the biceps. Further, the brachioradialis muscle can act with more force when the radioulnar joint is in a neutral position midway between pronation and supination. None of the elbow extensor muscles are affected by the position of the radioulnar joint. Triceps push-downs, in which elbow extension occurs with the radioulnar joints in the pronated position, require the wrist flexors to stabilize the wrist joint, whereas triceps pull-downs (supinated position) utilize the wrist extensors, which are usually much weaker than the flexors. Exercisers who want to concentrate on building the elbow extensors should perform triceps push-downs.

Wrist Joint

During wrist flexion and extension curls, the wrist muscles are affected by the position of the radioulnar joints. Gravity acts as resistance for wrist flexion when the radioulnar joints are in the supinated position and as resistance for extension when the radioulnar joints are in the pronated position.

Vertebral Column and Lumbosacral Joints

In general, neither neck hyperextension nor hyperflexion is desirable. The same pairs of muscles that act concentrically to cause flexion and extension can be strengthened or stretched, one side at a time, by cervical lateral flexion and rotation. Participants should tilt or turn the head from side to side rather than bend the neck forward or backward. Although hyperextension may not be contraindicated for the young, it teaches bad habits and is best avoided.

TABLE 3.2   Muscle Groups at Each Joint

Joint	Prime movers (assistant movers)
Shoulder girdle (scapulothoracic joint)	Protractors—serratus anterior, pectoralis minor Retractors—middle fibers of trapezius, rhomboids (upper and lower fibers of trapezius) Upward rotators—upper and lower fibers of trapezius, serratus anterior Downward rotators—rhomboids, pectoralis minor
Shoulder joint (glenohumeral joint)	Elevators—levator scapulae, upper fibers of trapezius rhomboids Depressors—lower fibers of trapezius, pectoralis minor Flexors—anterior deltoid, clavicular portion of pectoralis major (short head of biceps brachii) Extensors—sternal portion of pectoralis major, latissimus dorsi, teres major (posterior deltoid, long head of triceps brachii, infraspinatus/teres minor) Abductors—middle deltoid, supraspinatus (anterior deltoid, long head of biceps brachii) Adductors—latissimus dorsi, teres major, sternal portion of pectoralis major (short head of biceps brachii, long head of triceps brachii) External rotators—infraspinatus,* teres minor* (posterior deltoid) Internal rotators—pectoralis major, subscapularis,* latissimus dorsi, teres major (anterior deltoid, supraspinatus*) Horizontal adductors—both portions of pectoralis major, anterior deltoid Horizontal abductors—latissimus dorsi, teres major, infraspinatus, teres minor, posterior deltoid
Elbow joint	Flexors—brachialis, biceps brachii, brachioradialis (pronator teres, flexor carpi ulnaris and radialis) Extensors—triceps brachii (anconeus, extensor carpi ulnaris and radialis)
Radioulnar joint	Pronators—pronator quadratus, pronator teres, brachioradialis Supinators—supinator, biceps brachii, brachioradialis
Wrist joint	Flexors—flexor carpi ulnaris, flexor carpi radialis (flexor digitorum superficialis and profundus) Extensors—extensor carpi ulnaris, extensor carpi radialis longus and brevis (extensor digitorum) Abductors (radial flexors)—flexor carpi radialis, extensor carpi radialis longus and brevis (extensor pollicis) Adductors (ulnar flexors)—flexor carpi ulnaris, extensor carpi ulnaris
Lumbosacral joint	Anterior pelvic tilters—iliopsoas (rectus femoris) Posterior pelvic tilters—rectus abdominis, internal oblique (external oblique, gluteus maximus)
Spinal column (thoracic and lumbar areas)	Flexors—rectus abdominis, external oblique, internal oblique Extensors—erector spinae group Rotators—internal oblique, external oblique, erector spinae, rotatores, multifidus Lateral flexors—internal oblique, external oblique, quadratus, lumborum, multifidus, rotatores (erector spinae group)
Hip joint	Flexors—iliopsoas, pectineus, rectus femoris (sartorius, tensor fasciae latae, gracilis, adductor longus and brevis) Extensors—gluteus maximus, biceps femoris, semitendinosus, semimembranosus Abductors—gluteus medius (tensor fasciae latae, iliopsoas, sartorius) Internal rotators—gluteus maximus, the six deep external rotator muscles (iliopsoas, sartorius) External rotators—gluteus minimus, gluteus medius (tensor fasciae latae, pectineus)
Knee joint	Flexors—biceps femoris, semimembranosus, semitendinosus (sartorius, gracilis, gastrocnemius, plantaris) Extensors—rectus femoris, vastus medialis, vastus lateralis, vastus intermedius
Ankle joint	Plantarflexors—gastrocnemius, soleus (peroneus longus, peroneus brevis, tibialis posterior, flexor digitorum, flexor hallucis longus) Dorsiflexors—tibialis anterior, extensor digitorum longus, peroneus tertius (extensor hallucis longus)
Subtalar joint	Invertors—tibialis anterior, tibialis posterior (extensor and flexor hallucis longus, flexor digitorum longus) Evertors—extensor digitorum longus, peroneus brevis, peroneus longus, peroneus tertius

*Rotator cuff muscles

Many exercises require appropriate positioning of the lumbosacral joint and lumbar vertebrae and actions by the trunk muscles for either movement or stabilization. An abdominal curl-up or crunch should begin with a backward pelvic tilt that is maintained throughout the curl-up and return movement. If the backward pelvic tilt cannot be maintained or the exerciser feels tightness or an ache in the lumbar area, the exerciser should stop. If the problem is inadequate strength to maintain the backward tilt, the exercise should be modified to one that the exerciser has sufficient abdominal strength to perform correctly.

A full curl-up, in which the exerciser comes up to a sitting position, requires hip flexion by the hip flexor muscles during the last stages of the exercise. Initially, the abdominal muscles concentrically tilt the pelvis backward and then flex the vertebral column. Once flexion is achieved, these muscles act isometrically to keep the pelvis tilted backward and the trunk in a flexed position. During a full curl-up, the exerciser can feel a sticking point that occurs when the trunk flexion is complete and the hip flexors begin to bring the trunk to an upright position. Doing partial curl-ups or crunches helps eliminate the role of the hip flexors and maintain focus solely on strengthening the abdominal muscles.

The leg lift is considered an abdominal exercise, but often it is not taught correctly. From a supine position on the floor, the legs are lifted and held up by concentric and then isometric action of the hip flexors. Some of the hip flexors also pull the lumbosacral joint into a forward-tilted position. The abdominal muscles must prevent that forward tilt and maintain a flattened lumbar spine and posterior pelvic tilt. The backward pelvic tilt should precede the hip flexion, and, as in the case of the curl-up, if the proper tilt cannot be maintained, the exercise should not be done in that fashion.

The pelvis also tends to tilt forward during overhead upper-limb movements from a standing position. This can be prevented by keeping the arms in front of the ears and flexing the knees slightly.

When weights are lifted from a supine position, as in the bench press, there is a tendency to hyperextend the lumbar spine and tilt the pelvis forward. Although this tendency can allow the exerciser to lift a somewhat heavier weight, it does not increase the work of the upper limb and chest muscles, and it puts the low back into a compromising position. Bench presses are best done with the hips and knees in a flexed position and the feet on the bench or a bench extension to maintain a posterior pelvic tilt. Upright presses are best done seated with the back supported.

Hip Joint

A common error during side-lying leg raises for the hip abductors is the attempt to move the foot as high as possible. Because the ROM for true abduction is limited (about 45°), the exerciser will externally rotate the top limb, which turns the foot out and allows it to go higher. However, this rotation changes the muscle involvement more to the hip flexors. To exercise the primary abductor muscles, the limb should not be rotated and the toes should face forward, not upward.

In backward lower-limb movements for strengthening the gluteus muscles, hip extension is limited primarily by the tightness of the hip ligaments. A limb can appear to be more extended if it is accompanied by a forward pelvic tilt. The exerciser should be cautioned to keep the pelvis in its neutral position in order to focus on the gluteal muscles, even though some apparent hip extension is lost.

Knee Joint

Hyperflexion can strain and stretch knee ligaments and put pressure on the menisci. Therefore, a maximum squat depth to a 90° angle at the knee joint is recommended. During any lunging movements or forward–back stride positions in which the front knee is flexed, the knee should be over or in back of the foot and not in front. Any knee position that puts a twisting pressure on the knee joint should also be avoided. The hurdler position, with one limb out to the back and side with a flexed knee, should be avoided; instead, both legs should be out in front.

A common exercise position is standing with feet shoulder-width apart. The exerciser should have the feet turned slightly outward (7°-10°). The appropriate toe-out position is one that positions the kneecaps facing forward. During any squatting or standing movement, the knee should be in line directly above the foot (not moving to the outside or inside of the foot) to avoid straining the lateral and medial knee ligaments and to develop good lower-extremity positioning habits. Performing the exercise in front of a mirror is recommended to enable the exerciser to monitor the position of the knee relative to the foot.

Ankle Joint

If the squat exercise is performed with the heels of the feet resting on a low block, the soleus muscles are exercised more than they would be if the feet were flat. This position with the heels up shortens the gastrocnemius muscles even more (they are already shortened by the flexed knee), limiting their ability to generate force. The soleus muscles, which do not cross the knees, aren't shortened to the same extent. To increase the force production of the gastrocnemius muscles, the squat could be done with the balls of the feet on the block. A mountain climber especially would benefit from this modification because it mimics the knee and ankle positions in climbing. Individual limits to ROM at the ankle joint should also be taken into consideration during the squat. Exercisers with limited dorsiflexion benefit from placing the heels on a low block to prevent them from going onto tiptoes at the bottom of the squat. This ensures they maintain a stable base and can perform the exercise safely.

Subtalar Joint

The subtalar joint plays a role in adapting to uneven surfaces. A way of exercising the invertors and evertors is to walk across, instead of up and down, a ramp or hill.

KEY POINT

During exercises involving the vertebral column and lumbosacral joints, participants should remember to achieve a posterior (backward) pelvic tilt before initiating the exercise and should maintain the tilt throughout the exercise to protect the lumbar spine. For exercises involving the knee, participants should remember to keep the knee in line above the foot when observing themselves in a mirror. The knee should also stay behind or above the foot when observed from the side.

Basic Biomechanical Concepts for Human Movement

Biomechanics is the study of how the joints of the human body move and the forces that contribute to or hinder those movements. Understanding some key principles of biomechanics is necessary to fully understand human movement. Some of these concepts are described next.

Achieving Stability

Stability is a feature of the whole body and is influenced by the position of all parts of the body. It is the ability to maintain a stable, balanced position following a disruption such as being touched by an opposing player. In order to maintain balance, an individual's center of gravity must fall within the area of the base of support. In the simple case of standing on two feet with arms at the sides, there is a roughly rectangular base of support from the toes of each foot to the heels of each foot. With weight evenly distributed on both feet, the center of gravity will be in the middle of the base of support (see figure 3.18). Changing the foot position will change the shape and area of the base of support. Changing the position of the body or holding an object will alter the location of the center of gravity within the base of support.

Stability is proportional to the distance from the center of gravity to the edge of the base of support in the direction that an external force would propel the person. Figure 3.19 compares more and less stable positions relative to a force applied in a mediolateral direction. With the feet apart, if one leans so that the line of gravity falls directly over one foot and a pushing force is applied in the same direction of the lean, there is less stability than if the feet were together but with the line of gravity along the edge of the foot closer to the applied force. A wide base of support in the anticipated direction of perturbation typically provides greater stability. A lower body position and the accompanying lower center of gravity also contribute to a more stable position. For example, a football lineman may have a triangular base of support between one hand in contact with the ground and both feet. He will squat to lower his center of gravity and lean forward so that his center of gravity is as far as possible from the edge of the base of support in the direction he anticipates an opponent will try to move him. Stability is also directly proportional to body

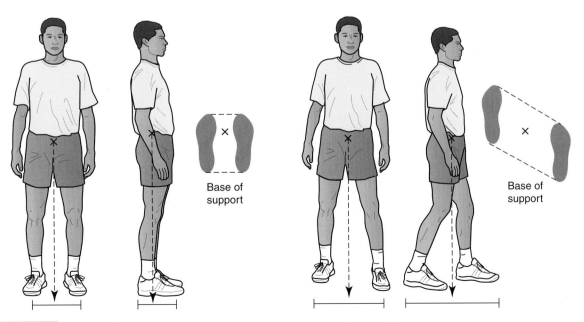

Base of support

Base of support

FIGURE 3.18 The relationships among center of gravity, body position, and base of support.

weight. With all other factors being equal, a heavy person is more stable than a lighter one. Thus, a 300 lb (136 kg) lineman in a three-point squat would be more stable than a 200 lb (91 kg) lineman in the same position.

Stability may be increased by moving the feet apart to widen the base of support and by flexing the knees and hips to lower the center of gravity. During standing exercises that require balance, stability can also be aided by holding or pushing against a nearby object such as a wall or chair. Many exercises can be executed from a sitting position, which increases the base of support and lowers the center of gravity. To help maintain stability against a potentially upsetting force, the weight should be shifted toward that force. Just before walking begins, a position close to instability is attained by shifting the center of gravity in the direction of the intended movement, closer to the anterior limits of the base of support. During walking, as the line of gravity moves outside the base of support, a new base of support is established when the other foot makes contact and stability is restored. In basketball, a guard who

takes a charge from a forward will fall quicker and easier if she is in an unstable position—standing erect with feet closer together and weight on the heels at the moment of the collision.

Torque (Moment of Force)

A force is any push or pull that is applied to a person or object. In the body, when a force is applied at a distance from a joint it produces a **torque (T)**, which will typically rotate the joint. Torque is the product of the magnitude of the force *(F)* and the **force arm *(FA)***, which is the perpendicular distance from the axis of rotation to the direction of application of that force. Torque can be expressed as follows:

$$T = F \times FA.$$

$$T_R = R \times RA.$$

When two opposing forces act to produce rotation in opposite directions, one of the forces is typically designated as the **resistance force (R)**, and its force arm is called the **resistance arm (RA)**, producing a resistance torque (TR). In considering torque produced by a muscle to cause movement against gravity or some other external force, *F* and *FA* are designated for the muscle and *R* and *RA* are designated for gravity or other opposing forces.

Applying Torque to Muscle Action

Muscle action is a force. The force arm is the perpendicular distance from the axis of rotation of the joint to the direction of the force from its point of application (where the muscle attaches to the bone being moved). Figure 3.20 illustrates the direction of pull of the biceps brachii on the radius with

KEY POINT

Stability is directly proportional to the distance of the center of gravity from the edge of the base of support. It is inversely proportional to the height of the center of gravity above the base of support, and it is directly proportional to the weight of the body. For greater stability during standing, the knees should be flexed, the feet spread apart in the direction of an oncoming force, and body weight shifted toward the force.

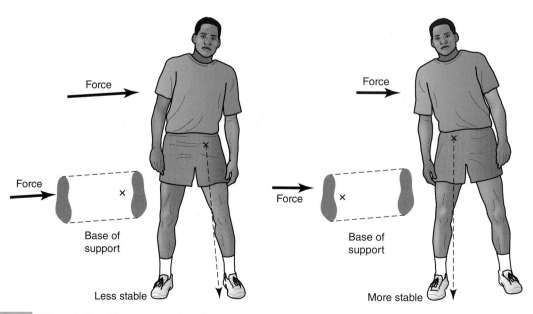

FIGURE 3.19 The relationships among the direction of a perturbing force, center of gravity, and base of support in more and less stable positions.

the elbow flexed to 90°. The force arm is the perpendicular distance from the elbow joint to this line of force. If the muscle insertion were closer to the joint, the force arm would be smaller, and the same force would produce less torque, or more muscle force would be required to produce the same torque. Joint position also affects torque. Figure 3.21 shows the direction of pull of the biceps brachii with the elbow in a more extended position. Note that the force arm is not always parallel to the bone. This shortens the force arm, so the same muscle force produces less torque at

that joint angle, or more muscle force is required to generate the same torque. This is why a dumbbell biceps curl feels harder at the start of the flexion movement compared with the middle of the flexion movement. It is crucial to remember that the force arm is the perpendicular distance from the line of action of the force to the axis of rotation, not the distance along the bone from the point of attachment of the muscle tendon on the bone to the joint axis.

Torque Resulting From Other Forces

The force of gravity directed vertically downward is treated as a resistance force. The resistance produced by gravity acting on a body part is the weight of the object. The resistance arm is the perpendicular distance from the axis of rotation to the point of the object that represents its center of gravity. The torque is the product of the resistance and the resistance arm. Figure 3.22 illustrates the torque produced by gravity acting on the forearm and hand, which acts to extend the elbow. This torque can be increased by adding mass to increase both the magnitude of force (total weight of forearm and hand plus the added mass) and the length of the resistance arm if the mass is added farther from the axis of rotation. The resistance arm of a force applied by someone pushing or pulling on a limb is the perpendicular distance from the axis of rotation to the point of application of the push or pull.

For muscle contraction to move a bone, the muscle force generated must produce a torque greater than the opposing or resistance torque. In this case, the muscle action is concentric and the joint moves in the direction of the muscle torque. If the resistance torque is greater than the muscle torque, the muscle acts eccentrically and lengthens under tension. In this case, the joint moves in the opposite direction of the muscle torque (in the direction of the resistance torque). When the muscular torque equals the resistance torque, no movement occurs and the muscle acts isometrically.

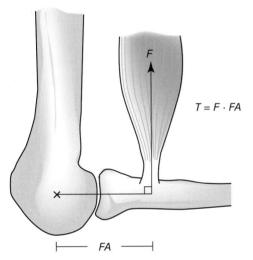

$$T = F \cdot FA$$

$$FA$$

FIGURE 3.20 Muscle force (F) and force arm (FA) of the biceps brachii with the elbow joint flexed to 90°.

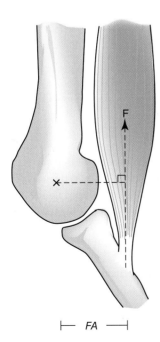

$$FA$$

FIGURE 3.21 The influence of elbow flexion less than 90° at the elbow joint on the force arm (FA) of biceps brachii. Note that FA is perpendicular to the muscle force (F).

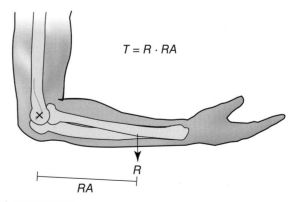

$$T = R \cdot RA$$

$$RA$$

FIGURE 3.22 Extensor torque (T) is the product of resistance force (R), located at the center of gravity of the forearm and hand, and the resistance arm (RA).

KEY POINT

Torque at a joint is the product of the force and the perpendicular distance to the axis of rotation, known as the force arm. Torque due to muscle force is often resisted by a resistance torque due to gravity of another force. The direction of joint movement depends on whether muscle torque or resistance torque is greater.

Applying Torque to Exercising

Knowledge of torque can be used to modify exercises for individuals. The amount of muscle force required by the exercise can be tailored to a person's needs by altering the amount of resistance, the resistance arm, or both in order to change the resistance torque. For example, resistance torque can be increased by adding external weight so that greater muscle force is required to overcome it. The resistance torque also can be changed by altering the position of the body parts. Figure 3.23 shows an exerciser reducing the required muscle force by not holding added weight and thus decreasing both the resistance and the resistance arm and then by flexing the elbow to shorten the resistance arm.

During an abdominal crunch, the position of the arms determines the length of the resistance arm and, therefore, the amount of resistance torque against which the abdominal muscles have to work to flex the trunk and lift the shoulders off the floor. The arms may be held at the sides of the body to bring the upper-body mass closer to the axis of rotation and reduce the required muscle force. To increase the challenge of this exercise, the arms can be raised with the hands on the back of the head. The resistance arm can be increased by holding the arms straight out overhead, which increases the resistance torque and therefore increases the muscle force required to perform the exercise.

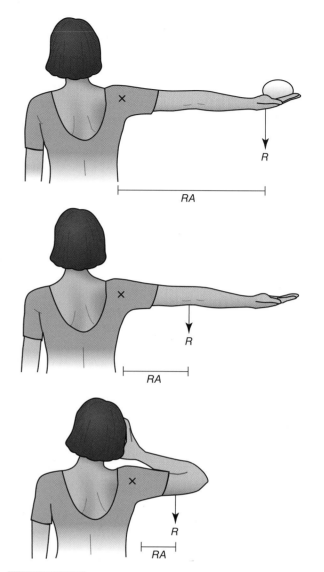

FIGURE 3.23 Modifying resistance torque by increasing the length of the resistance arm (*RA*) and by adding external mass in the form of an object to increase the resistance force (*R*).

KEY POINT

The torque that resists limb movements can be altered by modifying the amount of the resistance force and by changing the length of the resistance arm.

Rotational Inertia (Moment of Inertia)

Rotational inertia, or the resistance to change in the rotation of a body segment around a joint axis, depends on the mass of the segment and its distribution around the joint. A lower limb, for example, has more rotational inertia than an upper limb not only because it is heavier but also because its mass is concentrated a greater distance away from its axis of rotation. A swinging softball bat held by its fat, striking end has less rotational inertia than when held at the handle. When holding the bat by the striking end, most of its mass is close to the axis of rotation, which reduces its rotational inertia and makes it easier to swing. However, with less mass at the striking end, the bat will not move the ball very far. Optimal weight and weight distribution of the bat is a trade-off against how quickly the bat can be swung.

The rotational inertia of body segments before or during movement depends on the mass of the segments, which cannot be changed, and on the distribution of the mass around the joints, which can be manipulated. For example, an upper limb with the elbow extended has a greater rotational inertia than with the elbow flexed. Similarly, a lower limb with an extended knee has more rotational inertia than with the knee flexed. The amount of muscle force necessary to cause rapid limb movement is proportional to the rotational inertia of the limb to be moved. During jogging, the knee of the recovery limb is partially flexed to reduce the limb's rotational inertia around the hip joint. Less muscular force is needed to swing the recovery leg forward compared with a more extended knee, which reduces local fatigue of the hip flexors. In sprinting, on the other hand, the quicker the recovery limb is brought forward, the faster the running speed. Powerful actions of the hip flexors, along with maximal knee flexion, result in the recovery limb coming forward sooner and, thus, an increase in overall speed. Another example of rapid movement to which this principle can be applied is jumping jacks. Keeping the elbow flexed reduces the rotational inertia of the upper limb. This may reduce the amount of muscle force required from the shoulder abductor and adductor muscle groups to maintain a certain cadence, or, if greater muscle force is applied, it may result in faster movements.

Angular Momentum

Angular momentum, or the quantity of angular motion, is expressed as the product of angular velocity and rotational inertia. A moving body part possesses angular momentum; the faster it moves and the greater its rotational inertia, the greater the angular momentum. The amount of force necessary to change angular momentum is proportional to the amount of the momentum.

Applying Angular Momentum to Exercising

The concept of angular momentum can be applied to ballistic limb movements during exercise. A fast-moving body segment is decelerated by eccentric muscle actions; a faster movement, a greater mass, or a greater desired deceleration requires greater muscle force to decelerate the body segment. Care must be taken when performing rapid ballistic limb movements, especially when using added weight. The movements may generate great momentum, and considerable muscle strength may be required to decelerate and eventually stop them. This may result in damage to the muscle or the rotating joint.

Transfer of Angular Momentum

Transfer of angular momentum from one body segment to another can be achieved by stabilizing the initial moving body part at a joint, which causes angular movement of another body part. For example, when an exerciser performs an abdominal crunch to exercise the trunk flexors, flinging the arms forward from an overhead position transfers their momentum to the trunk. This decreases the amount of muscular force needed from the trunk flexors and makes the exercise easier. In another example, a jump with a turn in the air can be better achieved if, just before takeoff, the arms are swung forcibly across the body in the intended direction of the spin.

KEY POINT

Rotational inertia can be decreased by moving the mass of the limb closer to the joint axis and vice versa. The amount of eccentric force necessary to decelerate a moving body segment is proportional to its angular momentum (rotational inertia × angular velocity). Angular momentum can be transferred from one body segment to another.

Muscle-Group Involvement in Selected Activities

Human movement is caused or controlled by muscle forces. The following sections briefly review the involvement of muscle groups in some common physical activities.

Walking and Running

The phases and muscle groups involved in walking and running are similar, but more forceful muscle actions are needed during running as speed increases and greater joint ROMs are observed. The two basic phases of gait are the stance phase and the swing phase. The swing phase ends and the stance phase begins at foot contact; the stance phase ends at toe-off, when swing phase begins. The key difference between walking and running is that during walking either one or both feet are on the ground at all times, but during running only one foot is on the ground at a time. In between foot contacts during running there is a flight phase when neither foot is in contact with the ground.

Just before foot contact, the hip extensors act eccentrically to decelerate the forward limb swing. At foot contact with the ground, the knee extensors act eccentrically to control knee flexion against gravity and cushion the impact. The heel touches the ground first during walking and distance running. Following heel contact, the ankle dorsiflexors act eccentrically to control the lowering of the ball of the foot onto the ground. As running speed increases, the pattern of contact changes and the flat foot or the ball of the foot makes contact with the ground first. A small proportion of runners contact the ground with the flat foot or the ball of the foot at all speeds.

During the stance phase, the body moves forward over the stationary foot as the hip extends and the ankle dorsiflexes (see figure 3.24). Before push-off, the hip continues to extend as the knee extends and the ankle plantarflexes. At this point the swinging limb has moved forward in front of the body in preparation for the next foot contact. The push-off is accomplished by the concentric action of the hip extensors and ankle plantarflexors. The gluteus maximus assumes a greater role in hip extension as speed increases.

At the beginning of the swing phase, the hip flexors act concentrically to begin the forward limb swing. This is a ballistic movement, so the momentum initiated by the hip flexors continues the motion passively. Hip flexion is accompanied by pelvic rotation to bring the swinging limb in front of the body. The knee flexes at the beginning of the swing to reduce the rotational inertia of the swing limb. The knee extensors then initiate knee extension prior to foot contact, and the knee flexors work eccentrically to control knee extension at the end of the swing phase. The ankle joint is dorsiflexed to clear the foot from the ground and prepare for foot contact. Speed is a product of stride length and stride frequency; thus, one or both factors can be increased to increase speed. Greater hip ROM contributes to greater stride length. Rapid recovery of the swing leg via rapid hip flexion during the swing phase is vital to prepare for foot contact at the start of the next stance phase (see figure 3.25).

In the upper body, arm swing requires shoulder flexion and extension. As speed increases, the swing becomes more vigorous, and there is more elbow flexion. For the greatest efficiency, the arms should move in the sagittal plane. To increase the involvement of the upper limbs for exercise, a walker can exaggerate the shoulder flexion and extension movements.

Walking or running up an incline elicits greater action from the gluteus maximus muscle at the hip and from the knee extensors to raise the body against gravity. The ankle dorsiflexors are more active immediately before landing in order to match the position of the ankle joint to the angle of the incline. Because the ankle is in a more dorsiflexed position, the plantarflexors begin acting during push-off from a more stretched position. For these reasons, hill climbing requires greater flexibility in the plantarflexors, especially the soleus muscle, and greater strength in the dorsiflexors. During downhill running, there is more eccentric action by the knee extensors at foot contact compared with uphill running. As a result, these muscle groups are more apt to become fatigued and to be sore afterward.

Running in place requires the ankle plantarflexors to propel the body upward against gravity; thus, they work more than any of the other lower-extremity muscle groups

Gait Cycle

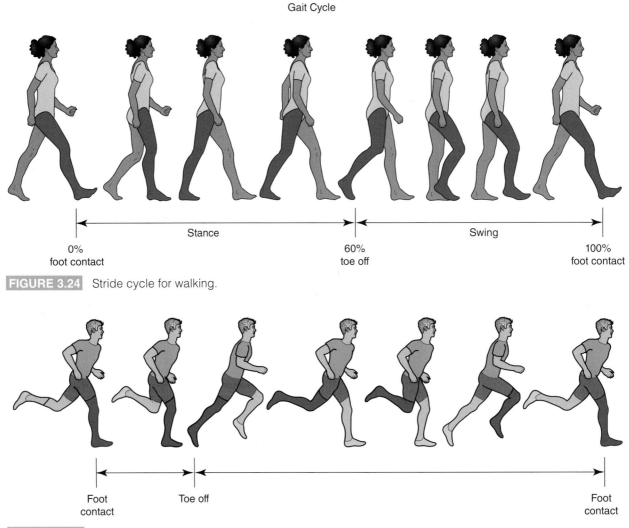

FIGURE 3.24 Stride cycle for walking.

FIGURE 3.25 Stride cycle for running.

in this activity. The knee extensors are primarily involved in eccentric action to cushion the landing at foot contact. During running in place, the ball of the foot touches the ground first. Therefore, the plantarflexors are active during the landing, acting eccentrically to control the speed and amount of ankle dorsiflexion. Additional muscles are involved in moving the limb immediately after push-off and before the foot lands again, including hip flexion and extension and knee flexion that brings the foot up to the front.

Cycling

The main force in cycling comes from the hip and knee extensors during the downward push. With toe clips, riders can use the hip flexors and ankle dorsiflexors to help return the pedal to the up position, but only if they make a conscious effort to do so.

Jumping

The hip and knee extensors, followed by the ankle plantarflexors, forcibly propel the body upward against gravity. The amount of trunk flexion primarily determines the angle of takeoff. The trunk extends, and the arms flex from an extended position just before the lower-limb joints extend. If the reach height of the arms is important, as in a jump ball in basketball or in a tennis smash, the scapulae elevate. During the landing, the hip and knee extensors and the ankle plantarflexors act eccentrically to control the rate of flexion of the lower-body joints.

Overarm Throwing

There are three phases in throwing: the windup, or preparation; the execution, or actual throw; and the follow-through,

or recovery. Figure 3.26 illustrates the sequence of the execution phase.

In preparation for throwing, the weight shifts to the back foot, the back hip internally rotates (because the foot is fixed on the ground, rotation is seen at the pelvis), and the trunk rotates with some lateral flexion and extension. In the upper limb, the shoulder externally rotates, and there is some horizontal abduction of the throwing arm accompanied by retraction of the scapula, flexion of the elbow, and extension of the wrist. The movements of the throwing arm are all ballistic. The external rotation at the shoulder is fast and powerful. Toward the end of the windup, the internal rotators begin to act eccentrically to decelerate the external rotation in preparation for the actual throw.

The weight shift forward is the initial movement in the execution of the throw. This is accomplished by the hip abductors, extensors, and external rotators; the ankle plantarflexors; and the subtalar evertors of the back limb. The front hip rotates externally. The trunk then flexes laterally in the direction opposite to that of the windup, rotates, and flexes. There is a forcible internal rotation of the shoulder, along with scapular protraction. Although there is some horizontal adduction, most of the contribution of the shoulder in an overhand throw comes from this internal rotation. The elbow extends, and the wrist moves toward flexion. Depending on the desired spin on the ball, the forearm pronators and the wrist abductors or adductors also may be involved.

Since the actions at the shoulder and elbow joints are vigorous ballistic movements, the shoulder external rotators and horizontal abductors act eccentrically to decelerate the movements during the follow-through, while the elbow flexors act eccentrically to prevent elbow hyperextension.

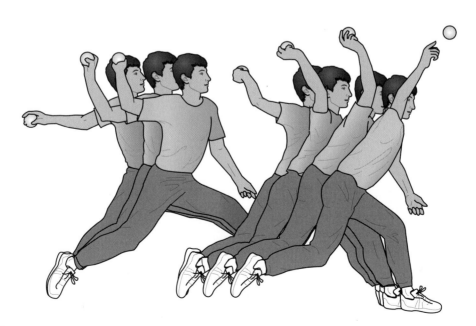

FIGURE 3.26 The execution phase of an overarm throw.

Swimming and Exercise in Water

Swimming is a unique activity because water resists movement of submerged body parts in all directions and at all speeds. Movements performed in water demand concentric muscle contractions. Since water is a dense medium, it provides some support for the weight-bearing joints against the force of gravity.

Lifting and Carrying Objects

The object to be lifted from the ground should be located close to the lifter's spread feet or even between them. The lifter squats, keeping the trunk as erect as possible. The lift should be accomplished by the powerful lower limbs rather than the spine or arms. Lifting begins by keeping the trunk in an upright position and then tilting the pelvis backward and keeping the abdominal muscles activated; the knee extensors along with the hip extensors then act concentrically. The lift should be slow and smooth, not jerky (see figure 3.27). Insufficient lower-limb strength can result in poor lifting technique. The weight should be carried close to the body, with the trunk assuming a position that allows the center of gravity to fall within the area of the base of support. The trunk lateral flexors are more active when the weight is carried on one side, the extensors are more active when the weight is in front, and the abdominal muscles are more active when the weight is carried across the top of the back, as in backpacking.

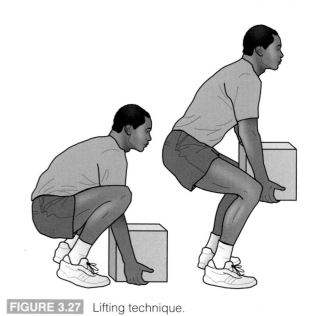

FIGURE 3.27 Lifting technique.

TABLE 3.3 Movements and Muscles Involved in Locomotion, Throwing, Cycling, Jumping, and Swimming

Major muscle group	Movement task
Hip extensors	Locomotion—push-off; cycling; jumping; swimming—front crawl, back crawl, sidestroke
Hip flexors	Locomotion—recovery; swimming—front crawl, back crawl, sidestroke
Hip abductors	Swimming—breaststroke; throwing
Hip adductors	Swimming—breaststroke
Hip external and internal rotators	Throwing
Knee extensors	Locomotion—landing; cycling; jumping
Knee flexors	Locomotion—recovery
Ankle plantarflexors	Locomotion—push-off, landing; jumping
Ankle dorsiflexors	Locomotion—recovery
Shoulder joint flexors	Underhand throwing
Shoulder joint extensors	Swimming—front crawl
Shoulder joint internal and external rotators	Throwing
Anterior shoulder joint muscles	Swimming—back crawl; sidestroke lead arm; throwing
Posterior shoulder joint muscles	Swimming—sidestroke trail arm, breaststroke; throwing—windup
Shoulder girdle upward and downward rotators	Swimming—breaststroke, sidestroke lead arm, front crawl, back crawl
Shoulder girdle protractors	Swimming—back crawl; throwing
Shoulder girdle retractors	Swimming—front crawl, breaststroke Throwing—windup
Shoulder girdle elevators	Swimming—front crawl, back crawl, sidestroke lead arm, breaststroke
Elbow flexors	Throwing
Elbow extensors	Throwing
Trunk flexors	Throwing
Trunk rotators	Throwing

Common Mechanical Errors in Walking and Running, Throwing, and Striking

Success in physical activities depends in part on properly executing movement. Some of the more common errors are discussed in the next sections.

Errors in Walking and Running

Some novice runners have a tendency to run with stiff legs, or with insufficient knee flexion of the recovery limb. This results in a greater rotational inertia of the limb, which means the hip flexors must exert greater force than they would if the knee were more flexed. Keeping the knees stiff during foot contact can also expose the stance limb to greater forces and increase the potential for injury.

Another potential error is the direction of upper- and lower-limb movements. All movements should be executed in the anterior and posterior directions. Excessively swinging the hands across the trunk rotates the upper trunk; in reaction, the lower trunk rotates in the opposite direction. This excess transverse-plane rotation does not contribute to forward motion of the runner.

Some joggers and runners propel themselves too high off the ground during the airborne phase. Again, excessive movement, this time in the vertical direction, does not contribute to forward motion of the runner. Typically, this bouncing style of running also shortens stride length. The runner must now increase stride frequency to maintain running speed.

Slapping the feet down onto the ground in a noisy running style can increase the impact forces that the limbs are exposed to every time they strike the ground. The tactile and aural cues of running softly and quietly may enable runners to reduce their impact forces.

Errors in Throwing and Striking

The speed of the ball in the hand just before release is the speed of the ball immediately after it leaves the hand. The more joints that are involved in the throwing motion, the greater the ball speed that can be achieved when it is released. Most throwing problems that result in low velocity, such as pushing the ball rather than throwing it, stem from a lack of trunk rotation or from poor timing of this rotation with the movements of the shoulder joint. The thrower should rotate the trunk and hips during the windup so that the pelvis is sideways to the intended direction of the throw and the shoulders are rotated even more to the back. As the hips and then the trunk rotate forward to begin the throw, the upper limb lags behind. This sets up a whiplike action of the upper limb and allows adequate time for the important shoulder internal rotation. Without the trunk rotation, the resulting inadequate shoulder rotation produces a pushing motion during the throw.

The same sequence of motion applies to striking events, such as tennis and badminton stroking and softball batting. A common fault in learning how to serve a tennis ball or smash a birdie is insufficient trunk rotation. It is easier to contact and hit an object without the added coordination requirements of trunk rotation, but less trunk rotation reduces the impact of the racket on the projectile. In batting, a common error is the lack of smooth, fluid timing among movements of the various body segments. The hip, trunk, and upper-limb movements follow one another so the bat is moving with great velocity on contact with the ball. Beginners often stop one motion before beginning the next.

STUDY QUESTIONS

1. Name the three cardinal planes and their associated axes.
2. Using the shoulder (glenohumeral) joint as an example, explain why a ball-and-socket joint is so mobile.
3. Explain how the trunk has such a large ROM even though each intervertebral joint within it has only a few degrees of motion.
4. Explain from an anatomical viewpoint why the knee is vulnerable to injury.
5. Identify the phase of a squat exercise in which quadriceps femoris is acting (a) concentrically and (b) eccentrically.

6. Explain in terms of torque how an abdominal crunch is more difficult when the arms are extended overhead compared with folded across the chest.

7. Using rotational inertia in your answer, explain why runners naturally flex the knee of the leg that is swinging forward.

8. Why is walking up an incline more challenging for the gluteal muscles than walking on level ground?

9. What type of muscle contractions are involved in exercises performed in water?

10. What is a common error made by novices in serving a tennis ball?

CASE STUDIES

You can check your answers by referring to appendix A.

1. You are supervising the resistance training area when you hear a lot of clanging noise coming from the vicinity of the seated leg press. You discover that the exerciser at that machine is not controlling the descent of the weights. You suggest that he slowly return the weights rather than letting them drop. He asks you why—he doesn't see any benefit in a controlled return other than reduced noise. What do you tell him?

2. Alice wants to know why she can move a heavier weight when she does wrist curls with her palms up than with her palms down and why she can do more pull-ups with her palms facing her than with her palms facing away. How do you answer her?

3. José complains that his lower back aches somewhat when he reaches overhead while standing in place during the cool-down portion of an aerobics class. What should he do during this movement to prevent the aching?

REFERENCES

1. Carr, G.A. 2004. *Sport mechanics for coaches.* 2nd ed. Champaign, IL: Human Kinetics.

2. Floyd, R.T. 2009. *Manual of structural kinesiology.* 17th ed. Boston: McGraw-Hill Higher Education.

3. Gray, H., P.L. Williams, & L.H. Bannister, eds. 1995. *Gray's anatomy: The anatomical basis of medicine and surgery.* New York: Churchill Livingstone.

4. Hall, S. J. 2007. *Basic biomechanics.* 5th ed. Boston: McGraw-Hill.

5. Hamill, J., & K. Knutzen. 2009. *Biomechanical basis of human movement.* 3rd ed. Philadelphia: Lippincott Williams & Wilkins.

6. Hay, J.G., & J.G. Reid. 1988. *Anatomy, mechanics and human motion.* 2nd ed. Englewood Cliffs, NJ: Prentice Hall.

7. Whittle, M. 2007. *Gait analysis: An introduction.* 4th ed. New York: Butterworth-Heinemann.

Exercise Physiology

OBJECTIVES

The reader will be able to do the following:

1. Explain how muscle produces energy aerobically and anaerobically and evaluate the importance of aerobic and anaerobic energy production in fitness and sport.

2. Describe the structure of skeletal muscle and the sliding-filament theory of muscle contraction.

3. Describe the power, speed, endurance, and metabolism of the types of muscle fibers.

4. Describe tension development in terms of twitch, summation, and tetanus, and describe the recruitment of muscle fiber types in exercise of increasing intensity.

5. Describe the various fuels for muscle work and how exercise intensity and duration affect the respiratory exchange ratio.

6. Describe how exercise tests, training, heredity, sex, age, altitude, carbon monoxide, and cardiovascular and pulmonary diseases influence $\dot{V}O_2$max.

7. Describe how ventilatory threshold and lactate threshold indicate fitness as well as predict performance in endurance events.

8. Explain how HR, stroke volume (SV), cardiac output, and oxygen extraction change during a graded exercise test (GXT) and during training, and link the variation in $\dot{V}O_2$max in the population to differences in maximal cardiac output and oxygen extraction.

9. Summarize the effects of endurance training on muscular, metabolic, and cardiorespiratory responses to submaximal work and on $\dot{V}O_2$max, and describe how reducing or ceasing training affects $\dot{V}O_2$max; describe the degree to which endurance training effects are specific to the muscles involved in the training.

10. Describe how men and women differ in their cardiovascular responses to graded exercise.

11. Contrast the importance of the various mechanisms for heat loss during heavy exercise and during submaximal exercise in a hot environment. Describe how training in a hot and humid environment affects heat tolerance.

Fitness professionals

Fitness professionals need to know basic exercise physiology to prescribe appropriate activities, deal with weight loss concerns, and explain to participants what happens when training in a hot and humid environment. This chapter can't possibly cover the extensive detail found in texts devoted to exercise physiology; instead, we summarize major topics and, where possible, apply the discussion to exercise testing and prescription. We refer the interested reader to the texts on exercise physiology listed in the references (2, 8, 22, 41, 46, 49, 52, 64).

Energy and Work

Energy is what makes the body go. Several kinds of energy exist in biological systems: electrical energy in nerves and muscles, chemical energy in the synthesis of molecules, mechanical energy in the contraction of muscle, and thermal energy, derived from all of these processes, that helps maintain body temperature. The ultimate source of the energy found in biological systems is the sun. The radiant energy from the sun is captured by plants and used to convert simple atoms and molecules into carbohydrates, fats, and proteins. The sun's energy is trapped within the chemical bonds of these food molecules.

For the cells to use this energy, they must break down the foodstuffs in a manner that conserves most of the energy contained in the bonds of the carbohydrates, fats, and proteins. In addition, the final product of the breakdown must be a molecule the cell can use—adenosine triphosphate (ATP). Cells use ATP as the primary energy source for biological work, whether this work is electrical, mechanical, or chemical. In ATP, three phosphates are linked by high-energy bonds. When a bond between the phosphates is broken, energy is released and may be used by the cell. At this point the ATP has been reduced to a lower energy state, becoming adenosine diphosphate (ADP) and inorganic phosphate (P_i).

During muscular activity, ATP is constantly converted to ADP and P_i in order to provide the energy needed for the work. The ATP must be replaced as fast as it is used if the muscle is to continue to generate force. The muscle cell has a great capacity to replace ATP under a variety of work circumstances, from a short dash to a marathon. Edington and Edgerton (18) devised a logical approach to help us understand how energy is supplied for muscle contraction—they divided the energy sources (ATP sources) into immediate, short term, and long term.

Immediate Sources of Energy

The very limited amount of ATP stored in a muscle might meet the energy demands of a maximal effort lasting about 1 sec. **Phosphocreatine (PC)**, another high-energy phosphate molecule stored in the muscle, is the most important immediate source of energy. PC can donate its phosphate molecule (and the energy therein) to ADP in order to make ATP, allowing the muscle to continue producing force.

$$PC + ADP \rightarrow ATP + C.$$

This reaction takes place as fast as the muscle forms ADP. Unfortunately, the PC store in muscle lasts only 3 to 5 sec when the muscle is working maximally. This process does not require oxygen and is one of the **anaerobic energy** (without oxygen) mechanisms for producing ATP. PC is the primary source of ATP during a shot put, a vertical jump, or the first seconds of a sprint.

Short-Term Sources of Energy

As the muscle's store of PC decreases, the muscle fibers break down glucose (a simple sugar) to produce ATP at a high rate. The glucose is obtained from blood or the muscle's glycogen store. The multienzyme pathway for glucose metabolism is called **glycolysis**, and it does not require oxygen to function (like the breakdown of PC, it too is an anaerobic process).

$$Glucose \rightarrow 2 \text{ pyruvic acid} + 2 \text{ ATP.}$$

In glycolysis, glucose is broken down into two molecules of pyruvic acid; in the process, ADP is converted to ATP, allowing the muscle to maintain a high rate of work. But glycolysis can only continue for a limited time. When glycolysis operates at high speed, pyruvic acid is converted to lactic acid, and lactic acid (lactate) accumulates in the muscle and the blood. This accumulation of lactic acid in the muscle slows the rate of glycogen metabolism and may interfere with the mechanism involved in muscle contraction. Supplying ATP via glycolysis has its shortcomings, but it does allow a person to run at fast speeds for short distances. This short-term energy source is of primary importance in events involving maximal work lasting about 2 min.

Long-Term Sources of Energy

Long-term sources of energy involve the production of ATP from a variety of fuels, but this method requires the utilization of oxygen—in other words, it is **aerobic energy**. The primary fuels include muscle glycogen, blood glucose, plasma free fatty acids, and intramuscular fats. Protein provides only a small percentage of energy for muscle contraction, so the focus is on carbohydrate and fat. Glucose is broken down in glycolysis (as described previously), but in this case the pyruvic acid is taken into the **mitochondria** of the cell, where it is converted to a 2-carbon fragment (acetyl CoA) that enters the Krebs cycle. Fats are taken into the mitochondria, where they are also broken down into acetyl CoA, which again enters the Krebs cycle. The energy originally contained in the glucose and fats is extracted from the acetyl CoA and is used to generate ATP in the electron transport chain in a process called *oxidative phosphorylation*, which requires oxygen.

$$\text{Carbohydrate and fat} + O_2 \rightarrow ATP.$$

ATP production via aerobic mechanisms is slower than production from immediate and short-term sources of energy, and during submaximal work it may be 2 or 3 min before the ATP needs of the cell are met completely by this aerobic process. One reason for this lag is the time it takes for the heart to increase the delivery of oxygen-enriched blood to the muscles at the rate needed to meet the ATP demands of the muscle. Another is the time it takes for oxidative phosphorylation to increase its rate of ATP production from resting levels to that needed to meet the exercise demand. Aerobic production of ATP is the primary means of supplying energy to the muscle in maximal work lasting more than 2 min and in all submaximal work.

Interaction of Exercise Intensity, Exercise Duration, and Energy Production

The proportion of energy coming from anaerobic sources (immediate and short-term energy) is influenced by the intensity and duration of the activity. Figure 4.1 shows that during an all-out activity lasting less than 1 min (e.g., a 400 m dash), the muscles obtain most of their ATP from anaerobic sources. In a 2 to 3 min maximal effort, approximately 50% of the energy comes from anaerobic sources and 50% comes from aerobic sources; in a 10 min maximal effort, the anaerobic component drops to 15%. For a 30 min all-out effort, the anaerobic component is about 5%, and it is even smaller in a typical submaximal 30 min training session.

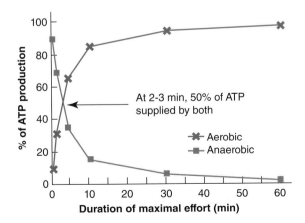

FIGURE 4.1 Percent of aerobic and anaerobic contributions to total energy supply during maximal work of various durations (49).

Understanding Muscle Structure and Function

Exercise means movement, and movement requires muscle action. To discuss human physiology related to exercise and endurance training, we must start with skeletal muscle, the tissue that converts the chemical energy of ATP to mechanical work. How does a muscle do this?

Figure 4.2 shows the structure of skeletal muscle, from the intact muscle to the smallest functional unit within the muscle. A **muscle fiber** is a cylindrical cell that has repeating light and dark bands, giving it the name *striated muscle*. The striations are attributable to a more basic structural component called the **myofibril**, which runs the length of the muscle. Each myofibril is composed of a long series of **sarcomeres**, the fundamental units of muscle contraction. Figure 4.2 shows that the sarcomere contains the thick filament **myosin** and the thin filament **actin** and is bounded by connective tissue called the **Z line** (63).

An enlargement of two sarcomeres in figure 4.2 shows the **A band, I band,** and **H zone** and the changes that take place when the sarcomere moves from the resting state to the contracted state. The I band is composed of actin and is bisected by the Z line, and the A band is composed of myosin and actin. According to the **sliding-filament theory** of muscle contraction, the thin actin filaments slide over the thick myosin filaments, pulling the Z lines toward the center of the sarcomere. In this way the entire muscle shortens, but the contractile proteins do not change size. So how does the muscle release the energy in ATP for shortening?

If ATP is the energy supply, then an ATPase (an enzyme) must exist in muscle to split ATP and release the potential energy contained within its bonds. ATPase is found in an extension of the thick myosin filament, the **crossbridge**, which also can bind to actin. Figure 4.3 shows how ATP, the crossbridge, and actin interact to shorten the sarcomere (63).

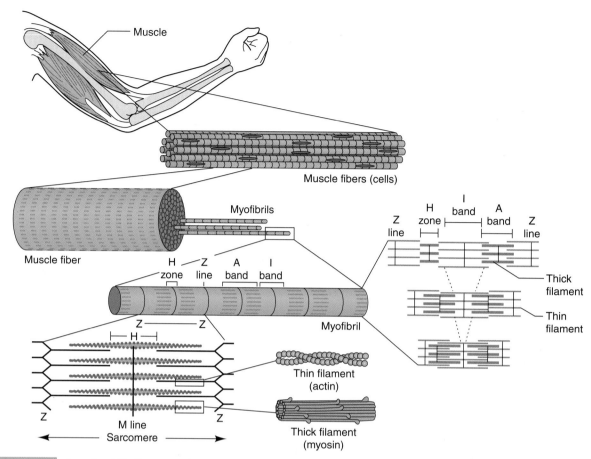

FIGURE 4.2 Levels of fibrillar organization within a skeletal muscle, and changes in filament alignment and banding pattern in a myofibril during shortening.

Reprinted, by permission, from A.J. Vander, J.H. Sherman and D.S. Luciano, 1980, *Human physiology*, 3rd ed. (New York, NY: McGraw-Hill, Inc.), 212, 216. ©The McGraw-Hill Companies.

Why aren't the crossbridges always moving and the muscles always in contraction? At rest, two proteins that are associated with actin block the interaction of myosin with actin: **troponin**, which has the capacity to bind calcium, and **tropomyosin**. Figure 4.4 shows that when a muscle is depolarized (excited) by a motor nerve, the action potential spreads over the surface of the muscle fiber and enters the fiber through special channels called **transverse tubules** (this process is step 1 in the figure). Once inside the muscle fiber, this wave of depolarization spreads over the **sarcoplasmic reticulum (SR)**, a membrane that surrounds the myofibril, and the SR releases calcium (Ca²⁺) into the sarcoplasm (step 2 in the figure). When the calcium binds with troponin, the tropomyosin aligns the crossbridge binding site on the actin so that the myosin crossbridge can interact with it (step 3 in the figure). When the crossbridge binds to actin, energy is released, the crossbridge moves, and the sarcomere shortens (step 4 in the figure). This sequence repeats as long as calcium is present and the muscle can replace the ATP it uses. The muscle relaxes when the calcium is pumped back into the SR and troponin and tropomyosin can again block the interaction of actin and myosin (steps 5 and 6 in the figure) (63). The muscle needs ATP for moving the crossbridge, pumping the calcium back to the SR, and

KEY POINT

A muscle contracts when ATP is split to form a high-energy myosin–ATP crossbridge, the myosin–ATP crossbridge binds to actin and releases energy, the crossbridge moves and pulls actin toward the center of the sarcomere, and, finally, ATP binds to and releases the crossbridge from actin to start contracting again. Calcium release from the SR blocks inhibitory proteins (troponin and tropomyosin) and allows the crossbridge to bind to actin to begin moving. Relaxation occurs when calcium is pumped back into the SR and ATP binds to the crossbridge.

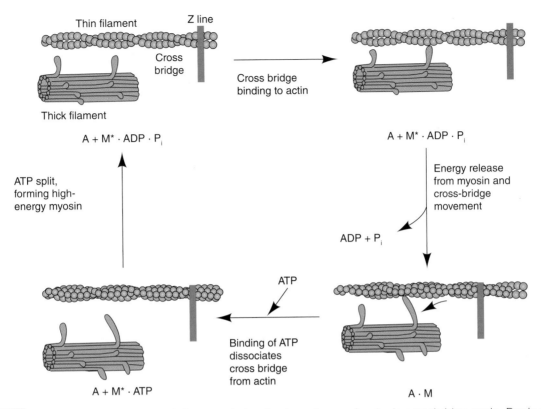

Thin filament

Z line

Cross bridge

Thick filament

$A + M^* \cdot ADP \cdot P_i$

Cross bridge binding to actin

$A + M^* \cdot ADP \cdot P_i$

ATP split, forming high-energy myosin

Energy release from myosin and cross-bridge movement

$ADP + P_i$

ATP

$A + M^* \cdot ATP$

Binding of ATP dissociates cross bridge from actin

$A \cdot M$

FIGURE 4.3 Chemical and mechanical changes during the four stages of a single crossbridge cycle. Begin reading the figure at the lower left. A = actin; M* = energized form of myosin; ATP = adenosine triphosphate; ADP = adenosine diphosphate; P_i = inorganic phosphate.

Reprinted, by permission, from A.J. Vander, J.H. Sherman and D.S. Luciano, 1985, *Human physiology,* 4th ed. (New York, NY: McGraw-Hill, Inc.), 263. ©The McGraw-Hill Companies.

maintaining the resting membrane potential that allows the muscle to be depolarized.

Muscle Fiber Types and Performance

Muscle fibers vary in their abilities to produce ATP by the aerobic and anaerobic mechanisms described earlier in the chapter. Some muscle fibers contract quickly and have an innate capacity to produce great force, but they fatigue quickly. These muscle fibers produce most of their ATP by PC breakdown and glycolysis, and they are called **fast glycolytic fibers** or **type IIx fibers**. Other muscle fibers contract slowly and produce little force, but they have great resistance to fatigue. These fibers produce most of their ATP aerobically in the mitochondria and are called **slow oxidative fibers** or **type I fibers**. These fibers have many mitochondria and a relatively large number of capillaries helping to deliver oxygen to the mitochondria. Last, there is a fiber with both type I and type IIx characteristics. It is a fast-contracting muscle fiber that not only produces great force when stimulated but also resists fatigue because of its large number of mitochondria and capillaries. These fibers are called **fast oxidative glycolytic fibers** or **type IIa fibers**.

KEY POINT

Muscle fibers differ in speed of contraction, force, and resistance to fatigue. Type I fibers are slow, generate low force, and resist fatigue. Type IIa fibers are fast, generate high force, and resist fatigue. Type IIx fibers are fast, generate high force, and easily fatigue.

Muscle Fiber Types: Genetics, Sex, and Training

In the average male and female, about 52% of the muscle fibers are type I, with the fast-twitch fibers divided into approximately 33% type IIa and 13% type IIx (57, 58). The distribution of fiber types in the overall population greatly varies, however. Studies comparing identical and fraternal twins suggest that the distribution of fast and slow fibers is genetic. In addition, fast-twitch fibers cannot be converted to slow-twitch fibers, or vice versa, with endurance training (3). In contrast, the capacity of the muscle fiber to produce ATP aerobically (its oxidative capacity) seems to be easily altered by endurance training. In fact,

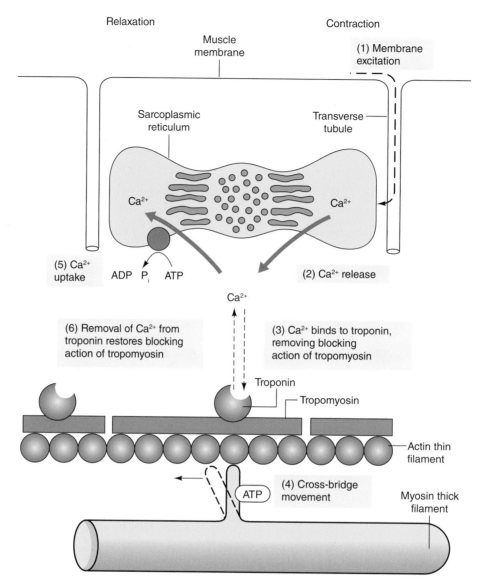

FIGURE 4.4 Role of calcium in muscle excitation–contraction coupling. ADP = adenosine diphosphate; P$_i$ = inorganic phosphate; ATP = adenosine triphosphate; Ca^{2+} = calcium ions.

in some elite endurance athletes, type IIx fibers can't be found; they have been converted to the oxidative version, type IIa (57). The increase in mitochondria and capillaries in endurance-trained muscles allows a person to meet ATP demands aerobically, with less glycogen depletion and lactate formation (30).

Tension (Force) Development in the Muscle

The tension, or force, generated by a muscle depends on more than the fiber type. When a single threshold-level stimulus excites a muscle fiber, a single, low-tension twitch results—a brief contraction followed by relaxation. If the frequency of stimulation increases, the muscle fiber can't

relax between stimuli, and the tension of one contraction adds to tension from the previous one. This addition process is called **summation**. A further increase in the frequency of stimulation results in the contractions fusing together into a smooth, sustained, high-tension contraction called **tetanus**. Muscle fibers typically develop tension through tetanic contractions. In addition to frequency of stimulation, the force of contraction depends on the degree to which the muscle fibers contract simultaneously (synchronous firing) and the number of muscle fibers recruited for the contraction. The latter factor, muscle fiber recruitment, is the most important.

Figure 4.5 shows the order in which the various muscle fiber types are recruited as the intensity of exercise increases. The order is from the most to the least oxidative,

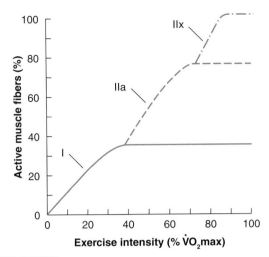

FIGURE 4.5 Recruitment of muscle fiber types in exercise of increasing intensity.

Reprinted, by permission, from D.G. Sale, 1987, "Influence of exercise and training on motor unit activation," *Exercise and Sport Sciences Reviews* 15: 99.

from the slowest to the fastest fiber (type I to type IIa to type IIx) (55). Consequently, at higher work rates when the type IIx fibers are recruited, there is a greater chance of producing lactic acid. Although chronic light exercise (less than 40% $\dot{V}O_2$max) only recruits and causes a training effect in type I fibers, exercise beyond 70% $\dot{V}O_2$max involves all fiber types. This fact has important implications in the specificity of training and the potential for transferring training effects from one activity to another. Obviously, if you don't use a muscle fiber, it can't become trained.

KEY POINT

Muscle tension depends on the frequency of the stimulation leading to a tetanus contraction, the synchronous firing of muscle fibers, and the recruitment of muscle fibers. The order of recruitment of muscle fibers is from the most to the least oxidative. Light to moderate exercise uses type I muscle fibers, whereas moderate to vigorous exercise requires type IIa fibers. Both favor the aerobic metabolism of carbohydrate and fat. Heavy exercise requires type IIx fibers that favor anaerobic glycolysis, which increases the likelihood of lactate production.

Metabolic, Cardiovascular, and Respiratory Responses to Exercise

A primary task of the fitness professional is to recommend physical activities that increase or maintain cardiorespira-

tory function. Activities that demand aerobic energy (ATP) production automatically cause the circulatory and respiratory systems to deliver oxygen to the muscle to meet the demand. The selected aerobic activities must be strenuous enough to challenge and thus improve the cardiorespiratory system. This crucial link between aerobic activities and cardiorespiratory function provides the basis for much of exercise programming. The following sections summarize selected metabolic, cardiovascular, and respiratory responses to submaximal work and to a maximal graded exercise test (GXT). We begin by discussing how oxygen uptake is measured.

Measuring Oxygen Uptake

How does oxygen get to the mitochondria? First, oxygen enters the lungs during inhalation; it then diffuses from the alveoli of the lungs into the blood. Oxygen is bound to hemoglobin in the red blood cells, and the heart delivers the oxygen-enriched blood to the muscles. Oxygen then diffuses into the muscle cells and reaches the mitochondria, where it is used (consumed) in the production of ATP.

Oxygen consumption ($\dot{V}O_2$) during exercise is measured by subtracting the volume of oxygen exhaled from the volume of oxygen inhaled.

$$\dot{V}O_2 = \text{volume } O_2 \text{ inhaled} - \text{volume } O_2 \text{ exhaled.}$$

To measure $\dot{V}O_2$, the subject breathes through a two-way valve that allows the lungs to inhale room air (containing 20.93% O_2 and 0.03% CO_2) while directing exhaled air to a device that measures the number of liters of air exhaled per minute, which is called **pulmonary ventilation**. In addition, a sample of the exhaled air is directed to gas analyzers to determine its oxygen and carbon dioxide content (see figure 4.6). Oxygen consumption (uptake) is calculated by multiplying the volume of air breathed by the percentage of oxygen extracted. Oxygen extraction is the percentage of oxygen extracted from the inhaled air, the difference between the 20.93% of O_2 in room air and the percentage of O_2 in exhaled air.

The following is a simplified presentation of the steps used to calculate $\dot{V}O_2$; a more detailed presentation is found in appendix B. Note that computer-controlled oxygen uptake equipment (see figure 4.6) does all of the calculations and prints out the results of the test.

$$\dot{V}O_2 = \text{pulmonary ventilation } (L \cdot min^{-1}) \cdot O_2 \text{ extraction.}$$

If ventilation = 60 L · min⁻¹, and exhaled O_2 = 16.93%, then

$$\dot{V}O_2 = 60 \text{ L} \cdot min^{-1} (20.93\% \, O_2 - 16.93\% \, O_2), \text{ and}$$

$$\dot{V}O_2 = 60 \text{ L} \cdot min^{-1} (4.00\% \, O_2) = 2.4 \text{ L} \cdot min^{-1}.$$

CO_2 is produced in the mitochondria and diffuses out of the muscle into the venous blood, where it is carried back to the lungs. There it diffuses into the alveoli and is exhaled. CO_2 production ($\dot{V}CO_2$) can be calculated as described for the $\dot{V}O_2$:

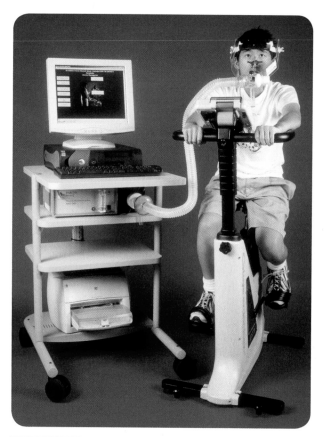

FIGURE 4.6 Computer-controlled equipment for measuring oxygen uptake and carbon dioxide production.

Photo courtesy of ParvoMedics.

If ventilation = 60 L · min^{-1}, and exhaled CO_2 = 3.03%, then

$$\dot{V}CO_2 = 60 \text{ L} \cdot \text{min}^{-1} (3.03\% \ CO_2 - 0.03\% \ CO_2), \text{ and}$$

$$\dot{V}CO_2 = 60 \text{ L} \cdot \text{min}^{-1} (3.00\% \ CO_2) = 1.8 \text{ L} \cdot \text{min}^{-1}.$$

The ratio of CO_2 production ($\dot{V}CO_2$) to oxygen consumption ($\dot{V}O_2$) at the cell is called the **respiratory quotient (RQ)**. Because $\dot{V}CO_2$ and $\dot{V}O_2$ are measured at the mouth rather than at the tissue, this ratio is called the **respiratory exchange ratio (R)**. This ratio tells us what type of fuel is being used during exercise (see the next section, Fuel Utilization During Exercise).

$$R = \dot{V}CO_2 \div \dot{V}O_2.$$

Using the values already calculated,

$$R = 1.8 \text{ L} \cdot \text{min}^{-1} \div 2.4 \text{ L} \cdot \text{min}^{-1} = 0.75.$$

Fuel Utilization During Exercise

In general, protein contributes less than 5% to total energy production during exercise, and for the purpose of our discussion it will be ignored (49). Ignoring protein leaves carbohydrate (muscle glycogen and blood glucose, which is derived from liver glycogen) and fat (adipose tissue and intramuscular fat) as the primary fuels for exercise. The ability of R to provide good information about the metabolism of fat and carbohydrate during exercise stems from the following observations about the metabolism of fat and glucose.

When $R = 1.0$, 100% of the energy is derived from carbohydrate, 0% from fat; when $R = 0.7$, the reverse is true. When $R = 0.85$, approximately 50% of the energy comes from carbohydrate and 50% comes from fat (see Respiratory Quotients for Carbohydrate and Fat sidebar). For the R measurement to be correct, the subject must be in a steady state. If lactic acid is increasing in the blood, the plasma bicarbonate (HCO_3^-) buffer store reacts with the acid (H^+) and produces CO_2, which must be exhaled so that the exerciser is stimulated to hyperventilate:

$$H^+ + HCO_3^- \rightarrow H_2CO_3 \rightarrow H_2O + CO_2.$$

This CO_2 does not come from the aerobic metabolism of carbohydrate and fat, so when it is exhaled, it results in an overestimation of the true value of R. During strenuous work, lactic acid is produced in great amounts, and R can exceed 1.0.

Effect of Exercise Intensity on Fuel Utilization

Figure 4.7 shows how R changes during progressive work up to $\dot{V}O_2$max. In the progressive test, R increases at about

Respiratory Quotients for Carbohydrate and Fat

For glucose ($C_6H_{12}O_6$),

$$C_6H_{12}O_6 + 6 O_2 \rightarrow 6 CO_2 + 6 H_2O + \text{energy}$$

$$R = \frac{6 \ CO_2}{6 \ O_2} = 1.0.$$

For palmitate ($C_{16}H_{32}O_2$, a fatty acid),

$$C_{16}H_{32}O_2 + 23 O_2 \rightarrow 16 CO_2 + 16 H_2O + \text{energy}$$

$$R = \frac{16 \ CO_2}{23 \ O_2} = 0.7.$$

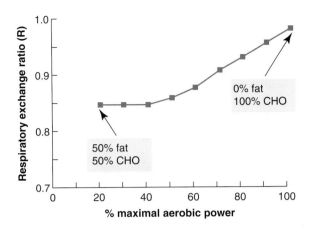

FIGURE 4.7 Changes in *R* (respiratory exchange ratio) with increasing exercise intensity (2).

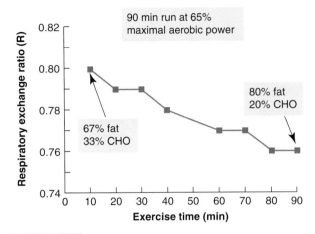

FIGURE 4.8 Changes in *R* (respiratory exchange ratio) during prolonged steady-state exercise (50).

40% to 50% $\dot{V}O_2$max, indicating that type IIa fibers are being recruited and carbohydrate (CHO) is becoming a more important fuel source. Using carbohydrate provides an adaptive advantage—the muscle obtains about 6% more energy from each liter of O_2 when carbohydrate is used (5 kcal $\cdot$ L^{-1}) compared with when fat is used (4.7 kcal $\cdot$ L^{-1}).

Carbohydrate fuels for muscular exercise include muscle glycogen and liver glycogen, which maintains the blood glucose concentration. Muscle glycogen is the primary carbohydrate fuel for heavy exercise lasting less than 2 hr, and inadequate muscle glycogen results in premature fatigue (11). As muscle glycogen is depleted during prolonged heavy exercise, blood glucose becomes more important in supplying the carbohydrate fuel. Toward the end of heavy exercise lasting 3 hr or more, blood glucose provides almost all the carbohydrate used by the muscles. Therefore, heavy exercise is limited by the availability of carbohydrate fuels, which must be either stored in abundance before exercise (muscle glycogen) or replaced through the ingestion of carbohydrate during exercise (blood glucose) (10).

Effect of Exercise Duration on Fuel Utilization

Figure 4.8 shows how *R* changes during a 90 min test performed at 65% of the subject's $\dot{V}O_2$max (50). *R* decreases over time, indicating a greater reliance on fat as a fuel. The fat is derived from both intramuscular fat stores and adipose tissue, which releases free fatty acids into the blood to be carried to the muscle. Using more fat spares the remaining carbohydrate stores and extends the time to exhaustion.

Effect of Diet and Training on Fuel Utilization

The type of fuel used during exercise depends on diet. It has been demonstrated clearly that a diet high in carbohydrate (versus an average diet) increases the muscle glycogen

content and extends the time to exhaustion (33). Further, the muscle gains a greater capacity to increase its glycogen store if a person performs strenuous exercise before eating high-carbohydrate meals (33, 61). Finally, during prolonged heavy exercise, carbohydrate drinks help to maintain the blood glucose concentration and extend the time to fatigue (10).

Endurance training increases the number of mitochondria in the muscles involved in the training program. Having more mitochondria increases the ability of the muscle to use fat as a fuel and to process the available carbohydrate aerobically. This ability spares the carbohydrate store and reduces lactate production, both of which favorably influence performance (30).

KEY POINT

The respiratory exchange ratio (*R*) tracks fuel use during steady-state exercise. When *R* = 1.0, 100% of the energy is derived from carbohydrate; when *R* = 0.7, 100% of the energy is derived from fat. When lactic acid increases in the blood during heavy exercise, the acid is buffered by plasma bicarbonate. This buffering produces CO_2 and invalidates using *R* as an indicator of fuel use during exercise. As exercise intensity increases, *R* increases, indicating that carbohydrate plays a bigger role in generating ATP. During prolonged moderately strenuous exercise, *R* decreases over time, indicating that fat is being used more and carbohydrate is being spared.

Transition From Rest to Steady-State Work

Some readers might mistakenly assume from our discussion up to this point that immediate, short-term, and long-term sources of energy (ATP) are used in distinct activities and do not work together to allow the body to make the transition from rest to exercise. When a person steps onto a treadmill belt moving at a velocity of 200 m · min⁻¹ (7.5 mi · hr⁻¹), the ATP requirement increases from the low level needed to stand alongside the treadmill to the new level required to run at 200 m · min⁻¹. This change in the ATP supply to the muscle must take place in the first step on the treadmill. If this change fails to occur, the person will drift off the back of the treadmill. What energy sources supply ATP during the first minutes of work?

Oxygen Uptake

The cardiovascular and respiratory systems cannot instantaneously increase the delivery of oxygen to the muscles to completely meet the ATP demands of aerobic processes. In the interval between the time a person steps onto the treadmill and the time the cardiovascular and respiratory systems deliver the required oxygen, the immediate and short-term sources of energy supply the needed ATP. The volume of oxygen missing in the first few minutes of work is the **oxygen deficit** (figure 4.9). PC supplies some of the needed ATP, and the anaerobic breakdown of glycogen to lactic acid provides the rest until the oxidative mechanisms meet the ATP requirement. When the uptake of oxygen levels off during submaximal work, the oxygen uptake value represents the **steady-state oxygen requirement** for the activity. At this point, the ATP need of the cell is being met by the aerobic production of ATP in the mitochondria of the muscle on a pay-as-you-go basis.

When the person stops running and steps off the treadmill, the ATP need of the muscles that were involved in the activity suddenly drops toward the resting value. The oxygen uptake decreases quickly at first and then more gradually approaches the resting value. This elevated oxygen uptake during recovery from exercise is the **excess postexercise oxygen consumption (EPOC)**; it also is called the *oxygen debt* and *oxygen repayment* (figure 4.9). In part, the elevated oxygen uptake is used to make

additional ATP to bring the PC store of the muscle back to normal (remember that it was depleted somewhat at the onset of work). Some of the extra oxygen taken in during recovery is used to pay the ATP requirement for the higher HR and breathing during recovery (compared with rest). The liver uses a small part of the oxygen repayment to convert some of the lactic acid produced at the onset of work into glucose (49).

If an individual reaches the steady-state oxygen requirement earlier during the first minutes of work, a smaller oxygen deficit is incurred. The body depletes less PC and produces less lactic acid. Endurance training speeds up the kinetics of oxygen transport; that is, it decreases the time needed to reach a steady state of oxygen uptake. People in poor condition, as well as people with cardiovascular or pulmonary disease, take longer to reach the steady-state oxygen requirement. They incur a larger oxygen deficit and must produce more ATP from the immediate and short-term sources of energy when beginning work or transitioning from one intensity to the next (26, 47).

Heart Rate and Pulmonary Ventilation

The link between the cardiorespiratory responses to work and the time it takes to reach the steady-state oxygen requirement should be no surprise. Figure 4.10 shows how HR and pulmonary ventilation typically respond to a submaximal run test. The shape of the curve in each case resembles the curve for oxygen uptake described earlier.

In addition, the muscle contributes to the lag in oxygen uptake at the onset of work. An untrained muscle has relatively few mitochondria available to produce ATP aerobically and relatively few capillaries per muscle fiber to bring the oxygen-enriched arterial blood to those mitochondria. Following endurance training, both of these factors increase so that the muscle can produce more ATP aerobically at the onset of work. In addition, less lactic acid is produced at the onset of work and the blood lactic acid concentration is lower for a fixed submaximal work rate (26, 30, 47).

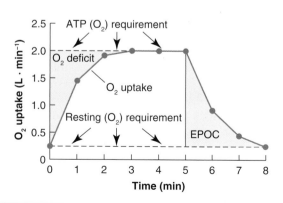

FIGURE 4.9 Oxygen (O₂) deficit and EPOC during a 5 min run on a treadmill.

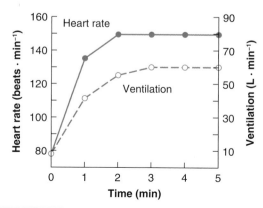

FIGURE 4.10 Response of HR and pulmonary ventilation during a 5 min run on a treadmill.

KEY POINT

At the onset of submaximal exercise, $\dot{V}O_2$ does not increase immediately (oxygen deficit), and some of the ATP must be supplied anaerobically by PC and glycolysis. At the end of exercise, $\dot{V}O_2$ remains elevated for some time to replenish PC stores, support the energy cost of the elevated HR and breathing, and synthesize glucose from lactic acid. Training reduces the oxygen deficit because it creates a more rapid increase in $\dot{V}O_2$ at the onset of work, allowing the steady-state oxygen requirement to be reached more quickly.

Graded Exercise Test

Oxygen consumption and CRF are clearly linked, because oxygen delivery to tissue depends on lung and heart function. One of the most common tests used to evaluate cardiorespiratory function is a GXT, in which participants exercise at progressively increasing work rates until they reach maximum work tolerance. During the test the participant may be monitored for cardiovascular variables (ECG, HR, BP), respiratory variables (pulmonary ventilation, respiratory frequency), and metabolic variables (oxygen uptake, blood lactic acid level). The way a person responds to the GXT provides important information about cardiorespiratory function and the capacity for prolonged work.

Oxygen Uptake and Maximal Aerobic Power

Oxygen uptake, measured as described earlier, is expressed per kilogram of body weight to facilitate comparisons between people or between tests for the same person over time. The $\dot{V}O_2$ value in liters per minute is simply multiplied by 1,000 to convert $\dot{V}O_2$ to ml · min^{-1}, and that value is divided by the subject's body weight in kilograms to yield a value expressed in milliliters per kilogram per minute.

$$\dot{V}O_2 = 2.4 \text{ L} \cdot \text{min}^{-1} \cdot 1{,}000 \text{ ml} \cdot \text{L}^{-1},$$

$$\dot{V}O_2 = 2{,}400 \text{ ml} \cdot \text{min}^{-1}.$$

For a 60 kg subject,

$$\dot{V}O_2 = 2{,}400 \text{ ml} \cdot \text{min}^{-1} \div 60 \text{ kg} = 40 \text{ ml} \cdot \text{kg}^{-1} \cdot \text{min}^{-1}.$$

Figure 4.11 shows a GXT conducted on a treadmill in which the speed is constant at 3 mi · hr^{-1} (4.8 km · hr^{-1}) and the grade changes 3% every 3 min. With each stage of the GXT, oxygen uptake increases to meet the ATP demand of the work rate. Also, the participant incurs a small oxygen deficit at each stage as the cardiovascular system tries to adjust to the new demand of the increased work rate.

Apparently healthy individuals reach the steady-state oxygen requirement by 1.5 min or so of each GXT stage up to moderately heavy work (44, 45). People who have low

$\dot{V}O_2$ increases with each stage of GXT. At the end of a maximal GXT the percent grade increases, but $\dot{V}O_2$ does not. $\dot{V}O_2$max has been reached.

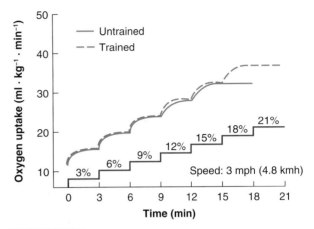

FIGURE 4.11 Oxygen uptake responses to a GXT (38).

CRF or who have cardiovascular and pulmonary diseases may not be able to reach the expected values in the same amount of time and might incur larger oxygen deficits with each stage of the test. For these individuals, the oxygen uptake measured at various stages of the test is lower than expected because they do not reach the expected steady-state demands of the test at each stage.

Toward the end of a GXT, a point is reached at which the work rate changes (i.e., the grade on the treadmill increases) but the oxygen uptake does not. In effect, the cardiovascular system has reached its limits for transporting oxygen to the muscle. This point is called **maximal aerobic power**, or **maximal oxygen uptake ($\dot{V}O_2$max)**. A complete leveling off in oxygen consumption is not seen in all cases because the subject must work one stage past the actual point at which $\dot{V}O_2$max is reached, requiring high motivation. In some GXT protocols, the plateau in oxygen uptake is judged against the criterion of less than 2.1 ml · kg^{-1} · min^{-1} increase in $\dot{V}O_2$ from one stage to the next (62). Other criteria for having achieved $\dot{V}O_2$max include an R greater than 1.15 (34) and a blood lactate concentration greater than 8 mmol · L^{-1}, about 8 times the resting value (1). These and other criteria have been used alone and in combination to establish whether or not the subject has achieved $\dot{V}O_2$max (32). Participation in a 10 to 20 wk endurance training program increases $\dot{V}O_2$max. When trained people retake the GXT, they reach the steady state sooner at light to moderate work rates and then go one or more stages further into the test, at which time the greater $\dot{V}O_2$max is measured.

Maximal aerobic power describes the greatest rate at which the body (primarily muscle) can produce ATP aerobically during dynamic exercise involving a large muscle mass (e.g., running, cycling). It is also the upper limit at which the cardiovascular system can deliver oxygen-enriched blood to the muscles. Thus, maximal aerobic power is not only a good index of CRF, it is also a good predictor of performance capability in aerobic events such as distance running, cycling, cross-country skiing, and swimming (4, 5). In the apparently healthy person, maximal aerobic power is the quantitative limit at which the cardiovascular system can deliver oxygen to tissues. This usual interpretation must be tempered by the mode of exercise (test type) used to impose the work rate on the subject.

Test Type

For the average person, the highest value for maximal aerobic power is measured when the subject completes a GXT involving uphill running. A GXT conducted at a walking speed usually results in a $\dot{V}O_2$max value 4% to 6% below the graded running value, and a test on a cycle ergometer may yield a value 10% to 12% lower than the graded running value (20, 42, 43). If a subject works to exhaustion using an arm ergometer, then the highest oxygen uptake value is less than 70% of that measured with the legs (23). Knowing these variations in maximal aerobic power is helpful in making recommendations about the intensity of various exercises needed to achieve the target or training HR. At any given submaximal work rate, most physiological responses (HR, BP, and blood lactic acid) are greater for arm work than for leg work (23, 60). Maximal aerobic power is influenced by more than the type of test used in its measurement. Other factors include endurance training, heredity, sex, age, altitude, pollution, and cardiovascular and pulmonary disease.

Training and Heredity

Endurance training increases $\dot{V}O_2$max by 5% to 25%, with the magnitude of the change depending, in part, on the initial level of fitness. A person with a low $\dot{V}O_2$max sees the largest change, but there is considerable individual variation in response (see chapter 11 for more on this). Eventually, a point is reached where further training does not increase $\dot{V}O_2$max. Approximately 40% of the extremely high values of maximal aerobic power found in elite cross-country skiers and distance runners relates to a genetic predisposition for having a superior cardiovascular system (6). Because typical endurance programs may increase $\dot{V}O_2$max by only 20% or so, it is unrealistic to expect a person with a $\dot{V}O_2$max of 40 ml · kg⁻¹ · min⁻¹ to increase to 80 ml · kg⁻¹ · min⁻¹, a value measured in some elite cross-country skiers and distance runners (56). On the other hand, those who do severe interval training can achieve gains of 44% in $\dot{V}O_2$max (25).

Sex and Age

Women's $\dot{V}O_2$max values (ml · kg⁻¹ · min⁻¹) are about 15% lower than men's, a difference that exists across ages 20 to 60. The primary reasons for the gender difference relate to differences in percent body fat and in hemoglobin levels (see later discussion). The 15% difference between men and women is an average, and $\dot{V}O_2$max values overlap considerably in these populations (2). In most people, aging gradually but systematically reduces $\dot{V}O_2$max by about 1% each year. $\dot{V}O_2$max is influenced by physical activity and percent body fat, so people who remain active and maintain body weight (which is not the usual case) have higher $\dot{V}O_2$max values across the age span. In fact, endurance training by middle-aged people gives the appearance of reversing the aging effect because it elevates $\dot{V}O_2$max to a level consistent with that of a younger, sedentary person (35-37).

Altitude and Pollution

$\dot{V}O_2$max decreases with increasing altitude. At 7,400 ft (2,300 m), $\dot{V}O_2$max is only 88% of the sea-level value. This decrease in $\dot{V}O_2$max is attributable primarily to the reduction in arterial oxygen content that occurs as the oxygen pressure in the air decreases with increasing altitude. When the arterial oxygen content is lower, the heart must pump more blood per minute to meet the oxygen needs of any task. As a result, the HR response is higher at submaximal intensities performed at greater altitudes (31).

Carbon monoxide, produced from the burning of fossil fuel as well as from cigarette smoke, binds readily to hemoglobin and can decrease oxygen transport to muscles. The critical concentration of carbon monoxide in blood needed to decrease $\dot{V}O_2$max is about 4%. After that, $\dot{V}O_2$max decreases approximately 1% for every 1% increase in the carbon monoxide concentration in the blood (51).

Cardiovascular and Pulmonary Diseases

Cardiovascular and pulmonary diseases decrease $\dot{V}O_2$max by diminishing the delivery of oxygen from the air to the blood and reducing the capacity of the heart to deliver blood to the muscles. Patients with CVD have some of the lowest $\dot{V}O_2$max (functional capacity) values, but they also experience the largest changes in $\dot{V}O_2$max from endurance

KEY POINT

Maximal oxygen uptake, $\dot{V}O_2$max, is the greatest rate at which O_2 can be delivered to working muscles during dynamic exercise. $\dot{V}O_2$max is influenced by heredity and training, decreases about 1% per year with age, and is about 15% lower in women compared with men. $\dot{V}O_2$max is lower at high altitudes, and carbon monoxide in the blood decreases $\dot{V}O_2$max because it binds to hemoglobin and limits oxygen transport. Cardiovascular and pulmonary diseases lower $\dot{V}O_2$max; however, people with CVD can attain large improvements in $\dot{V}O_2$max through endurance training.

training. Table 4.1 shows common values for $\dot{V}O_2$max in a variety of populations (2, 22, 64).

Blood Lactate and Pulmonary Ventilation

Muscle produces lactic acid, which is released into the blood. Figure 4.12 shows that during a GXT, blood lactate concentration changes little or not at all at the lower work rates; lactate is metabolized as fast as it is produced (7). As the GXT increases in intensity, a work rate is reached at which the blood lactate concentration suddenly increases. This work rate is referred to as the **lactate threshold**, and it typically occurs between 50% and 80% $\dot{V}O_2$max. This sudden increase in the blood lactate concentration is sometimes called the *anaerobic threshold,* but because several conditions other than a lack of oxygen (hypoxia)

at the muscle cell can result in lactate being produced and released into the blood, *lactate threshold* is the preferred term. Endurance training increases the number of mitochondria in the trained muscles, facilitating the aerobic metabolism of carbohydrate and the use of more fat as fuel. As a result, when the subject retakes the GXT following training, less lactate is produced and the lactate threshold occurs at a later stage of the test. Lactate threshold is a good indicator of endurance performance and has been used to predict performance in endurance races (4, 5).

Pulmonary ventilation is the volume of air inhaled or exhaled per minute and is calculated by multiplying the frequency (*f*) of breathing by the tidal volume *(TV),* the volume of air moved in one breath. For example,

$$\text{Ventilation (L} \cdot \text{min}^{-1}) = TV \text{ (L} \cdot \text{breath}^{-1}) \cdot f \text{ (breaths} \cdot \text{min}^{-1}),$$
and
$$30 \text{ (L} \cdot \text{min}^{-1}) = 1.5 \text{ L} \cdot \text{breath}^{-1} \cdot 20 \text{ breaths} \cdot \text{min}^{-1}.$$

Pulmonary ventilation increases linearly with work rate until 50% to 80% of $\dot{V}O_2$max, at which point a relative **hyperventilation** results (see figure 4.13). The inflection point in the pulmonary ventilation response is the **ventilatory threshold**. The ventilatory threshold has been used as a noninvasive indicator of the lactate threshold and as a predictor of performance (17, 48). The increase in pulmonary ventilation is mediated by changes in the frequency of breathing (from about 10-12 breaths $\cdot$ min^{-1} at rest to 40-50 breaths $\cdot$ min^{-1} during maximal work) and in the tidal volume (from 0.5 L $\cdot$ breath^{-1} at rest to 2-3 L $\cdot$ breath^{-1} in maximal work). Endurance training lowers pulmonary ventilation during submaximal work, so the ventilatory threshold occurs later in the GXT. The maximal value for pulmonary ventilation tends to change in the direction of $\dot{V}O_2$max.

TABLE 4.1 Maximal Aerobic Power in Healthy and Diseased Populations

Population	$\dot{V}O_2$MAX (ML $\cdot$ KG^{-1} $\cdot$ MIN^{-1})	
	Men	Women
Elite cross-country skiers	75-85	65-75
Elite distance runners	70-80	65-75
College students	40-50	30-40
Middle-aged adults	30-40	25-35
Post-MI patients	~22	~18
Patients with severe pulmonary disease	~13	~13

Data compiled from Åstrand, et al 2003; Fox, et al., 1998; Wilmore, et al., 2008; the Fort Sanders Cardiac Rehabilitation Program; and J.T. Daniels (personal communication).

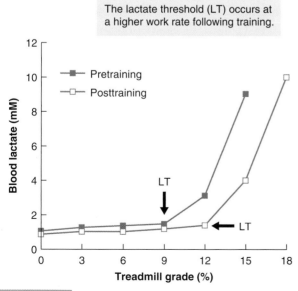

FIGURE 4.12 Training causes the lactate threshold (LT) to occur at a higher exercise intensity (19).

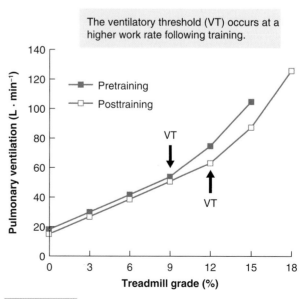

FIGURE 4.13 Following training, the ventilatory threshold (VT) occurs later in the GXT.

KEY POINT

The points at which the blood lactic acid concentration and the pulmonary ventilation increase suddenly during a GXT are called the *lactate* and *ventilatory thresholds,* respectively. These typically occur between 50% and 80% $\dot{V}O_2$max. The lactate and ventilatory thresholds are good predictors of performance in endurance events (e.g., 10K runs, marathons).

Heart Rate

Once the HR reaches about 110 beats · min⁻¹, it increases linearly with work rate during a GXT until near-maximal efforts. Figure 4.14 shows how training influences the subject's HR response at the same work rates. The lower HR at submaximal work rates is a beneficial effect because it decreases the oxygen needed by the heart muscle. Maximal HR shows no change or is slightly reduced as a result of endurance training.

Stroke Volume

The volume of blood pumped by the heart per beat (ml · beat⁻¹) is called the *stroke volume (SV).* For people doing work in the upright position (cycling, walking), SV increases in the early stages of the GXT until about 40% $\dot{V}O_2$max is reached and then it levels off (see figure 4.15) (2). Consequently, when $\dot{V}O_2$ is greater than 40% $\dot{V}O_2$max, HR is the sole factor responsible for the increased flow of blood from the heart to the working muscles. This is what makes HR a good indicator of the metabolic rate during exercise—it is linearly related to exercise intensity from

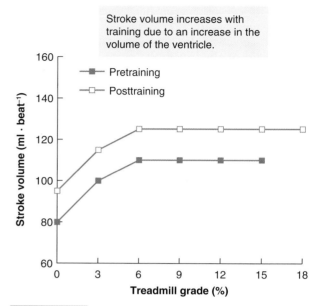

Stroke volume increases with training due to an increase in the volume of the ventricle.

FIGURE 4.15 SV increases with training due to larger volume of the ventricle (19).

light exercise to heavy exercise. One of the primary effects of endurance training is an increase in SV at rest and during work; this increase is due to a larger volume of the ventricle that is linked, in part, to a larger blood volume (19). This allows a greater **end-diastolic volume**, the volume of blood in the heart just before contraction. So, following endurance training, even if the same fraction of blood in the ventricle is pumped per beat (**ejection fraction**), the heart pumps more blood per minute at the same HR.

Cardiac Output

Cardiac output (*Q*) is the volume of blood pumped by the heart per minute and is calculated by multiplying the HR (beats · min⁻¹) by the SV (ml · beat⁻¹).

$$\text{Cardiac output} = \text{HR} \cdot \text{SV}$$
$$= 60 \text{ beats} \cdot \text{min}^{-1} \cdot 80 \text{ ml} \cdot \text{beat}^{-1}$$
$$= 4{,}800 \text{ ml} \cdot \text{min}^{-1}, \text{ or } 4.8 \text{ L} \cdot \text{min}^{-1}.$$

Cardiac output increases linearly with work rate. Generally, the cardiac output response to light and moderate work is not affected by endurance training. What changes is how the cardiac output is achieved: with a lower HR and higher SV.

Maximal cardiac output (highest value reached in a GXT) is the most important cardiovascular variable determining maximal aerobic power because the oxygen-enriched blood (carrying about 0.2 L of O_2 per liter of blood) must be delivered to the muscle for the mitochondria to use. If a person's maximal cardiac output is 10 L · min⁻¹, only 2 L of O_2 would leave the heart each minute (i.e., 0.2 L of O_2 per liter of blood times a cardiac output of 10 L · min⁻¹ = 2 L of O_2 · min⁻¹). A person with a maximal cardiac

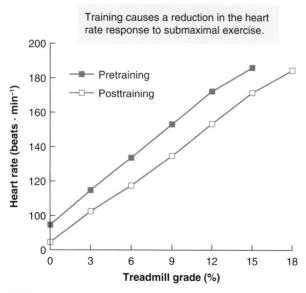

Training causes a reduction in the heart rate response to submaximal exercise.

FIGURE 4.14 Training reduces the HR response to submaximal exercise (19).

output of 30 L · min^{-1} would deliver 6 L of O$_2$ · min^{-1} to the tissues. Endurance training increases the maximal cardiac output and thus the delivery of oxygen to the muscles (see figure 4.16). This increase in maximal cardiac output is matched by greater capillary numbers in the muscle to allow the blood to move slowly enough through the muscle to maintain the time needed for oxygen to diffuse from the blood to the mitochondria (57). The increase in maximal cardiac output accounts for 50% of the increase in maximal oxygen uptake that occurs in previously sedentary people who engage in endurance training (54).

In the general population, SV is the major variable influencing maximal cardiac output. Differences in maximal cardiac output and maximal aerobic power that exist between females and males, between trained and untrained individuals, and between world-class endurance athletes and average fit individuals can be explained largely by differences in maximal SV. This is shown in table 4.2, where $\dot{V}O_2$max varies by a factor of 3 among three distinct groups, while maximal HR is almost the same for all three groups. Clearly, maximal SV is the primary factor related to the differences in $\dot{V}O_2$max that exist among individuals.

Oxygen Extraction

Two factors determine oxygen uptake at any time: the volume of blood delivered to the tissues per minute (cardiac output) and the volume of oxygen extracted from each liter of blood. Oxygen extraction is calculated by subtracting the oxygen content of mixed venous blood (as it returns to the heart) from the oxygen content of the arterial blood. This is the **arteriovenous oxygen difference**, or the *(a − $\bar{v}$) O$_2$ difference.*

$$\dot{V}O_2 = \text{cardiac output} \cdot (a - \bar{v})O_2 \text{ difference.}$$

At rest, cardiac output = 5 L · min^{-1},
arterial oxygen content = 200 ml of O$_2$ · L^{-1}, and
mixed venous oxygen content = 150 ml of O$_2$ · L^{-1}.

$$\dot{V}O_2 = 5 \text{ L} \cdot \text{min}^{-1} \cdot (200 - 150 \text{ ml of } O_2 \cdot L^{-1}),$$
$$\dot{V}O_2 = 5 \text{ L} \cdot \text{min}^{-1} \cdot 50 \text{ ml of } O_2 \cdot L^{-1}, \text{ and so}$$
$$\dot{V}O_2 = 250 \text{ ml} \cdot \text{min}^{-1}.$$

The $(a - \bar{v})O_2$ difference reflects the ability of the muscle to extract oxygen, and it increases with exercise intensity (see figure 4.17). The ability of tissue to extract oxygen is a function of the capillary-to-muscle-fiber ratio and the number of mitochondria in the muscle fiber. Endurance training increases both of these factors, thus increasing the maximal capacity to extract oxygen in the last stage of the GXT (57). This increase in the $(a - \bar{v})O_2$ difference accounts for about 50% of the increase in $\dot{V}O_2$max that occurs with endurance training in previously sedentary individuals (54).

Blood Pressure

BP is dependent on the balance between cardiac output and the resistance the blood vessels offer to blood flow (total peripheral resistance). The resistance to blood flow is altered by the constriction or dilation of **arterioles**, which are blood vessels located between the artery and the capillary.

$$\text{BP} = \text{cardiac output} \cdot \text{total peripheral resistance.}$$

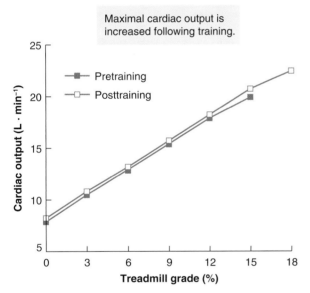

Maximal cardiac output is increased following training.

FIGURE 4.16 Maximal cardiac output increases following training (19).

TABLE 4.2 Maximal Values of $\dot{V}O_2$max, Heart Rate, Stroke Volume, and Arteriovenous Oxygen Difference in Three Groups With Very Low, Normal, and High Maximal $\dot{V}O_2$max

Group	$\dot{V}O_2$max (ml · min^{-1})	=	HR (beats · min^{-1})	×	SV (L · beat^{-1})	×	Arteriovenous (a − $\bar{v}$) oxygen difference (mL · L^{-1})
Mitral stenosis	1615	=	190	×	0.05	×	170
Sedentary	3200	=	200	×	0.10	×	160
Athlete	5200	=	190	×	0.16	×	170

Adapted, by permission, from L. Rowell, 1969, "Circulation," *Medicine and Science in Sports and Exercise* 1: 15-22.

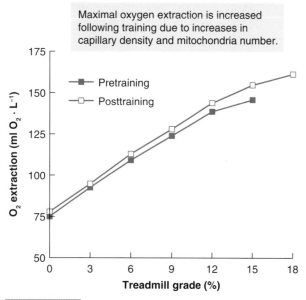

FIGURE 4.17 Following training, maximal O$_2$ extraction increases due to greater capillary and mitochondrial density in the trained muscles (19).

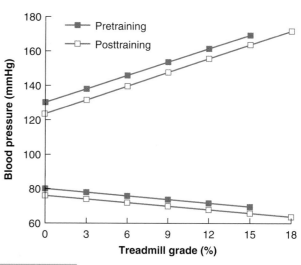

FIGURE 4.18 SBP increases until maximum work tolerance is reached. DBP remains steady or decreases.

BP is sensed by **baroreceptors** in the arch of the aorta and in the carotid arteries. When BP changes, the baroreceptors send signals to the cardiovascular control center in the brain, which in turn alters cardiac output or the diameter of arterioles. For example, if a person who has been lying supine suddenly stands, blood pools in the lower extremities, SV decreases, and BP drops. If BP is not restored, less blood flows to the brain and the person might faint. The baroreceptors monitor this decrease in BP, and the cardiovascular control center simultaneously increases the HR and reduces the diameter of the arterioles (to increase total peripheral resistance) to try to return BP to normal. During exercise, the arterioles dilate in the active muscle to increase blood flow and meet metabolic demands. This dilation is matched with a constriction of arterioles in the liver, kidneys, and gastrointestinal tract and an increase in HR and SV, as already mentioned. These coordinated changes maintain BP and direct most of the cardiac output to the working muscles.

BP is monitored at each stage of a GXT. Figure 4.18 shows how **systolic blood pressure (SBP)** increases with each stage until maximum work tolerance is reached. At that point, SBP might decrease. A fall in SBP with an increase in work rate is used as an indicator of maximal cardiovascular function and can aid in determining the end point for an exercise test. **Diastolic blood pressure (DBP)** tends to remain the same or decrease during a GXT. An increase in DBP toward the end of the test is another indicator that a subject has reached the limits of functional capacity. Endurance training reduces the BP responses at fixed submaximal work rates. See chapter 7 for criteria for terminating a GXT.

KEY POINT

During acute exercise, HR increases linearly with work rate once the HR reaches 110 beats · min^{-1}. During exercise in the upright position, SV increases until an intensity of about 40% $\dot{V}O_2$max is reached. Cardiac output (HR · SV) increases linearly with work rate. Endurance training reduces HR and increases SV at rest and during submaximal work; in addition, maximal cardiac output is greater, because SV increases with no change or a slight decrease in maximal HR. Variations in $\dot{V}O_2$max across the population are attributed primarily to differences in maximal SV. Half of the increase in $\dot{V}O_2$max attributable to endurance training is a result of an increase in maximal SV; the other half is attributable to an increase in oxygen extraction.

Two factors that determine the oxygen demand (work) of the heart during aerobic exercise are the HR and the SBP. The product of these two variables is called the **rate–pressure product**, or the **double product**, and is proportional to the myocardial oxygen demand (i.e., the volume of oxygen the heart muscle needs each minute to function properly). Factors that decrease the HR and BP responses to work increase the chance that the coronary blood supply to the heart muscle will adequately meet the oxygen demands of the heart. Endurance training decreases the HR and BP responses to fixed submaximal work and protects against any diminished blood supply (ischemia) to the myocardium. Drugs are also used to lower HR and BP to reduce the work of the heart (see chapter 25).

KEY POINT

SBP increases with each stage of a GXT, whereas DBP remains the same or decreases. The work of the heart is proportional to the product of the HR and the SBP. Training lowers both, making it easier for the coronary arteries to meet the oxygen demand of the heart. HR and BP are higher during arm work compared with leg work at the same work rate.

When a person does the same rate of work with the arms as with the legs, the HR and BP responses are considerably higher during the arm work. This is shown in figure 4.19, in which the rate–pressure product is plotted for various levels of arm and leg work. Given that the load on the heart and the potential for fatigue are greater for arm work, fitness professionals should choose activities that use the large muscle groups of the legs; such activities result in lower HR, BP, and perception of fatigue at the same work rate (23, 60). This will allow one to accomplish more work in a fixed time period than with arm exercise. That said, if participants need to increase their capacity for arm work

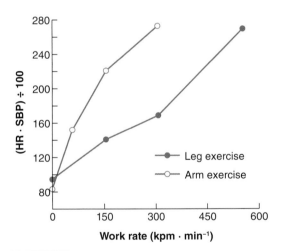

FIGURE 4.19 Rate–pressure product at rest and during arm and leg exercise.

Adapted from *American Heart Journal*, Vol. 94, J. Schwade, C.G. Blomqvist and W. Shapiro, "A comparison of the response in arm and leg work in patients with ischemic heart disease," pp. 203-208, Copyright 1977, with permission from Elsevier.

related to employment or sport, then structured progressive exercise programs should be implemented for that purpose.

Effects of Endurance Training and Detraining on Physiological Responses

Many observations have been made about the effects of endurance training on various physiological responses to exercise. In this section we show how some of these effects interrelate.

- Endurance training increases the number of mitochondria and capillaries in muscle, causing all active fibers to become more oxidative. This effect is manifested by the increase in type IIa fibers and decrease in type IIx fibers. These changes boost the endurance capacity of the muscle by allowing fat to be used for a greater percentage of energy production, sparing the muscle glycogen store and reducing lactate production. The lactate threshold shifts to the right, and performance times in endurance events improve.

- Endurance training decreases the time it takes to achieve a steady state in submaximal exercise. This reduces the oxygen deficit and reliance on PC and anaerobic glycolysis for energy.

- Endurance training enlarges the volume of the ventricle. This accommodates an increase in the end-diastolic volume such that more blood is pumped out per beat. The increased SV is accompanied by a decrease in HR during submaximal work, so the cardiac output remains the same. The heart works less to meet the oxygen needs of the tissues at the same work rate. Table 4.3 summarizes these changes that result from endurance training.

- Maximal aerobic power increases with endurance training, the increase being inversely related to the initial $\dot{V}O_2$max. In formerly sedentary individuals, about 50% of the increase in $\dot{V}O_2$max results from greater maximal cardiac output, a change brought about by an increase in maximal SV, given that maximal HR either remains the same or decreases

TABLE 4.3 Effects of Endurance Training on Cardiovascular Response to a Graded Exercise Test

Variable	Rest	At same relative $\dot{V}O_2$ (ml · kg^{-1} · min^{-1})	At maximal work
Cardiac output	Same	Same	Higher
SV	Higher	Higher	Higher
HR	Lower	Lower	No change/slightly lower

slightly. The other 50% of the increase in $\dot{V}O_2$max is attributable to an increase in oxygen extraction at the muscle, shown by an increase in the $(a - \bar{v})$ O_2 difference. This occurs as a result of higher numbers of capillaries and mitochondria in the trained muscles.

Transfer of Training

The training effects that have been discussed are observed only when the trained muscles are the muscles used in the exercise test. Although this may appear obvious for the decrease in blood lactate that is attributable to, in part, the greater numbers of mitochondria in the trained muscles, it is also linked to the changes that occur in the HR response to submaximal work following the training program. Figure 4.20 shows the results of repeated submaximal exercise tests conducted on subjects who trained only one leg on a cycle ergometer for 13 days. The HR response to a fixed submaximal work rate performed by the trained leg decreased as expected. At the end of the 13 days of training, the untrained leg was subjected to the same exercise test. The HR responded as if a training effect had not occurred. This indicates that part of the reason the HR response to submaximal exercise decreases following training is because of feedback from the trained muscles to the cardiovascular control center that, in turn, reduces sympathetic stimulation to the heart (9, 54). This finding has important implications for evaluating the effects of training programs. The expected training responses (lower lactate production, lower HR, more fat use) are linked to testing the same muscle groups that were involved in the training. The probability of the training effect carrying over to another activity depends on the degree to which the new activity uses the muscles that are already trained.

Detraining

How fast is a training effect lost? A number of investigations have explored this question by having subjects either reduce or completely cease training. Maximal oxygen uptake is typically used as the principal measure to evaluate physiological changes due to detraining, but an individual's response to a submaximal work rate also has been used to track these changes over time.

Ceasing Training

The following study used subjects who had trained for 10 ± 3 yr and agreed to cease training for 84 days (15). They were tested on days 12, 21, 56, and 84 of detraining. Figure 4.21 shows how their $\dot{V}O_2$max decreased 7% within the first 12 days. Remember that $\dot{V}O_2$max = cardiac output · $(a - \bar{v})$ O_2 difference. The decrease in $\dot{V}O_2$max was attributable entirely to a drop in maximal cardiac output because the maximal oxygen extraction, or $(a - \bar{v})O_2$ difference, was unchanged.

In turn, the lower maximal cardiac output was attributable entirely to a decrease in maximal SV, because maximal HR actually increased during detraining. A subsequent study showed that the reduced SV was caused by a reduction in plasma volume that occurred in the first 12 days of no training (13). In contrast, the drop in $\dot{V}O_2$max between days 21 and 84 was attributable to a decrease in the $(a - \bar{v})O_2$ difference because maximal cardiac output was unchanged (see figure 4.21). This lower oxygen extraction appeared to result from smaller numbers of mitochondria in the muscle, given that the number of capillaries surrounding each muscle fiber was unchanged (12).

The same subjects also completed a standard (fixed work rate) submaximal exercise test during the 84 days of no training (14). Figure 4.22 shows that HR and blood lactic acid responses to this work test increased throughout detraining. The higher responses relate to the fact that the same work rate required a greater percentage of $\dot{V}O_2$max because the latter variable decreased throughout the detraining. The magnitude of change in HR and blood lactic acid responses to this submaximal work, however, makes them sensitive indicators of a person's training state.

Reduced Training

To evaluate the effect of reducing training, Hickson and colleagues (27-29) trained subjects for 10 wk to increase $\dot{V}O_2$max. The training program was conducted 40 min · day^{-1}, 6 days · wk^{-1}. Three days involved running at near-maximum intensity for 40 min; the other 3 days required six 5 min bouts at near-maximum intensity on a cycle ergometer, with a 2 min rest between work bouts. Subjects expended about 600 kcal on each day of exercise, or 3,600 kcal each week. At the end of this 10 wk program, the subjects were divided into groups that trained at either a one-third or two-thirds reduction in the previous frequency (4 and 2 days · wk^{-1}, respectively), duration (26 and 13 min · day^{-1}, respectively), or intensity (a one-third or two-thirds reduction in work done or distance run per 40 min session). Data collected on the maximal treadmill tests showed that cutting duration from 40 to 26 or 13 min or frequency

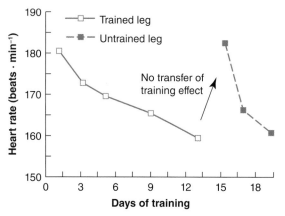

FIGURE 4.20 Lack of transfer of training effect (9).

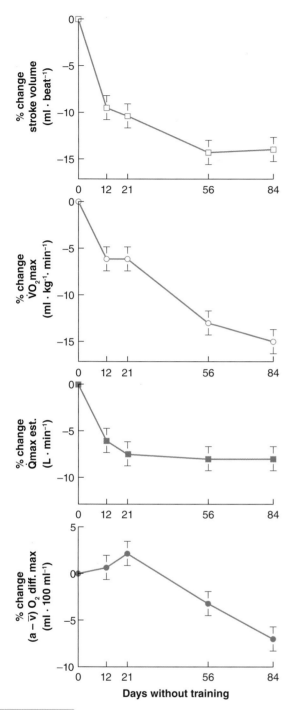

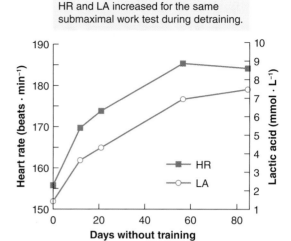

HR and LA increased for the same submaximal work test during detraining.

FIGURE 4.22 Changes in the HR and blood lactic acid (LA) responses to a standard exercise test taken during 84 days of detraining (14).

FIGURE 4.21 Effects of detraining on physiological responses during exercise. $\dot{V}O_2$max = maximal oxygen uptake; $\dot{Q}$max est. = maximal cardiac output; $(a - \bar{v})O_2$ diff. max = maximal arteriovenous oxygen difference.

Adapted from E.F. Coyle, 1984, "Time course of loss of adaptations after stopping prolonged intense endurance training" *Journal of Applied Physiology* 57: 1861. Used with permission.

KEY POINT

Endurance training increases the ability of a muscle to use fat as a fuel and to spare carbohydrate, decreases the time it takes to achieve a steady state during submaximal work, increases the size of the ventricle, and increases $\dot{V}O_2$max by increasing SV and oxygen extraction. Endurance training effects (lower HR, lower blood lactate) do not transfer when untrained muscles are used to perform the work. Maximal oxygen uptake decreases when training stops. The initial decrease is caused by a decrease in SV and, later, in oxygen extraction. Maximal oxygen uptake can be maintained by doing intense exercise, even when cutting exercise duration and frequency.

per week was cut from 3,600 to 1,200 kcal in the group whose exercise frequency and duration were reduced by two-thirds, but they were not able to maintain $\dot{V}O_2$max when the intensity was reduced, even though the subjects were still expending about 1,200 kcal · wk^{-1}. This shows that exercise intensity is critical in maintaining $\dot{V}O_2$max and that it takes less exercise to maintain than to achieve a specific level of $\dot{V}O_2$max.

Cardiovascular Responses to Exercise for Females and Males

Generally, **prepubescent** boys and girls differ little in $\dot{V}O_2$max or in their cardiovascular responses to submaximal

from 6 to 4 or 2 days did not affect $\dot{V}O_2$max. In contrast, $\dot{V}O_2$max clearly fell when the intensity of training was reduced by either one-third or two-thirds. The subjects were able to maintain $\dot{V}O_2$max when the total exercise

exercise. During puberty, differences between girls and boys appear because of girls's higher percentage of body fat, lower hemoglobin concentration, and smaller heart size relative to body weight (2). The two latter factors also affect a woman's cardiovascular responses to submaximal work. For example, if an 80 kg male walks on a 10% grade on a treadmill at 3 mi · hr^{-1} (4.8 km · hr^{-1}), his $\dot{V}O_2$ is 2.07 L · min^{-1}, or 25.9 ml · kg^{-1} · min^{-1}. His HR might be 140 beats · min $^{-1}$. If he carries a backpack weighing 15 kg, his $\dot{V}O_2$ expressed per kilogram does not change (25.9 ml · kg^{-1} · min^{-1}), but his total oxygen requirement increases 389 ml · min^{-1} (i.e., 15 kg · 25.9 ml · kg^{-1} · min^{-1}). His HR obviously is higher with this load than without it, even though the $\dot{V}O_2$ expressed per kilogram of body weight is the same. Likewise, performance in the 12 min run test to evaluate maximal aerobic power decreases by 89 m when body weight is experimentally increased to simulate a 5% gain in body fat (16). When a woman walks on a treadmill at a given grade and speed, her HR is higher than a comparable male's HR because of the additional fat weight she carries. Her lower hemoglobin concentration and smaller heart size also elevate the HR at the same oxygen uptake expressed per unit of body weight.

The differences between males and females in the cardiovascular response to submaximal work become more exaggerated when work is done on a cycle ergometer where a given work rate demands a similar $\dot{V}O_2$ in liters per minute, independent of sex or training. As previously mentioned, the average female has less hemoglobin and a smaller heart volume compared with the average male. To deliver the same volume of oxygen to the muscles, the woman must have a higher HR to compensate for the smaller SV and a slightly higher cardiac output to compensate for the slightly lower hemoglobin concentration (2). In addition, the average woman will typically have a smaller muscle mass with which to accomplish the work; this will increase the HR response (see arm versus leg work discussed previously). These differences between women's and men's cardiovascular responses to cycle ergometry are shown in figure 4.23. Table 4.4 summarizes the differences in cardiovascular responses between men and women in response to exercise.

KEY POINT

During submaximal exercise at the same relative $\dot{V}O_2$ (e.g., walking on a treadmill), women respond with a higher HR due to a higher percent fat, lower SV, and lower hemoglobin level. When exercising at the same work rate or absolute $\dot{V}O_2$ (e.g., riding a cycle ergometer), women respond with a higher HR to compensate for a lower SV and a lower hemoglobin level (and oxygen content) in the arterial blood.

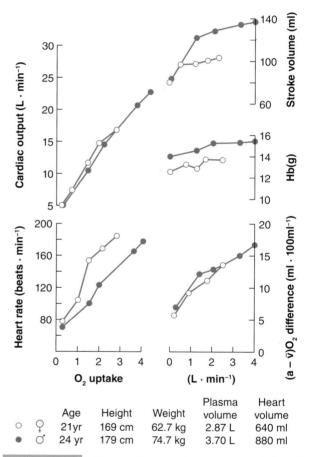

		Age	Height	Weight	Plasma volume	Heart volume
○	♀	21yr	169 cm	62.7 kg	2.87 L	640 ml
●	♂	24 yr	179 cm	74.7 kg	3.70 L	880 ml

FIGURE 4.23 The cardiovascular responses of well-trained men and women to cycle ergometry. Hb = hemoglobin.

Reprinted by permission, from P.-O. Åstrand and K. Rodahl, 2003, *Textbook of work physiology*, 4th ed. (Champaign, IL: Human Kinetics), 176.

TABLE 4.4 Cardiovascular Responses of Women Compared With Men

Variable	Rest	At same absolute $\dot{V}O_2$ (L · min^{-1})	At same relative $\dot{V}O_2$ (ml · kg^{-1} · min^{-1})	At maximal work
Cardiac output	Lower	Slightly higher	Same	Lower
SV	Lower	Lower	Lower	Lower
HR	Higher	Higher	Higher	Lower

Cardiovascular Responses to Isometric Exercise and Weightlifting

Most endurance exercise programs use dynamic activities involving large muscle masses to place loads on the cardiorespiratory system. The previous summary of the physiological responses to a GXT indicates that cardiovascular load is proportional to exercise intensity. But this is not necessarily the case for resistance training, in which a person can have a disproportionately high cardiovascular load relative to the exercise intensity. In a now classic study, a subject performed an isometric exercise test (sustained handgrip) at only 30% maximal voluntary contraction (MVC) strength while BP was monitored. In contrast to dynamic exercise, both the SBP and DBP increased over time, and SBP exceeded 220 mmHg. This kind of exercise puts a disproportionate load on the heart and is not recommended for older adults or people with heart disease (39). See chapter 13 for information on resistance training programs for patients with CVD.

Dynamic, heavy-resistance exercises can also cause extreme BP responses. Figure 4.24 shows the peak BP response achieved during exercise at 95% to 100% of the maximum weight that could be lifted one time (1RM). Both DBP and SBP are elevated, with average values

exceeding 300/200 mmHg for the two-leg leg press done to fatigue. The elevation in pressure was believed to be caused by the compression of the arteries by the muscles, a reflex response attributable to the static component associated with near-maximal dynamic lifts, and by the Valsalva maneuver, which can independently elevate BP (40). Another study reported peak values of about 190/140 mmHg for exercises of 50%, 70%, and 80% of 1-repetition max (1RM) done to fatigue in untrained lifters. Bodybuilders responded with lower BPs, indicating a cardiovascular adaptation to resistance training (21).

Regulating Body Temperature

Under resting conditions, the body's core temperature is 37 °C, and heat production and heat loss are balanced. Mechanisms of heat production include the basal metabolic rate, shivering, work, and exercise. During exercise, mechanical efficiency is about 20% or less, which means that 80% or more of energy production ($\dot{V}O_2$) is converted to heat. For example, if you are working on a cycle ergometer at a rate requiring a $\dot{V}O_2$ of 2.0 L · min⁻¹, your energy production is about 10 kcal · min⁻¹. At 20% efficiency, 2 kcal · min⁻¹ are used to do work, and 8 kcal · min⁻¹ are converted to heat. If most of this added heat is not lost, core temperature might quickly rise to dangerous levels. How does the body lose excess heat?

Heat-Loss Mechanisms

The body loses heat by four processes. In **radiation**, heat is transferred from the surface of one object to the surface of another, with no physical contact between the objects. Heat loss depends on the temperature gradient, that is, the temperature difference between the surfaces of the objects. When a person is seated at rest in a comfortable

KEY POINT

Isometric exercise and heavy-resistance exercise elicit high BP responses compared with dynamic endurance exercise. Both SBP and DBP increase with isometric and dynamic resistance training.

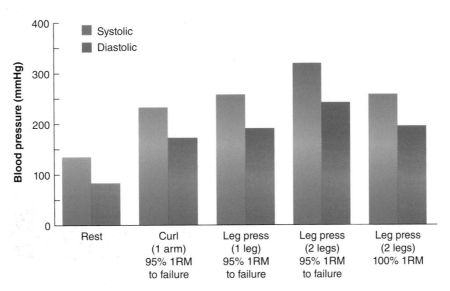

FIGURE 4.24 BP responses during weightlifting (40). RM = repetition maximum.

environment (21-22 °C), about 60% of body heat is lost through radiation to cooler objects. **Conduction** is the transfer of heat from one object to another by direct contact, and, like radiation, it depends on a temperature gradient. A person sitting on a cold marble bench loses body heat by conduction. **Convection** is a special case of conduction in which heat is transferred to air (or water) molecules, which become lighter and rise away from the body to be replaced by cold air (or water). Heat loss can be enhanced by increasing the movement of the air (or water) over the surface of the body. For example, a fan stimulates heat loss by placing more cold air molecules into contact with the skin.

All of these heat-loss mechanisms can be heat-gain mechanisms as well. We gain heat from the sun by radiation across 93 million mi (150 million km) of space, and we gain heat by conduction when we sit on hot sand at the beach. Similarly, if a fan were to place more hot air (warmer than skin temperature) into contact with the skin, we would gain heat. Heat gained from the environment adds to that generated by exercise and puts an additional strain on heat-loss mechanisms.

The fourth heat-loss mechanism is the evaporation of sweat. **Sweating** is the process of producing a watery solution over the surface of the body, and **evaporation** is a process in which liquid water converts to a gas. This conversion requires about 580 kcal of heat per liter of sweat evaporated. The heat for this comes from the body and, thus, the body is cooled. At rest, about 25% of heat loss is caused by evaporation, but during exercise evaporation becomes the primary mechanism for heat loss.

Evaporation depends on the **water vapor pressure gradient** between the skin and air and does not directly depend on temperature. The water vapor pressure of the air relates to the **relative humidity** and the **saturation pressure** at that air temperature. For example, the relative humidity can be 90% in winter, but because the saturation pressure of cold air is low, the water vapor pressure of the air is also low, and you can see water vapor rising from your body following exercise. In warm temperatures, however, the relative humidity is a good indicator of the water vapor pressure of the air. If the water vapor pressure of the air is too high, sweat will not evaporate, and sweat that does not evaporate does not cool the body (49).

Body Temperature Response to Exercise

Figure 4.25 shows that during exercise in a comfortable environment, the core temperature increases proportionally to the relative intensity (%$\dot{V}O_2$max) of the exercise and then levels off (59). The gain in body heat that occurs early in exercise triggers the heat-loss mechanisms discussed in the preceding section. After 10 to 20 min, heat loss equals heat production, and the core temperature remains steady

(24). What are the most important heat-loss mechanisms during exercise?

Heat Loss During Exercise

Exercise intensity and environmental temperature influence which heat-loss mechanism is primarily responsible for maintaining a steady core temperature during exercise. When a person participates in progressively difficult exercise tests in an environment that allows heat loss by all four mechanisms, the contribution that convection and radiation make to overall heat loss is modest. Because the temperature gradient between the skin and the room does not change much during exercise, the rate of heat loss is relatively constant. To compensate for this, evaporation picks up when heat losses by convection and radiation plateau, and evaporation is responsible for most of the heat loss in heavy exercise (figure 4.26).

When a person performs steady-state exercise in a warmer environment, the role that evaporation plays becomes even more important. Figure 4.27 shows that as environmental temperature increases, the gradient for heat loss by convection and radiation decreases, and the rate

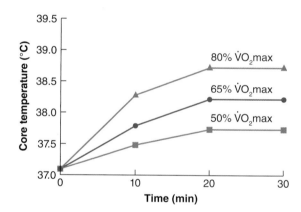

FIGURE 4.25 Core temperature increases over time as exercise intensity increases (2).

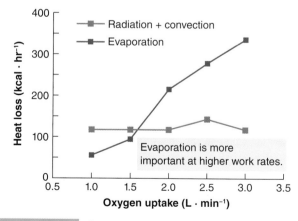

FIGURE 4.26 Importance of evaporation to relative work rate (59). Evaporation is more important at higher work rates.

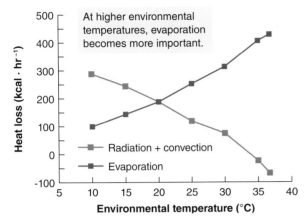

At higher environmental temperatures, evaporation becomes more important.

— Radiation + convection
— Evaporation

FIGURE 4.27 Importance of evaporation as a heat-loss mechanism during exercise as environmental temperature increases (2). At higher environmental temperatures, evaporation becomes more important.

of heat loss by these processes also decreases. As a result, evaporation must compensate to maintain core temperature.

In strenuous exercise or hot environments, evaporation is the most important process for losing heat and maintaining body temperature in a safe range. It should be no surprise, then, that factors affecting sweat production (such as dehydration) or sweat evaporation (such as impermeable clothing) are causes for concern. Chapter 11 provides details on dealing with heat and humidity when prescribing

exercise, and chapter 26 discusses how to prevent and treat heat-related disorders.

Training in a hot and humid environment for as few as 7 to 12 days results in specific adaptations that improve heat tolerance and, as a result, lower the trained person's body temperature during submaximal exercise (24). Adaptations that improve heat tolerance include the following:

- Increase in plasma volume
- Earlier onset of sweating
- Higher sweat rate
- Reduced salt loss through sweat
- Reduced blood flow to the skin

KEY POINT

Heat can be lost from the body by radiation and convection when a temperature gradient exists between the skin and the environment; however, evaporation is the primary mechanism of heat loss during high-intensity exercise or during exercise in a hot environment. Body temperature increases in proportion to the relative work rate (% $\dot{V}O_2$max) during submaximal exercise. Acclimatization to heat can be achieved in 7 to 12 days of training in a hot, humid environment and improves one's ability to exercise safely.

STUDY QUESTIONS

1. What are the two anaerobic sources of energy?
2. In an all-out run lasting 10 min, which energy system provides the greatest amount of energy?
3. Name the three fiber types, and indicate the order in which they are recruited as exercise intensity increases.
4. As exercise intensity increases, which substrate provides more energy—carbohydrate or fat?
5. Following an endurance training program, what changes in muscle allow more fat to be used as fuel during exercise?
6. Draw a graph showing how oxygen uptake increases at the beginning of a submaximal exercise bout, and label the oxygen deficit.
7. Define or describe (graphically) the lactate threshold (LT). What happens to the lactate threshold as a result of an endurance training program?
8. Draw a graph of the HR response to a GXT, and show the effect of an endurance training program on the response.
9. Since SV levels off at about 40% $\dot{V}O_2$max in a GXT, what explains the increase in cardiac output after that?
10. Which cardiovascular variable (maximal HR, SV, or oxygen extraction) explains the large differences in $\dot{V}O_2$max observed across the population?
11. What happens to BP when the arms perform at the same work rate as the legs?
12. What accounts for the decrease in $\dot{V}O_2$max with detraining?
13. Which is the most important training variable (intensity, frequency, duration) linked to maintaining $\dot{V}O_2$max when training level is reduced?
14. Why is the HR response of women higher at the same work rate compared with men?
15. What is the most important mechanism of heat loss during exercise?

You can check your answers by referring to appendix A.

1. A female competitive distance runner took a GXT on a motor-driven treadmill in which the speed of the run increased 0.5 mi · hr⁻¹ (0.8 km · hr⁻¹) each minute, with the test starting at 5 mi · hr⁻¹ (8 km · hr⁻¹). Blood samples for lactic acid determination were obtained each minute, and the lactate threshold was found to occur at the 8 mi · hr⁻¹ (13 km · hr⁻¹) stage of the test. Unfortunately, no one at the testing center knew what this meant relative to performance, and she has come to you for help. What do you tell her?

2. A client with whom you have been working retakes a maximal GXT following 10 wk of endurance training and finds that his HR is lower at each stage of the test. He is bothered by this because he thought his heart would be stronger and beat more times per minute. How do you help him understand what happened?

3. A female client is bothered by the fact that elite women runners who train as hard as elite male runners don't achieve the same performance times in distance races. She wants to know why and has come to you for the answer. How do you respond?

REFERENCES

1. Åstrand, P.-O. 1952. *Experimental studies of physical working capacity in relation to sex and age.* Copenhagen: Ejnar Munksgaard.
2. Åstrand, P.-O., K. Rodahl, H.A. Dahl, and S.B. Strømme. 2003. *Textbook of work physiology.* 4th ed. Champaign, IL: Human Kinetics.
3. Bassett Jr., D.R. 1994. Skeletal muscle characteristics: Relationships to cardiovascular risk factors. *Medicine and Science in Sports and Exercise* 26:957-966.
4. Bassett, D.R., and E.T. Howley. 1997. Maximal oxygen uptake: Classical versus contemporary viewpoints. *Medicine and Science in Sports and Exercise* 29:591-603.
5. Bassett, D.R., and E.T. Howley. 2000. Limiting factors for maximal oxygen uptake and determinants of endurance performance. *Medicine and Science in Sports and Exercise* 32:70-84.
6. Bouchard, C., R. Lesage, G. Lortie, J. Simoneau, P. Hamel, M. Boulay, L. Perusse, G. Theriault, and C. Leblank. 1986. Aerobic performance in brothers, dizygotic and monozygotic twins. *Medicine and Science in Sports and Exercise* 18:639-646.
7. Brooks, G.A. 1985. Anaerobic threshold: Review of the concept, and directions for future research. *Medicine and Science in Sports and Exercise* 17:22-31.
8. Brooks, G.A., T.D. Fahey, and T.P. White. 2005. *Exercise physiology: Human bioenergetics and its application.* 4th ed. New York: McGraw-Hill.
9. Claytor, R.P. 1985. *Selected cardiovascular, sympathoadrenal, and metabolic responses to one-leg exercise training.* Unpublished doctoral dissertation. University of Tennessee at Knoxville.
10. Coggan, A.R., and E.F. Coyle. 1991. Carbohydrate ingestion during prolonged exercise: Effects on metabolism and performance. *Exercise and Sport Sciences Reviews* 19:1-40.
11. Costill, D.L. 1988. Carbohydrates for exercise: Dietary demands of optimal performance. *International Journal of Sports Medicine* 9:1-18.
12. Coyle, E.F. 1988. Detraining and retention of training induced adaptations. In *Resource manual for guidelines for exercise testing and prescription,* ed. S.N. Blair, P. Painter, R.R. Pate, L.K. Smith, and C.B. Taylor, 83-89. Philadelphia: Lea & Febiger.
13. Coyle, E.F., M.K. Hemmert, and A.R. Coggan. 1986. Effects of detraining on cardiovascular responses to exercise: Role of blood volume. *Journal of Applied Physiology* 60:95-99.
14. Coyle, E.F., W.H. Martin III, S.A. Bloomfield, O.H. Lowry, and J.O. Holloszy. 1985. Effects of detraining on responses to submaximal exercise. *Journal of Applied Physiology* 59:853-859.
15. Coyle, E.F., W.H. Martin III, D.R. Sinacore, M.J. Joyner, J.M. Hagberg, and J.O. Holloszy. 1984. Time course of loss of adaptation after stopping prolonged intense endurance training. *Journal of Applied Physiology* 57:1857-1864.
16. Cureton, K.J., P.B. Sparling, B.W. Evans, S.M. Johnson, U.D. Kong, and J.W. Purvis. 1978. Effect of experimental alterations in excess weight on aerobic capacity and distance-running performance. *Medicine and Science in Sports* 10:194-199.
17. Davis, J.H. 1985. Anaerobic threshold: Review of the concept and directions for future research. *Medicine and Science in Sports and Exercise* 17:6-18.
18. Edington, D.W., and V.R. Edgerton. 1976. *The biology of physical activity.* Boston: Houghton Mifflin.
19. Ekblom, B., P.-O. Åstrand, B. Saltin, J. Stenberg, and B. Wallstrom. 1968. Effect of training on circulatory response to exercise. *Journal of Applied Physiology* 24:518-528.
20. Faulkner, J.A., D.E. Roberts, R.L. Elk, and J. Conway. 1971. Cardiovascular responses to submaximum and maximum effort cycling and running. *Journal of Applied Physiology* 30:457-461.
21. Fleck, S.J., and L.S. Dean. 1987. Resistance-training experience and the pressor response during resistance exercise. *Journal of Applied Physiology* 63:116-120.

22. Fox, E.L., R.W. Bowers, and M.L. Foss. 1998. *Fox's the physiological basis for exercise and sport.* 6th ed. Dubuque, IA: Brown.

23. Franklin, B.A. 1985. Exercise testing, training, and arm ergometry. *Sports Medicine* 2:100-119.

24. Gisolfi, C., and C.B. Wenger. 1984. Temperature regulation during exercise: Old concepts, new ideas. *Exercise and Sport Sciences Reviews* 12:339-372.

25. Hickson, R.C., H.A. Bomze, and J.O. Holloszy. 1977. Linear increase in aerobic power induced by a strenuous program of endurance exercise. *Journal of Applied Physiology: Respiratory, Environmental and Exercise Physiology* 42:372-376.

26. Hickson, R.C., H.A. Bomze, and J.O. Holloszy. 1978. Faster adjustment of O_2 uptake to the energy requirement of exercise in the trained state. *Journal of Applied Physiology: Respiratory, Environmental and Exercise Physiology* 44:877-881.

27. Hickson, R.C., C. Foster, M.L. Pollock, T.M. Galassi, and S. Rich. 1985. Reduced training intensities and loss of aerobic power, endurance, and cardiac growth. *Journal of Applied Physiology* 58:492-499.

28. Hickson, R.C., C. Kanakis Jr., J.R. Davis, A.M. Moore, and S. Rich. 1982. Reduced training duration effects on aerobic power, endurance, and cardiac growth. *Journal of Applied Physiology* 53:225-229.

29. Hickson, R.C., and M.A. Rosenkoetter. 1981. Reduced training frequencies and maintenance of increased aerobic power. *Medicine and Science in Sports and Exercise* 13:13-16.

30. Holloszy, J.O., and E.F. Coyle. 1984. Adaptations of skeletal muscle to endurance exercise and their metabolic consequences. *Journal of Applied Physiology: Respiratory, Environmental and Exercise Physiology* 56:831-838.

31. Howley, E.T. 1980. Effect of altitude on physical performance. In *Encyclopedia of physical education, fitness, and sports: Training, environment, nutrition, and fitness,* ed. G.A. Stull and T.K. Cureton, 177-187. Salt Lake City: Brighton.

32. Howley, E.T., D.R. Bassett Jr., and H.G. Welch. 1995. Criteria for maximal oxygen uptake—Review and commentary. *Medicine and Science in Sports and Exercise* 24:1055-1058.

33. Hultman, E. 1967. Physiological role of muscle glycogen in man, with special reference to exercise. *Circulation Research* 20-21(Suppl. 1): 99-114.

34. Issekutz, B., N.C. Birkhead, and K. Rodahl. 1962. The use of respiratory quotients in assessment of aerobic power capacity. *Journal of Applied Physiology* 17:47-50.

35. Kasch, F.W., J.L. Boyer, S.P. Van Camp, L.S. Verity, and J.P. Wallace. 1990. The effects of physical activity and inactivity on aerobic power in older men (a longitudinal study). *Physician and Sportsmedicine* 18(4): 73-83.

36. Kasch, F.W., J.P. Wallace, and S.P. Van Camp. 1985. Effects of 18 years of endurance exercise on the physical work capacity of older men. *Journal of Cardiopulmonary Rehabilitation* 5:308-312.

37. Kasch, F.W., J.P. Wallace, S.P. Van Camp, and L.S. Verity. 1988. A longitudinal study of cardiovascular stability in active men aged 45 to 65 yrs. *Physician and Sportsmedicine* 16(1): 117-126.

38. Katch, F.I., and W.D. McArdle. 1977. *Nutrition and weight control.* Boston: Houghton Mifflin.

39. Lind, A.R., and G.W. McNicol. 1967. Muscular factors which determine the cardiovascular responses to sustained and rhythmic exercise. *Canadian Medical Association Journal* 96:706-713.

40. MacDougall, J.D., D. Tuxen, D.G. Sale, J.R. Moroz, and J.R. Sutton. 1985. Arterial blood-pressure response to heavy resistance exercise. *Journal of Applied Physiology* 58:785-790.

41. McArdle, W.D., F.I. Katch, and V.L. Katch. 2010. *Exercise physiology, energy, nutrition, and human performance.* 7th ed. Baltimore: Lippincott Williams & Wilkins.

42. McArdle, W.D., F.I. Katch, and G.S. Pechar. 1973. Comparison of continuous and discontinuous treadmill and bicycle tests for max $\dot{V}O_2$. *Medicine and Science in Sports* 5(3):156-160.

43. McArdle, W.D., and J.R. Magel. 1970. Physical work capacity and maximum oxygen uptake in treadmill and bicycle exercise. *Medicine and Science in Sports* 2(3): 118-123.

44. Montoye, H.J., T. Ayen, F. Nagle, and E.T. Howley. 1986. The oxygen requirement for horizontal and grade walking on a motor-driven treadmill. *Medicine and Science in Sports and Exercise* 17:640-645.

45. Nagle, F.J., B. Balke, G. Baptista, J. Alleyia, and E. Howley. 1971. Compatibility of progressive treadmill, bicycle, and step tests based on oxygen-uptake responses. *Medicine and Science in Sports* 3:149-154.

46. Plowman, S.A., and D.L. Smith. 2008. *Exercise physiology for health, fitness and performance.* 3rd ed. New York: Benjamin Cummings.

47. Powers, S.K., S. Dodd, and R.E. Beadle. 1985. Oxygen-uptake kinetics in trained athletes differing in $\dot{V}O_2$max. *European Journal of Applied Physiology* 54:306-308.

48. Powers, S., S. Dodd, R. Deason, R. Byrd, and T. McKnight. 1983. Ventilatory threshold, running economy, and distance-running performance of trained athletes. *Research Quarterly for Exercise and Sport* 54:179-182.

49. Powers, S.K., and E.T. Howley. 2012. *Exercise physiology.* 8th ed. New York: McGraw-Hill.

50. Powers, S., W. Riley, and E. Howley. 1980. A comparison of fat metabolism in trained men and women during prolonged aerobic work. *Research Quarterly for Exercise and Sport* 52:427-431.

51. Raven, P.B., B.L. Drinkwater, R.O. Ruhling, N. Bolduan, S. Taguchi, J. Gliner, and S.M. Horvath. 1974. Effect of carbon monoxide and peroxyacetyl nitrate on man's maximal aerobic capacity. *Journal of Applied Physiology* 36:288-293.

52. Robergs, R.A., and S.J. Keteyian. 2003. *Fundamentals of exercise physiology: For fitness, performance and health.* 2nd ed. New York: McGraw-Hill.

53. Rowell, L.B. 1969. Circulation. *Medicine and Science in Sports* 1:15-22.

54. Rowell, L.B. 1986. *Human circulation-regulation during physical stress.* New York: Oxford University Press.

55. Sale, D.G. 1987. Influence of exercise and training on motor unit activation. *Exercise and Sport Sciences Reviews* 15:95-151.

56. Saltin, B. 1969. Physiological effects of physical conditioning. *Medicine and Science in Sports* 1:50-56.

57. Saltin, B., and P.D. Gollnick. 1983. Skeletal muscle adaptability: Significance for metabolism and performance. In *Handbook of physiology,* ed. L.D. Peachey, R.H. Adrian, and S.R. Geiger, 555-631. Baltimore: Williams & Wilkins.

58. Saltin, B., J. Henriksson, E. Nygaard, P. Anderson, and E. Jansson. 1977. Fiber types and metabolic potentials of skeletal muscles in sedentary man and endurance runners. *Annals of the New York Academy of Science* 301:3-29.

59. Saltin, B., and L. Hermansen. 1966. Esophageal, rectal, and muscle temperature during exercise. *Journal of Applied Physiology* 21:1757-1762.

60. Schwade, J., C.G. Blomqvist, and W. Shapiro. 1977. A comparison of the response to arm and leg work in patients with ischemic heart disease. *American Heart Journal* 94:203-208.

61. Sherman, W.M. 1983. Carbohydrates, muscle glycogen, and muscle glycogen supercompensation. In *Ergogenic aids in sports,* ed. M.H. Williams, 3-26. Champaign, IL: Human Kinetics.

62. Taylor, H.L., E.R. Buskirk, and A. Henschel. 1955. Maximal oxygen intake as an objective measure of cardiorespiratory performance. *Journal of Applied Physiology* 8:73-80.

63. Vander, A.J., J.H. Sherman, and D.S. Luciano. 1985. *Human physiology.* 4th ed. New York: McGraw-Hill.

64. Wilmore, J.H., D.L. Costill, and W. L. Kenney. 2008. *Physiology of sport and exercise.* 4th ed. Champaign, IL: Human Kinetics.

Nutrition

The reader will be able to do the following:

1. List the six classes of essential nutrients and describe their role in the proper functioning of the body.

2. List the recommended percentage of calories from carbohydrate, fat, and protein.

3. Understand the importance of vitamins and minerals and how to optimize them in a typical diet.

4. Describe assessment of dietary intake for healthy adults.

5. Understand the role of the U.S. Dietary Guidelines (2010) in making healthy nutritional choices.

6. Explain the relationship between blood lipid profile and cardiovascular disease and explain the role of diet and exercise in modifying blood lipids.

7. Know how to maintain hydration during exercise.

8. Discuss the protein, vitamin, and mineral needs of a physically active person.

9. Understand the basic principles behind increasing glycogen storage before competition.

10. List the three components of the female athlete triad.

Good nutrition

results from eating foods in the proper quantities and with the needed distribution of nutrients to maintain good health in the present and in the future. **Malnutrition**, on the other hand, is the outcome of a diet in which there is underconsumption, overconsumption, or unbalanced consumption of nutrients that leads to disease or increased susceptibility to disease. These definitions implicitly state that proper nutrition is essential to good health. A history of poor nutritional choices eventually leads to health consequences. Poor nutritional choices have been linked to chronic conditions including CVD and cancer.

The public is bombarded with messages about nutrition, and it is often difficult for the layperson to distinguish good information from bad. Fitness professionals can play an important role in conveying basic nutritional information. However, a registered dietitian is the appropriate health care professional to perform detailed dietary analysis and to counsel individuals with special nutrition needs.

Essential Nutrients

The body requires many **nutrients** for the maintenance, growth, and repair of tissues. Nutrients can be divided into six classes: carbohydrate, fat, protein, vitamins, minerals, and water. The Food and Nutrition Board of the Institute of Medicine has established **dietary reference intakes (DRIs)** to help people achieve a healthy intake of nutrients (12). The DRIs consist of recommended intakes for nutrients based on age and sex, including the **recommended dietary allowances (RDAs)**, or the amounts found to be adequate for approximately 97% of the population; **adequate intakes (AIs)**, or the amounts considered adequate although insufficient data exist to establish the appropriate RDA; and **tolerable upper intake levels (UL)**, or the highest intakes believed to pose no health risk. Additionally, **acceptable macronutrient distribution ranges (AMDRs)** have been established for fat, carbohydrate, and protein. The Institute of Medicine reports can be accessed at the National Academies Press website (www.nap.edu).

Carbohydrate

Carbohydrate is a nutrient composed of carbon, hydrogen, and oxygen and is an essential source of energy in the body. It can be divided into three categories: monosaccharides, disaccharides, and polysaccharides. Examples of monosaccharides are glucose and fructose. Lactose and sucrose are two of the disaccharides, which are carbohydrate that forms when monosaccharides combine. The monosaccharides and disaccharides are sometimes called **simple sugars**. Simple sugars contribute significantly to the caloric content of foods such as fruit juices, soft drinks, and candy. The most important simple sugar in the human body is **glucose**. The molecular formula for glucose is $C_6H_{12}O_6$.

Polysaccharides are **complex carbohydrate** formed by combining three or more sugar molecules. Starches and fiber are polysaccharides found in plants. Rice, pasta, and whole-grain breads are just a few examples of foods that are high in complex carbohydrate. When carbohydrate is stored in the body, glucose molecules join together to form large molecules called **glycogen**. Glycogen is stored in the liver and skeletal muscle.

Grains, vegetables, and fruits are excellent sources of carbohydrate. It is recommended that 45% to 65% of a person's daily calories come from carbohydrate (14) (see figure 5.1). The RDA for carbohydrate is 130 g · day^{-1} (14), but the average carbohydrate intake of Americans is well beyond this RDA. The majority of carbohydrate calories should come from complex carbohydrate; foods with added sugar should be limited (22). The reason for eating complex rather than simple carbohydrate is the higher **nutrient density** of complex carbohydrate. Nutrient density refers to the amount of essential nutrients in a food compared with the calories it contains. For example, a candy bar (containing simple sugars) has a low nutrient density, whereas a slice of whole-grain bread (containing complex carbohydrate) has a high nutrient density.

One of the benefits of consuming foods that are high in complex carbohydrate is that they also typically contain **dietary fiber**, a nonstarch polysaccharide that is found in plants and cannot be broken down by the human digestive system. Although fiber cannot be digested, it helps prevent hemorrhoids, constipation, and cancers of the digestive system because it helps food move quickly and easily through the digestive system. In addition, consuming water-soluble fiber has been shown to lower cholesterol

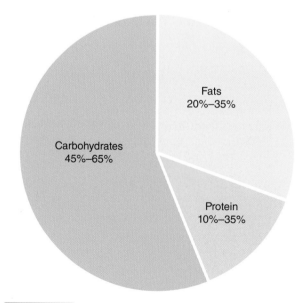

FIGURE 5.1 Acceptable macronutrient distribution for carbohydrate, fat, and protein (14).

Based on Food and Nutrition Board 2005.

levels (7). Unfortunately, the typical American diet is low in fiber, with the average intake being approximately 15 g · day^{-1} (22). The fiber AI for men and women aged 50 and younger is 38 g and 25 g · day^{-1}, respectively (14). For older men and women with lower calorie consumption, the daily recommended levels are 30 g and 21 g, respectively (14). *Dietary Guidelines for Americans, 2010* (22) recommends that adults consume approximately 14 g of fiber for every 1,000 kcal consumed. Excellent sources of dietary fiber are grains, vegetables, legumes, and fruits.

As mentioned earlier, carbohydrate is a vital source of energy in the human body. During high-intensity exercise, carbohydrate is the primary fuel source for ATP production. When carbohydrate is broken down in the human body, it yields approximately 4 kcal of energy per gram. This means that a person who eats 10 g of carbohydrate gains approximately 40 kcal of energy to use or store.

KEY POINT

The six classes of nutrients are carbohydrate, fat, protein, vitamins, minerals, and water. The metabolism of 1 g of carbohydrate yields 4 kcal of energy. Carbohydrate should contribute 45% to 65% of one's daily calories, with limited calories coming from simple sugars.

Fat

Fat is essential to a healthy diet and contributes to vital functions in the human body. Among the functions performed by fat are temperature regulation, protection of vital organs, distribution of some vitamins, energy production, and formation of cell membranes. Similar to carbohydrate, fat is composed of carbon, hydrogen, and oxygen; however, the chemical structure is different. **Triglycerides** are the primary storage form of fat in the body. These large molecules are composed of three fatty acid chains connected to a glycerol backbone. The majority of triglycerides are stored in adipose cells (i.e., fat cells), but these stored fats can also be found in other tissues (e.g., skeletal muscle). The aerobic metabolism of triglycerides provides much of the energy needed during rest and low-intensity exercise. When metabolized, 1 g of fat yields 9 kcal of energy. **Phospholipids** are another type of fat found in the body. As the name implies, these fats have phosphate groups attached to them. Phospholipids are important constituents of cell membranes. **Lipoproteins** are large molecules that allow fat to travel through the bloodstream. **Cholesterol** is a sterol, or a fatty substance in which carbon, hydrogen, and oxygen atoms are arranged in rings. In addition to the cholesterol we consume in our diet, the body constantly produces cholesterol, which is used in forming cell membranes and making steroidal hormones. Meat and eggs are the major sources of cholesterol in the typical American diet, and it is recommended that people consume no more than 300 mg of cholesterol each day (22). However, for those attempting to lower blood lipids, limiting daily cholesterol intake to 200 mg is recommended (11).

Sources of dietary fat come from both animals and plants. The AMDR for fat is 20% to 35% (14) (figure 5.1). Saturated fat comes primarily from animal sources and is typically solid at room temperature. Plant sources of saturated fat include palm oil, coconut oil, and cocoa butter. The chemical structure of saturated fat contains no double bonds between carbon atoms; in other words, the fat is saturated with hydrogen atoms. A high intake of saturated fat directly relates to increased CVD. Therefore, one should limit consumption of saturated fat to no more than 10% of total calories (22). Unsaturated fat contains fewer hydrogen

Focus on Glycemic Index

When carbohydrate is ingested, blood glucose rises and subsequently insulin is released from the pancreas. The rapidity with which blood glucose rises after food intake is represented by the **glycemic index**. Foods with a high glycemic index cause a rapid spike in blood glucose, whereas foods with a low glycemic index do not. A number of factors (e.g., biochemical composition, method of food preparation, fiber content) affect glycemic index. Examples of foods with a high glycemic index are baked potatoes, white rice, and soft drinks. Foods with a lower glycemic index include apples, kidney beans, and milk. For more information on the glycemic index of foods, see Walberg-Rankin (24).

Some evidence exists that a diet rich in foods with a low glycemic index helps fight CVD, obesity, and type 2 diabetes (19). Proposed benefits of this type of diet are increased satiety, lower triglycerides, higher HDL-C levels, and improved insulin sensitivity. Although some evidence exists that eating more foods with a lower glycemic index may improve health, this issue is still under investigation. In fact, recent dietary guidelines from the American Diabetes Association (ADA) do not emphasize using the glycemic index in making food choices. The ADA stresses attention to the total amount of carbohydrate rather than glycemic index; however, when consuming foods with a high glycemic index, it is wise to balance the meal with lower glycemic-index foods. The ADA suggests that a diet that promotes a healthy weight and is low in fat is preferable for preventing and treating type 2 diabetes and its comorbidities (7).

atoms because there are some double bonds between the carbon atoms. This type of fat is typically liquid at room temperature. Corn, peanut, canola, and soybean oil are sources of unsaturated fat. **Trans fat** is unsaturated fat that is common in many processed baked goods such as cookies and cakes. The intake of these fatty acids should be as low as possible because they are linked with negative health outcomes; in fact, various public health initiatives have focused on reducing the level of trans fat in the American diet. The effects of various kinds of fat on health risk are discussed later in the chapter (see Diet, Exercise, and the Blood Lipid Profile).

Monounsaturated fatty acids, found in olive and canola oil, have a single double bond between carbon atoms in the fatty acid chain. **Polyunsaturated fatty acids** (e.g., fish, corn, soybean, and peanut oils) have two or more double bonds between carbon atoms. Two polyunsaturated fatty acids, alpha-linolenic acid (a type of omega-3 fatty acid) and linoleic acid (an omega-6 fatty acid) cannot be made by the body and must be consumed in the diet. The AI for alpha-linolenic acid is $1.6 \text{ g} \cdot \text{day}^{-1}$ for men and $1.1 \text{ g} \cdot \text{day}^{-1}$ for women (14). Fish, walnuts, and canola oil are sources of this fatty acid. The AI for linolenic acid is 17 g and $12 \text{ g} \cdot \text{day}^{-1}$ for men and women, respectively (14). Sources include vegetable oils, nuts, avocados, and soybeans.

KEY POINT

The AMDR for fat is 20% to 35%, and no more than 10% of calories should come from saturated fat. Cholesterol intake should be limited to 300 $\text{mg} \cdot \text{day}^{-1}$. Intake of trans fat should be as low as possible. The breakdown of 1 g of fat yields 9 kcal of energy.

Protein

Protein is a substance composed of carbon, hydrogen, oxygen, and nitrogen. All forms of protein are combinations of **amino acids**. Amino acids are molecules composed of an amino group (NH_3), a carboxyl group (COO), a hydrogen atom, a central carbon atom, and a side chain. The differences in the side chains give unique characteristics to each amino acid. Amino acids can combine in innumerable ways to form proteins, and it is estimated that tens of thousands of protein types exist in the body. The order of the linked amino acids provides the unique structure and function of protein that allow it to serve many functions in the body. Some of the most common functions are the following:

- Carry oxygen (hemoglobin)
- Fight disease (antibodies)
- Catalyze reactions (enzymes)
- Allow muscle contraction (actin, myosin, and troponin)
- Act as connective tissue (collagen)
- Clot blood (prothrombin)
- Act as a messenger (protein hormones such as growth hormone)

Of the 20 amino acids required by the human body, most can be constructed from other substances in the body; however, there are eight **essential amino acids** (nine for children and some older adults) that the body cannot synthesize and so must be a part of one's regular diet. Eating a variety of protein-containing foods typically meets this need. Protein is found in both meat and plant products. Animal sources of protein such as meat, milk, and eggs contain the essential amino acids; however, plant sources of protein such as beans, starchy vegetables, nuts, and grains do not always contain all essential amino acids. Because of this, vegetarians must consume a variety of protein-containing foods. Examples of foods that contain complementary proteins are legumes and grains, vegetables and nuts, and legumes and seeds (9). For more information on planning vegetarian diets, see the summary of the vegetarian food guide established by the American Dietetic Association (ADA) and Dietitians of Canada (18).

The AMDR for protein is 10% to 35% (figure 5.1). This amount ensures adequate protein for the growth, maintenance, and repair of cells. The adult RDA is 0.8 g of protein for each kilogram of body weight (14). As discussed later in this chapter, individuals who are training intensely may have higher protein requirements. Additionally, children need more protein to support their continually growing bodies.

In addition to the functions listed previously, protein can be metabolized for energy production. The breakdown of 1 g of protein yields approximately 4 kcal of energy for the body. The contribution of protein to energy needs during exercise is usually quite small (<5%) in well-nourished individuals. However, during long bouts of exercise (>1 hr) or when a person is not well nourished, protein may supply up to 15% of the body's energy needs.

KEY POINT

Protein is made of amino acids and serves numerous functions. To ensure that all needed amino acids are adequately available, people should eat a variety of protein-containing foods each day. The AMDR for protein is 10% to 35%. The breakdown of 1 g of protein yields 4 kcal of energy.

Vitamins

Vitamins are organic substances that are essential to the normal functioning of the human body. Although vitamins do not contain energy for the body, they are essential in the metabolism of fat, carbohydrate, and protein. The body needs 14 vitamins for numerous processes, including blood clotting, protein synthesis, and bone formation. Because of the critical role vitamins play, they need to exist in proper quantities in the body. Major functions, important dietary sources, and recommended intakes of vitamins are listed in table 5.1. There are two major classifications of vitamins: fat soluble and water soluble.

The chemical structure of fat-soluble vitamins causes them to be transported and stored with lipids. The four fat-soluble vitamins are A, D, E, and K. Because these vitamins are stored in the body, it is not necessary to continually ingest large amounts of them; however, a small daily intake of each is recommended.

The B vitamins and vitamin C are water-soluble vitamins. These vitamins are not stored in large quantities in the body and therefore must be consumed daily. Deficiencies related to water-soluble vitamins such as scurvy (vitamin C deficiency) and beriberi (thiamin deficiency) may occur rather quickly. Overconsuming either fat-soluble or water-soluble vitamins can lead to toxic effects; however, because fat-soluble vitamins are stored in the body, the potential for overdose with these substances is greater (9).

Minerals

Minerals are inorganic elements that serve a variety of functions in the human body. The minerals that appear in the largest quantities (calcium, phosphorus, potassium, sulfur, sodium, chloride, and magnesium) are often called *macrominerals* or *major minerals*. Other minerals are also essential to normal functioning of the body, but because they exist in smaller quantities, they are called *microminerals* or *trace elements*. Functions, dietary sources, and recommended intakes of minerals are listed in table 5.2.

Calcium is often inadequately consumed by Americans. It is important in the mineralization of bone, in muscle contraction, and in transmission of nervous impulses. **Osteoporosis** is a disease characterized by a decrease in the total amount of bone mineral in the body and in the strength of the remaining bone. This condition is most common in the elderly but also may exist in younger people who have diets inadequate in calcium, vitamin D, or both. It is estimated that in the United States, osteoporosis results in approximately 1.5 million fractures per year with resultant health care costs of nearly $20 billion (23). Maximal bone density is achieved during the early adult years, and during older adult years, bone density declines in everyone. Those who achieve the highest bone density and maintain adequate intakes of calcium and vitamin D are most protected from osteoporosis. Recently, RDAs were released for calcium (see table 5.3) (16). The DRIs for vitamin D are contained in table 5.1. The calcium RDA for adults aged 19 to 50 is 1,000 mg · day^{-1}, with higher values for older adults and adolescents. Milk, dark green vegetables, and nuts are excellent sources of calcium. One cup (8 oz or 237 ml) of 1% milk has approximately 300 mg of calcium, which is almost one-third of the daily recommendation for a young adult.

Iron is another mineral that is often underconsumed by Americans, particularly women and children. In fact, the most prevalent nutrient deficiency in the United States is iron deficiency (9). In addition to being a critical component of hemoglobin and myoglobin, iron is necessary for the functioning of the immune system, the formation of brain neurotransmitters, and the functioning of the electron transport chain (9). The oxygen-carrying properties of hemoglobin depend on iron. There is a continual turnover of red blood cells in the body, and much of the iron used to form new hemoglobin comes from old red blood cells. However, there is a daily need for iron, and if iron reserves (liver, spleen, bone marrow) and intake are inadequate, hemoglobin cannot be formed and **iron-deficiency anemia** results. In this condition, the amount

Focus on Antioxidant Vitamins

During metabolic processes, molecules or fragments of molecules form that can damage the body's tissues. These **free radicals** have at least one unpaired electron in their outer shells; thus, they are very chemically reactive. Lipid-rich cell membranes and DNA are highly susceptible to free radicals, and cell damage can occur when free radicals accumulate; for example, atherosclerosis is linked with free radicals. Some vitamins can react with free radicals and diminish the damage they cause. These **antioxidant vitamins** are hypothesized to counteract the effects of aging and decrease the likelihood of developing CVD and cancer, and they have received a great deal of media attention in the past few years. **Beta-carotene** (a precursor of vitamin A), vitamin C, and vitamin E are highly touted antioxidants. Results from several large epidemiological studies suggest that the cardioprotective benefits of antioxidant vitamins are difficult to characterize. However, studies continue to explore the potential health benefits of these vitamins. Because of the toxic effects from an overdose of antioxidants, it is wise to avoid overconsuming these substances (see table 5.1).

TABLE 5.1 Vitamins: Functions, Sources, and Dietary Reference Intakes

Vitamin	Function	Sources	ADULT RDA[a] Men	ADULT RDA[a] Women	UL[b]
Thiamin (B$_1$)	Functions as part of a coenzyme to aid utilization of energy	Whole grains, nuts, lean pork	1.2 mg	1.1 mg	ND
Riboflavin (B$_2$)	Involved in energy metabolism as part of a coenzyme	Milk, yogurt, cheese	1.3 mg	1.1 mg	ND
Niacin	Facilitates energy production in cells	Lean meat, fish, poultry, grains	16 mg	14 mg	35 mg
B$_6$	Absorbs and metabolizes protein, aids in red blood cell formation	Lean meat, vegetables, whole grains	1.3 mg	1.3 mg	100 mg
Pantothenic acid	Aids in metabolism of carbohydrate, fat, and protein	Whole-grain cereals, bread, dark green vegetables	5 mg*	5 mg*	ND
Folic acid	Functions as coenzyme in synthesis of nucleic acids and protein	Green vegetables, beans, whole-wheat products	400 µg	400 µg	1,000 µg
B$_{12}$	Involved in synthesis of nucleic acids, red blood cell formation	Only in animal foods, not plant foods	2.4 µg	2.4 µg	ND
Biotin	Functions as coenzyme in synthesis of fatty acids and glycogen	Egg yolk, dark green vegetables	30 µg*	30 µg*	ND
Choline	Important in cell membrane integrity and signaling, nerve transmission	Beef liver, chicken, codfish, wheat germ, cauliflower	550 mg*	425 mg*	3.5 g
C	Aids intracellular maintenance of bone, capillaries, and teeth	Citrus fruits, green peppers, tomatoes	90 mg	75 mg	2,000 mg
A	Aids vision, formation and maintenance of skin and mucous membranes	Carrots, sweet potatoes, butter, liver	900 µg	700 µg	3,000 µg
D	Aids growth and formation of bones and teeth, aids calcium absorption	Eggs, tuna, liver, fortified milk	15 µg	15 µg	100 µg
E	Protects polyunsaturated fat, prevents damage to cell membrane	Whole-grain cereals and breads, green leafy vegetables	15 mg	15 mg	1,000 mg
K	Important in blood clotting	Green leafy vegetables, peas, potatoes	120 µg*	90 µg*	ND

[a]Values are recommended daily allowance (RDA) for adults aged 19 to 50, unless marked with an asterisk. The requirements may vary for children, older adults, and pregnant or lactating women.

[b]Tolerable upper intake levels (UL) for adults aged 19 to 50. Intakes above the UL may lead to negative health consequences.

*Values are adequate intakes (AIs), indicating that sufficient data to set the RDA are unavailable.

ND = not yet determined.

Adapted from Franks and Howley 1989; and various reports of the Food and Nutrition Board.

TABLE 5.2   Minerals: Functions, Sources, and Dietary Reference Intakes

Mineral	Functions	Sources	ADULT RDA[a] Men	ADULT RDA[a] Women	UL[b]
Calcium	Bones, teeth, blood clotting, nerve and muscle function	Milk, sardines, dark green vegetables, nuts	1,000 mg	1,000 mg	2,500 mg
Chloride	Nerve and muscle function, water balance (with sodium)	Salt	2.3 g*	2.3 g*	3.6 g
Magnesium	Bone growth, nerve, muscle, enzyme function	Nuts, seafood, whole grains, leafy green vegetables	420 mg	320 mg	350 mg[c]
Phosphorus	Bones, teeth, energy transfer	Meats, poultry, seafood, eggs, milk, beans	700 mg	700 mg	4,000 mg
Potassium	Nerve and muscle function	Fresh vegetables, bananas, citrus fruits, milk, meats, fish	4.7 g*	4.7 g*	ND
Sodium	Nerve and muscle function, water balance	Salt	1.5 g*	1.5 g*	2.3 g
Chromium	Glucose metabolism	Meats, liver, whole grains, dried beans	35 µg*	25 µg*	ND
Copper	Enzyme function, energy production	Meats, seafood, nuts, grains	900 µg	900 µg	10,000 µg
Fluoride	Bone and teeth growth	Fluoridated drinking water, fish, milk	4 mg	3 mg	10 mg
Iodine	Thyroid hormone formation	Iodized salt, seafood	150 µg	150 µg	1,100 µg
Iron	O_2 transport in red blood cells, enzyme function	Red meat, liver, eggs, beans, leafy vegetables, shellfish	8 mg	18 mg	45 mg
Manganese	Enzyme function	Whole grains, nuts, fruits, vegetables	2.3 mg*	1.8 mg*	11 mg
Molybdenum	Energy metabolism	Whole grains, organ meats, peas, beans	45 µg	45 µg	2,000 µg
Selenium	Works with vitamin E	Meat, fish, whole grains, eggs	55 µg	55 µg	400 µg
Zinc	Enzyme function, growth	Meat, shellfish, yeast, whole grains	11 mg	8 mg	40 mg

[a]Values are recommended daily allowance (RDA) for adults aged 19 to 50, unless marked with an asterisk. The requirements may vary for children, older adults, and pregnant or lactating women.

[b]Tolerable upper intake levels (UL) for adults aged 19 to 50. Intakes above the UL may lead to negative health consequences.

[c]Refers to pharmacological agents only and not to amounts contained in food and water. No evidence of ill effects from ingesting naturally occurring amounts in food and water.

*Values are adequate intakes (AIs), indicating that sufficient data to set the RDA are unavailable.

ND = not yet determined.

Adapted from Franks and Howley 1989; and various reports of the Food and Nutrition Board.

of hemoglobin in red blood cells falls, which decreases the capacity of the blood to transport oxygen. The recommended intake of iron for males and postmenopausal women is 8 mg · day⁻¹ (13). For females during the childbearing years, the recommended daily intake is 18 mg · day⁻¹ (13). Red meat and eggs are excellent sources of iron. Additionally, spinach, lima and navy beans, and prune juice are excellent vegetarian sources of iron. Consuming vitamin C with meals increases the ability to absorb iron.

TABLE 5.3 Guidelines for Daily Calcium Intake

Age	RDA (mg)
0-6 mo	200*
6-12 mo	260*
1-3 yr	700
4-8 yr	1,000
9-18 yr	1,300
19-50 yr	1,000
51-70 yr men	1,000
51-70 yr women	1,200
71 yr and older	1,200
Pregnant or lactating 18 yr or younger	1,300
Pregnant or lactating 19 yr or older	1,000

*These values are AIs because insufficient evidence exists to clearly establish RDA for infants.

From E.T. Howley and D.L. Thompson, 2012, *Fitness professional's handbook*, 6th ed. (Champaign, IL: Human Kinetics). Data from Institute of Medicine 2011.

Sodium, on the other hand, is a mineral that many Americans overconsume. High sodium intake has been linked with hypertension. The adult AI for sodium is 1.5 g · day^{-1} (15). Adults should limit their daily sodium intake to no more than 2.3 g (15, 22). People can substantially reduce their sodium intake by consuming fewer processed foods and adding less salt to foods when cooking.

Water

Water is considered an essential nutrient because of its vital role in the normal functioning of the body. It constitutes approximately 60% of the total body weight (15) and is essential in creating the environment in which all metabolic processes occur. Water is necessary to regulate temperature and transport substances throughout the body.

AI for total water is 3.7 L · day^{-1} for men and 2.7 L · day^{-1} for women (15). Approximately 80% of this amount comes from beverages. As discussed later in this chapter, the amount needed for good health may be higher for individuals exercising intensely. Environmental conditions may also increase the need for water. It is recommended that people limit the intake of caffeinated beverages because of their diuretic effects.

Assessing Dietary Intake

The U.S. Dietary Guidelines (22) suggest engaging in regular physical activity and eating a balanced diet that contains the calories needed to achieve and sustain a

KEY POINT

Vitamins, minerals, and water do not provide energy but are essential to healthy functioning of the body. In general, most Americans would benefit from limiting sodium consumption (to decrease BP), increasing calcium intake (to improve bone strength), and increasing iron ingestion (to prevent anemia).

healthy body weight. Keeping a food log (i.e., food diary or diet record) can help individuals to reflect on their calorie intake and eating habits. For this activity to yield valid results, the client should record everything that is consumed over a certain period of time. These records typically are kept for 3 to 7 days and provide a general idea of a person's nutritional habits (17). If the food diary is kept for 3 days, one of those days should be a weekend day because many people eat differently on weekends than they do on weekdays. Once the records are completed, there are several software packages that can be used to analyze the diet. A free resource available to analyze one's diet can be found at www.choosemyplate.gov. **MyPlate** provides dietary guidance based on age, sex, level of activity, and so on. This new guide replaces MyPyramid and is designed to help individuals choose foods that promote health and assist with achieving and maintaining a healthy weight. The MyPlate website allows the user to enter foods eaten and receive an analysis that compares them to recommended intake levels. This useful tool can help individuals determine whether they are in caloric balance and consuming various nutrients in healthy amounts.

Although food diaries provide important information, they may pose some problems (25):

- People tend to underreport what they eat.
- People do not keep records that are specific enough to provide quality information.
- People often temporarily change how they eat when they record their food intake.

The fitness professional can take steps to minimize these problems. First, make sure that the clients understand the importance of completely and honestly recording what they eat. Emphasize to clients that the accuracy and usefulness of the feedback depend on the information provided. Additionally, provide clients with models or descriptions of how to accurately report food consumption. For more information on instructing clients on completing food diaries, see *ACSM's Resource Manual for Guidelines for Exercise Testing and Prescription* (17). Providing explicit instructions will allow the client to provide a more useful and accurate record. Additionally, the food diary should be user friendly and include cues to elicit complete responses.

A sample food log with instructions is provided on form 5.1. For the typical client, the following intakes should be included in a nutritional profile:

- Total calories
- Percentage of calories from fat, carbohydrate, and protein

- Saturated fat, trans fat, and cholesterol
- Sodium
- Iron
- Calcium
- Fiber

FORM 5.1 Sample Food Log

Instructions

1. Record everything you eat, including foods and beverages eaten at meals and snacks.
2. Record carefully how the food was prepared. Be as descriptive as possible (e.g., fried in corn oil, broiled in 1 tbsp of margarine).
3. Be sure to indicate the amount of food eaten. Use typical household measures when possible (tsp = teaspoon; tbsp = tablespoon; c = cup; oz = ounce; g = gram).
4. Provide brand names and labels for packaged foods.
5. For composite foods such as sandwiches, casseroles, and soups, indicate the ingredients contained in the food. For example, a turkey sandwich might be described as 2 slices of whole wheat bread, 1 oz of baked turkey breast without skin, 1 slice of tomato, 2 leaves of iceberg lettuce, and 1 tbsp light mayonnaise.
6. Indicate where and with whom you were when you ate. Describe your feelings at the time—were you worried, content, lonely, stressed, hungry? (Be honest.)
7. Carry this form with you so that you can write down foods as you eat them. Do not wait until the end of the day to record your food intake.

Food and drink	Description (e.g., amount, cooking method, brand name)	Location (e.g., place, with people or alone)	Feelings (e.g., hunger, anger, joy)	Time

From E.T. Howley and D.L. Thompson, 2012, *Fitness professional's handbook, 6th ed.* (Champaign, IL: Human Kinetics).

It also can be useful to examine the food diary for emotional or social cues to eating behaviors. For example, some people eat when depressed or only eat when alone. Such information can be helpful in making behavior changes needed for weight loss and maintenance. More information on weight management is covered in chapter 12.

It is important to consider what information fitness professionals can provide to clients who seek nutritional advice (21). The Dietary Guidelines for Americans (22) contain general nutrition information that can be shared with clients. The following section, Recommendations for Dietary Intake, provides more information about these guidelines. Additionally, it is within the scope of practice for fitness professionals to suggest healthy recipes, provide information on nutrients and their role in good health, and so on. Sass and colleagues (21) provide an overview of the scope of practice for fitness professionals and registered dietitians. Clients with special metabolic conditions such as diabetes mellitus should always be referred to a registered dietitian for nutrition advice.

KEY POINT

Food diaries can be a useful tool in helping clients develop healthy dietary practices. The client must provide detailed information for the dietary assessment to be accurate.

Recommendations for Dietary Intake

Dietary Guidelines for Americans, 2010 (22) is a joint effort of the U.S. Department of Health and Human Services (HHS) and the U.S. Department of Agriculture (USDA). These recommendations can help people make healthy food choices, and they focus on lowering the risk of chronic disease and promoting health. They point out common nutritional inadequacies and suggest ways to improve health outcomes through nutritional changes. For example, most Americans are too sedentary and weigh too much; thus, the guidelines suggest increasing physical activity and reducing calorie intake to a level that will lead to a healthy weight. The guidelines provide both general and specific recommendations. For example, a general recommendation is to limit "intake of sodium, solid fats, added sugars, and refined grains and emphasizes nutrient-dense foods and beverages—vegetables, fruits, whole grains, fat-free or low-fat milk and milk products, seafood, lean meats and poultry, eggs, beans and peas, and nuts and seeds" (22). An example of specific information provided in the guidelines is the recommendation to pregnant women to consume adequate amounts of folic acid

($600 \ \mu g \cdot day^{-1}$). A complete copy of *Dietary Guidelines for Americans* (22) can be found at www.cnpp.usda.gov/DietaryGuidelines.htm.

These guidelines point out that many Americans fall short of healthy dietary practices. Commonly, Americans underconsume some foods (e.g., fruits, whole grains, calcium-containing foods) while overconsuming others (e.g., solid fat, added sugar, sodium-containing foods). Table 5.4 summarizes general dietary practices suggested in the guidelines.

People can choose a variety of eating plans to help achieve the goals set forward in the Dietary Guidelines for Americans. Table 5.5 outlines three viable approaches to healthy eating: the USDA Food Patterns, DASH diet, and Mediterranean diet patterns. The **USDA Food Patterns** suggest daily amounts that people should consume from five major food groups (vegetables, fruits, grains, dairy products, and protein). These correspond with the five elements found in the MyPlate materials mentioned previously. Suggested limits on intake of certain products (e.g., solid fat) are also included. This plan is based on the established DRIs for nutrients and the Dietary Guidelines for Americans. This approach allows a great deal of flexibility in choosing foods and is adaptable to a vegetarian lifestyle.

The **DASH** (Dietary Approaches to Stop Hypertension) **diet** was originally designed to help people control their BP. This diet is characterized by sodium restriction; an emphasis on vegetables, fruits, low-fat milk products, whole grains, and lean meats; and elimination or minimization of added sugars and processed meats. Several studies have shown this dietary approach can be helpful in reducing BP and weight.

Mediterranean diet patterns have become popular in recent years. These patterns vary somewhat based on region but generally emphasize grains (particularly whole grains), fruits, vegetables, olive oil, and nuts. More monounsaturated fatty acids than saturated fatty acids are consumed in this pattern. Wine consumption with meals is also common. This eating pattern has been linked with a lower prevalence of CVD. Table 5.5 compares the typical dietary intake of Americans with these healthy eating plans.

The U.S. Food and Drug Administration (FDA) requires that all food be labeled with nutrition information. These labels, titled Nutrition Facts (see figure 5.2), list the serving size, total calories, fat (including saturated fat), cholesterol, sodium, carbohydrate (including dietary fiber), protein, and various vitamins and minerals contained in the food. **Daily values (DVs)** indicate the percentage of daily recommended levels of nutrients that are contained in a food. The DVs were developed in an attempt to inform the public about the nutritional content of the foods they buy and are based on a daily intake of 2,000 kcal. The nutrition label contains the percentage of the recommended DVs provided

TABLE 5.4 General Recommendations From the Dietary Guidelines for Americans

Areas where reductions are needed*	Areas where increases are needed**
Reduce daily sodium intake to 2,300 mg. For African Americans; people with high BP, diabetes, or chronic kidney disease; and individuals 51 yr or older, intake should be reduced to 1,500 mg.	Increase fruit and vegetable intake.
Consume less than 10% of calories from saturated fatty acids.	Eat a variety of vegetables, especially red, orange, and dark green vegetables. Also consume a variety of beans and peas.
Daily dietary cholesterol should be less than 300 mg.	At least half of all grains consumed should be whole grains. Replace consumption of refined grains with whole grains.
Limit trans-fatty acids as much as possible.	Increase intake of fat-free or low-fat milk and milk products (e.g., yogurt, cheese).
Reduce intake of solid fat and added sugar.	Eat a variety of protein-containing foods (seafood, lean meat and poultry, eggs, beans, peas, soy products, unsalted nuts and seeds).
Limit consumption of foods with refined grains, particularly foods that also contain solid fat, added sugar, and sodium.	Increase the amount and variety of seafood consumed (eat instead of some meat and poultry).
If alcohol is consumed, limit to 1 drink per day for women and 2 drinks per day for men.	Replace protein foods high in solid fat with those that are lower in solid fat and calories.
	Use oils to replace solid fat when possible.
	Choose foods that provide more potassium, dietary fiber, calcium, and vitamin D.

*For the typical U.S. adult, these are areas where overconsumption is common. Each person should be considered on an individual basis to determine if these apply.

**Follow these eating patterns while staying within the calorie range needed to maintain a healthy weight.

Adapted from U.S. Department of Agriculture and U.S. Department of Health and Human Services 2010.

KEY POINT

The Dietary Guidelines for Americans (22) encourage most people to eat fewer calories, be more active, and make wiser food choices. USDA Food Patterns (MyPlate), the DASH diet, and Mediterranean diet patterns are approaches to healthy food consumption. Food labeling allows consumers to evaluate the nutritional content of foods.

by nutrients found in the food. For example, the suggested DV for cholesterol is 300 mg; therefore, if a food contains 15 mg of cholesterol, it will constitute 5% of the recommended daily intake of cholesterol. Additional information on food labels can be found at www.fda.gov/Food/LabelingNutrition/ConsumerInformation/ucm078889.htm.

Diet, Exercise, and the Blood Lipid Profile

CVD is the leading cause of death in the United States. One of the primary risk factors for CVD is a poor blood lipid profile. Both diet and exercise can positively affect this crucial risk factor.

Lipoproteins and Risk of Cardiovascular Disease

Because lipids are hydrophobic (i.e., not water soluble), they need to bind with some other substance to be transported in the blood. Lipoproteins are macromolecules composed of cholesterol, triglycerides, protein, and phospholipids. Classifications for these molecules are based on their size and makeup. The two classes of lipoproteins most closely linked with CVD are low-density lipoprotein

TABLE 5.5 Eating Patterns Comparison: Usual U.S. Intake, Mediterranean, DASH, and USDA Food Patterns, Average Daily Intake at or Adjusted to a 2,000-Calorie Level

Pattern	Usual U.S. intake (adults)[a]	Mediterranean patterns[b] Greece (G) Spain (S)	DASH[b]	USDA Food Pattern
Food groups:				
Vegetables: total (c)	1.6	1.2 (S) - 4.1 (G)	2.1	2.5
Dark green (c)	0.1	nd[c]	nd	0.2
Beans and peas (c)	0.1	<0.1 (G) - 0.4 (S)	See protein foods	0.2
Red and orange (c)	0.4	nd	nd	0.8
Other (c)	0.5	nd	nd	0.6
Starchy (c)	0.5	nd - 0.6 (G)	nd	0.7
Fruits and juices (c)	1.0	1.4 (S) - 2.5 (G) (including nuts)	2.5	2.0
Grains: total (oz)	6.4	2.0 (S) - 5.4 (G)	7.3	6.0
Whole grains (oz)	0.6	nd	3.9	≥3.0
Milk and milk products (dairy products) (c)	1.5	1.0 (G) - 2.1 (S)	2.6	3.0
Protein foods:				
Meat (oz)	2.5	3.5 (G) - 3.6 (S) (including poultry)	1.4	1.8
Poultry (oz)	1.2	nd	1.7	1.5
Eggs (oz)	0.4	nd - 1.9 (S)	nd	0.4
Fish/seafood (oz)	0.5	0.8 (G) - 2.4 (S)	1.4	1.2
Beans and peas (oz)	See vegetables	See vegetables	0.4 (0.1 cup)	See vegetables
Nuts, seeds, and soy products (oz)	0.5	See fruits	0.9	0.6
Oils (g)	18	19 (S) - 40 (G)	25	27
Solid fat (g)	43	nd	nd	16[d]
Added sugars (g)	79	nd - 24 (G)	12	32[d]
Alcohol (g)	9.9	7.1 (S) - 7.9 (G)	nd	nd[e]

[a]Source: U.S. Department of Agriculture, Agriculture Research Service and U.S. Department of Health and Human Services, and Centers for Disease Control and Prevention. What We Eat In America, NHANES 2001-2004. 1 day mean intake for adult males and females, adjusted to 2,000 calories and averaged.

[b]See the DGAC report for additional information and references at www.dietaryguidelines.gov.

[c]nd = not determined.

[d]Amounts of solid fat and added sugar are examples only of how calories from solid fat and added sugars in the USDA Food Patterns could be divided.

[e]In the USDA Food Patterns, some of the calories assigned to limits for solid fat and added sugar may be used for alcohol consumption instead.

Reprinted from U.S. Department of Agriculture; U.S. Department of Health and Human Services 2010.

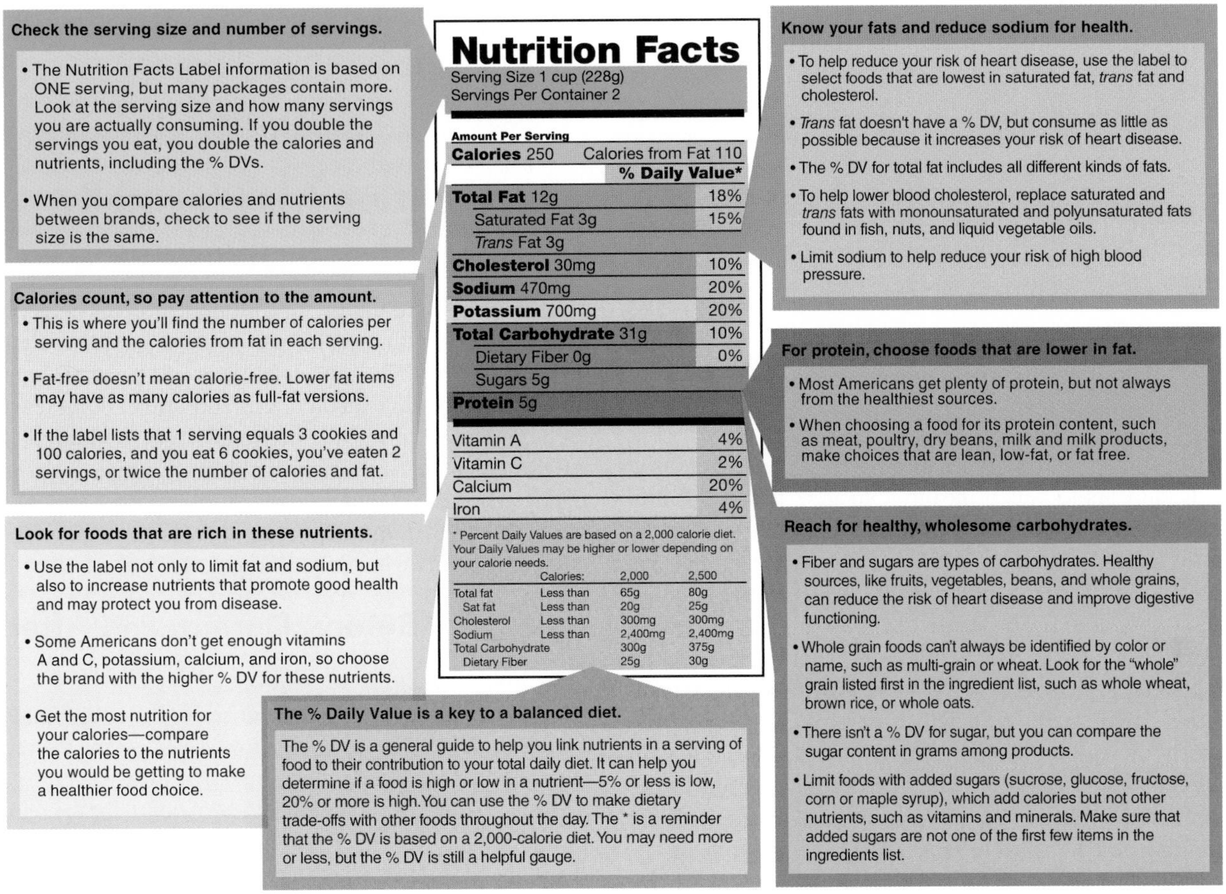

Check the serving size and number of servings.

- The Nutrition Facts Label information is based on ONE serving, but many packages contain more. Look at the serving size and how many servings you are actually consuming. If you double the servings you eat, you double the calories and nutrients, including the % DVs.

- When you compare calories and nutrients between brands, check to see if the serving size is the same.

Calories count, so pay attention to the amount.

- This is where you'll find the number of calories per serving and the calories from fat in each serving.

- Fat-free doesn't mean calorie-free. Lower fat items may have as many calories as full-fat versions.

- If the label lists that 1 serving equals 3 cookies and 100 calories, and you eat 6 cookies, you've eaten 2 servings, or twice the number of calories and fat.

Look for foods that are rich in these nutrients.

- Use the label not only to limit fat and sodium, but also to increase nutrients that promote good health and may protect you from disease.

- Some Americans don't get enough vitamins A and C, potassium, calcium, and iron, so choose the brand with the higher % DV for these nutrients.

- Get the most nutrition for your calories—compare the calories to the nutrients you would be getting to make a healthier food choice.

Nutrition Facts

Serving Size 1 cup (228g)
Servings Per Container 2

Amount Per Serving

Calories 250   Calories from Fat 110

	% Daily Value*
Total Fat 12g	18%
Saturated Fat 3g	15%
Trans Fat 3g	
Cholesterol 30mg	10%
Sodium 470mg	20%
Potassium 700mg	20%
Total Carbohydrate 31g	10%
Dietary Fiber 0g	0%
Sugars 5g	
Protein 5g	
Vitamin A	4%
Vitamin C	2%
Calcium	20%
Iron	4%

* Percent Daily Values are based on a 2,000 calorie diet. Your Daily Values may be higher or lower depending on your calorie needs.

	Calories:	2,000	2,500
Total fat	Less than	65g	80g
Sat fat	Less than	20g	25g
Cholesterol	Less than	300mg	300mg
Sodium	Less than	2,400mg	2,400mg
Total Carbohydrate		300g	375g
Dietary Fiber		25g	30g

The % Daily Value is a key to a balanced diet.

The % DV is a general guide to help you link nutrients in a serving of food to their contribution to your total daily diet. It can help you determine if a food is high or low in a nutrient—5% or less is low, 20% or more is high. You can use the % DV to make dietary trade-offs with other foods throughout the day. The * is a reminder that the % DV is based on a 2,000-calorie diet. You may need more or less, but the % DV is still a helpful gauge.

Know your fats and reduce sodium for health.

- To help reduce your risk of heart disease, use the label to select foods that are lowest in saturated fat, *trans* fat and cholesterol.

- *Trans* fat doesn't have a % DV, but consume as little as possible because it increases your risk of heart disease.

- The % DV for total fat includes all different kinds of fats.

- To help lower blood cholesterol, replace saturated and *trans* fats with monounsaturated and polyunsaturated fats found in fish, nuts, and liquid vegetable oils.

- Limit sodium to help reduce your risk of high blood pressure.

For protein, choose foods that are lower in fat.

- Most Americans get plenty of protein, but not always from the healthiest sources.

- When choosing a food for its protein content, such as meat, poultry, dry beans, milk and milk products, make choices that are lean, low-fat, or fat free.

Reach for healthy, wholesome carbohydrates.

- Fiber and sugars are types of carbohydrates. Healthy sources, like fruits, vegetables, beans, and whole grains, can reduce the risk of heart disease and improve digestive functioning.

- Whole grain foods can't always be identified by color or name, such as multi-grain or wheat. Look for the "whole" grain listed first in the ingredient list, such as whole wheat, brown rice, or whole oats.

- There isn't a % DV for sugar, but you can compare the sugar content in grams among products.

- Limit foods with added sugars (sucrose, glucose, fructose, corn or maple syrup), which add calories but not other nutrients, such as vitamins and minerals. Make sure that added sugars are not one of the first few items in the ingredients list.

FIGURE 5.2 Nutrition facts label.

Based on Federal Food and Drug Administration.

(LDL) and high-density lipoprotein (HDL). LDL transports cholesterol and triglycerides from the liver to be used in various cellular processes. HDL retrieves cholesterol from the cells and returns it to the liver to be metabolized.

Elevated levels of **total cholesterol** (the sum of all forms of cholesterol) and **low-density lipoprotein cholesterol (LDL-C)** are linked with the development of atherosclerotic plaque in the arteries. Increased levels of **high-density lipoprotein cholesterol (HDL-C)** help prevent the atherosclerotic process. According to the 2001 National Cholesterol Education Program (NCEP) guidelines, total cholesterol levels below 200 mg · dl^{-1} and LDL-C values below 100 mg · dl^{-1} are desirable (11). Total cholesterol of 240 mg · dl^{-1} or higher and LDL-C of 160 mg · dl^{-1} or higher are considered high and are associated with greater risk of CVD (see table 5.6). In addition, HDL-C below 40 mg · dl^{-1} is considered too low and HDL-C levels of 60 mg · dl^{-1} or higher are considered ideal (11).

Effects of Diet and Exercise on the Blood Lipid Profile

Consuming a diet low in saturated fat and cholesterol, losing weight, and participating in regular aerobic exercise

TABLE 5.6   Blood Lipid Classifications

Lipid level	Level rating
Total cholesterol	
<200	Desirable
200-239	Borderline high
≥240	High
HDL-C	
<40	Low
≥60	High
LDL-C	
<100	Optimal
100-129	Near or above optimal
130-159	Borderline high
160-189	High
≥190	Very high
Triglycerides	
<150	Normal
150-199	Borderline high
200-499	High
≥500	Very high

All values are mg · dl^{-1}.

Expert Panel on Detection, Evaluation, and Treatment of High Blood Cholesterol in Adults. 2001.

all have been linked to positive changes in the blood lipid profile. The 2001 NCEP guidelines (11) recommend a therapeutic lifestyle changes (TLC) diet to improve the blood lipid profile. The TLC diet includes the following dietary practices:

- Limiting total fat intake to 25% to 35% of calories (if at the higher end of the range, care should be taken to ensure that most fat is monounsaturated)

- Limiting saturated fat to 7%, polyunsaturated fat to 10%, and monounsaturated fat to 20% of calories

- Limiting cholesterol intake to <200 mg · day^{-1}

- Limiting intake of trans fat

Consuming certain types of fat, such as omega-3 fatty acids, appears to benefit health. Omega-3 fatty acids are found in canola oil as well as in fish such as salmon and tuna. Omega-3 fatty acids are a type of polyunsaturated fat that get their name from the site of the first double bond in the fatty acid chain. American diets are typically low in omega-3 fatty acids and higher in omega-6 fatty acids (e.g., peanut, corn, and soybean oils). Bringing the intake of these two types of fat into better balance appears to improve the lipoprotein profile and lower the risk of CVD.

People who engage in regular aerobic exercise and maintain a healthy weight typically have a better blood lipid profile compared to their sedentary counterparts. It is difficult to ascertain which of these changes are attributable to the exercise and which relate to a healthy body weight. It appears that the primary blood lipid changes

KEY POINT

Elevated total cholesterol and LDL-C and depressed HDL-C are risk factors for CVD. Aerobic exercise, weight loss, and low intake of saturated fat, trans fat, and cholesterol improve the blood lipid profile. A diet high in omega-3 fatty acids also has cardioprotective benefits.

resulting from aerobic exercise are increases in HDL-C and decreases in blood levels of triglycerides (10). Weight loss has been linked with lower total cholesterol, LDL-C, and triglycerides as well as with higher HDL-C.

Nutrition for Physically Active Individuals

Nutrition plays an important role in health, and it is also essential for optimal performance during physical activity. ACSM, the ADA, and Dietitians of Canada released an updated position statement in 2009 that addresses the dietary needs of physically active adults (4). Additionally, ACSM released a position stand on exercise and fluid replacement in 2007 (1). Fitness professionals should be familiar with these guidelines to provide basic nutritional advice to clients who exercise regularly.

Hydration Before, During, and After Exercise

Sweating is the primary mechanism for heat dissipation during exercise. The amount of sweat lost during exercise depends on environmental heat and humidity, the type and intensity of exercise, and the characteristics of the exerciser. Dehydration reduces the body's capacity for sweating and can impair performance by decreasing strength, endurance, and coordination. In addition, dehydration increases the risk of heat cramps, heat exhaustion, and heat stroke (see chapter 26).

Athletes should consume 5 to 7 ml · kg^{-1} body weight of water or a sport beverage at least 4 hr prior to competition (1, 4). If this fluid consumption does not yield urine output (or urine is dark), consume additional water (3-5 ml · kg^{-1}) 2 hr before the event (1). Fluid replacement during exercise is essential in activities that last an hour or longer, especially if they take place in hot, humid environments. Preventing excessive dehydration (>2% of body weight) should be the goal during exercise (practice or competition). Sweat

Focus on Trans Fat

Recent attention has focused on the health risks of trans-fatty acids (i.e., trans fat). Although small amounts of trans fat are found in animal products, the majority of this hydrogenated fat is found in processed foods produced from fat in plants. The hydrogenation process chemically transforms the spatial orientation of hydrogen atoms in the fat. This hardens the liquid plant oil and leads to a more stable product that is better suited for cooking. Consequently, many processed foods (e.g., cookies, chips, doughnuts, french fries) are prepared with trans fat. Foods high in trans fat will have partially hydrogenated vegetable oils as a primary ingredient listed on their food label. The problem with trans fat is that, as saturated fat, it can harm the blood lipid profile. Trans fat elevates LDL-C and lowers HDL-C; therefore, it should be avoided to improve the lipid profile (22). One of the most aggressive and public battles against trans fat occurred in New York City, where city government officials voted to ban trans fat from foods served in the city's restaurants. Although many restaurant owners fought this ordinance, the ban has now been successfully implemented across the city.

rates vary dramatically based on environmental conditions, intensity of exercise, and individual characteristics; thus, fluid consumption must be based on each specific case. Consuming 400 to 800 ml of water during endurance exercise is adequate for many individuals (1).

In activities where large amounts of sweat are lost, fluid should be fully replaced. Weighing oneself before and after these types of activities is recommended. The participant should drink approximately 16 to 24 oz (450-675 ml) of water for each pound (0.5 kg) of weight lost (4). If body weight has not returned to normal in the following days, additional water should be consumed before beginning exercise.

Protein Intake for Athletes

Athletes who are training intensely may benefit from increasing their protein intake above the level recommended for a sedentary person (i.e., $0.8 \text{ g} \cdot \text{kg}^{-1}$). An athlete training intensively in primarily endurance activities may benefit from consuming 1.2 to 1.4 g of protein per kilogram of body weight. For athletes engaging in high-intensity, high-volume resistance training, a protein intake of 1.2 to $1.7 \text{ g} \cdot \text{kg}^{-1}$ may be needed (4). To this point, most of the studies in this area have focused on male athletes, so little is known about the protein needs of female athletes.

Athletes should generally meet additional protein requirements through food choices, not through supplements. There is an upper limit to the rate at which muscle mass can be increased; therefore, excessive protein intake (i.e., above the recommendations) does not enhance performance or increase muscle mass (4). Because of the higher caloric intake of intensively training athletes, a diet with the normal distribution of macronutrients typically contains adequate amounts of protein, so purposefully consuming additional protein is usually not necessary (4, 26).

Another issue that sometimes arises is the adequacy of protein intake for vegetarian athletes. Because plant protein is not digested as well as animal protein, it is suggested that athletes following a strict vegetarian diet consume 1.3 to 1.8 g of protein per kilogram of body weight (4). The unique nutritional needs of the vegetarian athlete mean that consultation with a registered dietitian or sports dietitian may be needed (4).

Ergogenic Aids

The search for nutritional and pharmacological agents that improve performance has led to the marketing of numerous products touted as **ergogenic aids**. Some of these products (e.g., bee pollen, brewer's yeast) provide no scientifically proven physiological advantage. Other products, such as caffeine, may improve performance in some instances (26) and have been regulated by various sporting agen-

cies such as the International Olympic Committee. Some ergogenic aids must be strictly avoided, such as anabolic steroids, because of severe and sometimes fatal side effects (20). For more information on rules regarding the use of egrogenic aids during competition, see the websites of the United States Anti-Doping Agency (www.usantidoping. org) and the World Anti-Doping Agency (www.wada-ama. org). Additionally, ACSM (www.acsm.org) has released a number of Current Comments (official statements concerning topics of interest) on potential ergogenic aids.

Athletes often consume vitamins and minerals in amounts higher than the RDA in an attempt to improve performance. There is no evidence that this practice enhances performance; however, if an athlete's diet provides inadequate amounts of any nutrient, health and performance could suffer (26). The two minerals that often need to be increased in the diet are iron and calcium (8), and the most common mineral deficiency among athletes is iron deficiency (26). For athletes with anemia, increased iron consumption is advised and in many cases will improve performance (26). For female athletes with menstrual cycle irregularities, calcium supplementation often is prescribed to promote bone health. See chapter 17 for more information on issues specific to female athletes.

KEY POINT

Adequate hydration is essential to performance. Water should be consumed before, during, and after extended bouts of exercise. The typical protein RDA for adults ($0.8 \text{ g} \cdot \text{kg}^{-1}$) may be inadequate for athletes. People who are training intensely should consume 1 to 1.5 g of protein per kilogram of body weight. Ergogenic aids are pharmacological or nutritional agents thought to improve athletic performance. Although some products may enhance performance, there are many highly touted products with unproven results. In healthy, well-nourished athletes, extra vitamins and minerals (i.e., above the RDAs) do not improve performance.

Carbohydrate Loading and Intake During Exercise

Adequate intake of carbohydrate is necessary for optimal athletic performance in endurance events. Glucose is the major source of energy during exercise; when blood glucose levels decline, the ability to continue exercise is limited. A physically active person should routinely consume a diet in which 60% to 65% of the calories are from carbohydrate. For an athlete who trains heavily on

Focus on Creatine Supplementation

Phosphocreatine, a high-energy compound found in skeletal muscle, is a critical source of energy during bursts of high-intensity exercise. Athletes use creatine supplementation to increase the amount of phosphocreatine in muscle in an effort to enhance high-intensity exercise performance. Studies demonstrate that creatine supplementation does improve high-intensity exercise performance, particularly repeated bouts of high-intensity cycling, under laboratory conditions. Less is known about its effect on performance under competitive conditions. Creatine supplementation also is associated with weight gain (~1 kg) as a result of water retention. It is unclear if this extra weight could impede, rather than enhance, performance in weight-bearing activities such as sprinting. There are also reports of muscle cramping and gastrointestinal distress with creatine use. No studies have examined the side effects of long-term creatine use. For more information on creatine supplementation, refer to the ACSM roundtable report (3) and the review by Williams (26).

consecutive days or who engages in frequent exhaustive exercise bouts, a diet providing 6 to 10 g of carbohydrate per kilogram of body weight is recommended (4).

Carbohydrate loading is used to maximize glycogen storage before competition. This practice is most beneficial for athletes who compete in events requiring continuous activity lasting longer than an hour, such as marathon running. The ADA recommends the following practices to enhance glycogen storage (5):

- Consume a diet in which 65% to 70% of the total calories are from carbohydrate.
- Decrease the duration of exercise bouts during the week before competition.
- Rest completely on the day before competition.

During events that involve continuous vigorous activity, it is beneficial to consume easily absorbed forms of carbohydrate. In events lasting up to an hour, a solution containing 6% to 8% carbohydrate is recommended to balance the need for blood glucose maintenance and fluid replacement (4). The solution should be consumed in small to moderate amounts (150-350 ml) every 15 to 20 min. In events beyond an hour, it is even more important to consume carbohydrate. Beverages, gels, and easily digested foods (e.g., bananas) can be used. Research has shown that ingesting 0.7 g of carbohydrate per kilogram of body weight extends endurance exercise performance (4).

Female Athlete Triad

The **female athlete triad** is a condition characterized by inadequate calorie intake, menstrual irregularities, and loss of bone mineral density (BMD) (2). As discussed in chapter 17, disordered eating is more common in female athletes than in the general population. It is thought that the pressure to succeed and the drive to be thin lead many female athletes to begin unhealthy eating practices such as severe caloric restriction (anorexia), purging of food after eating (bulimia), and compulsive overexercising. These unhealthy patterns interfere with normal hormone secretion and eventually can lead to **oligomenorrhea** (irregular menses) or **amenorrhea** (lack of menses altogether). Because estrogen is essential in maintaining strong bones in women, the low estrogen levels observed in athletes with menstrual cycle irregularities can lead to bone loss. Weakening of the bones makes athletes more susceptible to stress fractures and can lead to an early and severe onset of osteoporosis.

Fitness professionals should encourage all physically active people to consume adequate calories and nutrients to support their energy expenditure. Active females who begin to miss menstrual periods should be referred to a physician. Some signs of disordered eating are listed in chapter 12. Athletes who exhibit these signs should be referred to a nutritionist or psychologist (or both) who is qualified to counsel people with eating disorders. See chapter 17 for a more detailed discussion of the female athlete triad.

KEY POINT

Adequate glycogen is necessary for optimal performance. Carbohydrate loading benefits extended bouts of exercise. Glucose intake during vigorous-intensity exercise can be beneficial, especially when exercise lasts 60 min or more.

KEY POINT

The female athlete triad (disordered eating, amenorrhea, and osteoporosis) can lead to serious health consequences. Athletes who exhibit signs of an eating disorder should be referred to a qualified nutritionist, psychologist, or both.

STUDY QUESTIONS

1. What three nutrients provide energy for the body? How many calories come from the breakdown of each gram of these nutrients?

2. What is the acceptable macronutrient distribution range for carbohydrate, protein, and fat?

3. What is the adequate intake for dietary fiber? How does this compare to the typical American intake?

4. What are trans-fatty acids? Why should they be avoided?

5. What is the RDA for iron for women of childbearing age? For men?

6. What nutrients do Americans typically overconsume? Underconsume?

7. According to NCEP, what are desirable values of HDL-C, LDL-C, and total cholesterol?

8. What are general recommendations regarding fluid intake during exercise?

9. What is the protein need for an intensely training endurance athlete? Strength athlete?

10. What are general recommendations to ensure adequate glycogen storage before competition?

CASE STUDIES

You can check your answers by referring to appendix A.

1. A male college basketball player (weight = 190 lb, or 86.2 kg) with a daily caloric intake of 3,500 kcal is considering additional protein supplements. He currently consumes approximately 15% of his calories from protein. Is his protein intake adequate? Would you recommend that he increase his protein intake?

2. Mr. Flanagan, a healthy 35-yr-old male, recently became your client for fitness training. He is gradually improving his fitness and is becoming more interested in his overall wellness. He is beginning to ask questions about how he should eat. What advice do you provide to Mr. Flanagan?

3. Mrs. Ortez is an obese 55-yr-old female with type 2 diabetes. She recently received physician clearance to join your fitness center. Her goals are to become regularly active, lose weight, and manage her diabetes with as little medication as possible. What dietary advice, if any, do you provide to Mrs. Ortez?

REFERENCES

1. American College of Sports Medicine (ACSM). 2007. Exercise and fluid replacement—position stand. *Medicine and Science in Sports and Exercise* 39(2):377-390.

2. American College of Sports Medicine (ACSM). 2007. The female athlete triad—position stand. *Medicine and Science in Sports and Exercise* 39(10):1867-1882.

3. American College of Sports Medicine (ACSM). 2000. The physiological and health effects of oral creatine supplementation. *Medicine and Science in Sports and Exercise* 32(3):706-717.

4. American College of Sports Medicine (ACSM), American Dietetic Association (ADA), and Dietitians of Canada. 2009. Nutrition and athletic performance. *Medicine and Science in Sports and Exercise* 31(3):709-731.

5. American Dietetic Association (ADA) and Canadian Dietetic Association. 1993. Nutrition for physical fitness and athletic performance for adults. *Journal of the American Dietetic Association* 93:691-696.

6. American Dietetic Association (ADA). 1997. Health implications of dietary fiber—Position of the ADA. *Journal of the American Dietetic Association* 97:1157-1159.

7. American Dietetic Association (ADA). 2008. Nutrition recommendations and interventions for diabetes: A position statement of the American Diabetes Association. Diabetes Care 31(Suppl. 1):S61-S78.

8. Berning, J.R. 1995. Nutritional concerns of recreational endurance athletes with an emphasis on swimming. In *Nutrition for the recreational athlete,* ed. C.G.R. Jackson, 55-68. Boca Raton, FL: CRC Press.

9. Driskell, J.A. 2000. *Sports nutrition.* Boca Raton, FL: CRC Press.

10. Durstine, J.L., and W.L. Haskell. 1994. Effects of exercise training on plasma lipids and lipoproteins. *Exercise and Sport Sciences Reviews* 22:477-521.

11. Expert Panel on Detection, Evaluation, and Treatment of High Blood Cholesterol in Adults. 2001. Executive Summary of the Third Report of the National Cholesterol Education Program (NCEP) Expert Panel on detection, evaluation, and treatment of high blood cholesterol in adults (Adult Treatment Panel III). *Journal of the American Medical Association* 285(19):2486-2497.

12. Food and Nutrition Board, Institute of Medicine. 2000. *Dietary reference intakes: Applications in dietary assessment.* Washington, DC: National Academy Press.

13. Food and Nutrition Board, Institute of Medicine. 2001. *Dietary reference intakes for vitamin A, vitamin K, arsenic, boron, chromium, copper, iodine, iron, manganese, molybdenum, nickel, silicon, vanadium, and zinc.* Washington, DC: National Academy Press.

14. Food and Nutrition Board, Institute of Medicine. 2002/2005. *Dietary reference intakes for energy, carbohydrate, fiber, fat, fatty acids, cholesterol, protein, and amino acids.* Washington, DC: National Academies Press.

15. Food and Nutrition Board, Institute of Medicine. 2005. *Dietary reference intakes for water, potassium, sodium, chloride, and sulfate.* Washington, DC: National Academies Press.

16. Food and Nutrition Board, Institute of Medicine. 2011. *Dietary reference intakes for calcium and vitamin D.* Washington, DC: National Academies Press.

17. Hagerman, P. 2010. Assessment of nutritional status. In *ACSM's resource manual for guidelines for exercise testing and prescription.* 6th ed. Ed. J.K. Ehrman, 214-226. Baltimore: Lippincott Williams & Wilkins.

18. Messina, V., V. Melina, and A.R. Mangels. 2003. A new food guide for North American vegetarians. *Canadian Journal of Dietetic Practice and Research* 64:82-86.

19. Morris, K.L., and M.B. Zemel. 1999. Glycemic index, cardiovascular disease, and obesity. *Nutrition Reviews* 57(9):273-276.

20. Ruud, J.S., and I. Wolinsky. 1995. Nutritional concerns of recreational strength athletes. In *Nutrition for the recreational athlete,* ed. C.G.R. Jackson, 55-68. Boca Raton, FL: CRC Press.

21. Sass, C., J.M. Eickhoff-Shemek, M.M. Manore, and L.J. Kruskall. 2007. Crossing the line: understanding the scope of practice between registered dietitians and health/fitness professionals. *ACSM's Health and Fitness Journal* 11(3):12-19.

22. U.S. Department of Agriculture (USDA) and U.S. Department of Health and Human Services (HHS). 2010. *Dietary Guidelines for Americans, 2010.* 7th ed. Washington, DC: U.S. Government Printing Office.

23. U.S. Department of Health and Human Services (HHS). 2004. *Bone health and osteoporosis: A report of the Surgeon General.* Rockville, MD: HHS, Office of the Surgeon General.

24. Walberg-Rankin, J. 1997. Glycemic index and exercise metabolism. *Gatorade Sports Science Institute: Sports Science Exchange* 10(1):1-7.

25. Westerterp, K.R. 2000. The assessment of energy and nutrient intake in humans. In *Physical activity and obesity,* ed. C. Bouchard, 133-149. Champaign, IL: Human Kinetics.

26. Williams, M.H. 1998. Nutritional ergogenics and sports performance. *PCPFS Physical Activity and Fitness Research Digest* 3(2):1-14.

Energy Costs of Physical Activity

The reader will be able to do the following:

1. Describe common techniques used to measure and track physical activity.

2. Describe how measurements of oxygen consumption can be used to estimate energy production, and list the number of calories derived per liter of oxygen and per gram of carbohydrate, fat, and protein.

3. Express energy expenditure as $L \cdot min^{-1}$, $kcal \cdot min^{-1}$, $ml \cdot kg^{-1} \cdot min^{-1}$, METs, and $kcal \cdot kg^{-1} \cdot hr^{-1}$.

4. Estimate the oxygen cost of walking, jogging, and running, including the cost of walking and running 1 mi (1.6 km).

5. Estimate the oxygen cost of cycle ergometry for both arm and leg work.

6. Estimate the oxygen cost of bench stepping.

7. Identify the approximate energy cost of recreational activities, sport, and other activities, and describe the effect of environmental factors on the HR response to a fixed work rate.

Fitness professionals usually ask the following three questions when they work with their clients:

1. What kinds and amounts of physical activities is the person currently doing?
2. Are the activities of the appropriate intensity to achieve the THR (see chapter 11)?
3. Is the combination of intensity and duration appropriate for achieving an energy expenditure that results in health-related benefits (see chapter 11) and balances or exceeds caloric intake to maintain or lose body weight (see chapter 12)?

To answer these questions, the fitness professional should become familiar with methods of measuring and tracking physical activity and estimating the energy costs of various activities. This chapter offers basic information to accomplish those goals.

Measuring Physical Activity

In chapter 1 we described the health-related benefits associated with regular participation in physical activity. In order to make such statements, investigators had to be able to measure the physical activity of the population under study (e.g., adults, older adults, children). This section provides a brief overview of the techniques used to monitor physical activity. Some of these techniques are used by fitness professionals to track their clients' activity over time, as discussed in chapter 22.

Various techniques have been used to obtain information about activity levels, and each has strengths and weaknesses (11). The following list provides details about common approaches to tracking physical activity.

- Self-report. Participants might be asked to fill out a questionnaire or talk with an interviewer about recent (weeks or months) patterns of physical activity. This is a relatively quick and inexpensive process, but people might misinterpret the questions or have difficulty recalling information about the intensity of the activity or how long it was done.

- Accelerometers. These devices are worn on the arm, hip, leg, or foot to track the acceleration of the body and thus provide information about the intensity, duration, and frequency of physical activity. Data are easily downloaded and the device can store days or weeks of information. Downsides include the cost of the device and computer interface, and the fact that accelerometers are unable to accurately assign energy expenditure to certain kinds of activities (e.g., upper-body movements, walking up an incline).

- Pedometers. These devices track the number of steps a person takes and can give information about the distance walked when stride length is programmed into the device. They are relatively inexpensive and easy to use; however, they do not provide information about the intensity or rate of walking, and nonlocomotor activities (e.g., biking) are not recorded. Because walking is the most prevalent form of physical activity, pedometers are used in activity intervention programs and by fitness professionals who help clients begin and maintain a walking program (see chapter 22).

- HR monitoring. HR is a good measure of the intensity of physical activity (see chapter 11). HR monitors can store data over the course of days, and the data can be easily downloaded for analysis of intensity, duration, and frequency of bouts of activity. However, HR is affected by variables such as meals, heat and humidity, dehydration, and training status. Further, there is a lag in the time it takes for HR to increase and decrease at the start and end of the activity session (see chapter 4).

Each of these techniques has strengths and weaknesses, with the weaknesses leading to inaccuracy in the estimations of physical activity. To discuss the relationship between physical activity and health across these diverse techniques, many investigators convert the measured activity into energy expenditure values (e.g., kilocalories used per minute). Let's now examine how energy expenditure is measured.

Measuring Energy Expenditure

Energy expenditure can be measured by direct and indirect calorimetry. **Direct calorimetry** requires that the person perform an activity within a specially constructed chamber that is insulated and has water flowing through its walls. The water is warmed by the heat given off by the subject, and heat production can be calculated by knowing the volume of water flowing through the chamber per minute and the change in the water temperature from entry to exit. For example, a person in the chamber does bench stepping at the rate of 30 steps · min^{-1} using a 20 cm bench. The water flows through the walls of the chamber at 20 L · min $^{-1}$, and the increase in water temperature from entry to exit is 0.5 °C. Because it takes approximately 1 kcal to raise the temperature of 1 L of water 1 °C, the following calculation yields the approximate energy expenditure.

$$\frac{20\ L}{min} \cdot \frac{1\ kcal}{°C} \cdot 0.5\ °C = \frac{10\ kcal}{min}$$

The subject loses additional heat through evaporation of water from the skin and respiratory passages. This heat loss can be measured and added to that picked up by the water in the chamber walls to yield the rate of energy the person produced for that task.

Indirect calorimetry estimates energy production by measuring oxygen consumption; the procedures for these measurements are described in chapter 4. These calculations use certain constants for converting liters of oxygen consumption to calories expended. The constants are derived from measurements made in a bomb calorimeter, a heavy metal chamber into which carbohydrate, fat, or protein can be placed with 100% oxygen under pressure. The chamber is immersed in a water bath, and the foodstuff is oxidized to CO_2 and H_2O when an electric spark sets this combustion reaction in motion. The heat given off by the combustion warms the water, and it has been determined that carbohydrate, fat, and protein give off approximately 4.0, 9.0, and 5.6 kcal of heat per gram, respectively. Because the nitrogen in protein cannot be completely oxidized in the body and is excreted as urea, the physiological value for protein is actually 4.0 kcal · g^{-1}.

Knowing how much oxygen is required to oxidize 1 g of carbohydrate, fat, and protein allows one to calculate the number of calories of energy produced when 1 L of oxygen is consumed. This is called the **caloric equivalent of oxygen**. Values for carbohydrate, fat, and protein are listed in table 6.1. The table shows that carbohydrate gives about 6% more energy per liter of oxygen than fat gives (5.0 versus 4.7 kcal · L^{-1}), whereas fat gives more than twice as much energy per gram than carbohydrate gives (9 versus 4 kcal · g^{-1}). If a person is deriving energy from a 50–50 mixture of carbohydrate and fat during exercise, the caloric equivalent is approximately 4.85 kcal · L^{-1}, halfway between the value of 4.7 for fat and 5.0 for carbohydrate (21). The ratio of carbon dioxide produced to oxygen consumed at the cell is called the *respiratory quotient (RQ)*. The same ratio, when measured by conventional gas exchange procedures, is called the *respiratory exchange ratio (R)* and is used to indicate fuel use (carbohydrate versus fat) during exercise (see chapter 4).

TABLE 6.1 Caloric Density, Caloric Equivalent, and Respiratory Quotient Associated With Oxidation of Carbohydrate, Fat, and Protein

Measurement	Carbohydrate	Fat	Protein[a]
Caloric density (kcal · g^{-1})	4.0	9.0	4.0
Caloric equivalent of 1 L of O_2 (kcal · L^{-1})	5.0	4.7	4.5
Respiratory quotient	1.0	0.7	0.8

[a]Does not include energy derived from the oxidation of nitrogen in the amino acids because the body excretes this as urea.

Adapted from Koebel 1984.

RESEARCH INSIGHT

Carbohydrate yields about 6% more energy (5 kcal) per liter of oxygen than fat (4.7 kcal), making carbohydrate a better fuel for high-intensity exercise when oxygen delivery to the working muscles is limited. However, with rare exceptions, carbohydrate makes up at least 50% of the fuel used during a workout in the intensity range of 60% to 80% of maximal oxygen uptake, a typical range for individuals with average levels of CRF (see chapter 11). Consequently, the range of values that might be used to convert oxygen uptake to kilocalories is reduced to 4.85 to 5.0 $kcal \cdot L^{-1}$ (with about a 3% difference between the low and high ends of the range). Therefore, using a constant value of 5 $kcal \cdot L^{-1}$ to convert oxygen uptake to kilocalories involves little error.

Indirect calorimetry employs two techniques to measure oxygen consumption: **closed-circuit** and **open-circuit spirometry**. In the closed-circuit technique, the subject breathes 100% oxygen from a spirometer, and the exhaled air passes through a chemical that absorbs the carbon dioxide. Over time, the volume of oxygen contained in the spirometer decreases, giving a measure of the oxygen consumption in milliliters per minute ($ml \cdot min^{-1}$). Because the carbon dioxide is absorbed, R cannot be calculated, so a caloric equivalent of 4.82 $kcal \cdot L^{-1}$ is used to indicate that a mixture of carbohydrate, fat, and protein is used to produce the energy. This closed-circuit technique was used extensively to measure basal metabolic rate but has been replaced with modern open-circuit methods (21).

The open-circuit technique for measuring oxygen consumption and carbon dioxide production is the most common indirect calorimetry technique. In this procedure, oxygen consumption is calculated by simply subtracting the volume of oxygen exhaled from the volume of oxygen inhaled. The difference is taken as the oxygen uptake, or oxygen consumption (see chapter 4). Carbon dioxide production is calculated in the same manner. Knowing carbon dioxide production makes it possible to calculate R. Knowing R allows you to determine which substrate, fat or carbohydrate, provided the most energy during work and also what value to use for the caloric equivalent of 1 L of oxygen in the calculation of energy expenditure (i.e., 5.0 $kcal \cdot L^{-1}$ for carbohydrate and 4.7 $kcal \cdot L^{-1}$ for fat). However, as described in the Research Insight, an average value of 5.0 $kcal \cdot L^{-1}$ is typically used to convert oxygen uptake to kilocalories.

KEY POINT

Oxygen consumption ($\dot{V}O_2$) is a measure of how much energy (calories) is produced by the body. The bomb calorimeter provides the number of calories gained per gram of food: 4 $kcal \cdot g^{-1}$ for carbohydrate, 9 $kcal \cdot g^{-1}$ for fat, and 4 $kcal \cdot g^{-1}$ for protein. Knowing how much oxygen is used to metabolize the food, we know that we obtain 4.7 $kcal \cdot L^{-1}$ when fat is oxidized and 5.0 $kcal \cdot L^{-1}$ when carbohydrate is oxidized. When a 50–50 mixture of carbohydrate and fat is used for energy, we obtain 4.85 $kcal \cdot L^{-1}$.

Expressing Energy Expenditure

The energy requirement for an activity is calculated from the subject's steady-state oxygen uptake ($\dot{V}O_2$) measured during an activity. Once the subject reaches steady-state oxygen uptake, we know that the energy (ATP) supplied to the muscles is derived from aerobic metabolism. See chapter 4 for more information on steady-state oxygen uptake. The measured oxygen uptake then can be used to express energy expenditure in various ways. The five most common expressions follow.

1. $\dot{V}O_2$ ($L \cdot min^{-1}$). The calculation of oxygen uptake (see chapter 4) yields a value expressed in liters of oxygen used per minute, sometimes called the *absolute* $\dot{V}O_2$. For example, the follow-

ing data were collected for an 80 kg man performing a submaximal run on a treadmill: Ventilation (STPD) = 60 L $\cdot$ min^{-1}, inspired O_2 = 20.93%, and expired O_2 = 16.93%.

$$\dot{V}O_2(L \cdot min^{-1}) = 60 \text{ L} \cdot min^{-1}(20.93\% \text{ } O_2 - 16.93\% \text{ } O_2) = 2.4 \text{ L} \cdot min^{-1}.$$

2. kcal $\cdot$ min^{-1}. Oxygen uptake can be expressed in kilocalories used per minute. The caloric equivalent of 1 L of O_2 ranges from 4.7 kcal $\cdot$ L^{-1} for fat to 5.0 kcal $\cdot$ L^{-1} for carbohydrate. For practical reasons, and with little loss in precision, 5 kcal per liter of O_2 is used to convert the oxygen uptake to kilocalories per minute (see Research Insight). Energy expenditure is calculated by multiplying the kilocalories expended per minute (kcal $\cdot$ min^{-1}) by the duration of the activity in minutes. For example, if the 80 kg man mentioned previously running on the treadmill for 30 min at a $\dot{V}O_2$ of 2.4 L $\cdot$ min^{-1}, the total energy expenditure can be calculated as follows.

$$\frac{2.4 \text{ L } O_2}{min} \cdot \frac{5 \text{ kcal}}{\text{L } O_2} = \frac{12 \text{ kcal}}{min}$$

$$\frac{12 \text{ kcal}}{min} \cdot 30 \text{ min} = 360 \text{ kcal}$$

3. $\dot{V}O_2$ (ml $\cdot$ kg^{-1} $\cdot$ min^{-1}). If the measured oxygen uptake, expressed in liters per minute, is multiplied by 1,000 to yield milliliters per minute and then divided by the subject's body weight in kilograms, the value is expressed in milliliters of O_2 per kilogram of body weight per minute, or ml $\cdot$ kg^{-1} $\cdot$ min^{-1}. This expression, sometimes called the *relative $\dot{V}O_2$*, helps in comparing values for people of different body sizes. For example, for the 80 kg man with a $\dot{V}O_2$ of 2.4 L $\cdot$ min^{-1},

$$\frac{2.4 \text{ L}}{min} \cdot \frac{1000 \text{ ml}}{L} \div 80 \text{ kg} = 30 \text{ ml} \cdot kg^{-1} \cdot min^{-1}.$$

4. METs. *MET* is a term used to describe a standard or reference resting metabolic rate. Because the actual resting metabolic rate varies with age and gender, being smaller in females than in males and decreasing with age (21), the MET is taken, by convention, to be 3.5 ml $\cdot$ kg^{-1} $\cdot$ min^{-1}. This is called *1 MET*. Activities are expressed in terms of multiples of the MET unit. For example, using the $\dot{V}O_2$ values presented previously in number 3,

$$30 \text{ ml} \cdot kg^{-1} \cdot min^{-1} \div 3.5 \text{ ml} \cdot kg^{-1} \cdot min^{-1} = 8.6 \text{ METs}.$$

5. kcal $\cdot$ kg^{-1} $\cdot$ hr^{-1}. The MET expression of energy expenditure carries a special bonus: It also indicates the number of calories the subject uses per kilogram of body weight per hour. In the example mentioned previously, the subject is working at 8.6 METs, or about 30 ml $\cdot$ kg^{-1} $\cdot$ min^{-1}. When this value is multiplied by 60 min $\cdot$ hr^{-1}, it equals 1,800 ml $\cdot$ kg^{-1} $\cdot$ hr^{-1}, or 1.8 L $\cdot$ kg^{-1} $\cdot$ hr^{-1}. If the person is using a mixture of carbohydrate and fat as fuel, then this oxygen consumption is multiplied by 4.85 kcal per liter of O_2 to give 8.7 kcal $\cdot$ kg^{-1} $\cdot$ hr^{-1}. The following steps show the details of this calculation.

$$8.6 \text{ METs} \cdot \frac{3.5 \text{ ml} \cdot kg^{-1} \cdot min^{-1}}{\text{MET}} = 30 \text{ ml} \cdot kg^{-1} \cdot min^{-1}$$

$$30 \text{ ml} \cdot kg^{-1} \cdot min^{-1} \cdot 60 \text{ min} \cdot hr^{-1} = 1{,}800 \text{ ml} \cdot kg^{-1} \cdot hr^{-1} = 1.8 \text{ L} \cdot kg^{-1} \cdot hr^{-1}$$

$$1.8 \text{ L} \cdot kg^{-1} \cdot hr^{-1} \cdot 4.85 \text{ kcal} \cdot \text{L } O_2^{-1} = 8.7 \text{ kcal} \cdot kg^{-1} \cdot hr^{-1}$$

As indicated in chapter 1, the volume of physical activity is linked to numerous health outcomes. The volume or amount of physical activity is easily calculated from the rate of energy expenditure and the duration of the activity. For example, if someone is exercising at an energy expenditure of 10 kcal $\cdot$ min^{-1} for 30 min, 300 kcal of energy are expended. The MET scale can also be used to calculate the volume of energy expenditure. If a person is exercising at 7 METs for 30 min, 210 MET-min of energy expenditure is accomplished. The U.S. Physical Activity Guidelines indicate that when people regularly accomplish 500 to 1,000 MET-min of physical activity per week, substantial health benefits are realized. In the case of the person working at 7 METs for 30 min sessions, only three sessions a week would be needed to meet the low end of that physical activity range, and five sessions would allow the person to reach the top end of the range, where more health benefits are realized (29).

KEY POINT

Energy expenditure can be expressed in $L \cdot min^{-1}$, $kcal \cdot min^{-1}$, $ml \cdot kg^{-1} \cdot min^{-1}$, METs, and $kcal \cdot kg^{-1} \cdot hr^{-1}$:

- To convert $L \cdot min^{-1}$ to $kcal \cdot min^{-1}$, multiply by $5.0 \, kcal \cdot L^{-1}$.
- To convert $L \cdot min^{-1}$ to $ml \cdot kg^{-1} \cdot min^{-1}$, multiply by 1,000 and divide by body weight in kilograms.
- To convert $ml \cdot kg^{-1} \cdot min^{-1}$ to METs or $kcal \cdot kg^{-1} \cdot hr^{-1}$, divide by $3.5 \, ml \cdot kg^{-1} \cdot min^{-1}$.

Equations for Estimating the Energy Cost of Activities

In the mid-1970s, ACSM identified some simple equations to estimate the steady-state energy requirement associated with common modes of activities used in GXTs, including walking, stepping, running, and cycle ergometry (2). Over the years the equations have been modified to reflect the best information available, and this chapter discusses the current thinking in estimating energy costs (3). The oxygen uptake calculated from these equations is an estimate, and a typical **standard deviation** associated with the actual measured average value is about 7% to 9% (3, 10). Remember this normal variation in the energy costs of activities when using these equations in prescribing exercise.

The ACSM equations have been applied to GXTs to estimate maximal aerobic power. This application gives reasonable estimates when the subjects are healthy and the rate at which the GXT progresses is slow enough to allow the subject to achieve steady-state oxygen uptake at each stage (24, 25). When the increments between the stages of the GXT are large or the person is somewhat unfit, oxygen uptake will not keep pace with each stage of the test. In these cases, the equations overestimate the actual measured oxygen uptake (17), because the equations are designed to estimate steady-state energy requirements. This overestimation is more likely to happen in populations with disease (e.g., cardiac patients), suggesting that the GXTs used to test these populations may be too aggressive (see Research Insight on how investigators have dealt with this problem). A test that progresses at a slower rate and allows the subject to reach the steady-state $\dot{V}O_2$ at each stage reduces the chance of overestimating functional capacity (see chapter 11).

RESEARCH INSIGHT

All of the equations presented in this chapter estimate the energy cost of activities based on steady-state considerations. However, when a person completes a maximal GXT to volitional exhaustion (see chapter 7), the person is clearly *not* in a steady state in the last stage of the test. It has been shown that when $\dot{V}O_2$max is estimated based on the steady-state equations, it is systematically higher than what is actually measured. To deal with this, investigators have developed unique equations for predicting $\dot{V}O_2$max for the treadmill (14) and cycle (28). Additionally, if the patient or client holds onto the treadmill railing during the test, the overestimation is even greater (15), which is no surprise since the patient is off-loading some of the work by holding onto the railing and can complete more stages of the test. Thus, investigators have developed specialized equations to account for holding onto the railing (23). An interesting approach was taken by Foster et al. (15) in which they used the steady-state equations (presented in this chapter) to predict the oxygen cost of the last stage of the treadmill test and then developed a prediction equation to estimate $\dot{V}O_2$max. It worked both for patients who held onto the treadmill railing and those who did not.

When the ACSM equations were developed, an attempt was made to use a true physiological oxygen cost for each type of work. Each activity is broken down into the energy components. That is, in estimating the total oxygen cost of walking up a grade, you add the net oxygen cost of the horizontal walk (one component) to the net oxygen cost of the vertical (grade) walk (one component) to the resting metabolic rate (one component), which is taken to be 1 MET (3.5 ml $\cdot$ kg^{-1} $\cdot$ min^{-1}).

$$\text{Total O}_2 \text{ cost} = \text{net oxygen cost of activity} + 3.5 \text{ ml} \cdot \text{kg}^{-1} \cdot \text{min}^{-1}.$$

For the equations to properly estimate the oxygen cost of the activity, the subject must follow instructions carefully (e.g., not hold onto the treadmill railing, maintain the pedal cadence) and the work instruments (i.e., treadmill, cycle ergometer) must be calibrated so the settings are correct (see chapter 7).

Energy Requirements of Walking, Running, Cycle Ergometry, and Stepping

The following sections provide equations to estimate the energy cost of walking, running, cycle ergometry, and stepping. These activities are common in cardiac rehabilitation and adult fitness programs. Examples are provided to show how the equations are used in designing exercise programs.

Oxygen Cost of Walking

The oxygen cost of walking is determined by walking speed and whether the walker is on a horizontal or a graded surface. Prediction equations address all of these factors.

Horizontal Surface

One of the most common activities in exercise programs and GXTs is walking. The following equation can be used to estimate the energy requirement between the walking speeds of 50 and 100 m $\cdot$ min^{-1}, or 1.9 and 3.7 mi $\cdot$ hr^{-1}. (Multiply miles per hour by 26.8 to obtain meters per minute. Divide meters per minute by 26.8 to obtain miles per hour.) Dill (13) showed that the net cost of walking 1 m $\cdot$ min^{-1} on a horizontal surface is about 0.1 ml $\cdot$ kg^{-1} $\cdot$ min^{-1}, and this value is used in the ACSM equation. The ACSM equation for calculating the oxygen cost (ml $\cdot$ kg^{-1} $\cdot$ min^{-1}) of walking on a flat surface is as follows:

$$\dot{V}O_2 = 0.1 \text{ ml} \cdot \text{kg}^{-1} \cdot \text{min}^{-1}(\text{horizontal velocity}) + 3.5 \text{ ml} \cdot \text{kg}^{-1} \cdot \text{min}^{-1}.$$

QUESTION: What are the estimated steady-state $\dot{V}O_2$ and METs for a walking speed of 90 m $\cdot$ min^{-1} (3.4 mi $\cdot$ hr^{-1})?

ANSWER:

$$\dot{V}O_2 = 90 \text{ m} \cdot \text{min}^{-1} \cdot \frac{0.1 \text{ ml} \cdot \text{kg}^{-1} \cdot \text{min}^{-1}}{\text{m} \cdot \text{min}^{-1}} + 3.5 \text{ ml} \cdot \text{kg}^{-1} \cdot \text{min}^{-1}$$

$$\dot{V}O_2 = 9.0 \text{ ml} \cdot \text{kg}^{-1} \cdot \text{min}^{-1} + 3.5 \text{ ml} \cdot \text{kg}^{-1} \cdot \text{min}^{-1} = 12.5 \text{ ml} \cdot \text{kg}^{-1} \cdot \text{min}^{-1}$$

$$12.5 \text{ ml} \cdot \text{kg}^{-1} \cdot \text{min}^{-1} \div 3.5 \text{ ml} \cdot \text{kg}^{-1} \cdot \text{min}^{-1} = 3.6 \text{ METs or } 3.6 \text{ kcal} \cdot \text{kg}^{-1} \cdot \text{hr}^{-1}$$

The equations also can be used to predict the level of activity required to elicit a specific energy expenditure.

QUESTION: An unfit participant is told to exercise at 11.5 ml $\cdot$ kg^{-1} $\cdot$ min^{-1} to achieve the proper exercise intensity. What walking speed would you recommend?

ANSWER:

$$11.5 \text{ ml} \cdot \text{kg}^{-1} \cdot \text{min}^{-1} = ? \text{ m} \cdot \text{min}^{-1} \cdot \frac{0.1 \text{ ml} \cdot \text{kg}^{-1} \cdot \text{min}^{-1}}{\text{m} \cdot \text{min}^{-1}} + 3.5 \text{ ml} \cdot \text{kg}^{-1} \cdot \text{min}^{-1}$$

Subtract the resting metabolic rate of 3.5 ml · kg⁻¹ · min⁻¹ from both sides of the equation. Subtracting 3.5 ml · kg⁻¹ · min⁻¹ from 11.5 ml · kg⁻¹ · min⁻¹ gives the net oxygen cost of the activity (8.0 ml · kg⁻¹ · min⁻¹):

$$8 \text{ ml} \cdot \text{kg}^{-1} \cdot \text{min}^{-1} = ? \, \text{m} \cdot \text{min}^{-1} \cdot \frac{0.1 \text{ ml} \cdot \text{kg}^{-1} \cdot \text{min}^{-1}}{\text{m} \cdot \text{min}^{-1}}$$

The net cost (8 ml · kg⁻¹ · min⁻¹) is divided by 0.1 ml · kg⁻¹ · min⁻¹ per m · min⁻¹ to yield 80 m · min⁻¹. To obtain miles per hour, divide meters per minute by 26.8 to get 3 mi · hr⁻¹:

$$80 \text{ m} \cdot \text{min}^{-1} = 8 \text{ ml} \cdot \text{kg}^{-1} \cdot \text{min}^{-1} \div \frac{0.1 \text{ ml} \cdot \text{kg}^{-1} \cdot \text{min}^{-1}}{\text{m} \cdot \text{min}^{-1}}$$

$$3.0 \text{ mi} \cdot \text{hr}^{-1} = 80 \text{ m} \cdot \text{min}^{-1} \div \frac{26.8 \text{ m} \cdot \text{min}^{-1}}{\text{mi} \cdot \text{hr}^{-1}}$$

Walking Up a Grade

The oxygen cost of walking up a grade is the sum of the oxygen cost of horizontal walking, the oxygen cost of the vertical component of walking on a grade, and the resting metabolic rate of 3.5 ml · kg⁻¹ · min⁻¹. Studies have shown that the oxygen cost of moving (walking or stepping) 1 m · min⁻¹ vertically is 1.8 ml · kg⁻¹ · min⁻¹ (7, 26). The vertical component (vertical velocity) is calculated by multiplying the grade (expressed as a fraction) times the speed in meters per minute. A person walking at 80 m · min⁻¹ on a 10% grade is walking 8 m · min⁻¹ vertically (0.10 · 80 m · min⁻¹). The equation for calculating the oxygen cost (ml · kg⁻¹ · min⁻¹) of walking on a grade is as follows:

$$\dot{V}O_2 = 0.1 \text{ ml} \cdot \text{kg}^{-1} \cdot \text{min}^{-1}(\text{horizontal velocity}) +$$

$$1.8 \text{ ml} \cdot \text{kg}^{-1} \cdot \text{min}^{-1}(\text{vertical velocity}) + 3.5 \text{ ml} \cdot \text{kg}^{-1} \cdot \text{min}^{-1}.$$

QUESTION: What is the total oxygen cost of walking 90 m · min⁻¹ up a 12% grade?

ANSWER:

The horizontal component is calculated as in the preceding equation for walking on a horizontal surface and equals 9 ml · kg⁻¹ · min⁻¹. The following equations show how to calculate the vertical component and finally the total oxygen cost for walking 90 m · min⁻¹ up a 12% grade:

$$\dot{V}O_2 = 0.12 \, (\text{grade}) \cdot 90 \text{ m} \cdot \text{min}^{-1} \cdot \frac{1.8 \text{ ml} \cdot \text{kg}^{-1} \cdot \text{min}^{-1}}{\text{m} \cdot \text{min}^{-1}} = 19.4 \text{ ml} \cdot \text{kg}^{-1} \cdot \text{min}^{-1}$$

$$\dot{V}O_2 \, (\text{ml} \cdot \text{kg}^{-1} \cdot \text{min}^{-1}) = 9.0 \, (\text{horizontal}) + 19.4 \, (\text{vertical}) + 3.5 \, (\text{rest}) =$$

$$31.9 \text{ ml} \cdot \text{kg}^{-1} \cdot \text{min}^{-1} \text{ or } 9.1 \text{ METs or } 9.1 \text{ kcal} \cdot \text{kg}^{-1} \cdot \text{hr}^{-1}$$

As indicated earlier, the equations can be used to estimate the treadmill settings needed to elicit a specific oxygen uptake.

QUESTION: How would you set the treadmill grade to achieve an energy requirement of 6 METs (21.0 ml · kg⁻¹ · min⁻¹) when walking at 60 m · min⁻¹?

ANSWER:

The net oxygen cost of the activity is 21 − 3.5, or 17.5 ml · kg⁻¹ · min⁻¹. Now we must calculate the vertical and horizontal energy components to reach the final answer:

$$\text{Horizontal component} = 60 \text{ m} \cdot \text{min}^{-1} \cdot \frac{0.1 \text{ ml} \cdot \text{kg}^{-1} \cdot \text{min}^{-1}}{\text{m} \cdot \text{min}^{-1}}$$

$$= 6.0 \text{ ml} \cdot \text{kg}^{-1} \cdot \text{min}^{-1}$$

$$\text{Vertical component} = 17.5 - 6.0 = 11.5 \text{ ml} \cdot \text{kg}^{-1} \cdot \text{min}^{-1}$$

$$11.5 \text{ ml} \cdot \text{kg}^{-1} \cdot \text{min}^{-1} = \text{fractional grade} \cdot 60 \text{ m} \cdot \text{min}^{-1} \cdot \frac{1.8 \text{ ml} \cdot \text{kg}^{-1} \cdot \text{min}^{-1}}{\text{m} \cdot \text{min}^{-1}}$$

$$11.5 \text{ ml} \cdot \text{kg}^{-1} \cdot \text{min}^{-1} = \text{fractional grade} \cdot 108 \text{ ml} \cdot \text{kg}^{-1} \cdot \text{min}^{-1}$$

$$\text{Fractional grade} = 11.5 \div 108 = 0.106 \cdot 100\% = 10.6\% \text{ grade}$$

Walking at Various Speeds

The preceding equations are useful for walking speeds of 50 to 100 m · min^{-1} (1.9-3.7 mi · hr^{-1}); beyond that, the oxygen requirement for walking increases curvilinearly (10). Because many people choose to walk quickly rather than jog, knowing the energy requirements for walking at these higher speeds is useful in prescribing exercise. Values for the energy requirements for walking horizontally and at various grades at these faster speeds (4.0-5.0 mi · hr^{-1}, or 107-134 m · min^{-1}) are included in table 6.2.

One of the most common and useful ways to express the energy cost of walking is in kilocalories per minute. In this way, the fitness professional can simply locate the walking speed in a table, identify the number of calories used per minute, and calculate the total energy expenditure based on the duration of the walk. Table 6.3 presents the energy cost (in kcal · min^{-1}) for walking at speeds of 2 to 5 mi · hr^{-1} (54-134 m · min^{-1}) and includes values for various body weights. The

TABLE 6.2 Energy Requirement in METs for Walking at Various Speeds and Grades

Grade (%)	SPEED (MI · HR^{-1}/M · MIN^{-1}) 2.0/54	2.5/67	3.0/80	3.5/94	4.0/107	4.5/121	5.0/134
0	2.5	2.9	3.3	3.7	4.9	6.2	7.9
2	3.1	3.6	4.1	4.7	5.9	7.4	9.3
4	3.6	4.3	4.9	5.6	7.1	8.7	10.6
6	4.2	5.0	5.8	6.6	8.1	9.9	12.0
8	4.7	5.7	6.6	7.5	9.3	11.1	13.4
10	5.3	6.3	7.4	8.5	10.4	12.4	14.8
12	5.8	7.1	8.3	9.5	11.4	13.6	16.6
14	6.4	7.7	9.1	10.4	12.6	14.9	17.5
16	6.9	8.4	9.9	11.4	13.6	16.1	18.9
18	7.5	9.1	10.7	12.4	14.8	17.4	20.3
20	8.1	9.8	11.6	13.3	15.9	18.6	21.7
22	8.6	10.3	12.4	14.3	17.0	19.9	23.1
24	9.1	11.1	13.2	15.3	18.1	21.1	
26	9.7	11.9	14.0	16.2	19.2	22.3	
28	10.3	12.5	14.9	17.2	20.3	23.6	
30	10.8	13.2	15.7	18.2	21.4		

Based on American College of Sports Medicine 2010; Bubb et al. 1985.

TABLE 6.3 Energy Costs of Walking (kcal · min^{-1})

BODY WEIGHT kg	lb	SPEED (MI · HR^{-1}/M · MIN^{-1}) 2.0/54	2.5/67	3.0/80	3.5/94	4.0/107	4.5/121	5.0/134
50.0	110	2.1	2.4	2.8	3.1	4.1	5.2	6.6
54.5	120	2.3	2.6	3.0	3.4	4.4	5.6	7.2
59.1	130	2.5	2.9	3.2	3.6	4.8	6.1	7.8
63.6	140	2.7	3.1	3.5	3.9	5.2	6.6	8.4
68.2	150	2.8	3.3	3.7	4.2	5.6	7.0	9.0
72.7	160	3.0	3.5	4.0	4.5	5.9	7.5	9.6
77.3	170	3.2	3.7	4.2	4.8	6.3	8.0	10.2
81.8	180	3.4	4.0	4.5	5.0	6.7	8.4	10.8
86.4	190	3.6	4.2	4.7	5.3	7.0	8.9	11.4
90.9	200	3.8	4.4	5.0	5.6	7.4	9.4	12.0
95.4	210	4.0	4.6	5.2	5.9	7.8	9.9	12.6
100.0	220	4.2	4.8	5.5	6.2	8.2	10.3	13.2

Multiply value by duration of the activity to obtain total calories expended.

Based on American College of Sports Medicine 2010; Bubb et al. 1985.

energy cost of walking increases with the speed of the walk; however, the rate of increase is larger at higher speeds. For example, when a 170 lb (77.3 kg) participant increases walking speed from 2 to 3 mi · hr^{-1} (from 54 to 80 m · min^{-1}), the energy cost increases from 3.2 to 4.2 kcal · min^{-1}. But going from 4 to 5 mi · hr^{-1} (from 107 to 134 m · min^{-1}), the energy cost increases from 6.3 to 10.2 kcal · min^{-1}. A sedentary person can walk at slow speeds and achieve the desired exercise intensity, and a relatively fit person can walk at higher speeds at which the elevated energy requirement provides the necessary stimulus for a training effect. As a participant loses weight, the energy cost of walking at a certain speed decreases because the energy cost of walking depends on body weight. The participant can compensate for the lower energy cost by walking for a longer duration or for a greater distance.

Oxygen Cost of Jogging and Running

Jogging and running are common in fitness programs for apparently healthy individuals. It is possible to use the ACSM equations to estimate the oxygen cost of these activities for a broad range of speeds, generally from 130 to 350 m · min^{-1}. The equations are also useful at speeds below 130 m · min^{-1} as long as the person is actually jogging. The fact that a person can walk or jog at speeds below 130 m · min^{-1} complicates the issue. The oxygen cost of walking is less than that of jogging at slow speeds; however, at approximately 140 m · min^{-1} (5.2 mi · hr^{-1}), the oxygen costs of jogging and walking are about the same. Above this speed, the oxygen cost of walking exceeds that of jogging (5).

Jogging and Running on a Horizontal Surface

The net oxygen cost of jogging or running 1 m · min^{-1} on a horizontal surface is about twice that of walking, 0.2 ml · kg^{-1} · min^{-1} per m · min^{-1} (6, 9, 22). Remember that the equation gives reasonable estimates of the oxygen cost of running for the average person. However, it is well known that trained runners are more economical (in terms of energy expenditure) than the average person and that running economy varies within any group, trained or untrained (9, 12, 25). The equation for estimating the oxygen cost (ml · kg^{-1} · min^{-1}) of running on a flat surface is as follows:

$$\dot{V}O_2 = 0.2 \text{ ml} \cdot \text{kg}^{-1} \cdot \text{min}^{-1} \text{ (horizontal velocity)} + 3.5 \text{ ml} \cdot \text{kg}^{-1} \cdot \text{min}^{-1}.$$

QUESTION: What is the oxygen requirement for running a 10K (10,000 m) race on a track in 60 min?

ANSWER:

$$10,000 \text{ m} \div 60 \text{ min} = 167 \text{ m} \cdot \text{min}^{-1}$$

$$\dot{V}O_2 = 167 \text{ m} \cdot \text{min}^{-1} \cdot \frac{0.2 \text{ ml} \cdot \text{kg}^{-1} \cdot \text{min}^{-1}}{\text{m} \cdot \text{min}^{-1}} + 3.5 \text{ ml} \cdot \text{kg}^{-1} \cdot \text{min}^{-1}$$

$$= 36.9 \text{ ml} \cdot \text{kg}^{-1} \cdot \text{min}^{-1} \text{ or } 10.5 \text{ METs or } 10.5 \text{ kcal} \cdot \text{kg}^{-1} \cdot \text{hr}^{-1}$$

QUESTION: A 20-yr-old female distance runner with a $\dot{V}O_2$max of 50 ml · kg^{-1} · min^{-1} wants to run intervals at 90% of $\dot{V}O_2$max. At what speed should she run on a track given that 1 mi equals 1,610 m?

ANSWER:
90% of 50 = 45 ml · kg^{-1} · min^{-1}, and the net cost of the run equals 45 ml · kg^{-1} · min^{-1} − 3.5 ml · kg^{-1} · min^{-1}, or 41.5 ml · kg^{-1} · min^{-1}.

$$41.5 \text{ ml} \cdot \text{kg}^{-1} \cdot \text{min}^{-1} \div \frac{0.2 \text{ ml} \cdot \text{kg}^{-1} \cdot \text{min}^{-1}}{\text{m} \cdot \text{min}^{-1}} = 207 \text{ m} \cdot \text{min}^{-1}$$

$$1610 \text{ m} \cdot \text{mi}^{-1} \div 207 \text{ m} \cdot \text{min}^{-1} = 7.78 \text{ min, or } 7:47 \text{ (min:s) mile pace}$$

Jogging and Running Up a Grade

There is not as much information about the oxygen cost of running up a grade as there is about the cost of walking up a grade or running on a flat track. But one thing is clear—the oxygen cost of running up a grade is about half that of walking up a grade (8, 22). Some of the vertical lift associated with running on a flat surface is used to accomplish some of the grade work during inclined running, lowering the net oxygen requirement for the vertical work. The oxygen cost of running

$1 \text{ m} \cdot \text{min}^{-1}$ vertically is about $0.9 \text{ ml} \cdot \text{kg}^{-1} \cdot \text{min}^{-1}$. As in the calculations for uphill walking, the vertical velocity is calculated by multiplying the fractional grade times the horizontal velocity. The following equation is used for calculating the oxygen cost of running up a grade.

$$\dot{V}O_2 = 0.2 \text{ ml} \cdot \text{kg}^{-1} \cdot \text{min}^{-1} \text{ (horiz. velocity)} + 0.9 \text{ ml} \cdot \text{kg}^{-1} \cdot \text{min}^{-1} \text{ (vert. velocity)} + 3.5 \text{ ml} \cdot \text{kg}^{-1} \cdot \text{min}^{-1}.$$

QUESTION: What is the oxygen cost of running $150 \text{ m} \cdot \text{min}^{-1}$ up a 10% grade?

ANSWER:
Horizontal component:

$$\dot{V}O_2 = 150 \text{ m} \cdot \text{min}^{-1} \cdot \frac{0.2 \text{ ml} \cdot \text{kg}^{-1} \cdot \text{min}^{-1}}{\text{m} \cdot \text{min}^{-1}} = 30 \text{ ml} \cdot \text{kg}^{-1} \cdot \text{min}^{-1}$$

Vertical component:

$$\dot{V}O_2 = 0.10 \text{ (fractional grade)} \cdot 150 \text{ m} \cdot \text{min}^{-1} \cdot \frac{0.9 \text{ ml} \cdot \text{kg}^{-1} \cdot \text{min}^{-1}}{\text{m} \cdot \text{min}^{-1}}$$
$$= 13.5 \text{ ml} \cdot \text{kg}^{-1} \cdot \text{min}^{-1}$$
$$\dot{V}O_2 = 30.0 \text{ (horizontal)} + 13.5 \text{ (vertical)} + 3.5 \text{ (rest)} = 47 \text{ ml} \cdot \text{kg}^{-1} \cdot \text{min}^{-1}$$
$$= 13.4 \text{ METs or } 13.4 \text{ kcal} \cdot \text{kg}^{-1} \cdot \text{hr}^{-1}$$

QUESTION: The oxygen cost of running $350 \text{ m} \cdot \text{min}^{-1}$ on a flat surface is about $73.5 \text{ ml} \cdot \text{kg}^{-1} \cdot \text{min}^{-1}$. What grade should be set on a treadmill for a speed of $300 \text{ m} \cdot \text{min}^{-1}$ to achieve the same $\dot{V}O_2$?

ANSWER:
Horizontal component:

$$\dot{V}O_2 = 300 \text{ m} \cdot \text{min}^{-1} \cdot \frac{0.2 \text{ ml} \cdot \text{kg}^{-1} \cdot \text{min}^{-1}}{\text{m} \cdot \text{min}^{-1}} = 60 \text{ ml} \cdot \text{kg}^{-1} \cdot \text{min}^{-1}$$

Vertical component:

$$\text{Net } \dot{V}O_2 = 73.5 \text{ (total)} - 60 \text{ (horizontal)} - 3.5 \text{ (rest)} = 10.0 \text{ ml} \cdot \text{kg}^{-1} \cdot \text{min}^{-1}$$
$$10.0 \text{ ml} \cdot \text{kg}^{-1} \cdot \text{min}^{-1} = \text{fractional grade} \cdot 300 \text{ m} \cdot \text{min}^{-1} \cdot \frac{0.9 \text{ ml} \cdot \text{kg}^{-1} \cdot \text{min}^{-1}}{\text{m} \cdot \text{min}^{-1}}$$
$$\text{Fractional grade} = 10 \text{ ml} \cdot \text{kg}^{-1} \cdot \text{min}^{-1} \div 270 \text{ ml} \cdot \text{kg}^{-1} \cdot \text{min}^{-1}$$
$$= .037, \text{ or } 3.7\% \text{ grade}$$

Table 6.4 summarizes oxygen costs of running on a level surface and up a grade.

TABLE 6.4 Energy Requirement in METs for Jogging or Running at Various Speeds and Grades

Grade (%)	SPEED (MI · HR⁻¹/M · MIN⁻¹)							
	3/80	4/107	5/134	6/161	7/188	8/215	9/241	10/268
0	5.6	7.1	8.7	10.2	11.7	13.3	14.8	16.3
1	5.8	7.4	9.0	10.6	12.2	13.8	15.4	17.0
2	6.0	7.7	9.3	11.0	12.7	14.4	16.0	17.7
3	6.2	7.9	9.7	11.4	13.2	14.9	16.6	18.4
4	6.4	8.2	10.0	11.9	13.7	15.5	17.3	19.1
5	6.6	8.5	10.4	12.3	14.2	16.1	17.9	19.8
6	6.8	8.8	10.7	12.7	14.6	16.6	18.5	20.4
7	7.0	9.0	11.0	13.1	15.1	17.1	19.1	21.1
8	7.2	9.3	11.4	13.5	15.6	17.7	19.7	21.8
9	7.4	9.6	11.7	13.9	16.1	18.3	20.3	22.5
10	7.6	9.9	12.1	14.3	16.6	18.8	21.0	23.2

Based on American College of Sports Medicine 2010.

Jogging and Running at Various Speeds

In contrast to the energy cost of walking, the energy cost of jogging and running increases linearly with increasing speed. Table 6.5 shows the caloric cost of running, in kilocalories per minute, for runners of various body weights. For the 170 lb (77.3 kg) participant, the energy cost increases from 7.2 to 11.2 kcal · min^{-1} when speed jumps from 3 to 5 mi · hr^{-1} (from 80 to 134 m · min^{-1}); the increase is also 4 kcal · min^{-1} when speed increases from 7 to 9 mi · hr^{-1} (from 188 to 241 m · min^{-1}). As with walking, the energy cost is higher for heavier individuals.

Oxygen Cost of Walking and Running a Mile

Despite the vast amount of information regarding the costs of walking and running, a good deal of misunderstanding still exists. We hear claims that the energy cost of walking 1 mi (1.6 km) is equal to that of running the same distance. In general, this is not the case (19). The equations for estimating the energy cost of walking and running can be used to estimate the caloric cost of walking and running 1 mi (1.6 km), information that is useful in achieving energy expenditure goals.

If a person walks at 3 mi · hr^{-1} (80 m · min^{-1}), he completes 1 mi (1.6 km) in 20 min. The caloric cost for walking 1 mi (1.6 km) for a 70 kg person is calculated as follows:

$$\dot{V}O_2 = 80 \text{ m} \cdot \text{min}^{-1} (0.1 \text{ ml} \cdot \text{kg}^{-1} \cdot \text{min}^{-1}) + 3.5 \text{ ml} \cdot \text{kg}^{-1} \cdot \text{min}^{-1}$$

$$= 11.5 \text{ ml} \cdot \text{kg}^{-1} \cdot \text{min}^{-1},$$

$$\dot{V}O_2 \text{ (ml} \cdot \text{mile}^{-1}) = 11.5 \text{ ml} \cdot \text{kg}^{-1} \cdot \text{min}^{-1} \cdot 70 \text{ kg} \cdot 20 \text{ min} \cdot \text{mile}^{-1} = 16{,}100 \text{ ml} \cdot \text{mi}^{-1}, \text{ and so}$$

$$\dot{V}O_2 \text{ (L} \cdot \text{min}^{-1}) = 16{,}100 \text{ ml} \cdot \text{mi}^{-1} \div 1{,}000 \text{ ml} \cdot \text{L}^{-1} = 16.1 \text{ L} \cdot \text{mi}^{-1}.$$

At about 5.0 kcal per liter of O_2, the gross caloric cost per mile of walking is 80.5 kcal (5 kcal · L^{-1} · 16.1 L · mi^{-1}). The net caloric cost for the mile walk can be calculated by subtracting the oxygen cost of 20 min of rest from the gross cost of the 3 mi · hr^{-1} walk. For this individual:

* Resting oxygen uptake = 3.5 ml · kg^{-1} · min^{-1} · 70 kg = 245 ml · min^{-1}.
* 20 min of rest (20 min · 245 ml · min^{-1}) = 4,900 ml, or 4.9 L O_2.
* At 5 kcal · L^{-1}, 4. 9 L O_2 equals 24.5 kcal for 20 min of rest.
* The net cost of the mile walk is 80.5 kcal − 24.5 kcal, or 56 kcal for each mile.

If the same 70 kg man ran the mile at 6 mile · hr^{-1} (161 m · min^{-1}), his oxygen cost could be calculated by the following method.

TABLE 6.5 Energy Costs of Jogging and Running (kcal · min^{-1})

BODY WEIGHT		SPEED (MI · HR^{-1}/M · MIN^{-1})							
kg	lb	3.0/80	4.0/107	5.0/134	6.0/161	7.0/188	8.0/215	9.0/241	10.0/268
50.0	110	4.7	5.9	7.2	8.5	9.8	11.1	12.3	13.6
54.5	120	5.1	6.4	7.9	9.3	10.6	12.1	13.4	14.8
59.1	130	5.5	7.0	8.6	10.0	11.5	13.1	14.6	16.1
63.6	140	5.9	7.5	9.2	10.8	12.4	14.1	15.7	17.3
68.2	150	6.4	8.1	9.9	11.6	13.3	15.1	16.8	18.5
72.7	160	6.8	8.6	10.5	12.4	14.2	16.1	17.9	19.8
77.3	170	7.2	9.1	11.2	13.1	15.1	17.1	19.1	21.0
81.8	180	7.6	9.7	11.8	13.9	15.9	18.1	20.2	22.2
86.4	190	8.1	10.2	12.5	14.7	16.8	19.1	21.3	23.5
90.9	200	8.5	10.8	13.2	15.4	17.7	20.1	22.4	24.7
95.4	210	8.9	11.3	13.8	16.2	18.6	21.1	23.5	25.9
100.0	220	9.3	11.8	14.5	17.0	19.5	22.2	24.7	27.2

Multiply value by duration of the activity to obtain total calories expended.

$$\dot{V}O_2 = 161 \text{ m} \cdot \text{min}^{-1} (0.2 \text{ ml} \cdot \text{kg}^{-1} \cdot \text{min}^{-1}) + 3.5 \text{ ml} \cdot \text{kg}^{-1} \cdot \text{min}^{-1}$$

$$= 35.7 \text{ ml} \cdot \text{kg}^{-1} \cdot \text{min}^{-1},$$

$$\dot{V}O_2 \text{ (ml} \cdot \text{mi}^{-1}) = 35.7 \text{ ml} \cdot \text{kg}^{-1} \cdot \text{min}^{-1} \cdot 70 \text{ kg} \cdot 10 \text{ min} \cdot \text{mi}^{-1} = 25,000 \text{ ml} \cdot \text{mi}^{-1}, \text{ and so}$$

$$\dot{V}O_2 \text{ (L} \cdot \text{min}^{-1}) = 25,000 \text{ ml} \cdot \text{mi}^{-1} \div 1,000 \text{ ml} \cdot \text{L}^{-1} = 25 \text{ L} \cdot \text{mi}^{-1}.$$

At about 5 kcal per liter of O_2, 125 kcal are used to jog or run 1 mi ($5 \text{ kcal} \cdot \text{L}^{-1} \cdot 25 \text{ L} \cdot \text{mi}^{-1}$). The gross caloric cost per 1 mi (or per 1.6 km) is about 50% higher for jogging than for walking (125 versus 80 kcal). The net caloric cost of jogging or running 1 mi or 1.6 km (calories used above resting), however, is independent of speed and is about twice that of walking. For example, when we subtract the caloric cost for 10 min of rest (12 kcal) from the gross caloric cost of the run (125 kcal), the net cost is 113 kcal, or twice that for the walk (56 kcal). This follows from the net cost of running versus walking: $0.2 \text{ ml} \cdot \text{kg}^{-1} \cdot \text{min}^{-1}$ per m $\cdot$ min^{-1} versus $0.1 \text{ ml} \cdot \text{kg}^{-1} \cdot \text{min}^{-1}$ per m $\cdot$ min^{-1}. Table 6.6 lists values for the net and gross caloric costs of walking and running 1 mi (1.6 km) for a variety of body weights, with the values expressed in kilocalories per mile.

For weight control, it is important to use the net cost of the activity, because it measures the energy used above that used for sitting. When a person walks at slow to moderate speeds (2-3.5 mi $\cdot$ hr^{-1}, or 54-94 m $\cdot$ min^{-1}), the net cost of walking a mile (1.6 km) is about half that of jogging or running the mile. This means that a person who jogs a mile at 3 mi $\cdot$ hr^{-1} (80 m $\cdot$ min^{-1}) expends twice as many calories as someone who walks at the same speed. Because many people walk at these slower speeds, it is important to remember that the net energy cost of the mile is half that of running. If we look at high walking speeds such as 5 mi $\cdot$ hr^{-1} (134 m $\cdot$ min^{-1}), or 1 mi in 12 min, however, we see that the net energy cost of walking 1 mi is similar to that of running.

KEY POINT

The oxygen cost of walking increases linearly between the speeds of 50 and 100 m $\cdot$ min^{-1}; it increases faster at higher walking speeds. The oxygen cost of jogging or running increases linearly with speed from slow jogging (3 mi $\cdot$ hr^{-1}, or 80 m $\cdot$ min^{-1}) to fast running. The net caloric cost of jogging or running a mile (1.6 km) is twice that of walking a mile at a moderate pace.

Table 6.6 shows that the net cost of running a mile (1.6 km) is independent of speed. It does not matter whether participants jog at 3 mi $\cdot$ hr^{-1} (80 m $\cdot$ min^{-1}) or run at 6 mi $\cdot$ hr^{-1} (161 m $\cdot$ min^{-1})—the net caloric cost for running a mile is the same. At 6 mi $\cdot$ hr^{-1}, the participant expends energy at about twice the rate measured at 3 mi $\cdot$ hr^{-1} (161 m $\cdot$ min^{-1}), but because the mile is finished in half the time, the net energy expenditure is about the same. HR will, of course, be higher in the 6 mi $\cdot$ hr^{-1} (161 m $\cdot$ min^{-1}) run in order to deliver the oxygen to the muscles at the higher rate.

Oxygen Cost of Cycle Ergometry

Cycle ergometry is a popular exercise done at a sport club, at home, or as part of a rehabilitation program. Generally, cycle ergometry expends energy while causing less trauma to the ankle, knee, and hip joints compared with jogging. Cycle ergometers are used for conventional leg-exercise programs, but they are also adapted for arm exercise (by placing the ergometer on a table). The following sections describe how to estimate the energy costs of leg and arm cycle ergometry.

Leg Ergometry

In the previous activities the participants were carrying their body weight, and the oxygen requirement was therefore proportional to body weight (ml $\cdot$ kg$^{-1} \cdot$ min^{-1}). This is not the case in cycle ergometry, in which body weight is supported by the cycle seat and the work rate is determined primarily by the pedal rate and the resistance on the wheel. The oxygen requirement, in liters per minute, is approximately the same for people of all sizes for the same work rate. Thus, when a light person is doing the same work rate as a heavy person, the relative $\dot{V}O_2$ (ml $\cdot$ kg$^{-1} \cdot$ min^{-1}), or MET level, is higher for the lighter person.

TABLE 6.6   Gross and Net (Gross/Net) Cost for Walking and Running One Mile (kcal · mi⁻¹)

WALKING

BODY WEIGHT		SPEED (MI · HR⁻¹/M · MIN⁻¹)						
kg	lb	2.0/54	2.5/67	3.0/80	3.5/94	4.0/107	4.5/121	5.0/134
50.0	110	64/39	58/39	54/39	53/39	60/48	68/57	79/67
54.5	120	69/42	63/42	59/42	57/42	66/52	75/63	86/81
59.1	130	75/45	68/45	64/45	62/45	71/57	81/68	93/81
63.6	140	80/49	73/49	69/49	67/49	77/61	87/73	100/88
68.2	150	87/52	79/52	74/52	72/52	82/65	93/78	108/94
72.7	160	92/56	84/56	79/56	76/56	88/70	100/84	115/100
77.3	170	98/59	90/59	84/59	81/59	93/74	106/89	122/107
81.8	180	104/63	95/63	89/63	86/63	99/78	112/94	139/113
86.4	190	110/66	100/66	94/66	91/66	104/83	118/99	136/119
90.9	200	115/70	105/70	99/70	95/70	110/87	124/104	144/125
95.4	210	121/73	111/73	104/73	100/73	115/92	131/110	151/132
100.0	220	127/77	116/77	109/77	105/77	121/96	137/115	158/138

RUNNING

BODY WEIGHT		SPEED (MI · HR⁻¹/M · MIN⁻¹)						
kg	lb	3.0/80	4.0/107	5.0/134	6.0/161	7.0/188	8.0/215	9.0/241	10.0/268
50.0	110	93/77	89/77	86/77	84/77	84/77	82/77	82/77	81/77
54.5	120	101/83	97/83	94/83	92/83	92/83	89/83	89/83	89/83
59.1	130	110/90	105/90	102/90	100/90	99/90	97/90	97/90	96/90
63.6	140	118/97	113/97	110/97	108/97	107/97	104/97	104/97	104/97
68.2	150	127/104	121/104	118/104	115/104	114/104	112/104	112/104	111/104
72.7	160	135/111	129/111	125/111	123/111	122/111	119/111	119/111	119/111
77.3	170	144/118	137/118	133/118	131/118	130/118	127/118	127/118	126/118
81.8	180	152/125	146/125	141/125	138/125	137/125	134/125	134/125	133/125
86.4	190	161/132	154/132	149/132	146/132	145/132	141/132	141/132	141/132
90.9	200	169/139	162/139	157/139	154/139	153/139	149/139	149/139	148/139
95.4	210	177/146	170/146	165/146	161/146	160/146	156/146	156/146	155/146
100.0	220	186/153	178/153	173/153	169/153	168/153	164/153	164/153	163/153

Multiply value by the number of miles walked or run to obtain the total (gross/net) calories expended.

The work rate is set on the simple, mechanically braked cycle ergometers by varying the force (weight, or load) on the wheel and the number of pedal revolutions per minute (rev · min⁻¹). On the Monark cycle ergometer, the wheel travels 6 m per pedal revolution. At a pedal rate of 50 rev · min⁻¹, the wheel moves a distance of 300 m (6 m · 50 rev · min⁻¹). If a 1 kg weight (force) is applied to the wheel, the work rate is 300 kgm · min⁻¹ (kilogram-meters per minute). Work rates also are expressed in watts (W), where 6.1 kgm · min⁻¹ equals 1 W; the 300 kgm · min⁻¹ work rate would be expressed as 50 W. The work rate can be doubled by changing the force from 1 to 2 kg or by changing the pedal rate from 50 to 100 rev · min⁻¹. In contrast, some cycle ergometers are electronically controlled to deliver a specific work rate somewhat independent of pedal rate; as the pedal rate decreases, the load on the wheel is increased proportionally to maintain the work rate (4).

The total oxygen cost of leg cycle ergometry is the sum of the resting oxygen uptake, the cost of unloaded cycling (movement of the legs against no resistance), and the cost of the work itself. The oxygen cost of doing 1 kgm of work is 1.8 ml. The energy required to move the pedals against no resistance has been estimated to be 1 MET, or 3.5 ml · kg⁻¹ · min⁻¹. As with the other equations, resting oxygen uptake is 3.5 ml · kg⁻¹ · min⁻¹ (3). The latter two terms are combined in the equation to yield 7 ml · kg⁻¹ · min⁻¹. The estimates from the following equations are reasonable for work rates between approximately 150 and 1,200 kgm · min⁻¹ (see table 6.7). The equations for work rates expressed in kgm · min⁻¹ and watts follow.

$$\dot{V}O_2 \text{ (ml · kg}^{-1}\text{ · min}^{-1}\text{)} = \text{(kgm · min}^{-1}\text{ · 1.8 ml O}_2\text{ · kgm}^{-1}\text{)} \div \text{body weight (kg)} + 7 \text{ ml · kg}^{-1}\text{ · min}^{-1},$$
$$\dot{V}O_2 \text{ (ml · kg}^{-1}\text{ · min}^{-1}\text{)} = \text{(W · 10.8 ml O}_2\text{ · W}^{-1}\text{)} \div \text{body weight (kg)} + 7 \text{ ml · kg}^{-1}\text{ · min}^{-1}.$$

QUESTION: What is the oxygen cost of doing 600 kgm · min⁻¹ (100 W) on a cycle ergometer for 50 kg and 100 kg subjects?

ANSWER:

For the 50 kg subject:

$$\dot{V}O_2 \text{ (ml · kg}^{-1}\text{ · min}^{-1}\text{)} = \text{(600 kgm · min}^{-1}\text{ · 1.8 ml O}_2\text{ · kgm}^{-1}\text{)} \div 50 \text{ kg} + 7 \text{ ml · kg}^{-1}\text{ · min}^{-1}$$
$$= 28.6 \text{ ml · kg}^{-1}\text{ · min}^{-1}, \text{ or } 8.2 \text{ METs (8.2 kcal · kg}^{-1}\text{ · hr}^{-1}\text{)}.$$

For the 100 kg subject:

$$\dot{V}O_2 \text{ (ml · kg}^{-1}\text{ · min}^{-1}\text{)} = \text{(600 kgm · min}^{-1}\text{ · 1.8 ml O}_2\text{ · kgm}^{-1}\text{)} \div 100 \text{ kg} + 7 \text{ ml · kg}^{-1}\text{ · min}^{-1}$$
$$= 17.8 \text{ ml · kg}^{-1}\text{ · min}^{-1}, \text{ or } 5.1 \text{ METs (5.1 kcal · kg}^{-1}\text{ · hr}^{-1}\text{)}.$$

In some exercise programs, a participant might use a variety of exercise equipment to achieve a training effect and might want to set about the same intensity on each machine. The equation for the cycle ergometer can be used to set the load to achieve a particular MET value on the cycle ergometer and bring it in balance with what is done during walking or jogging.

QUESTION: A 70 kg participant must work at 6 METs (21 ml · kg⁻¹ · min⁻¹) to match the intensity of his walking program. What force (load) should be set on a Monark cycle ergometer at a pedal rate of 50 rev · min⁻¹?

ANSWER:

$$21 \text{ ml · kg}^{-1}\text{ · min}^{-1} = \text{(? kgm · min}^{-1}\text{ · 1.8 ml O}_2\text{ · kgm}^{-1}\text{)} \div 70 \text{ kg} + 7 \text{ ml · kg}^{-1}\text{ · min}^{-1},$$
$$\text{Net cost of cycling} = 21 - 7 \text{ ml · kg}^{-1}\text{ · min}^{-1} = 14 \text{ ml · kg}^{-1}\text{ · min}^{-1},$$
$$14 \text{ ml · kg}^{-1}\text{ · min}^{-1} = \text{(? kgm · min}^{-1}\text{ · 1.8 ml O}_2\text{ · kgm}^{-1}\text{)} \div 70 \text{ kg}.$$

Multiply each side by 70 kg.

$$980 \text{ ml · min}^{-1} = \text{? kgm · min}^{-1}\text{ · 1.8 ml O}_2\text{ · kgm}^{-1}.$$

Divide each side by 1.8 ml O₂ · kgm⁻¹ to obtain the work rate.

$$\text{Work rate} = 544 \text{ kgm · min}^{-1}.$$

Because the Monark wheel travels 300 m · min⁻¹ at 50 rev · min⁻¹, the load on the wheel should be 544 kgm · min⁻¹ ÷ 300 m · min⁻¹, or 1.8 kg.

Arm Ergometry

A cycle ergometer can be used to exercise the muscles of the arms and shoulder girdle by modifying the pedals and placing the cycle on a table. Arm ergometry is used on a limited basis as a GXT to evaluate cardiovascular function. It is used more generally as a routine exercise in rehabilitation programs (16). There are a variety of factors to keep in mind when considering arm ergometry:

- $\dot{V}O_2$max for the arms is only 70% of that measured with the legs in a normal healthy population and is less in an unfit, elderly, or diseased population.
- The natural endurance of the muscles used in this work is less than that of the legs.
- The HR and BP responses are higher for arm work compared with leg work at the same $\dot{V}O_2$.
- There is no need to account for unloaded arm cycling, but the oxygen cost of doing 1 kgm is about 3 ml O₂ · kgm⁻¹ for arm work because of the inefficiency of the action (3).

The equations for estimating the oxygen cost of arm work for work rates expressed in kgm · min⁻¹ or watts are as follows:

$$\dot{V}O_2 (ml \cdot kg^{-1} \cdot min^{-1}) = (kgm \cdot min^{-1} \cdot 3\ ml\ O_2 \cdot kgm^{-1}) \div body\ weight\ (kg) + 3.5\ ml \cdot kg^{-1} \cdot min^{-1},$$
$$\dot{V}O_2 (ml \cdot kg^{-1} \cdot min^{-1}) = (W \cdot 18\ ml\ O_2 \cdot W^{-1}) \div body\ weight\ (kg) + 3.5\ ml \cdot kg^{-1} \cdot min^{-1}.$$

See table 6.7 for estimates of the oxygen cost of arm work on a cycle ergometer.

QUESTION: What is the oxygen requirement for a 70 kg man doing 150 kgm $\cdot$ min^{-1} on an arm ergometer?

ANSWER:

$$\dot{V}O_2 (ml \cdot kg^{-1} \cdot min^{-1}) = (150\ kgm \cdot min^{-1} \cdot 3\ ml\ O_2 \cdot kgm^{-1}) \div 70\ kg + 3.5\ ml \cdot kg^{-1} \cdot min^{-1}$$
$$= 9.9\ ml \cdot kg^{-1} \cdot min^{-1},\ or\ 2.8\ METs\ (2.8\ kcal \cdot kg^{-1} \cdot hr^{-1}).$$

TABLE 6.7 Energy Expenditure in METs for Cycle Ergometry for Legs and Arms

BODY WEIGHT		WORK RATE (KGM $\cdot$ MIN^{-1}/W)						
kg	lb	300/50	450/75	600/100	750/125	900/150	1,050/175	1,200/200
50	110	5.1(6.1)	6.6(8.7)	8.2(11.3)	9.7(13.9)	11.3(–)	12.8(–)	14.3(–)
60	132	4.6(5.3)	5.9(7.4)	7.1(9.6)	8.4(11.7)	9.7(–)	11.0(–)	12.3(–)
70	154	4.2(4.7)	5.3(6.5)	6.4(8.3)	7.5(10.2)	8.6(12.0)	9.7(–)	10.8(–)
80	176	3.9(4.2)	4.9(5.8)	5.9(7.4)	6.8(9.0)	7.8(10.6)	8.8(12.3)	9.7(–)
90	198	3.7(3.9)	4.6(5.3)	5.4(6.7)	6.3(8.1)	7.1(9.6)	8.0(11.0)	8.9(12.4)
100	220	3.5(3.6)	4.3(4.9)	5.1(6.1)	5.9(7.4)	6.6(8.7)	7.4(10.0)	8.2(11.3)

Values in ( ) are for arm work.

Based on American College of Sports Medicine 2010.

KEY POINT

The oxygen cost of cycle ergometry primarily depends on the work rate because body weight is supported. The net oxygen cost of leg ergometry is 1.8 ml $\cdot$ kgm^{-1} versus 3 ml $\cdot$ kgm^{-1} for arm ergometry. Physiological responses (HR, BP) are exaggerated for arm work compared with leg work at the same work rate because the oxygen cost is higher and represents a higher percentage of the arm $\dot{V}O_2$max.

Oxygen Cost of Bench Stepping

One of the most useful and inexpensive forms of exercise is bench stepping; it can be done at home and requires little or no equipment. The work rate is adjusted easily by simply increasing step height or cadence (number of lifts per minute). The total oxygen cost of this exercise is the sum of the costs of (a) stepping up, (b) stepping down, (c) moving back and forth on a level surface at the specified cadence, and (d) resting oxygen uptake (3.5 ml $\cdot$ kg^{-1} $\cdot$ min^{-1}). The oxygen cost of stepping up is 1.8 ml $\cdot$ kg^{-1} $\cdot$ min^{-1} per m $\cdot$ min^{-1}, as in walking (26). The oxygen cost of stepping down is a third of the cost of stepping up; therefore, the oxygen cost of stepping up and down is 1.33 times the cost of stepping up. The oxygen cost of stepping back and forth on a flat surface is equal to 0.2 ml O_2 per kilogram of body mass for each four-cycle step (3). The number of meters moved up or down per minute is calculated by multiplying the number of lifts per minute by the height of the step; for example, if the step height is 0.2 m (20 cm) and the cadence is 30 steps $\cdot$ min^{-1}, then the total lift or descent per minute is 30 times 0.2 m, or 6 m $\cdot$ min^{-1}. To determine step height, multiply inches by 2.54 to obtain centimeters, and divide centimeters by 100 to obtain meters. The equation for estimating the energy requirement for stepping follows:

$$\dot{V}O_2 (ml \cdot kg^{-1} \cdot min^{-1}) = (0.2 \cdot step\ rate) +$$
$$(1.8 \cdot 1.33 \cdot step\ rate \cdot step\ height\ in\ meters) + 3.5\ ml \cdot kg^{-1} \cdot min^{-1}.$$

QUESTION: What is the oxygen requirement for stepping at a rate of 20 steps $\cdot$ min^{-1} on a 20 cm bench?

ANSWER:

$$\dot{V}O_2 = \left(\frac{0.2 \text{ ml} \cdot \text{kg}^{-1} \cdot \text{min}^{-1}}{\text{steps} \cdot \text{min}^{-1}} \cdot 20 \text{ steps} \cdot \text{min}^{-1} \right) +$$

$$\left(\frac{1.8 \text{ ml}}{\text{kgm}} \cdot 1.33 \cdot \frac{0.2 \text{ m}}{\text{step}} \cdot \frac{20 \text{ steps}}{\text{min}} \right) + 3.5 \text{ ml} \cdot \text{kg}^{-1} \cdot \text{min}^{-1}$$

$$= 4.0 \text{ ml} \cdot \text{kg}^{-1} \cdot \text{min}^{-1} + 9.6 \text{ ml} \cdot \text{kg}^{-1} \cdot \text{min}^{-1} + 3.5 \text{ ml} \cdot \text{kg}^{-1} \cdot \text{min}^{-1}$$

$$= 17.1 \text{ ml} \cdot \text{kg}^{-1} \cdot \text{min}^{-1}, \text{ or } 4.9 \text{ METs } (4.9 \text{ kcal} \cdot \text{kg}^{-1} \cdot \text{hr}^{-1})$$

Table 6.8 summarizes the energy requirement of stepping at various rates.

KEY POINT

The oxygen cost of bench stepping includes the cost of stepping up and down, moving horizontally back and forth, and resting oxygen uptake. The oxygen cost of stepping up is the same as in walking. The oxygen cost of stepping up and down is 1.33 times the cost of stepping up. The oxygen cost of stepping back and forth is $0.2 \text{ ml} \cdot \text{kg}^{-1} \cdot \text{min}^{-1}$ times the step rate.

Energy Requirements of Other Activities

Many activities are available for designing a fitness program (see chapter 22). These include exercising to music, rope skipping, swimming, and playing games. Not surprisingly, the energy expenditure associated with these activities is difficult to predict compared with walking or running, in which the energy cost between people is similar because of the natural movements associated with those activities. In contrast, these other activities have variable energy costs depending on the skill level of the participants and the motivation they bring to the activity, as will be clear in the following examples. Estimates of the energy requirements of some common aerobic activities also are presented.

Exercising to Music

Exercising to music is a fun alternative to walking and running. The energy requirement depends on whether the session is high or low impact; done at a low, medium, or high intensity; and done with or without hand weights (30). A person who is starting out might simply walk through the movements, whereas an experienced person might go through the full motion with each step. Thus,

TABLE 6.8 Energy Expenditure in METs During Stepping at Various Rates and Step Heights

STEP HEIGHT		STEPS · MIN⁻¹			
cm	in.	12	18	24	30
0	0	1.7	2.0	2.4	2.7
4	1.6	2.0	2.5	3.0	3.5
8	3.2	2.3	3.0	3.7	4.4
12	4.7	2.7	3.5	4.3	5.2
16	6.3	3.0	4.0	5.0	6.0
20	7.9	3.3	4.5	5.7	6.8
24	9.4	3.7	5.0	6.3	7.6
28	11.0	4.0	5.5	7.0	8.5
32	12.6	4.3	6.0	7.6	9.3
36	14.2	4.6	6.5	8.3	10.1
40	15.8	5.0	7.0	8.9	10.9

Based on American College of Sports Medicine 2010.

the energy cost of this activity varies considerably, from as low as 4 METs for someone walking through the routine to 10 METs for the experienced participant working at a high intensity (30). This activity often involves small muscle groups and includes some static (stabilizing) muscle contractions; as a result, HR response is higher for the same oxygen uptake measured in walking and running. Table 6.9 summarizes the caloric expenditure associated with exercise to music at low, moderate, and high intensities.

TABLE 6.9 Gross Energy Cost of Exercise to Music (kcal · min⁻¹)

Body weight (kg)	Body weight (lb)	Low intensity, or 4 METs	Moderate intensity, or 7 METs	High intensity, or 10 METs
50.0	110	3.3	5.8	8.3
54.5	120	3.6	6.4	9.1
59.1	130	3.9	6.9	9.8
63.6	140	4.2	7.4	10.6
68.2	150	4.5	7.9	11.3
72.7	160	4.8	8.5	12.1
77.3	170	5.1	9.0	12.8
81.8	180	5.4	9.5	13.6
86.4	190	5.7	10.1	14.3
90.9	200	6.0	10.6	15.1
95.4	210	6.3	11.1	15.9
100.0	220	6.6	11.7	16.7

Multiply value by duration of the aerobic phase to obtain total calories expended.

Rope Skipping

In walking and running, the energy requirement is proportional to the rate at which the person moves. But the energy requirement for rope skipping at only 60 to 80 turns · min⁻¹ (as slowly as the rope can be turned) is about 9 METs. At 120 turns · min⁻¹, the energy cost increases to only 11 METs (20). Consequently, rope skipping is not a graded activity, unlike walking and running. Second, the HR response is higher than expected from the oxygen cost of the activity. This may be because a small muscle mass (lower leg) is the primary muscle group involved in the activity. Despite this, rope skipping can be included as a part of a fitness session when done intermittently using THR as the guide (see chapters 11 and 22). Rope skipping should not be used, however, in the early phase of a fitness program because the energy cost and the loading on the ankle, knee, and hip joints are relatively high. Table 6.10 summarizes the energy costs of skipping rope at two speeds.

TABLE 6.10 Gross Energy Cost of Rope Skipping (kcal · min⁻¹)

Body weight (kg)	Body weight (lb)	Slow skipping (60-80 turns · min⁻¹)	Fast skipping (120 turns · min⁻¹)
50.0	110	3.3	5.8
54.5	120	3.6	6.4
59.1	130	8.9	10.9
63.6	140	9.5	11.7
68.2	150	10.2	12.5
72.7	160	10.9	13.4
77.3	170	11.6	14.2
81.8	180	12.3	15.0
86.4	190	13.0	15.9
90.9	200	13.6	16.7
95.4	210	14.3	17.5
100.0	220	15.0	18.4

Multiply value by duration of rope skipping to obtain total calories expended.

Swimming

Swimming is a preferred activity for many people because it is dynamic, uses large muscle groups, and causes little joint trauma. The limitation is in finding a convenient facility that allows lap swimming and, of course, in having enough skill to swim. The energy requirement depends on the swimming velocity, the stroke being used, and the swimmer's skill. A skilled swimmer requires less energy to move through the water and thus must swim a greater distance to achieve the same caloric expenditure.

The energy cost of simply treading water can be as high as $1.5 \text{ L} \cdot \text{min}^{-1}$ ($7.5 \text{ kcal} \cdot \text{min}^{-1}$). Elite swimmers use this same number of kilocalories per minute to swim at $36 \text{ m} \cdot \text{min}^{-1}$, whereas an unskilled swimmer might require twice that to maintain the same velocity. For elite swimmers, the front and back crawl are the most economical strokes and the butterfly is the least economical stroke. The net caloric cost per mile (1.6 km) of swimming has been estimated to be more than 400 kcal, or about 4 times that of running the mile and about 8 times that of walking the mile. However, the actual caloric cost per mile of swimming depends greatly on skill and gender: It is lower for highly skilled swimmers and for women (because of the greater buoyancy due to a higher percent body fat). Table 6.11 summarizes the caloric costs presented by Holmer (18) for men and women.

The HR response measured during swimming at a specific $\dot{V}O_2$ is lower than that measured during running at the same $\dot{V}O_2$. In fact, the maximal HR response is about $14 \text{ beats} \cdot \text{min}^{-1}$ lower for swimming (see chapter 18). With this in mind, fitness professionals should instruct participants to decrease the THR range for swimming activities.

TABLE 6.11 Caloric Cost per Mile (kcal · mi⁻¹) of Swimming the Front Crawl

Skill level	Women	Men
Competitive	180	280
Skilled	260	360
Average	300	440
Unskilled	360	560
Poor	440	720

1 mi = 1.6 km.

Adapted from Holmér 1979.

Using the Compendium of Physical Activities

Appendix C contains information about the Compendium of Physical Activities, an excellent source of information about the energy cost of a wide variety of physical activities, including leisure time and occupational activities (1). This list, originally published in 1993 and updated in 2000, now resides on a website where the values can be updated more frequently. In appendix C, we present a brief historical overview of the compendium and provide two examples of how to use it to calculate the energy cost of activities.

Estimation of Energy Expenditure Without Equations

If you did not have access to the compendium of physical activities but only had information about the client's HR response to exercise and $\dot{V}O_2$max, could you still estimate energy expenditure? The following is another approach to estimating the energy costs of an exercise session.

The fitness professional selects activities that cause participants to exercise at 40% to 84% of their $\dot{V}O_2$max, the intensity range needed to improve or maintain CRF and realize health benefits (see chapter 11). It should be possible, therefore, to estimate the energy expenditure for each individual on the basis of the subject's $\dot{V}O_2$max and the portion of the THR range at which the individual is working. If a person has a $\dot{V}O_2$max of 10 METs, energy expenditure can be estimated in the following way.

- 10 METs = 10 kcal · kg^{-1} · hr^{-1}.
- If a person exercises at the low end of the vigorous-intensity range, at about 60% $\dot{V}O_2$max, then the energy expenditure should be about 6 kcal · kg^{-1} · hr^{-1} (60% of 10 METs).
- If the person weighs 70 kg, then 420 kcal are expended per hour (70 kg · 6 kcal · kg^{-1} · hr^{-1}).
- A 30 min workout expends half this amount, or about 210 kcal.

These simple calculations assume that the person is performing an activity that uses large muscle groups. Table 6.12 shows the estimated calorie expenditure for a 30 min workout at 70% $\dot{V}O_2$max for a variety of fitness levels ($\dot{V}O_2$max expressed as METs) and body weights (27).

TABLE 6.12 Estimated Gross Energy Expenditure for a 30 Min Workout at 70% Functional Capacity for People of Various Fitness Levels ($\dot{V}O_2$max) and Body Weights

$\dot{V}O_2$max, in METs (kcal · kg^{-1} · hr^{-1})	70% max, in METs (kcal · kg^{-1} · hr^{-1})	50 kg/110 lb	70 kg/154 lb	90 kg/198 lb
20	14.0	350	490	630
18	12.6	315	441	567
16	11.2	280	392	504
14	9.8	245	343	441
12	8.4	210	294	378
10	7.0	175	245	315
8	5.6	140	196	252
6	4.2	105	147	189

MET = metabolic equivalent.

Environmental Concerns

Although changes in temperature, relative humidity, pollution, and altitude do not change the energy requirements for submaximal exercise, they do change the participant's response to the exercise. Remember that a person's HR response is the best indicator of the relative stress being experienced due to the interaction of exercise intensity, exercise duration, and environmental factors. The participant should cut back on the intensity of the activity when environmental factors increase the HR response. The duration of the activity can be increased to accommodate any energy expenditure goal.

KEY POINT

The energy cost of exercising to music varies from 4 to 10 METs, depending on effort and whether the exercise is high or low impact. Rope skipping requires about 10 METs, whereas the oxygen cost of swimming is inversely related to skill. Energy expenditure can be estimated without equations. If a person works at 60% of $\dot{V}O_2$max and has a $\dot{V}O_2$max of 10 METs, the energy expenditure is 6 METs, or 6 kcal · kg^{-1} · hr^{-1}. If the person weighs 80 kg, 480 kcal are expended per hour. Environmental factors such as heat, humidity, altitude, and pollution can increase the HR response to work while not really affecting the energy cost. HR should be monitored more frequently in these settings to adjust the intensity of the activity downward to keep the person in the appropriate HR range (see chapter 11 for more on this issue).

STUDY QUESTIONS

1. What can an accelerometer measure that a pedometer cannot when monitoring physical activity?
2. How do you convert oxygen uptake in $L \cdot min^{-1}$ to $kcal \cdot min^{-1}$?
3. What is a MET equal to in $ml \cdot kg^{-1} \cdot min^{-1}$ and $kcal \cdot kg^{-1} \cdot hr^{-1}$?
4. How much greater is the net oxygen cost of running $1\ m \cdot min^{-1}$ on a flat surface compared with walking?
5. When a 50 kg person and an 80 kg person exercise at $600\ kgm \cdot min^{-1}$ on a cycle ergometer, how do the oxygen uptakes compare in $L \cdot min^{-1}$ and $ml \cdot kg^{-1} \cdot min^{-1}$?
6. If a woman has a $\dot{V}O_2max$ of 10 METs and she is working at 70% $\dot{V}O_2max$, how many calories is she expending in $kcal \cdot kg^{-1} \cdot hr^{-1}$?

CASE STUDIES

You can check your answers by referring to Appendix A.

1. A 75 kg man walks at $3.5\ mi \cdot hr^{-1}$ for 30 min. How many calories does he expend?
2. A 60 kg woman rides a cycle ergometer at a work rate of 100 W. What is her oxygen uptake?
3. A 70 kg college student runs 3 mi (4.8 km) in 24 min. How many calories does he expend?
4. An 85 kg man with a $\dot{V}O_2max$ of 12 METs works at 70% $\dot{V}O_2max$ for 30 min. How many calories does he expend?
5. A client mentions he has read that he can expend the same number of calories per mile whether he walks it at $3\ mi \cdot hr^{-1}$ $(4.8\ km \cdot hr^{-1})$ or jogs it at $6\ mi \cdot hr^{-1}$ $(9.7\ km \cdot hr^{-1})$. How do you respond?

REFERENCES

1. Ainsworth B.E., W.L. Haskell, S.D. Herrmann, N. Meckes, D.R. Bassett Jr., C. Tudor-Locke, J.L. Greer, J. Vezina, M.C. Whitt-Glover, A.S. Leon. 2011 Compendium of Physical Activities: a second update of codes and MET values. *Medicine and Science in Sports and Exercise,* 2011;43(8):1575-1581.

2. American College of Sports Medicine (ACSM). 1980. *Guidelines for graded exercise testing and exercise prescription.* 2nd ed. Philadelphia: Lea & Febiger.

3. American College of Sports Medicine (ACSM). 2010. *ACSM's guidelines for exercise testing and prescription.* 8th ed. Baltimore: Lippincott Williams & Wilkins.

4. Åstrand, P.-O. 1979. *Work tests with the bicycle ergometer.* Verberg, Sweden: Monark-Crescent AB.

5. Åstrand, P.-O., and K. Rodahl. 1986. *Textbook of work physiology.* 3rd ed. New York: McGraw-Hill.

6. Balke, B. 1963. A simple field test for assessment of physical fitness. In *Civil Aeromedical Research Institute report,* 63-66. Oklahoma City: Civil Aeromedical Research Institute.

7. Balke, B., and R.W. Ware. 1959. An experimental study of "physical fitness" of Air Force personnel. *Armed Forces Medical Journal* 10:675-688.

8. Bassett Jr., D.R., M.D. Giese, F.J. Nagle, A. Ward, D.M. Raab, and B. Balke. 1985. Aerobic requirements of overground versus treadmill running. *Medicine and Science in Sports and Exercise* 17:477-481.

9. Bransford, D.R., and E.T. Howley. 1977. The oxygen cost of running in trained and untrained men and women. *Medicine and Science in Sports* 9:41-44.

10. Bubb, W.J., A.D. Martin, and E.T. Howley. 1985. Predicting oxygen uptake during level walking at speeds of 80 to 130 meters per minute. *Journal of Cardiac Rehabilitation* 5(10): 462-465.

11. Dale, D., G.J. Welk, and C.E. Matthews. 2002. Methods of assessing physical activity and challenges for research. In *Physical activity assessments for health-related research,* ed. G.J. Welk, 19-34. Champaign, IL: Human Kinetics.

12. Daniels, J.T. 1985. A physiologist's view of running economy. *Medicine and Science in Sports and Exercise* 17:332-338.

13. Dill, D.B. 1965. Oxygen cost of horizontal and grade walking and running on the treadmill. *Journal of Applied Physiology* 20:19-22.

14. Foster, C., A.S. Jackson, M.L. Pollock, M.M. Taylor, J. Hare, S.M. Sennett, J.L. Rod, M. Sarwar, and D.H. Schmidt. 1984. Generalized equations for predicting functional capacity from treadmill performance. *American Heart Journal* 107:1229-1234.

15. Foster, C., A.J. Crowe, E. Daines, M. Dumit, M.A. Green, S. Lettau, N.N. Thompson, and J. Weymier. 1996. Predicting functional capacity during treadmill testing independent of exercise protocol. *Medicine and Science in Sports and Exercise* 6:752-756.

16. Franklin, B.A. 1985. Exercise testing, training, and arm ergometry. *Sports Medicine* 2:100-119.

17. Haskell, W.L., W. Savin, N. Oldridge, and R. DeBusk. 1982. Factors influencing estimated oxygen uptake during exercise testing soon after myocardial infarction. *American Journal of Cardiology* 50:299-304.

18. Holmer, I. 1979. Physiology of swimming man. *Exercise and Sport Sciences Reviews* 7:87-123.

19. Howley, E.T., and M.E. Glover. 1974. The caloric costs of running and walking 1 mile for men and women. *Medicine and Science in Sports* 6:235-237.

20. Howley, E.T., and D. Martin. 1978. Oxygen uptake and heart-rate responses measured during rope skipping. *Tennessee Journal of Health, Physical Education and Recreation* 16:7-8.

21. Knoebel, L.K. 1984. Energy metabolism. In *Physiology*, 5th ed. Ed. E. Selkurt, 635-650. Boston: Little, Brown.

22. Margaria, R., P. Cerretelli, P. Aghemo, and J. Sassi. 1963. Energy cost of running. *Journal of Applied Physiology* 18:367-370.

23. McConnell, T.R., and B.A. Clark. 1987. Prediction of maximal oxygen consumption during handrail-supported treadmill exercise. *Journal of Cardiopulmonary Rehabilitation* 7:324-331.

24. Montoye, H.J., T. Ayen, F. Nagle, and E.T. Howley. 1986. The oxygen requirement for horizontal and grade walking on a motor-driven treadmill. *Medicine and Science in Sports and Exercise* 17:640-645.

25. Nagle, F.J., B. Balke, G. Baptista, J. Alleyia, and E. Howley. 1971. Compatibility of progressive treadmill, bicycle, and step tests based on oxygen-uptake responses. *Medicine and Science in Sport* 3:149-154.

26. Nagle, F.J., B. Balke, and J.P. Naughton. 1965. Gradational step tests for assessing work capacity. *Journal of Applied Physiology* 20:745-748.

27. Sharkey, B.J. 1990. *Physiology of fitness.* 3rd ed. Champaign, IL: Human Kinetics.

28. Storer, T.W., J.A. Davis, and V.J. Caiozzo. 1990. Accurate prediction of $\dot{V}O_2$max in cycle ergometry. *Medicine and Science in Sports and Exercise* 22:704-712.

29. U.S. Department of Health and Human Services (HHS). 2008. *2008 physcial activity guidelines for Americans.* www.health.gov/paguidelines/guidelines/default.aspx.

30. Williford, H.N., M. Scharff-Olson, and D.L. Blessing. 1989. The physiological effects of aerobic dance—A review. *Sports Medicine* 8:335-345.

Fitness Assessment

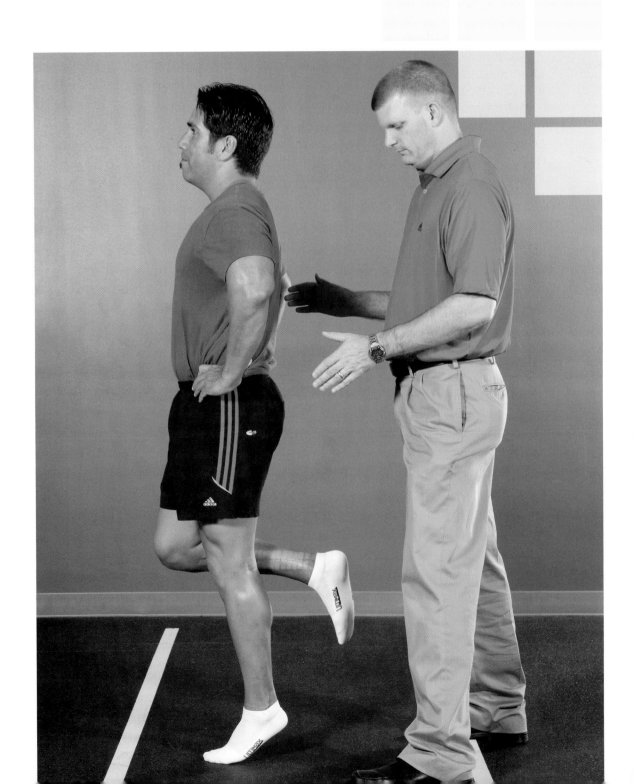

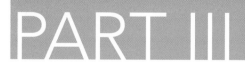

PART III

Fitness professionals must know how to measure each of the components of fitness and interpret the scores for the clients. In the chapters in part III, we examine the assessment of cardiorespiratory fitness (CRF) (chapter 7), body composition (chapter 8), muscular strength and endurance (chapter 9), and flexibility and low-back function (chapter 10).

Before you begin, you may want to review the general principles of fitness testing. How do you select appropriate tests? How can you obtain more accurate results? For a more complete introduction to the topic of fitness assessment, please see appendix E.

Assessment of Cardiorespiratory Fitness

The reader will be able to do the following:

1. Describe how CRF relates to health and list reasons for testing CRF as well as risks associated with CRF testing.

2. Present a logical sequence of testing.

3. Describe procedures for walking and jogging or running field tests to estimate CRF.

4. Contrast the treadmill, cycle ergometer, and bench step as instruments for GXTs.

5. List variables measured during a GXT.

6. Describe procedures used before, during, and after testing.

7. Contrast submaximal and maximal GXTs.

8. Describe the HR extrapolation procedures to estimate $\dot{V}O_2max$ using submaximal treadmill, cycle, and bench-step GXTs.

9. Calibrate a treadmill, a Monark cycle ergometer, and a sphygmomanometer.

As described in chapter 1, there is no question that higher levels of physical activity and CRF are associated with reduced risks of chronic diseases and death from all causes. Consequently, it is important to focus on a healthy level of CRF as a lifelong goal that makes life more enjoyable as well as healthy. Those benefits alone merit the inclusion of CRF in any discussion about positive health. CRF, also called *cardiovascular* or *aerobic fitness,* is a good measure of the heart's ability to pump oxygen-rich blood to the muscles. Although the terms *cardio* (heart), *vascular* (blood vessels), *respiratory* (lungs and ventilation), and *aerobic* (working with oxygen) differ technically, they all reflect aspects of CRF. A person with a healthy heart that can pump great volumes of blood with each beat has a high level of CRF. CRF values are expressed in the following ways (see chapter 6):

- Liters of oxygen used by the body per minute ($L \cdot min^{-1}$)
- Milliliters of oxygen used per kilogram of body weight per minute ($ml \cdot kg^{-1} \cdot min^{-1}$)
- METs, multiples of resting metabolic rate, where $1 \text{ MET} = 3.5 \ ml \cdot kg^{-1} \cdot min^{-1}$

A person with the ability to use $35 \ ml \cdot kg^{-1} \cdot min^{-1}$ during maximal exercise is said to have a CRF equal to 10 METs ($35 \div 3.5 = 10$). Aerobic training programs increase the heart's ability to pump blood, so it is no surprise that such programs improve CRF.

Chapter 4 describes how a wide variety of physiological variables (HR, BP, and so on) respond to acute or short-term exercise and how endurance training affects those responses. Chapter 11 explains how to recommend activities to clients to improve their CRF. This chapter emphasizes how to evaluate CRF. The reader is referred to other resources for additional details (2, 3).

Historically, HR, BP, and electrocardiogram (ECG) measurements taken at rest were used to evaluate CRF. In addition, some static pulmonary function tests (e.g., vital capacity) were used to characterize respiratory function. It became clear, however, that measurements taken at rest reveal little about the way a person's cardiorespiratory system responds to physical activity. We are now familiar with using GXTs to evaluate HR, ECG, BP, ventilation, and oxygen uptake responses during work.

Why Test Cardiorespiratory Fitness?

Results from CRF tests are used to write exercise recommendations and allow the fitness professional or physician to evaluate positive or negative changes in CRF resulting from physical conditioning, aging, illness, or inactivity. Given the current increase in obesity and inactivity in people of all ages, it makes sense to evaluate CRF throughout life, from early childhood to old age. This information can indicate where individuals stand on health-criterion tests, and it alerts them to subtle changes in lifestyle that may compromise positive health. The nature of the tests and the level of monitoring should vary across age groups to reflect the information that is needed.

CRF testing depends on the purposes of the test, the type of person to be evaluated, and the work tasks available. Reasons for testing include

- determining physiological responses at rest and during **submaximal** or maximal work,
- providing a basis for exercise programming,
- evaluating the effectiveness of one's training program,
- screening for CHD, and
- determining a person's ability to perform a specific work task.

Choosing an appropriate test depends on several factors. People differ in age, fitness level, known health problems, and risks of CHD. Also, financial considerations determine the amount of time that can be devoted to each person (e.g., physician versus fitness professional administering the test) and the work tasks available.

Risks of Cardiorespiratory Fitness Testing

As indicated in chapter 1, the risks associated with exercise testing are quite low. Health professionals should emphasize that the overall CHD risk is greater for those who remain sedentary than for those who take an exercise test and then embark on a regular exercise program (2). This is consistent with evidence showing that low CRF directly relates to a higher risk of heart disease and death (13).

> ### KEY POINT
>
> CRF is an important aspect of quality of life as well as a risk factor for CHD. The ability to use oxygen during exercise is the basis for CRF and can be expressed in $L \cdot min^{-1}$, $ml \cdot kg^{-1} \cdot min^{-1}$, and METs. CRF testing is used for programming exercise, screening for heart disease, and determining a person's ability to do a specific task. The risk of death attributable to exercise testing is very low.

Testing Sequence

A logical sequence for fitness testing (and activities) can be followed when people attend the same fitness center over

Sequence of Testing and Activity Prescription

1. Informed consent
2. Health history
3. Screening
4. Resting cardiovascular tests (e.g., BP) and body composition assessment
5. Submaximal CRF tests
6. Tests for low-back function
7. Beginning of moderate-intensity physical activity program
8. Tests for muscular strength and endurance
9. Maximal CRF tests
10. Activity program revision (including games and sports)
11. Periodic retest and activity revision

time. This sequence progresses from the initial screening to fitness testing and programming, with opportunities for periodic retesting and revision of the program as fitness gains are made. The sequence of testing and activity prescription is shown in the sidebar Sequence of Testing and Activity Prescription. The rest of this section details the process. For people who request fitness testing but are not continually involved with the fitness center, the submaximal and maximal tests are usually part of the same GXT protocol.

Informed Consent

Fitness participants should be informed volunteers. The informed-consent form should clearly describe all of the procedures and potential risks and benefits. Participants should understand that their data are confidential and that they can terminate any test or activity at any time should they feel uncomfortable. They should sign a written informed-consent form after reading a description of the program and having all questions answered. A sample consent form is included in the appendix at the end of this chapter.

Health History

Chapter 2 describes procedures for conducting a health screening and assigning the category of risk based on age, known diseases, and risk factors associated with chronic disease. If you have not already done so, please read chapter 2 to become familiar with the process of making these decisions that affect testing, exercise programming, and referral to medical or allied health personnel.

Screening

We recommended in chapter 2 that individuals undergo regular medical examinations and health screenings and engage in moderate-intensity exercise. Fitness programs must determine whether a person needs medical permis-

sion to begin programs involving vigorous activities. Older adults and people with CHD or other known major health problems must have medical supervision or clearance before embarking on any fitness testing or program that goes beyond moderate-intensity exercise.

In the sidebar Contraindications to Exercise Testing, we list the conditions (absolute contraindications) that ACSM has identified in which the risk of testing outweighs the possible benefits. Other conditions (relative contraindications) may increase the risk of exercise testing; people with these conditions should only be tested if a doctor determines that the need for the test outweighs the potential risk.

Apparently healthy people who have no known major health problems or symptoms can be tested or begin the type of fitness program recommended in this book with minimal risk. Chapter 2 identifies people who need medical clearance for exercising, carefully supervised programs, and educational information about health problems and behaviors.

Resting Measurements

Typical resting tests may include CRF measures (e.g., 12-lead ECG, HR, BP, blood chemistry profile) as well as other fitness variables such as body composition. Evaluation of the ECG by a physician determines whether any abnormalities require further medical attention. People with extreme BP or blood chemistry values (see chapter 2) should also be referred to their physicians.

Submaximal Tests to Estimate Cardiorespiratory Fitness

If the resting tests reflect normal values, then a submaximal test is administered. The submaximal test usually provides the HR and BP responses to various intensities of work ranging from light intensity up to a predetermined point (usually 85% of predicted maximum HR). This test can use

Contraindications to Exercise Testing

Absolute Contraindications

- A recent significant change in the resting ECG suggesting significant ischemia, recent myocardial infarction (MI) (within 2 days), or other acute event
- Unstable angina
- Uncontrolled cardiac dysrhythmias causing symptoms or hemodynamic compromise
- Symptomatic severe aortic stenosis
- Uncontrolled symptomatic heart failure
- Acute pulmonary embolus or pulmonary infarction
- Acute myocarditis or pericarditis
- Suspected or known dissecting aneurysm
- Acute systemic infection accompanied by fever, body aches, or swollen lymph glands

Relative Contraindications[†]

- Left main coronary stenosis
- Moderate stenotic valvular heart disease
- Electrolyte abnormalities (i.e., hypokalemia, hypomagnesemia)
- Severe arterial hypertension (i.e., systolic pressure of >200 mmHg or diastolic pressure of >100 mmHg at rest)
- Tachydysrhythmia or bradydysrhythmia
- Hypertrophic cardiomyopathy and other forms of outflow tract obstruction
- Neuromuscular, musculoskeletal, or rheumatoid disorders that are exacerbated by exercise
- High-degree atrioventricular (AV) block
- Ventricular aneurysm
- Uncontrolled metabolic disease (i.e., diabetes, thyrotoxicosis, myxedema)
- Chronic infectious disease (i.e., mononucleosis, hepatitis, AIDS)
- Mental or physical impairment leading to inability to exercise adequately

[†]Relative contraindications can be superseded if benefits outweigh risks of exercise. In some instances, these individuals can exercise with caution using low-level end points, especially if they are asymptomatic at rest.

Reprinted, by permission, from American College of Sports Medicine, 2010, *ACSM's guidelines for exercise testing and prescription,* 8th ed. (Philadelphia, PA: Lippincott, Williams & Wilkins), 54. Modified from R.J. Gibbons, G.J. Balady, J. Bricker et al., 2002, ACC/AHA 2002 guideline update for exercise testing: A report of the American College of Cardiology/American Heart Association Task Force on Practice Guidelines (Committee on Exercise Testing).

a bench step, cycle ergometer, or treadmill. Once again, if unusual responses to the submaximal test appear, the person is referred for further medical tests. If the results appear normal, then the person begins an activity program at intensities less than those reached on the test (e.g., a person goes to 85% of maximum HR on the test and starts the fitness program at 70%). After the person has become accustomed to regular exercise and appears to be adjusting to fitness activities, a maximal test can be administered.

Submaximal tests also can be used to estimate maximal oxygen uptake by extrapolating HR to a predicted maximum and then using the linear relationship between HR and oxygen uptake to estimate maximal oxygen uptake. Although this estimated maximum is useful for evaluating a person's current CRF status and prescribing or revising

exercise, the estimation involves considerable error (15%). In addition to submaximal CRF, flexibility and muscular strength and endurance (especially for low-back function) are often measured at this stage (see chapters 9 and 10).

Maximal Tests to Estimate or Measure Cardiorespiratory Fitness

If no problems occur up to this point, a maximal test can be administered. Two types of maximal tests are used to estimate CRF: laboratory tests that measure physiological responses (e.g., HR, BP) to increasing workloads and field tests that measure all-out endurance performance tests (e.g., time on a 1 mi, or 1.6 km, run). The results of the maximal test can be used to revise the activity program (i.e., the person's maximal oxygen uptake provides a new basis for selecting fitness activities). The person's measured maximal HR (instead of estimated maximal HR) should be used to determine the target or training HR when it is available (see chapter 11).

Program Modification and Periodic Retests

After the program participant achieves a minimum level of fitness, a wider variety of activities (e.g., games and sports) can be included in the fitness program. All of the fitness tests should be readministered periodically to determine the progress being made and to revise the program in areas where the gains are not as great as desired.

KEY POINT

A logical sequence of steps to follow in fitness testing includes informed consent, health history, screening, resting CRF, submaximal CRF and other tests, moderate-intensity activity prescription, maximal CRF, program modification, and periodic retesting (see the sidebar Sequence of Testing and Activity Prescription).

Field Tests

A variety of field tests can be used to estimate CRF. They are called *field tests* because they require little equipment, can be done just about anywhere, and use the simple activities of walking and running. Because these tests involve running or walking as fast as possible over a set distance, they are not recommended at the start of an exercise program. Instead, participants should complete the graduated walking program before taking the walking test and the graduated jogging program before taking the running test. The walking and jogging programs are found in chapter 22. The graduated nature of the fitness programs allows participants to start at a low, safe level of activity and gradually improve. It is then appropriate to administer an endurance run test to evaluate fitness status.

Field tests rely on the observation that for a person to walk or run at high speeds over long distances, the heart must pump great volumes of oxygen to the muscles. In this way, the average speed maintained in these walk or run tests gives an estimate of CRF. The higher the CRF score, the greater the heart's capacity to transport oxygen. An endurance run of a set distance for a given time or of a set time for a given distance provides information about a person's cardiorespiratory endurance as long as the run is 1 mi (1.6 km) or longer. The advantages of an endurance run test include its moderately high correlation to maximum oxygen uptake, the use of a natural activity, and the large numbers of participants who can be tested

in a short time. The disadvantages of endurance running are that it is difficult to monitor physiological responses, other factors affect the outcome (e.g., motivation, environment), and endurance running cannot be used for graded or submaximal testing.

RESEARCH INSIGHT

Estimating $\dot{V}O_2$max by any of the methods described in this chapter is associated with an inherent error compared with the directly measured $\dot{V}O_2$max. To determine the validity of an exercise test to estimate $\dot{V}O_2$max, investigators must first test large numbers of subjects in the laboratory to measure each subject's $\dot{V}O_2$max. On another day, the investigators may have the subjects complete a distance run for time or a standardized graded treadmill or cycle ergometer test to determine the highest percent grade and speed or work rate that the subject can achieve. That information is then used to develop an equation to predict the measured $\dot{V}O_2$max from the time of the distance run, the last grade and speed achieved on a treadmill test, or the final work rate on the cycle ergometer test.

The predicted value will not usually equal the measured $\dot{V}O_2$max value, and the standard error of estimate (SEE) describes how far off (higher or lower) the predicted value might be from the true value when using the prediction equation. One SEE describes where 68% of the estimates are compared to the true value. If the SEE were 1 ml · kg^{-1} · min^{-1}, then 68% of the predicted $\dot{V}O_2$max values would fall within ±1 ml · kg^{-1} · min^{-1} of the true value. Typically, the SEE is larger than that, approaching 5 ml · kg^{-1} · min^{-1} in some cases (44).

The relatively large standard errors might suggest that these exercise tests have little value, but that is not the case. The tests are reliable, and when the same person takes the same test over time, the change in estimated $\dot{V}O_2$max monitored by the test is a reasonable reflection of improvements in CRF. This can serve as both a motivational and an educational tool when working with fitness clients.

Mile Walk Test

A 1 mi (1.6 km) walk test to predict CRF accommodates individuals of different ages and fitness levels. Follow the steps in the sidebar Steps to Administer the Mile Walk Test to administer the 1 mi walk test.

In this test, the person walks as fast as possible on a measured track, and HR is measured at the end of the mile.

The following equation is used to calculate $\dot{V}O_2max$ (ml $\cdot$ kg^{-1} $\cdot$ min^{-1}):

$$\dot{V}O_2max = 132.853 - 0.0769 \text{ (weight)} - 0.3877 \text{ (age)} + 6.315 \text{ (sex)} - 3.2649 \text{ (time)} - 0.1565 \text{ (HR)},$$

where weight is body weight in pounds, age is in years, sex equals 0 for females and 1 for males, time is in minutes and hundredths of minutes, and HR is in beats per minute. The formula was developed and validated on men and women aged 30 to 69 yr (32), and the SEE is about 5 ml $\cdot$ kg^{-1} $\cdot$ min^{-1} (2, 32).

QUESTION: What is the CRF of a 25-yr-old, 170 lb (77.1 kg) man who walks the mile in 20 min and has an immediate postexercise HR of 140 beats $\cdot$ min^{-1}?

ANSWER:

$$\dot{V}O_2max = 132.853 - 0.0769 \text{ (weight)} - 0.3877 \text{ (age)} + 6.315 \text{ (sex)} - 3.2649 \text{ (time)} - 0.1565 \text{ (HR)} =$$
$$132.853 - 0.0769 (170) - 0.3877 (25) + 6.315 (1)$$
$$3.2649 (20.0) - 0.1565 (140) = 29.2 \text{ ml} \cdot \text{kg}^{-1} \cdot \text{min}^{-1}.$$

To simplify the calculations for this 1 mi (1.6 km) walk test, table 7.1 was generated on the basis of the preceding formula for men weighing 170 lb (77.1 kg) and women weighing 125 lb (56.7 kg). For each 15 lb (6.8 kg) above (or below) these weights, subtract (or add) 1 ml $\cdot$ kg^{-1} $\cdot$ min^{-1}.

To use table 7.1, find the part of the table for the person's sex and age, go across the top until you find the time (to the nearest minute) that person took to walk a mile (1.6 km), and then go down that column until it intersects with the person's postexercise HR (listed on the left side). The number at which the mile time and postexercise HR meet is the CRF value in terms of ml $\cdot$ kg^{-1} $\cdot$ min^{-1}. For example, a 25-yr-old man who walked the mile in 20 min and had a postexercise HR of 140 has an estimated maximal oxygen uptake of 29.2 ml $\cdot$ kg^{-1} $\cdot$ min^{-1}. You can evaluate CRF by comparing that number with the standards presented in table 7.2. In the example of the 25-yr-old man, his maximal oxygen uptake is below the 20th percentile, indicating a considerable need for improvement. This low value places him at a much higher risk for heart disease. The percentile

Steps to Administer the Mile Walk Test

Before Test Day

1. Arrange to have the following elements at the test site:
   - A person to start and read the time from a stopwatch
   - A partner with a watch (with a second hand) for each walker (perhaps with a sheet to mark off laps)
   - A stopwatch for the timer (with a spare ready)
   - A score sheet or scorecard
2. Explain the purpose of the test (i.e., to determine how fast the participants can walk 1 mi [1.6 km], which reflects the endurance of the cardiovascular system).
3. Select and mark off (if needed) a level area for the walk.
4. Explain to people being tested that they are to walk the mile in the fastest time possible. Only walking is allowed, and the goal is to cover the distance as fast as possible.

Test Day

1. Participants warm up with stretching and slow walking.
2. Several people will walk at the same time.
3. Explain the procedure again. Remind the participants not to speed up at the end of the walk but to maintain a fast, steady pace throughout.
4. The timer says, "Ready, go," and starts the stopwatch.
5. Each participant has a partner standing at the start and finish line with a watch with a second hand.
6. The partner counts the laps and tells the participant at the end of each lap how many more laps to walk.
7. The timer calls out the minutes and seconds as each person finishes the mile walk.
8. The partner listens for the time when the walker finishes the mile and records it (to the nearest second) immediately on a scorecard.
9. The walker takes a 10 sec HR immediately after the end of the mile walk, with the partner timing it.

Note: These directions were written for test administration in a class setting; however, this test can be used in a one-on-one setting as well.

TABLE 7.1 Estimated Maximal Oxygen Uptake (ml · kg⁻¹ · min⁻¹) for Men and Women Aged 20 to 69

					MIN · MI⁻¹						
HR	10	11	12	13	14	15	16	17	18	19	20
MEN (20-29)											
120	65.0	61.7	58.4	55.2	51.9	48.6	45.4	42.1	38.9	35.6	32.3
130	63.4	60.1	56.9	53.6	50.3	47.1	43.8	40.6	37.3	34.0	30.8
140	61.8	58.6	55.3	52.0	48.8	45.5	42.2	39.0	35.7	32.5	29.2
150	60.3	57.0	53.7	50.5	47.2	43.9	40.7	37.4	34.2	30.9	27.6
160	58.7	55.4	52.2	48.9	45.6	42.4	39.1	35.9	32.6	29.3	26.1
170	57.1	53.9	50.6	47.3	44.1	40.8	37.6	34.3	31.0	27.8	24.5
180	55.6	52.3	49.0	45.8	42.5	39.3	36.0	32.7	29.5	26.2	22.9
190	54.0	50.7	47.5	44.2	41.0	37.7	34.4	31.2	27.9	24.6	21.4
200	52.4	49.2	45.9	42.7	39.4	36.1	32.9	29.6	26.3	23.1	19.8
WOMEN (20-29)											
120	62.1	58.9	55.6	52.3	49.1	45.8	42.5	39.3	36.0	32.7	29.5
130	60.6	57.3	54.0	50.8	47.5	44.2	41.0	37.7	34.4	31.2	27.9
140	59.0	55.7	52.5	49.2	45.9	42.7	39.4	36.1	32.9	29.6	26.3
150	57.4	54.2	50.9	47.6	44.4	41.1	37.8	34.6	31.3	28.0	24.8
160	55.9	52.6	49.3	46.7	42.8	39.5	36.3	33.0	29.7	26.5	23.2
170	54.3	51.0	47.8	44.5	41.2	38.0	34.7	31.4	28.2	24.9	21.6
180	52.7	49.5	46.2	42.9	39.7	36.4	33.1	29.9	26.6	23.3	20.1
190	51.2	47.9	44.6	41.4	38.1	34.8	31.6	28.3	25.0	21.8	18.5
200	49.6	46.3	43.1	39.8	36.5	33.3	30.0	26.7	23.5	20.2	16.9
MEN (30-39)											
120	61.1	57.8	54.6	51.3	48.0	44.8	41.5	38.2	35.0	31.7	28.4
130	59.5	56.3	53.0	49.7	46.5	43.2	39.9	36.7	33.4	30.1	26.9
140	58.0	54.7	51.4	48.2	44.9	41.6	38.4	35.1	31.8	28.6	25.3
150	56.4	53.1	49.9	46.6	43.3	40.1	36.8	33.5	30.3	27.0	23.8
160	54.8	51.6	48.3	45.0	41.8	38.5	35.2	32.0	28.7	25.5	22.2
170	53.3	50.0	46.7	43.5	40.2	36.9	33.7	30.4	27.1	23.9	20.6
180	51.7	48.4	45.2	41.9	38.6	35.4	32.1	28.8	25.6	22.3	19.1
190	50.1	46.9	43.6	40.3	37.1	33.8	30.5	27.3	24.0	20.8	17.5
WOMEN (30-39)											
120	58.2	55.0	51.7	48.4	45.2	41.9	38.7	35.4	32.1	28.9	25.6
130	56.7	53.4	50.1	46.9	43.6	40.4	37.1	33.8	30.6	27.3	24.0
140	55.1	51.8	48.6	45.3	42.1	38.8	35.5	32.3	29.0	24.7	22.5
150	53.5	50.3	47.0	43.8	40.5	37.2	34.0	30.7	27.4	24.2	20.9
160	52.0	48.7	45.4	42.2	38.9	35.7	32.4	29.1	25.9	22.6	19.3
170	50.4	47.1	43.9	40.6	37.4	34.1	30.8	27.6	24.3	21.0	17.8
180	48.8	45.6	42.3	39.1	35.8	32.5	29.3	26.0	22.7	19.5	16.2
190	47.3	44.0	40.8	37.5	34.2	31.0	27.7	24.4	21.2	17.9	14.6
MEN (40-49)											
120	57.2	54.0	50.7	47.4	44.2	40.9	37.6	34.4	31.1	27.8	24.6
130	55.7	52.4	49.1	45.9	42.6	39.3	36.1	32.8	29.5	26.3	23.0
140	54.1	50.8	47.6	44.3	41.0	37.8	34.5	31.2	28.0	24.7	21.4
150	52.5	49.3	46.0	42.7	39.5	36.2	32.9	29.7	26.4	23.1	19.9
160	51.0	47.7	44.4	41.2	37.9	34.6	31.4	28.1	24.8	21.6	18.3
170	49.4	46.1	42.9	39.6	36.3	33.1	29.8	26.5	23.3	20.0	16.7
180	47.8	44.6	41.3	38.0	34.8	31.5	28.2	25.0	21.7	18.4	15.2

(continued)

TABLE 7.1 *(continued)*

	MIN · MI⁻¹										

HR	10	11	12	13	14	15	16	17	18	19	20
WOMEN (40-49)											
120	54.4	51.1	47.8	44.6	41.3	38.0	34.8	31.5	28.2	25.0	21.7
130	52.8	49.5	46.3	43.0	39.7	36.5	33.2	29.9	26.7	23.4	20.1
140	51.2	48.0	44.7	41.4	38.2	34.9	31.6	28.4	25.1	21.8	18.6
150	49.7	46.4	43.1	39.9	36.6	33.3	30.1	26.8	23.5	20.3	17.0
160	48.1	44.8	41.6	38.3	35.0	31.8	28.5	25.2	22.0	18.7	15.5
170	46.5	43.3	40.0	36.7	33.5	30.2	26.9	23.7	20.4	17.2	13.9
MEN (50-59)											
120	53.3	50.0	46.8	43.5	40.3	37.0	33.7	30.5	27.2	23.9	20.7
130	51.7	48.5	45.2	42.0	38.7	35.4	32.2	28.9	25.6	22.4	19.1
140	50.2	46.9	43.7	40.4	37.1	33.9	30.6	27.3	24.1	20.8	17.5
150	48.6	45.4	42.1	38.8	35.6	32.3	29.0	25.8	22.5	19.2	16.0
160	47.1	43.8	40.5	37.3	34.0	30.7	27.5	24.2	20.9	17.7	14.4
170	45.5	42.2	39.0	35.7	32.4	29.2	25.9	22.6	19.4	16.1	12.8
WOMEN (50-59)											
120	50.5	47.2	43.9	40.7	37.4	34.1	30.9	27.6	24.3	21.1	17.8
130	48.9	45.6	42.4	39.1	35.8	32.6	29.3	26.0	22.8	19.5	16.2
140	47.3	44.1	40.8	37.5	34.3	31.0	27.7	24.5	21.2	17.9	14.7
150	45.8	42.5	39.2	36.0	32.7	29.4	26.2	22.9	19.6	16.4	13.1
160	44.2	40.9	37.7	34.4	31.1	27.9	24.6	21.3	18.1	14.8	11.5
170	42.6	39.4	36.1	32.8	29.6	26.3	23.0	19.8	16.5	13.2	10.0
MEN (60-69)											
120	49.4	46.2	42.9	39.6	36.4	33.1	29.8	26.6	23.3	20.0	16.8
130	47.9	44.6	41.3	38.1	34.8	31.5	28.3	25.0	21.7	18.5	15.2
140	46.3	43.0	39.8	36.5	33.2	30.0	26.7	23.4	20.2	16.9	13.6
150	44.7	41.5	38.2	34.9	31.7	28.4	25.1	21.9	18.6	15.3	12.1
160	43.2	39.9	36.6	33.4	30.1	26.8	23.6	20.3	17.0	13.8	10.5
WOMEN (60-69)											
120	46.6	43.3	40.0	36.8	33.5	30.2	27.0	23.7	20.5	17.2	13.9
130	45.0	41.7	38.5	35.2	31.9	28.7	25.4	22.2	18.9	15.6	12.4
140	43.4	40.2	36.9	33.6	30.4	27.1	23.8	20.6	17.3	14.1	10.8
150	41.9	38.6	35.3	32.1	28.8	25.5	22.3	19.0	15.8	12.5	9.2
160	40.3	37.0	33.8	30.5	27.2	24.0	20.7	17.5	14.2	10.9	7.7

Note: Calculations assume 170 lb (77.1 kg) for men and 125 lb (56.7 kg) for women. For each 15 lb (6.8 kg) beyond these values, subtract 1 ml · kg⁻¹ · min⁻¹. HR = heart rate.

Based on Kline et al. 1987.

values in table 7.2 provide reference points for comparison with members of a group. However, the client is best served by using the value as a reference point for personal change when an exercise program is introduced (see appendix E).

Jog or Run Test

One of the most common CRF field tests is the 12 min or 1.5 mi (2.4 km) run popularized by Cooper (18). This test is similar to the walk test mentioned previously: Participants jog or run as fast as possible for 12 min or for 1.5 mi (2.4

km). This test is based on work by Balke (10), who showed that 10 to 20 min running tests could be used to estimate $\dot{V}O_2$max. Balke found the optimal duration for the run test to be 15 min. The test relies on the relationship between running velocity and the oxygen uptake required to run at that velocity (figure 7.1). The greater the running speed, the greater the oxygen uptake required. The reason for the duration of 12 to 15 min is that the running test has to be long enough to diminish the contribution of anaerobic energy (immediate and short-term sources of energy) to the average velocity. The average velocity that can be maintained in a 5 or 6 min run overestimates $\dot{V}O_2$max because anaerobic energy sources contribute substantially to total energy production in a 5 min run compared with a 12 to 15 min run. If the run lasts too long, the person is not able to run close to 100% of $\dot{V}O_2$max and the estimate is too low (figure 7.2).

The $\dot{V}O_2$ associated with a specific running speed can be calculated from the following formula (see chapter 6 for details):

$$\dot{V}O_2 = \text{horizontal velocity (m} \cdot \text{min}^{-1}) \cdot$$
$$\frac{0.2\ \text{ml} \cdot \text{kg}^{-1} \cdot \text{min}^{-1}}{(\text{m} \cdot \text{min}^{-1})} + 3.5\ \text{ml} \cdot \text{kg}^{-1} \cdot \text{min}^{-1}$$

These estimates are reasonable for adults who jog or run the entire 12 min or 1.5 mi (2.4 km). The formula underestimates $\dot{V}O_2$max in children because they have a higher oxygen cost of running (21). In contrast, the formula overestimates $\dot{V}O_2$max in trained runners because of their better running economy (20) and in those who walk the test because the net oxygen cost of walking is half that of running (see chapter 6).

QUESTION: A 20-yr-old woman takes the Cooper 12 min run test following a 15 wk walk and jog program and completes 6 laps on a 440 yd (402.3 m) track. What is her $\dot{V}O_2$max?

ANSWER:

$$402.3\ \text{m} \cdot \text{lap}^{-1} \cdot 6\ \text{laps} = 2{,}414\ \text{m, and}$$
$$2{,}414\ \text{m} \div 12\ \text{min} = 201\ \text{m} \cdot \text{min}^{-1},\ \text{so}$$
$$\dot{V}O_2 = 201\ \text{m} \cdot \text{min}^{-1} \cdot \frac{0.2\ \text{ml} \cdot \text{kg}^{-1} \cdot \text{min}^{-1}}{(\text{m} \cdot \text{min}^{-1})} +$$
$$3.5\ \text{ml} \cdot \text{kg}^{-1} \cdot \text{min}^{-1}$$
$$\dot{V}O_2\text{max} = 40.2 + 3.5 = 43.7\ \text{ml} \cdot \text{kg}^{-1} \cdot \text{min}^{-1}.$$

Applying the 12 Min Run Test

The advantage of the 12 min run is that it can be used to regularly evaluate CRF without expensive equipment. It is easily adapted to cyclists and swimmers, who can evaluate their CRF progress by determining how far they can ride or swim in 12 min. Although no equations exist that relate cyclists' and swimmers' respective performances to $\dot{V}O_2$max, participants can personally judge their current CRF and improvement attributable to training by monitoring the distance they can cover in 12 min.

As Cooper (18) and others agree, an endurance run should not be used for testing CRF at the beginning of an exercise program. A person new to exercise should progress through the walking and jogging programs (see chapter 22) to make fitness improvements before taking an endurance run test.

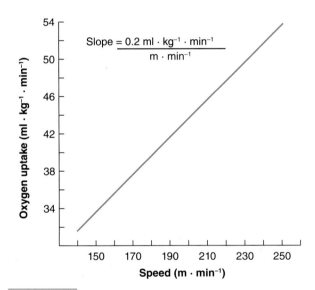

FIGURE 7.1 Relationship between steady-state oxygen uptake and running speed (15).

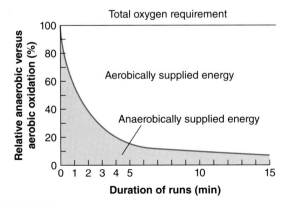

FIGURE 7.2 The relative role of aerobic and anaerobic energy sources in best-effort runs of various durations.
Reprinted from Balke 1963.

KEY POINT

A 1 mi (1.6 km) walking test can be used to estimate CRF. The time of the walk and the HR measured at the end of the walk are used to calculate $\dot{V}O_2$max. A 1.5 mi (2.4 km) run test also can be used to estimate CRF. The time for the 1.5 mi (2.4 km) is used to determine average velocity, and a formula (see chapter 4) is used to calculate $\dot{V}O_2$max.

Canadian Aerobic Fitness Test

In contrast to the Cooper 1.5 mi (2.4 km) run test and the 1 mi (1.6 km) walk test, which require an all-out effort, the Canadian Aerobic Fitness Test (CAFT) is a submaximal field test. Originally called the *Canadian Home Fitness Test*, it uses the lowest two 8 in. (20.3 cm) steps found in a

Progressive Aerobic Cardiovascular Endurance Run (PACER)

An alternative CRF field test is the Progressive Aerobic Cardiovascular Endurance Run, or PACER. This test, developed by Leger et al. (34, 35), is a 20 m shuttle run test done to the sound of a beep as the individual moves between the boundary lines. The speed required at the start is 5.3 mi · hr⁻¹ (8.5 km · hr⁻¹) and it increases 0.3 mi · hr⁻¹ (0.5 km · hr⁻¹) with each level. Three rapid beeps signal progression to the next level, where the time between beeps becomes shorter. The test is terminated when the individual cannot keep up with the beeps, and the number of 20 m laps completed is used to estimate CRF. The PACER test is part of the fitness testing battery in the Fitnessgram, developed by the Cooper Institute (see www.fitnessgram.net for more information) (19). Criterion-referenced standards for CRF (see chapter 15) have been validated for this test (17). This protocol has also been used to estimate $\dot{V}O_2$max in adults (39, 51); however, a practice trial may be needed to establish a stable baseline to use as a reference for monitoring changes over time (33).

conventional staircase in a home (9). The stepping cadence (6 counts per step cycle) is maintained by an audio tape. Before the test, participants complete the PAR-Q (see chapter 2) to determine if they should proceed. In the CAFT, the first stage of the test requires the person to step for 3 min at a rate equivalent to 65% to 70% of the average $\dot{V}O_2$max of the next oldest age group (remember, $\dot{V}O_2$max generally decreases with age). An immediate 10 sec recovery pulse is counted between 5 and 15 sec postexercise, and if it does not exceed the maximum allowable, another 3 min step test at 65% to 70% of the average $\dot{V}O_2$max of the person's own age group is completed. Based on the HR response and the final stage of the test completed, fitness could be classified as undesirable, minimum, and recommended. However, when HR is measured (not palpated) for greater accuracy, as would be done in a laboratory, $\dot{V}O_2$max can be estimated from the CAFT results (31).

The CAFT has been done by millions of people with few problems (49); however, concerns have been raised about the accuracy of the test as an estimate of $\dot{V}O_2$max, especially in fit subjects (53). In 1993, Weller et al. (54) provided a modified version of the CAFT (mCAFT) to address these concerns. One of the primary changes was to have the subjects work until they achieved a HR of 85% of age-predicted maximal HR (220 – age). The other was to add two more stages to challenge the most-fit subjects.

The improved prediction equation was validated in a later study (55), with a SEE of 6 ml · kg⁻¹ · min⁻¹. However, as with all submaximal GXTs, the simple HR response to the last stage of the test, independent of its conversion to a $\dot{V}O_2$max value, can be used to educate and motivate clients, one of the original intents of the CAFT (47, 48, 50). Details and materials for the administration of this test can be obtained at www.csep.ca.

Table 7.2 lists percentile values for maximal aerobic power. The table takes age and sex into consideration. For example, a 20-yr-old woman who ran 6 laps in the 12 min run and had an estimated $\dot{V}O_2$max of 43.7 ml · kg⁻¹ · min⁻¹ is just short of the 80th percentile, possessing good CRF. Encourage participants to achieve and maintain healthy levels of CRF. Blair et al. (13) found that values of 9 METs (31.5 ml · kg⁻¹ · min⁻¹) for women and 10 METs (35 ml · kg⁻¹ · min⁻¹) for men were associated with low risks of chronic disease and death from all causes. If people are not at that level, help them make small, systematic progress toward that goal by using the walking and jogging programs in chapter 22.

Administrating an Endurance Run Test

The 1 mi (1.6 km) run is used in many youth fitness programs (19, 45). The steps to administering this run are listed in the sidebar Steps to Administer the Mile Run.

TABLE 7.2 Percentile Values for Maximal Oxygen Uptake

AGE	20-29		30-39		40-49		50-59		60-69		70-79	
Rating (percentile)	M	W	M	W	M	W	M	W	M	W	M	W
Superior (95th)	56	50	54	47	53	45	50	40	46	37	42	37
Excellent (80th)	51	44	48	41	47	39	43	35	40	32	36	30
Good (60th)	46	40	44	37	42	35	38	31	35	29	31	27
Average (50th)	44	37	42	35	40	33	37	30	33	28	29	25
Fail (40th)	42	36	41	34	38	32	35	29	31	27	28	24
Poor (20th)	38	32	37	30	35	28	31	26	27	24	24	21

Values are in ml · kg⁻¹ · min⁻¹ and are rounded to nearest whole number. M = men; W = women.

Based on tables in *ACSM's guidelines for exercise testing and prescription* that were provided by the Cooper Institute.

They can be used for other endurance runs (e.g., 1.5 mi or 12 min run); the 1 mi (1.6 km) run is used as an example.

Graded Exercise Tests

Many fitness programs use **graded exercise tests (GXTs)** to evaluate CRF. These multilevel tests can be administered with a bench, cycle ergometer, or treadmill.

Bench Step

Bench stepping is very economical and can be used for both submaximal and maximal testing. The disadvantages include the limited number of stages that can be included for any one bench height and individual fitness level and the difficulty of taking certain measurements during the test (e.g., BP). The oxygen costs for stepping at various rates on steps of various heights are presented in chapter 6.

Cycle Ergometer

Cycle ergometers are portable, moderately priced work instruments that allow easy measurement of HR and BP because the participant's upper body is essentially stationary. Their disadvantages, however, are that the exercise load is self-paced and that fatigued leg muscle may be a limiting factor. On mechanically braked cycle ergometers such as the Monark models, altering the pedal rate or the resistance on the flywheel changes the work rate. Generally, the pedal rate is constant during a GXT at a rate appropriate to the person being tested: 50 to 60 rev · min⁻¹ for those of low to average fitness and 70 to 100 rev · min⁻¹ for highly fit and competitive cyclists (27). A metronome or some other source of feedback such as a speedometer helps the person maintain the pedal rate. The resistance (load) on the wheel is increased sequentially to systematically overload the cardiovascular system. The starting work rate and the

---

Steps to Administer the Mile Run

Before Test Day

1. Arrange to have the following elements at the test site:
   - A person to start and read the time from a stopwatch
   - A partner for each runner (perhaps with a sheet to mark off laps)
   - A stopwatch for the tester (with a spare ready)
   - A score sheet or scorecard
2. Explain the purpose of the test (i.e., to determine how fast participants can run 1 mi [1.6 km], which reflects the endurance of the cardiovascular system).
3. Do not administer the test until participants have had several fitness sessions, including some with running.
4. Have participants practice running at a set submaximal pace for 1 lap, then 2, and so on, several times before the test day.
5. Select and mark off (if needed) a level area for the run.
6. Explain to people being tested that they are to run the mile in the fastest time possible. Walking is allowed, but the goal is to cover the distance as quickly as possible.

Test Day

1. Participants warm up with stretching, walking, and slow jogging.
2. Several people will run at the same time.
3. Explain the procedure again.
4. The timer says, "Ready, go," and starts the stopwatch.
5. Each participant has a partner with a watch with a second hand.
6. The partner counts the laps and tells the participant at the end of each lap how many more laps to run.
7. The timer calls out the minutes and seconds as the runner finishes the mile run.
8. The partner listens for the time when the runner finishes the mile and records it (to the nearest second) immediately on a scorecard.
9. The runner continues to walk 1 lap after finishing the run.

increment from one stage to the next depend on the fitness of the person being tested and the purpose of the test. $\dot{V}O_2$ can be estimated from a formula (2) that gives reasonable estimates of $\dot{V}O_2$ up to work rates of about 1,200 kgm · min^{-1} or 200 W (see chapter 6 for details):

$$\dot{V}O_2 \ (ml \cdot kg^{-1} \cdot min^{-1}) = (work\ rate\ [kgm \cdot min^{-1}] \cdot 1.8\ ml\ O_2 \cdot kgm^{-1}) \div body\ weight\ (kg) + 7\ ml \cdot kg^{-1} \cdot min^{-1}, or$$

$$\dot{V}O_2 \ (ml \cdot kg^{-1} \cdot min^{-1}) = (work\ rate\ [W] \cdot 10.8\ ml\ O_2 \cdot W^{-1}) \div body\ weight\ (kg) + 7\ ml \cdot kg^{-1} \cdot min^{-1}.$$

The cycle ergometer differs from the treadmill in that the seat supports the body weight and the work rate depends primarily on pedal rate and the load on the wheel. This means that the relative $\dot{V}O_2$ at any work rate is higher for a smaller person than for a bigger person.

QUESTION: What is the MET value for two individuals, one weighing 60 kg and the other 90 kg, who exercise at the same work rate (900 kgm · min^{-1}) on a cycle ergometer?

ANSWER:
For the 60 kg subject,

$$\dot{V}O_2 \ (ml \cdot kg^{-1} \cdot min^{-1})$$
$$= (900\ kgm \cdot min^{-1} \cdot 1.8\ ml\ O_2 \cdot kgm^{-1})$$
$$\div 60\ kg + 7\ ml \cdot kg^{-1} \cdot min^{-1}, and$$
$$\dot{V}O_2 \ (ml \cdot kg^{-1} \cdot min^{-1}) = 34\ ml \cdot kg^{-1} \cdot min^{-1}, or\ 9.7\ METs.$$

For the 90 kg subject,

$$\dot{V}O_2 \ (ml \cdot kg^{-1} \cdot min^{-1})$$
$$= (900\ kgm \cdot min^{-1} \cdot 1.8\ ml\ O_2 \cdot kgm^{-1})$$
$$\div 90\ kg + 7\ ml \cdot kg^{-1} \cdot min^{-1}, and$$

$$\dot{V}O_2 \ (ml \cdot kg^{-1} \cdot min^{-1}) = 25\ ml \cdot kg^{-1} \cdot min^{-1}, or\ 7.1\ METs.$$

In addition, the increments in the work rate demand a fixed increase in the $\dot{V}O_2$ (e.g., an increment of 150 kgm · min^{-1} equals a $\dot{V}O_2$ change of 270 ml · min^{-1}), forcing the small or unfit subject to make cardiovascular adjustments greater than those of a large or highly fit subject. As we will see, these factors are considered in selecting work rates for a cycle ergometer test used to evaluate CRF. Table 7.3 summarizes how differences in body weight affect the metabolic responses to weight-supported (e.g., cycle ergometry) and weight-carrying (e.g., bench stepping, jogging) work tasks. Thus, for tasks in which body weight provides the resistance (weight-carrying tasks), a larger person achieves a greater absolute $\dot{V}O_2$ (L · min^{-1}) than a smaller person achieves, but both work at the same MET level. In cycling (a weight-supported task), the two people achieve a similar absolute $\dot{V}O_2$, but the larger person has a lower MET level.

Treadmill

Treadmill protocols are very reproducible because they set the pace for the subject, whereas the subject may go too slow or too fast on the bench step or the cycle ergometer. Treadmill tests can accommodate people of any fitness level and use the natural activities of walking and running, with the running tests placing the greatest potential load on the cardiovascular system. Treadmills, however, are expensive, are not portable, and make some measurements (e.g., BP and blood sampling) difficult. The type of treadmill test influences the measured $\dot{V}O_2$max, with the graded running test giving the highest value, the running test at 0% grade giving the next highest value, and the walking test giving the lowest value (8, 38).

To estimate $\dot{V}O_2$ by varying grade and speed, the grade and speed settings on the treadmill must be calibrated correctly (see details on how to calibrate a treadmill and other equipment at the end of this chapter). Further, the subject cannot hold onto the treadmill railing during the test if the estimated $\dot{V}O_2$ values are going to be correct. For example, it was observed that HR decreased 17 beats · min^{-1} when a subject who was walking on a treadmill at 3.4 mi · hr^{-1} (5.5 km · hr^{-1}) and at a 14% grade held onto the treadmill railing (6). Holding onto the railing results in an overestimation of the $\dot{V}O_2$max because the HR is lower at any stage of the test and so the test lasts longer. With the

TABLE 7.3 Work Differences Based on Body Weight in Work Tasks

Work task	$\dot{V}O_2$MAX		Total work (kcal)	METs
	L · min^{-1}	ml · kg^{-1} · min^{-1}		
A heavier person will respond with the following differences compared with a lighter person when both are doing the same task at the same rate.				
Bench	↑	=	↑	=
Walk	↑	=	↑	=
Jog	↑	=	↑	=
Bodyweight-supported cycle	=	↓	=	↓

MET = metabolic equivalent.

treadmill test, there is no need to adjust the $\dot{V}O_2$ calculation for differences in body weight because the person being tested carries her own weight; therefore, the $\dot{V}O_2$ (ml $\cdot$ kg^{-1} $\cdot$ min^{-1}) is independent of body weight (40).

KEY POINT

CRF can be determined with bench stepping, cycle ergometers, or treadmills. The oxygen uptake values (expressed in ml $\cdot$ kg^{-1} $\cdot$ min^{-1}) are similar for most adults at specific stages of a treadmill or step test because the energy cost is proportional to body weight, which is carried by the test participant. In contrast, the absolute oxygen uptake (expressed in L $\cdot$ min^{-1}) is similar for most adults at each stage of a cycle ergometer test; however, the relative oxygen cost (ml $\cdot$ kg^{-1} $\cdot$ min^{-1}) is higher for lighter participants.

Common Variables Measured During a Graded Exercise Test

The variables commonly measured for resting and submaximal tests include HR, BP, and RPE. For maximal testing, $\dot{V}O_2$ max and the final stage achieved on a GXT are often measured.

Heart Rate

Heart rate (HR) often is used as a fitness indicator at rest and during a standard submaximal-work task. Maximal HR is useful for determining the THR for fitness workouts (see chapter 11), but it is not a good fitness indicator because it changes very little with training. Table 7.4 summarizes how endurance training affects HR in various situations.

When an ECG is recorded, the HR can be taken from the ECG strip (see chapter 25). Without an ECG, HR can be taken with an HR watch, a stethoscope, or manual palpation of an artery at the wrist or neck. HR watches are accurate and are the easiest way to measure HR. When

TABLE 7.4 Effects of Endurance Training on Heart Rate

Condition	Effects of fitness on HR
Rest	↓
Standard submaximal work (same external work rate)	↓
Maximal work	No change
Set % of maximal	No change

HR = heart rate.

palpating, fingers (not the thumb) should be used, preferably at the wrist (radial artery). Taking the HR at the neck (carotid artery) requires caution because applying too much pressure can trigger a reflex that slows the HR. Reliable measures are obtained, however, when people are trained in this procedure (43). The HR at rest or during steady-state exercise should be taken for 30 sec for higher reliability. When HR is taken after exercise, measurement should begin soon after exercise ends (e.g., within 5 sec) and should be taken for 10 or 15 sec because the HR changes so rapidly. The 10 or 15 sec rate is multiplied by 6 or 4, respectively, to calculate beats per minute. For example, if a 10 sec postexercise HR is 20 beats $\cdot$ min^{-1}, the HR is 120 beats $\cdot$ min^{-1} (6 $\cdot$ 20).

Blood Pressure

SBP and DBP are often determined at rest, during work, and after work. Proper cuff size (in which the bladder overlaps two-thirds of the arm) and a sensitive stethoscope are required to get accurate values at rest and during work. At rest, the person should have both feet flat on the floor and be in a relaxed position with the arm supported. The cuff should be wrapped securely around the arm at heart level, usually with the tube on the inside of the arm. The stethoscope should be below (not under) the cuff; placement depends on where the sound can be most easily heard, often toward the inside of the arm (24). The first and fourth Korotkoff sounds (the first sound heard and the sound when the tone changes or becomes muffled) should be used for SBP and DBP, respectively, during exercise. The fifth Korotkoff sound (disappearance of sound) is used to classify BP at rest (2).

Rating of Perceived Exertion

Borg introduced the **rating of perceived exertion (RPE)**, that is, how hard a client or patient perceives the exercise to be, using a scale from 6 to 20 (roughly based on resting to maximal HR, i.e., 60-200 beats $\cdot$ min^{-1}) (14). For many years the Borg Rating of Perceived Exertion (RPE) scale has been used to judge the degree of effort (intensity) experienced during an exercise test or an exercise session. For example, using the classic 6-20 scale, the intensity (of effort) can be classified in the following way (see also table 11.2):

- Very light <10
- Light 10-11
- Moderate 12-13
- Vigorous 14-16
- Very hard 17-19
- Maximal 20

The RPE scale can be used with a GXT to provide useful information during the test as the person approaches exhaustion and to serve as a reference for exercise prescription. In the latter case, RPE values of 12-13 are taken as moderate-intensity physical activity and 14-16 as vigorous or hard physical activity. We will see more on how to use the RPE scale in exercise prescriptions in chapter 11. When administering the RPE scale during a GXT, we recommend that fitness professionals provide the following instructions (1, p. 78):

> During the exercise test we want you to pay close attention to how hard you feel the exercise work rate is. This feeling should reflect your total amount of exertion and fatigue, combining all sensations and feelings of physical stress, effort, and fatigue. Don't concern yourself with any one factor such as leg pain, shortness of breath, or exercise intensity, but try to concentrate on your total, inner feeling of exertion. Try not to underestimate or overestimate your feelings of exertion; be as accurate as you can.

Estimating Versus Measuring Functional Capacity ($\dot{V}O_2$max)

Functional capacity is defined as the highest work rate (oxygen uptake) reached in a GXT during which HR, BP, and ECG responses are within the normal range for heavy work. For cardiac patients, the highest work rate normally does not reflect the maximal capacity of their cardiorespiratory systems because the GXT might be stopped for ECG changes, angina, claudication pain, and so on. For the apparently healthy person, functional capacity can be called *maximal aerobic power* or *maximal oxygen uptake, or* $\dot{V}O_2$max (see chapter 4 for procedures for measuring oxygen uptake).

Oxygen uptake increases with each stage of the GXT until it reaches its upper limit. At that point, $\dot{V}O_2$ does not increase when the test moves to the next stage; the person's $\dot{V}O_2$max has been reached. Given the complexity and cost of procedures for directly measuring $\dot{V}O_2$max, it is usually estimated with equations relating the stage of the GXT to a specific oxygen uptake.

As discussed in chapter 6, many formulas may be used to estimate oxygen uptake from the stage reached in a GXT. In general, these formulas reasonably estimate $\dot{V}O_2$ if the GXT is suited to the individual. However, if the increments in the GXT stages are too large relative to the person's CRF, or if the time spent at each stage is too short, then the person might not reach the steady-state oxygen requirement associated with that stage (41). Failure to achieve the oxygen requirement for a GXT stage results in overestimating $\dot{V}O_2$ at each stage of the test, with the overestimation growing larger with each stage. The inability to reach the oxygen

requirement is a common problem with people who are less fit (e.g., cardiac patients). This inability suggests that more conservative (i.e., smaller increments between stages) GXT protocols should be used to allow these individuals to reach the oxygen demand at each stage. This problem is explained more completely in chapter 4, and the use of non-steady-state formulas to deal with this concern is presented in chapter 6.

In contrast, shorter stages and larger increments between stages in a GXT can be used if the purpose of the tests is to screen for ECG abnormalities (rather than to estimate $\dot{V}O_2$max). In addition, changes in a participant's CRF over time can be determined by periodically using the same GXT.

> ### KEY POINT
> Common variables measured during a resting or submaximal GXT include HR, BP, and RPE. Oxygen uptake can be measured at each stage of a test and at maximal exertion; however, $\dot{V}O_2$max usually is estimated (using the formulas described in chapter 4) from the final stage achieved during the GXT.

Procedures for Graded Exercise Tests

This section explains how to administer a GXT and uses examples of various testing protocols. Before administering any GXT, the tester should

- calibrate the equipment;
- check supplies and data forms;
- select the appropriate test protocol for the participant;
- obtain informed consent;
- instruct the participant about the task, including the cool-down;
- have the participant practice the task (if needed); and
- check to see that the participant followed pretest instructions.

Because HR, BP, and RPE responses to submaximal work are influenced by several factors, variation in each factor from test to test should be carefully minimized. Some of these factors include

- temperature and relative humidity of the room;
- number of hours of sleep before testing;

- emotional state;
- hydration state;
- medication;
- time of day;
- time since last meal, cigarette smoking, caffeine intake, and exercise; and
- psychological environment of the test (i.e., the participant's comfort level with the surroundings during testing).

Attention to these factors increases the likelihood that changes in HR, BP, or RPE from one test to the next actually reflect changes in physical fitness and physical activity habits. A form such as the Pretest Instructions for a Fitness Test (see form 7.1) helps ensure that the client is ready for testing.

Typical procedures to follow during GXTs are shown in the sidebar Steps to Administering a Graded Exercise Test. A series of end points should be used to stop a GXT (1).

KEY POINT

Equipment for measuring and recording CRF variables should be calibrated and checked for availability before testing. Carefully attending to procedures before and during a test enhances safety and accuracy. The tester should know when to stop a test given certain signs, symptoms, or CRF measurements.

These guidelines are for nondiagnostic testing performed without direct physician involvement or ECG monitoring.

When to Use Submaximal and Maximal Tests

GXTs have been used to evaluate CRF in fitness programs for healthy populations and in the clinical assessment of ischemic heart disease, a condition in which an inadequate blood flow to the heart muscle can alter the ECG. Exercise is used to place a load on the heart to determine the cardiovascular response and to see if the ECG changes (22).

Some controversy has arisen concerning whether to use submaximal or maximal GXTs. On the basis of thousands of exercise stress tests conducted since the mid-1950s, a maximal or sign- and symptom-limited exercise test is generally recommended for finding ischemic heart disease in asymptomatic individuals. Although submaximal exercise tests are not as effective in identifying disease, they are appropriate for making activity recommendations, adjusting the medical regimen, and identifying the need for additional diagnostic tests (2).

When a fitness center is responsible for both fitness testing and the fitness program, the sequence of testing and activity recommended earlier provides the advantages of each while minimizing their disadvantages. The main objection to using maximal tests is that they stress people who have been inactive. Although the health risk of a maximal GXT is very small with adequate screening and qualified testing personnel, the discomfort of performing

---

FORM 7.1   Pretest Instructions for a Fitness Test

Name_____   Test date _____ Time_____

Report to _____

INSTRUCTIONS

Please observe the following:

1. Wear running shoes, shorts, and a loose-fitting shirt.
2. No food, drink (except water), tobacco, or caffeine for 3 hr before test.
3. Minimal physical activity on day of test.

CANCELLATION

If you cannot keep this appointment, please call _____ or _____.

From E.T. Howley and D.L. Thompson, 2012, *Fitness professional's handbook, 6th ed.* (Champaign, IL: Human Kinetics).

Steps to Administering a Graded Exercise Test

1. Greet participant.
2. Obtain consent (oral and written).
3. Record age and measure height and weight. Calculate and record estimated HRmax and 70% to 85% HRmax.
4. Obtain resting HR and BP.
5. Instruct participant on how to do a step test.
   - Instruct participant to step all the way up and all the way down.
   - Tell participant to keep pace with the metronome.

or

Instruct participant in how to use the cycle ergometer.
   - Tell participant to adjust seat height so the knee is slightly flexed when the foot is at the bottom of the pedal swing and parallel to the floor.
   - Instruct participant to keep pace with the metronome.
   - Tell participant not to tightly hold onto the handlebars; tell participant to release hold when BP is taken.

or

Instruct participant in how to walk on the treadmill.
   - Have participant hold onto railing and get the feel of the belt speed by putting one foot on the belt, keeping up with belt speed.
   - Instruct participant to step on, keeping eyes ahead and back straight, and to walk relaxed with arms swinging.
   - Initially, the person can hold on for balance and then touch the railing lightly with just a finger or the back of the hand.

6. Follow test protocol.
   - Advise participant to talk about how he or she feels during the test.
   - Follow criteria for terminating the test.

For fitness evaluations, HR, BP, and RPE are the usual variables measured.

Reprinted, by permission, from E.T. Howley, 1988, The exercise testing laboratory. In *Resource manual for guidelines for exercise testing and prescription*, edited by S.N. Blair et al. (Philadelphia, PA: Lea & Febiger), 406-413.

at maximum exertion without previous conditioning may discourage some people from participating in a fitness program. Objections to the submaximal test include finding fewer abnormal responses to exercise and inaccurately estimating $\dot{V}O_2$max from submaximal data. In a fitness program for apparently healthy people, the objections against giving either maximal or submaximal tests are overcome by administering the submaximal test early in the fitness program and the maximal test after the participant has been involved in regular exercise. Any of the GXT protocols can be used for submaximal or maximal testing—the only difference is the criteria for stopping the test. Either test is stopped if any of the abnormal responses listed in the box General Indications for Stopping an Exercise Test in Low-Risk Adults occur. In the absence of abnormal responses,

KEY POINT

GXT protocols can be used for submaximal tests (early in the testing sequence) or maximal tests (for active people who have reached a minimal fitness level). Submaximal and maximal tests can use the same GXT protocol; however, their criteria for test termination differ. Maximal tests are more effective in identifying ischemic heart disease. Submaximal tests are useful in assessing fitness and are relatively inexpensive to administer. Although the $\dot{V}O_2$max estimated from a submaximal test is not as accurate as that obtained from a maximal test, it is useful in evaluating changes in CRF due to an exercise program.

the submaximal test is usually terminated when the person reaches a certain HR (often 85% of maximum HR), and the maximal test is stopped when the person reaches voluntary exhaustion.

Maximal Exercise Test Protocols

No one GXT protocol is appropriate for all people. The durations, starting points, and increments between stages vary from person to person. Young active people, normal sedentary people, and people with questionable health status should start at 6, 4, and 2 METs, respectively. The same three groups should increase by 2 to 3, 1 to 2, and 0.5 to 1 METs, respectively, for progressive stages of the test. If the test is for comparing CRF at different times, then 1 or 2 min per stage can be used. If it is for predicting $\dot{V}O_2$max, however, the time per stage should be 2 to 3 min. Table 7.5 illustrates how these criteria might be used for a bench, cycle, or treadmill test administered to individuals of different fitness levels.

The following testing protocols are examples of tests used for different populations. The first protocol, shown in table 7.6, could be used with deconditioned subjects, who would start at a very low MET level, walk slowly, and increase 1 MET per 3 min stage (42). The Balke standard protocol (11) could be used for typical inactive adults by having them start at a higher MET level and progress 1 MET per 2 min stage. More active or younger people could be tested on the Bruce protocol (16), which starts at a moderate MET level and goes up 2 or 3 METs per 3 min stage. Unfortunately, some testing centers use the same testing protocol for all people, with the result that the initial stage is often too high or too low and the work increments for each stage are too small or too large for the individual

being tested. Estimating $\dot{V}O_2$max from the final stage of a maximal GXT has a SEE of about 3 ml $\cdot$ kg^{-1} $\cdot$ min^{-1} (44).

Submaximal Exercise Test Protocols

Any GXT protocol can be used for submaximal or maximal testing. The fitness professional typically uses a submaximal GXT to estimate $\dot{V}O_2$max or to simply show how the exercise program changes selected variables. Predicting maximal oxygen uptake from any submaximal test involves substantial error. However, it can provide useful information for estimating a person's functional capacity and for determining the person's fitness category and what exercise programming is most appropriate. The only way to determine a participant's true functional capacity is to measure it during a maximal test. However, submaximal tests are reliable, and changes in HR, BP, and RPE resulting from exercise conditioning make submaximal tests a good mechanism for showing improvements in CRF. Estimation of $\dot{V}O_2$max from submaximal exercise tests has a SEE of about 5 ml $\cdot$ kg^{-1} $\cdot$ min^{-1} (44).

Submaximal Treadmill Test Protocol

The initial stage and rate of progression of the GXT should be selected using the criteria mentioned earlier. In the following example, a Balke standard protocol (3 mi $\cdot$ hr^{-1}, or 4.8 km $\cdot$ hr^{-1}, 2.5% grade increase every 2 min) was used; HR was monitored in the last 30 sec of each stage. The test was terminated at 85% of the age-predicted maximal HR (with the equation 220 − age). Maximal aerobic power was estimated by extrapolating the HR response to the person's estimated maximal HR. Figure 7.3 presents the results of this test with a graph showing the HR response at each work rate. The HR response is rather flat between the 0%

General Indications for Stopping an Exercise Test in Low-Risk Adults*

- Onset of angina or angina-like symptoms
- Drop in SBP of >10 mmHg from baseline BP despite an increase in workload
- Excessive rise in BP: systolic pressure of >250 mmHg or diastolic pressure of >115 mmHg
- Shortness of breath, wheezing, leg cramps, or claudication
- Signs of poor perfusion: light-headedness, confusion, ataxia, pallor, cyanosis, nausea, or cold and clammy skin
- Failure of HR to increase with increased exercise intensity
- Noticeable change in heart rhythm
- Request by subject to stop
- Physical or verbal manifestations of severe fatigue
- Failure of the testing equipment

*Assumes that testing is nondiagnostic and is being performed without direct physician involvement or ECG monitoring.

Reprinted, by permission, from American College of Sports Medicine, 2010, *ACSM's guidelines for exercise testing and prescription*, 8th ed. (Philadelphia, PA: Lippincott, Williams & Wilkins), 83.

TABLE 7.5 Testing Protocol for Various Groups

		BENCH		CYCLE		TREADMILL	
Stage	METs	Height (cm)	Steps · min⁻¹	Work rate (kpm · min⁻¹)	RPM	Speed (km · hr⁻¹)	Grade (%)
INDIVIDUALS WITH QUESTIONABLE HEALTH							
1	2	0	24	0	50	3.2	0
2	3	16	12	150	50	4.8	0
3	4	16	18	300	50	4.8	2.5
4	5	16	24	450	50	4.8	5.0
5	6	16	30	600	50	4.8	7.5
NORMAL SEDENTARY INDIVIDUALS							
1	4	16	18	360	60	4.8	2.5
2	6	16	30	540	60	4.8	7.5
3	7-8	36	18-24	720-900	60	4.8-5.5	10.0
4	9	36	27	900-1,080	60	5.5	12.0
5	10-11	36	30-33	1,080-1,260	60	9.7	0-1.75
YOUNG ACTIVE INDIVIDUALS							
1	6	16	30	630	70	4.8	7.5
2	9	36	27	1,060	70	5.5	12.0
3	12	36	36	1,270	70	9.7	3.5
4	15	50	33	1,900	70	11.3	7.0
5	17	50	39	2,110	70	11.3	11.0

MET = metabolic equivalent.

Reprinted, by permission, from B.D. Franks, 1979, Methodology of the exercise ECG test. In *Exercise electrocardiography: Practical approach,* edited by E.K. Chung (Baltimore, MD: Lippincott, Williams & Wilkins), 46-61.

and 5% grades. This is not uncommon (see the discussion that follows the YMCA test); perhaps the subject is too excited, or perhaps the SV changes are accounting for the changes in cardiac output at these low work rates. The HR response is usually quite linear between 110 beats · min⁻¹ and the subject's 85% HRmax.

To estimate $\dot{V}O_2$max, the procedures of Maritz and colleagues (36) are followed. A line is drawn through the HR points from the 7.5% grade to the final work rate. This line is extended (extrapolated) to the person's estimated maximal HR (183 beats · min⁻¹). A vertical line is dropped from the last point to the baseline to estimate the subject's maximal aerobic power, which in this example is 11.8 METs, or 41.3 ml · kg⁻¹ · min⁻¹. Any formula (e.g., 220 – age) used to estimate maximal HR has a SEE of about 10 beats · min⁻¹. Consequently, this possible inaccuracy influences any estimate of maximal oxygen uptake derived from extrapolating HR to an estimated maximal HR. If this person's true (measured) maximal HR is 173 or 193 beats · min⁻¹, the estimated maximal MET level is 11.0 METs or 12.6 METs, respectively.

Submaximal Cycle Ergometer Test Protocol

The steps in administering submaximal cycle ergometer tests are provided in the sidebar Steps to Administering a Submaximal Cycle Ergometer Test. One of the most common submaximal cycle ergometer protocols (figure 7.4) comes from the *YMCA Fitness Testing and Assessment Manual* (26). This protocol relies on the linear relationship between HR and work rate ($\dot{V}O_2$) that occurs once an HR of approximately 110 beats · min⁻¹ is reached. The test requires the person to complete one more stage beyond the one that induces an HR of 110 beats · min⁻¹. The line describing the HR–work rate relationship is extrapolated to the person's age-predicted maximal HR (as was done for the treadmill protocol) to estimate the person's $\dot{V}O_2$max. Each stage of the test lasts 3 min, unless a person's HR has not yet reached a steady state (there is >5 beats · min⁻¹ difference between 2nd and 3rd min HR). In that case, an extra minute is added to that stage. The pedal rate is maintained at 50 rev · min⁻¹ so that, on a Monark cycle ergometer, a 0.5 kg increase in

TABLE 7.6 Treadmill Protocols for Various Categories

Stage	METs	Speed (km · hr⁻¹)	Grade (%)	Time (min)
DECONDITIONED INDIVIDUALS[a]				
1	2.5	3.2	0	3
2	3.5	3.2	3.5	3
3	4.5	3.2	7	3
4	5.4	3.2	10.5	3
5	6.4	3.2	14	3
6	7.3	3.2	17.5	3
7	8.5	4.8	12.5	3
8	9.5	4.8	15	3
9	10.5	4.8	17.5	3
NORMAL INACTIVE INDIVIDUALS[b]				
1	4.3	4.8	2.5	2
2	5.4	4.8	5	2
3	6.4	4.8	7.5	2
4	7.4	4.8	10	2
5	8.5	4.8	12.5	2
6	9.5	4.8	15	2
7	10.5	4.8	17.5	2
8	11.6	4.8	20	2
9	12.6	4.8	22.5	2
10	13.6	4.8	25	2
YOUNG ACTIVE INDIVIDUALS[c]				
1	5	2.7	10	3
2	7	4	12	3
3	9.5	5.4	14	3
4	13	6.7	16	3
5	16	8	18	3

MET = metabolic equivalent.

[a]From Naughton and Haider 1973. [b]From Balke 1970. [c]From Bruce 1972.

load equals 150 kgm · min⁻¹ (25 W). Seat height is adjusted so that the knee is slightly bent (7) when the pedal is at the bottom of the swing through 1 revolution. The seat height is recorded for future reference. HR is monitored during the latter half of the second and third minutes of each stage.

Selection of the initial work rate and the rate of progression on the cycle ergometer should consider body weight, sex, age, and physical activity level. In general, absolute $\dot{V}O_2max$ (L · min⁻¹) is lower in smaller people; women have lower absolute $\dot{V}O_2max$ values than men; $\dot{V}O_2max$ decreases with age; and inactivity is associated with low $\dot{V}O_2max$ values. The YMCA test addresses body weight, fitness, and so on by starting everyone at 150 kgm · min⁻¹ and using the HR response to that specified work rate to set subsequent stages in the test (see figure 7.4). Large or

fit subjects would have a low HR response to this work rate and would use the most strenuous sequence of work rates (far left boxes in the figure). A small or unfit subject would have a high HR response to the 150 kgm · min⁻¹ work rate and would follow the sequence with the smallest increments in the power output. Subjects should complete only one additional work rate beyond the one demanding an HR of 110 beats · min⁻¹.

The HR values for the second and third minutes of each work rate are recorded, and directions are followed to estimate $\dot{V}O_2max$ in liters per minute. Figure 7.5 presents the YMCA protocol directions and an example of a test for a 50-yr-old woman who weighs 59 kg. The stages followed the pattern dictated by the HR response to the initial work rate of 150 kgm · min⁻¹. A line was drawn through the last two HR values and extrapolated to the estimated maximal HR. A vertical line, dropped from the last point of the extrapolated line to the baseline, estimated the subject's maximal work rate to be 750 kgm · min⁻¹. With the formula described earlier (and in chapter 6) for the cycle ergometer, $\dot{V}O_2max$ for this woman was estimated to be about 30 ml · kg⁻¹ · min⁻¹, or 1.77 L · min⁻¹.

In contrast to the YMCA test, the Åstrand and Rhyming cycle ergometer test (7) requires the subject to complete only one 6 min work rate demanding an HR between 125 and 170 beats · min⁻¹. These investigators observed that for young (18-30 yr) subjects, the average HR was 128 beats · min⁻¹ for males and 138 beats · min⁻¹ for females at 50% $\dot{V}O_2max$, while at 70% $\dot{V}O_2max$ the average HRs were 154 and 164 beats · min⁻¹, respectively. So if you know from an HR response that a person is at 50% $\dot{V}O_2max$ at a work rate equal to 1.5 L · min⁻¹, then you know the estimated $\dot{V}O_2max$ is twice that, or 3.0 L · min⁻¹. Table 7.7 is used to estimate $\dot{V}O_2max$ from the subject's HR response to one 6 min work rate (5).

Using the data from the previous example of the woman taking the YMCA test, we can see how $\dot{V}O_2max$ is estimated in the Åstrand and Rhyming protocol. The 50-yr-old woman had an HR of 140 beats · min⁻¹ at a work rate of 450 kgm · min⁻¹. Using table 7.7, look down the leftmost column of values for women to an HR of 140, and look across to the second column of values (for a work rate of 450 kgm · min⁻¹).

The estimated $\dot{V}O_2max$ is 2.4 L · min⁻¹. Because maximal HR decreases with increasing age, however, and the data in table 7.7 were collected on young subjects, I. and P.-O. Åstrand (4, 5) established the following age-correction factors to correct for the lower maximal HR:

Age	Factor	Age	Factor	Age	Factor
55	0.71	15	1.10	40	0.83
60	0.68	25	1.00	45	0.78
65	0.65	35	0.87	50	0.75

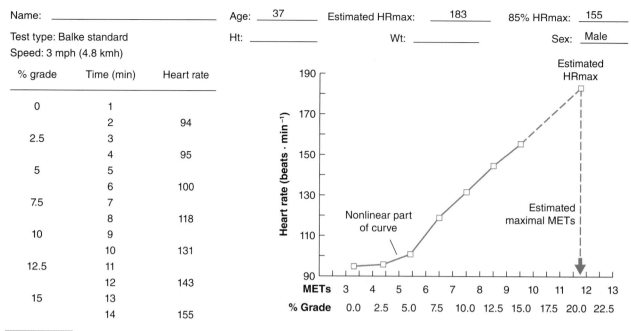

Name: _____	Age: __37__	Estimated HRmax: __183__	85% HRmax: __155__
Test type: Balke standard	Ht: _____	Wt: _____	Sex: __Male__
Speed: 3 mph (4.8 kmh)			

% grade	Time (min)	Heart rate
0	1	
	2	94
2.5	3	
	4	95
5	5	
	6	100
7.5	7	
	8	118
10	9	
	10	131
12.5	11	
	12	143
15	13	
	14	155

FIGURE 7.3 Maximal aerobic power estimated by measuring the HR response to a submaximal GXT on a treadmill.

Steps to Administering a Submaximal Cycle Ergometer Test

1. Complete the pretest items.
2. Select the test protocol.
3. Estimate the participant's HRmax (220 − age = HRmax in beats · min^{-1}).
4. Determine 85% of the participant's HRmax (HRmax · 0.85 = 85% HRmax).
5. Review the procedure with participant.
6. Set and record the seat height (leg should be slightly bent at the knee when the foot is at the bottom of the pedaling stroke).
7. Start the metronome (set at 100 beats · min^{-1} so that one foot is at the bottom of the pedaling stroke on each beat, resulting in 50 complete rev · min^{-1}).
8. Have the participant begin pedaling in rhythm with the metronome.
9. As soon as the correct pace is achieved, set the resistance according to the protocol chosen.
10. Start the timer for the beginning of the 3 min stage.
11. Check the resistance setting (it may drift) and observe the participant for signs or symptoms that require termination of the test.
12. At 1:30 into the stage, measure and record BP and HR.
13. At 2:30, measure and record HR.
14. At 2:50, ask for and record the participant's RPE.
15. At 2:55, ask the participant, "How are you doing?"
16. At 3:00, if HR is less than 85% of HRmax, BP is responding normally, and the participant is all right, increase resistance to the next stage. If the two HR values (from minutes 2 and 3) are not within 5 beats · min^{-1}, the YMCA protocol calls for adding another minute to the stage to obtain a steady-state value.
17. Repeat steps 10 through 16 until the participant reaches 85% of HRmax or there is another reason to stop the test. Go back to stage 1 (for cool-down) and repeat steps 10 through 15, stopping at 3:00 in the cool-down stage.
18. Talk with the participant and check for any problems.

From B.D. Franks and E.T. Howley, 1989, *Fitness leader's handbook* (Champaign, IL: Human Kinetics), 87.

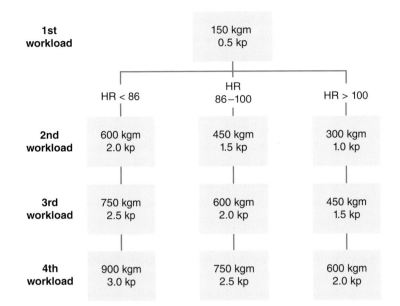

1st workload		150 kgm 0.5 kp		
	HR < 86	HR 86–100	HR > 100	
2nd workload	600 kgm 2.0 kp	450 kgm 1.5 kp	300 kgm 1.0 kp	
3rd workload	750 kgm 2.5 kp	600 kgm 2.0 kp	450 kgm 1.5 kp	
4th workload	900 kgm 3.0 kp	750 kgm 2.5 kp	600 kgm 2.0 kp	

Directions:

1. Set the first workload at 150 kgm · min⁻¹ (0.5 kp).

2. If the HR in the third minute is
   - less than 86, set the second load at 600 kgm (2.0 kp);
   - 86 to 100, set the second load at 450 kgm (1.5 kp);
   - greater than 100, set the second load at 300 kgm (1.0 kp).

3. Set the third and fourth (if required) loads according to the loads in the boxes below the second loads.

FIGURE 7.4 Guide for setting power outputs (workloads) on YMCA submaximal cycle ergometer test.

Name: _____

Sex: _Female_ Age: _50_

Estimated HRmax: _170_ Ht: _____ in. Wt: _____ lb

85% HRmax: _145_ _____ cm _59_ kg

Work rate kpm · min⁻¹	Heart rate 2nd min	3rd min
150	95	96
300		
450	138	140
600	153	154

YMCA Protocol

1. Plot 3rd min HR for each work rate.
2. Draw line though points starting at HR . 110.
3. Extrapolate line to subject's estimated HRmax.
4. Drop vertical line from HRmax to baseline.
5. Record estimated maximal work rate.

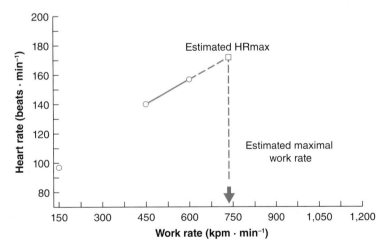

FIGURE 7.5 Maximal aerobic power estimated by measuring the HR response to a submaximal GXT on a cycle ergometer using the protocol from the *YMCA Fitness Testing and Assessment Manual*.

To calculate the corrected $\dot{V}O_2$max, the estimated $\dot{V}O_2$max is multiplied by the appropriate correction factor. For our 50-yr-old subject, the correction factor is 0.75, and the corrected $\dot{V}O_2$max is $0.75 \cdot 2.4$ L $\cdot$ min^{-1} = 1.8 L $\cdot$ min^{-1}. This value compares well with that estimated by the YMCA protocol. The Åstrand and Rhyming calculations can be simplified by using formulas developed by Shephard (46).

Submaximal Step-Test Protocol

A multistage step test can be used to estimate $\dot{V}O_2$max and to show changes in CRF resulting from training or detraining. As always, the initial stage and rate of progression of the stages must be suited to the individual. Table 7.5 presented three examples of step-test protocols. The subject must follow the metronome (4 counts per cycle, i.e., up-up-down-down) and step all the way up and all the way down. Each stage should last at least 2 min, with HR monitored in the last 30 sec of each 2 min.

HR is more difficult to monitor during a step test if the palpation technique is used. An HR watch simplifies the process, but when one is not available, a BP cuff can be used. When an HR measure is needed, pump the cuff

TABLE 7.7 Predicting Maximal Oxygen Uptake From Heart Rate and Workload During a 6 Min Cycle Ergometer Test

	$\dot{V}O_2$MAX (L $\cdot$ MIN^{-1}) VALUES FOR WOMEN						$\dot{V}O_2$MAX (L $\cdot$ MIN^{-1}) VALUES FOR MEN				
HR	300 kgm $\cdot$ min^{-1}	450 kgm $\cdot$ min^{-1}	600 kgm $\cdot$ min^{-1}	750 kgm $\cdot$ min^{-1}	900 kgm $\cdot$ min^{-1}	HR	300 kgm $\cdot$ min^{-1}	600 kgm $\cdot$ min^{-1}	900 kgm $\cdot$ min^{-1}	1,200 kgm $\cdot$ min^{-1}	1,500 kgm $\cdot$ min^{-1}
120	2.6	3.4	4.1	4.8		120	2.2	3.5	4.8		
121	2.5	3.3	4.0	4.8		121	2.2	3.4	4.7		
122	2.5	3.2	3.9	4.7		122	2.2	3.4	4.6		
123	2.4	3.1	3.9	4.6		123	2.1	3.4	4.6		
124	2.4	3.1	3.8	4.5		124	2.1	3.3	4.5	6.0	
125	2.3	3.0	3.7	4.4		125	2.0	3.2	4.4	5.9	
126	2.3	3.0	3.6	4.3		126	2.0	3.2	4.4	5.8	
127	2.2	2.9	3.5	4.2		127	2.0	3.1	4.3	5.7	
128	2.2	2.8	3.5	4.2	4.8	128	2.0	3.1	4.2	5.6	
129	2.2	2.8	3.4	4.1	4.8	129	1.9	3.0	4.2	5.6	
130	2.1	2.7	3.4	4.0	4.7	130	1.9	3.0	4.1	5.5	
131	2.1	2.7	3.4	4.0	4.6	131	1.9	2.9	4.0	5.4	
132	2.0	2.7	3.3	3.9	4.5	132	1.8	2.9	4.0	5.3	
133	2.0	2.6	3.2	3.8	4.4	133	1.8	2.8	3.9	5.3	
134	2.0	2.6	3.2	3.8	4.4	134	1.8	2.8	3.9	5.2	
135	2.0	2.6	3.1	3.7	4.3	135	1.7	2.8	3.8	5.1	
136	1.9	2.5	3.1	3.6	4.2	136	1.7	2.7	3.8	5.0	
137	1.9	2.5	3.0	3.6	4.2	137	1.7	2.7	3.7	5.0	
138	1.8	2.4	3.0	3.5	4.1	138	1.6	2.7	3.7	4.9	
139	1.8	2.4	2.9	3.5	4.0	139	1.6	2.6	3.6	4.8	

| | VO₂MAX (L · MIN⁻¹) VALUES FOR WOMEN | | | | | | VO₂MAX (L · MIN⁻¹) VALUES FOR MEN | | | | |
HR	300 kgm · min⁻¹	450 kgm · min⁻¹	600 kgm · min⁻¹	750 kgm · min⁻¹	900 kgm · min⁻¹	HR	300 kgm · min⁻¹	600 kgm · min⁻¹	900 kgm · min⁻¹	1,200 kgm · min⁻¹	1,500 kgm · min⁻¹
140	1.8	2.4	2.8	3.4	4.0	140	1.6	2.6	3.6	4.8	6.0
141	1.8	2.3	2.8	3.4	3.9	141		2.6	3.5	4.7	5.9
142	1.7	2.3	2.8	3.3	3.9	142		2.5	3.5	4.6	5.8
143	1.7	2.2	2.7	3.3	3.8	143		2.5	3.4	4.6	5.7
144	1.7	2.2	2.7	3.2	3.8	144		2.5	3.4	4.5	5.7
145	1.6	2.2	2.7	3.2	3.7	145		2.4	3.4	4.5	5.6
146	1.6	2.2	2.6	3.2	3.7	146		2.4	3.3	4.4	5.6
147	1.6	2.1	2.6	3.1	3.6	147		2.4	3.3	4.4	5.5
148	1.6	2.1	2.6	3.1	3.6	148		2.4	3.2	4.3	5.4
149		2.1	2.6	3.0	3.5	149		2.3	3.2	4.3	5.4
150		2.0	2.5	3.0	3.5	150		2.3	3.2	4.2	5.3
151		2.0	2.5	3.0	3.4	151		2.3	3.1	4.2	5.2
152		2.0	2.5	2.9	3.4	152		2.3	3.1	4.1	5.2
153		2.0	2.4	2.9	3.3	153		2.2	3.0	4.1	5.1
154		2.0	2.4	2.8	3.3	154		2.2	3.0	4.0	5.1
155		1.9	2.4	2.8	3.2	155		2.2	3.0	4.0	5.0
156		1.9	2.3	2.8	3.2	156		2.2	2.9	4.0	5.0
157		1.9	2.3	2.7	3.2	157		2.1	2.9	3.9	4.9
158		1.8	2.3	2.7	3.1	158		2.1	2.9	3.9	4.9
159		1.8	2.2	2.7	3.1	159		2.1	2.8	3.8	4.8
160		1.8	2.2	2.6	3.0	160		2.1	2.8	3.8	4.8
161		1.8	2.2	2.6	3.0	161		2.0	2.8	3.7	4.7
162		1.8	2.2	2.6	3.0	162		2.0	2.8	3.7	4.6
163		1.7	2.2	2.6	2.9	163		2.0	2.8	3.7	4.6
164		1.7	2.1	2.5	2.9	164		2.0	2.7	3.6	4.5
165		1.7	2.1	2.5	2.9	165		2.0	2.7	3.6	4.5
166		1.7	2.1	2.5	2.8	166		1.9	2.7	3.6	4.5
167		1.6	2.1	2.4	2.8	167		1.9	2.6	3.5	4.4
168		1.6	2.0	2.4	2.8	168		1.9	2.6	3.5	4.4
169		1.6	2.0	2.4	2.8	169		1.9	2.6	3.5	4.3
170		1.6	2.0	2.4	2.7	170		1.8	2.6	3.4	4.3

Reprinted, by permission, from P.-O. Åstrand, 1979, *Work tests with the bicycle ergometer* (Varberg, Sweden: Monark Exercise AB), 24.

Name: _____ Age: __55__ Estimated HRmax: __165__ 85% HRmax: __140__

Step test protocol
Step height = 16 cm

Ht: _____

Wt: _____

Step rate	Heart rate
12	100
18	115
24	128
30	142

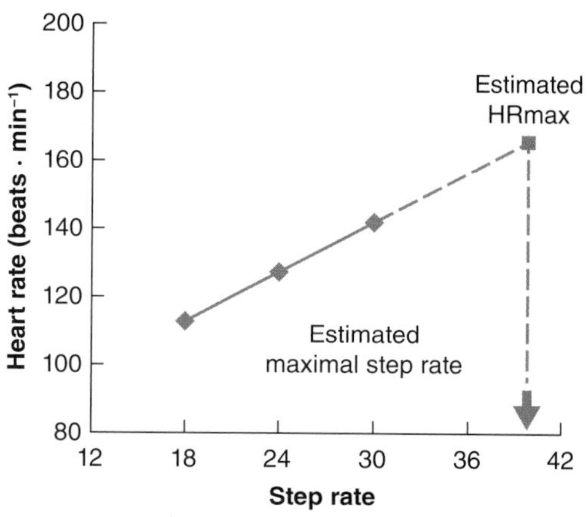

Sex: __Male__

FIGURE 7.6 Maximal aerobic power estimated by measuring HR response to a submaximal graded exercise step test.

up just above diastolic pressure (around 80-100 mmHg). With the stethoscope, count the pulse rate for 15 to 30 sec. Release the pressure after each measurement. An alternative is for the participant to stop stepping after each stage, taking the HR for a 10 sec count 5 sec after completing the stage.

As in most submaximal GXT protocols, HR is plotted against work rate or $\dot{V}O_2$ for each stage, and a line is drawn through the points to the estimated maximal HR. A vertical line is then drawn to the baseline to estimate the step rate that would have been achieved if the subject had completed a maximal test. Figure 7.6 shows the results of a step test for a sedentary 55-yr-old man. His estimated maximal step rate was 40 steps $\cdot$ min^{-1}. The $\dot{V}O_2$max, calculated with the formula for stepping given in chapter 6, was 7.7 METs, or about 27 ml $\cdot$ kg^{-1} $\cdot$ min^{-1}.

KEY POINT

A plot of HR responses (>110 beats $\cdot$ min^{-1}) to a GXT on a treadmill, cycle ergometer, or bench step can be used to estimate $\dot{V}O_2$max. A line is drawn through the HR values and is extrapolated to the subject's age-predicted estimate of maximal HR. A vertical line is drawn to the x-axis to estimate the work rate and $\dot{V}O_2$ the person would have achieved if the test had been a maximal test.

Posttest Procedures

When the test is over, the tester should conduct a cooldown, monitor test variables, and give posttest instructions. The tester should also organize the test data (see Posttest Protocol).

RESEARCH INSIGHT

Can $\dot{V}O_2$max be estimated without doing an exercise test?

This may seem like a strange question given the focus of this chapter on exercise testing. However, if it were possible, it would allow investigators (primarily epidemiologists) to easily classify large numbers of people into CRF categories (e.g., bottom 20%, middle 20%, and top 20%) and determine if CRF is linked to various chronic diseases. Doing exercise testing on such large populations would be impossible due to time, cost, personnel, and so on.

In one of the earliest investigations, Jackson and colleagues (30) showed that by using the simple variables of age, gender, body fatness or BMI, and self-reported physical activity, $\dot{V}O_2$max could be estimated with a SEE of ~5 ml $\cdot$ kg^{-1} $\cdot$ min^{-1}, an error similar to what we observe with field tests and submaximal GXT estimates of $\dot{V}O_2$max. The accuracy of the prediction (SEE ~4-6 ml $\cdot$ kg^{-1} $\cdot$ min^{-1}) has been confirmed in several other studies (25, 28, 37, 52, 56, 57). These models have been useful in placing subjects into fitness categories; however, the prediction is less accurate in the most and least fit subjects (52).

What does this say about doing exercise tests? As we mentioned at the outset, even though the SEE is relatively large for field tests and submaximal GXTs, the tests are reliable, and when the same person takes the same test over time, the change in estimated $\dot{V}O_2$max monitored by the test is a reasonable reflection of improvements in CRF. This can serve as both a motivational and educational tool when working with fitness clients.

Posttest Protocol

1. Use a cool-down as programmed per physician or other guidelines:
   - Have subject sit down or lie down depending on the follow-up tests to be used.
   - Monitor HR, BP, and ECG immediately and after 1, 2, 4, and 6 min.
   - Remove cuff and electrodes when HR and BP are close to pretest value.
2. Provide instructions for showering:
   - Ask subject to wait about 30 min before showering.
   - Ask subject to move around in the shower and use warm (not hot) water. Wait for subject to return from the shower.
3. Organize test data and discuss test results with subject.

Adapted, by permission, from E.T. Howley, 1988, The exercise testing laboratory. In *Resource manual for guidelines for exercise testing and prescription*, edited by S.N. Blair et al. (Philadelphia, PA: Lea & Febiger), 413.

STUDY QUESTIONS

1. What is the general relationship between CRF and chronic disease?
2. What is the logical sequence of steps to take leading up to a GXT?
3. You are using the 1 mi (1.6 km) walk test to track CRF over time, but you are not concerned with generating a $\dot{V}O_2$max value. If you wanted to provide good feedback to your client about fitness improvements being made, what two variables would you measure from this test? What would you expect to happen to them as fitness improves?
4. Why are running tests to estimate $\dot{V}O_2$max usually done for 12 min or so for adults? What would happen to the estimated $\dot{V}O_2$max value if an all-out 3 min run test were used?
5. What are some advantages and disadvantages of cycle ergometer tests compared with treadmill tests?
6. Why are clients asked to not eat, smoke, or drink caffeinated beverages in the hours before a submaximal GXT?
7. What is the difference between a submaximal and maximal GXT?
8. If submaximal GXT protocols have an inherent error associated with estimating $\dot{V}O_2$max, why do the test?
9. What investigators would be interested in estimating $\dot{V}O_2$max without exercise testing?

CASE STUDIES

You can check your answers by referring to appendix A.

1. You are contacted by a fitness club to review the test it uses to evaluate CRF in middle-aged participants. The club requires the participants to perform the 1.5 mi (2.4 km) run test during their first exercise session. The club director says he uses this test because so many data exist for it—the test has been used for more than 10 yr. What is your reaction?
2. You conduct the 1 mi (1.6 km) walk test with a 45-yr-old male client and record the following information: Time = 15 min, HR = 140 beats · min⁻¹, weight = 170 lb (77.1 kg). Calculate and evaluate his estimated $\dot{V}O_2$max.
3. A 50-yr-old male weighing 180 lb (81.7 kg) completes a submaximal GXT on a cycle ergometer, and the following data are obtained:

kgm · min⁻¹	HR	kgm · min⁻¹	HR
300	100	600	125
450	110	750	140

Estimate the subject's $\dot{V}O_2$max using the extrapolation procedure. Express the value in METs.

4. A 30-yr-old woman weighing 120 lb (54.4 kg) completes four stages of a submaximal Balke treadmill test at 3 mi · hr⁻¹ (4.8 km · hr⁻¹), and the following data are obtained:

% Grade	HR	% Grade	HR
2.5	96	7.5	135
5	120	10	150

Estimate the subject's $\dot{V}O_2$max using the extrapolation method and express it in $ml \cdot kg^{-1} \cdot min^{-1}$, $L \cdot min^{-1}$, and METs.

5. A Monark cycle ergometer is calibrated with 0.5, 1.0, 1.5, and 2.0 kg weights, and each of the values is 0.25 kg too high on the scale. What could have caused this?

REFERENCES

1. American College of Sports Medicine (ACSM). 2006. *ACSM's guidelines for exercise testing and prescription.* 7th ed. Philadelphia: Lippincott Williams & Wilkins.

2. American College of Sports Medicine (ACSM). 2010. *ACSM's guidelines for exercise testing and prescription.* 8th ed. Philadelphia: Lippincott Williams & Wilkins.

3. American College of Sports Medicine (ACSM). 2010. *ACSM's resource manual for guidelines for exercise testing and prescription.* 6th ed. Baltimore: Lippincott Williams & Wilkins.

4. Åstrand, I. 1960. Aerobic work capacity in men and women with special reference to age. *Acta Physiologica Scandinavica* 49(Suppl. 169): 1-92.

5. Åstrand, P.-O. 1979. *Work tests with the bicycle ergometer.* Varberg, Sweden: Monark-Crescent AB.

6. Åstrand, P.-O. 1984. Principles of ergometry and their implications in sport practice. *International Journal of Sports Medicine* 5:102-105.

7. Åstrand, P.-O., and I. Rhyming. 1954. A nomogram for calculation of aerobic capacity (physical fitness) from pulse rate during submaximal work. *Journal of Applied Physiology* 7:218-221.

8. Åstrand, P.-O., and B. Saltin. 1961. Maximal oxygen uptake and heart rate in various types of muscular activity. *Journal of Applied Physiology* 16:977-981.

9. Bailey, D.A., R.J. Shephard, and R.L. Mirwald. 1976. Validation of a self-administered home test of cardiorespiratory fitness. *Canadian Journal of Applied Sports Sciences* 1:67-78.

10. Balke, B. 1963. A simple field test for assessment of physical fitness. In *Civil Aeromedical Research Institute report,* 63-66. Oklahoma City: Civil Aeromedical Research Institute.

11. Balke, B. 1970. *Advanced exercise procedures for evaluation of the cardiovascular system* (Monograph). Milton, WI: Burdick.

12. Baum, W.A. 1961. *Sphygmomanometers, principles and precepts.* New York: Baum.

13. Blair, S.N., H.W. Kohl III, R.S. Paffenbarger Jr., D.G. Clark, K.H. Cooper, and L.W. Gibbons. 1989. Physical fitness and all-cause mortality. *Journal of the American Medical Association* 262:2395-2401.

14. Borg, G. 1998. *Borg's perceived exertion and pain scales.* Champaign, IL: Human Kinetics.

15. Bransford, D.R., and E.T. Howley. 1977. The oxygen cost of running in trained and untrained men and women. *Medicine and Science in Sports* 9:41-44.

16. Bruce, R.A. 1972. Multistage treadmill test of submaximal and maximal exercise. In *Exercise testing and training of apparently healthy individuals: A handbook for physicians,* ed. American Heart Association, 32-34. New York: American Heart Association.

17. Chun, D.M., C.B. Corbin, and R.P. Pangrazi. 2000. Validation of criterion-referenced standards for the mile run and progressive aerobic cardiovascular endurance tests. *Research Quarterly for Exercise and Sport* 71:125-134.

18. Cooper, K.H. 1977. *The aerobics way.* New York: Bantam Books.

19. Cooper Institute for Aerobics Research. 1999. *Fitnessgram test administration manual.* Champaign, IL: Human Kinetics.

20. Daniels, J.T. 1985. A physiologist's view of running economy. *Medicine and Science in Sports and Exercise* 17:332-338.

21. Daniels, J., N. Oldridge, F. Nagle, and B. White. 1978. Differences and changes in $\dot{V}O_2$ among young runners 10-18 years of age. *Medicine and Science in Sports* 10:200-203.

22. Ellestad, M. 1994. *Stress testing: Principles and practice.* Philadelphia: Davis.

23. Franks, B.D. 1979. Methodology of the exercise ECG test. In *Exercise electrocardiography: Practical approach,* ed. E.K. Chung, 46-61. Baltimore: Williams & Wilkins.

24. Frohlich, E.D., C. Grim, D.R. Labarthe, M.H. Maxwell, D. Perloff, and W.H. Weidman. 1988. Recommendations for human blood-pressure determination by sphygmomanometers. *Circulation* 77:501A-514A.

25. George, J.D., W.J. Stone, and L.N. Burkett. 1997. Nonexercise $\dot{V}O_2$max estimation for physically active college students. *Medicine and Science in Sports and Exercise* 29:415-423.

26. Golding, L.A. 2000. *YMCA fitness testing and assessment manual.* 4th ed. Champaign, IL: Human Kinetics.

27. Hagberg, J.M., J.P. Mullin, M.D. Giese, and E. Spitznagel. 1981. Effect of pedaling rate on submaximal exercise responses of competitive cyclists. *Journal of Applied Physiology* 51:447-451.

28. Heil, D.P., P.S. Freedson, L.E. Ahlquist, J. Price, and J.M. Rippe. 1995. Nonexercise regression models to estimate

peak oxygen consumption. *Medicine and Science in Sports and Exercise* 27:599-606.

29. Howley, E.T. 1988. The exercise testing laboratory. In *Resource manual for guidelines for exercise testing and prescription,* ed. S.N. Blair, P. Painter, R.R. Pate, L.K. Smith, and C.B. Taylor, 406-413. Philadelphia: Lea & Febiger.

30. Jackson, A.S., S.N. Blair, M.T. Mahar, L.T. Wier, R.M. Ross, and J.E. Stuteville. Prediction of functional aerobic capacity without exercise testing. *Medicine and Science in Sports and Exercise* 22:863-870.

31. Jette, M., J. Campbell, J. Mongeon, and R. Routhier.1976. The Canadian Home Fitness Test as a predictor for aerobic capacity. *Canadian Medical Association Journal* 114:680-682.

32. Kline, G.M., J.P. Porcari, R. Hintermeister, P.S. Freedson, A. Ward, R.F. McCarron, J. Ross, and J.M. Rippe. 1987. Estimation of $\dot{V}O_2$max from a 1-mile track walk, gender, age, and body weight. *Medicine and Science in Sports and Exercise* 19:253-259.

33. Lamb, K.L., and L. Rogers. 2007. A reappraisal of the reliability of the 20 m multistage shuttle run test. *European Journal of Applied Physiology* 100:287-292.

34. Leger, L.A., and J. Lambert. 1982. A maximal multistage 20 m shuttle run test to predict $\dot{V}O_2$max. *European Journal of Applied Physiology* 49:1-12.
35. Leger, L.A., D. Mercier, C. Gadoury, and J. Lambert. 1982. The multistage 20-meter shuttle run test for aerobic fitness. *Journal of Sport Science* 6:93-101.

36. Maritz, J.S., J.F. Morrison, J. Peter, N.B. Strydom, and C.H. Wyndham. 1961. A practical method of estimating an individual's maximal oxygen uptake. *Ergonomics* 4:97-122.

37. Matthews, C.E., D.P. Heil, P.S. Freedson, and H. Pastides. 1999. Classification of cardiorespiratory fitness without exercise testing. *Medicine and Science in Sports and Exercise* 31:486-493.

38. McArdle, W.D., F.I. Katch, and G.S. Pechar. 1973. Comparison of continuous and discontinuous treadmill and bicycle tests for max $\dot{V}O_2$. *Medicine and Science in Sports* 5(3): 156-160.

39. McNaughton, L., P. Hall, and D. Cooley. 1998. Validation of several methods of estimating maximal oxygen uptake in young men. *Perceptual and Motor Skills* 87:575-584.

40. Montoye, H.J., and T. Ayen. 1986. Body-size adjustment for oxygen requirement in treadmill walking. *Research Quarterly for Exercise and Sport* 57:82-84.

41. Montoye, H.J., T. Ayen, F. Nagle, and E.T. Howley. 1985. The oxygen requirement for horizontal and grade walking on a motor-driven treadmill. *Medicine and Science in Sports and Exercise* 17:640-645.

42. Naughton, J.P., and R. Haider. 1973. Methods of exercise testing. In *Exercise testing and exercise training in coronary heart disease,* ed. J.P. Naughton, H.R. Hellerstein, and L.C. Mohler, 79-91. New York: Academic Press.

43. Oldridge, N.B., W.L. Haskell, and P. Single. 1981. Carotid palpation, coronary heart disease, and exercise rehabilitation. *Medicine and Science in Sports and Exercise* 13:6-8.

44. Pollock, M.L., and J.H. Wilmore. 1990. *Exercise in health and disease.* 2nd ed. Philadelphia: Saunders.

45. President's Council on Physical Fitness and Sports. 2002. *President's Challenge Physical Activity and Fitness Award Program.* Washington, DC: Author.

46. Shephard, R.J. 1970. Computer programs for solution of the Åstrand nomogram and the calculation of body surface area. *Journal of Sports Medicine and Physical Fitness* 10:206-210.

47. Shephard, R.J. 1980. The current status of the Canadian Home Fitness Test. *British Journal of Sports Medicine* 14:114-125.

48. Shephard, R.J., M. Cox, P. Corley, and R. Smyth. 1979. Some factors affecting accuracy of the Canadian Home Fitness Test scores. *Canadian Journal of Applied Sport Science* 4:205-209.

49. Shephard, R.J., S. Thomas, and I. Weller. 1991. The Canadian Home Fitness Test—1991 update. *Sports Medicine* 11:358-366.

50. Shephard, R.J., D.A. Bailey, and R.L. Mirwald. 1976. Development of the Canadian Home Fitness Test. *Canadian Medical Association Journal* 114:675-679.

51. Strickland, M.K., S.R. Petersen., and M. Bouffard. 2003. Prediction of maximal aerobic power from the 20 m multistage shuttle run test. *Canadian Journal of Applied Physiology* 28:272-282.

52. Weir, L.T., A.S. Jackson, G.W. Ayers, and B. Arenare. 2006. Nonexercise models for estimating $\dot{V}O_2$max with waist girth, percent fat, or BMI. *Medicine and Science in Sports and Exercise* 38:555-561.

53. Weller, I.M.R., S.G. Thomas, M.H. Cox, and P.N. Corey. 1992. A study to validate the Canadian Aerobic Fitness Test. *Canadian Journal of Public Health* 83:120-124.

54. Weller, I.M.R., S. Thomas, N. Gledhill, D. Paterson, and A. Quinney. 1995. A study to validate the modified Canadian Aerobic Fitness Test. *Canadian Journal of Applied Physiology* 20:211-221.

55. Weller, I.M.R., S. Thomas, P.N. Corey, and M.H. Cox. 1993. Prediction of maximal oxygen uptake from a modified Canadian aerobic fitness test. *Canadian Journal of Applied Physiology* 18:175-188.

56. Whaley, M.H., L.A. Kaminsky, G.B. Dwyer, and L.H. Getchell. 1995. Failure of predicted $\dot{V}O_2$peak to discriminate physical fitness in epidemiological studies. *Medicine and Science in Sports and Exercise* 27:85-91.

57. Williford, H.N., M. Scharff-Olson, N. Wang, D.L. Blessing, F.H. Smith, and W.J. Duey. 1996. Cross-validation of nonexercise predictions of $\dot{V}O_2$peak in women. *Medicine and Science in Sports and Exercise,* 28:926-930.

Consent Form

The following is an example of a general consent form for exercise testing. The consent form you use should be developed and approved by administrative personnel associated with the setting in which you work (see chapter 27)

FORM 7.2   Sample Informed Consent for Fitness Test Participation

Testing objectives: In order to more safely participate in an exercise program, I hereby consent, voluntarily, to a series of exercise tests. Each test will assist in the determination of my overall physical fitness and will assess the following: cardiorespiratory fitness, body composition, muscular strength and endurance, and flexibility. I shall perform a graded exercise test (GXT) by walking on a treadmill or riding a cycle ergometer. The GXT will begin at a low level and gradually increase in difficulty until my target heart rate is achieved. The test may be stopped at any time because of feelings of significant fatigue or for any other personal reason. Body composition will be determined using skinfold tests. Muscular strength and endurance will be assessed with proper resistance training equipment. A sit-and-reach test will ascertain the flexibility of the hip joint.

Risk and discomforts: I understand that the risks of the GXT or other test procedures may include abnormal heart rhythms, abnormal blood pressure response, fainting, and very rarely a heart attack. Every professional effort will be made to minimize these risks through proper administration of a completed health status questionnaire (HSQ) as well as assessment of relevant health questions and supervision during the tests.

Responsibilities of the participant: I acknowledge that I have completed the HSQ and answered any attendant health questions accurately. During the GXT or other tests, I will report any heart-related symptom (i.e., pain, pressure, tightness, or heaviness in the chest, neck, jaw, back, or arms) immediately. I have reported all medications (including nonprescription medications) taken on a regular basis, including today, to the appropriate staff member.

Benefits to be expected: I desire to pursue a GXT and additional fitness tests so that I may obtain better advice regarding my present level of cardiorespiratory fitness and overall physical fitness. This information will be used to prescribe an appropriate individualized exercise program. I understand that this test does not entirely eliminate risk in the proposed exercise program.

Inquiries: I understand that I can withdraw my consent or discontinue participation in any aspect of the fitness testing at any time without penalty or prejudice toward me. I have read the above statements and have had all of my questions answered to my satisfaction.

Use of medical records: I have been informed that the information obtained from the fitness tests is privileged and confidential as described in the Health Insurance Portability and Accountability Act of 1996 (HIPAA). It will not be disclosed to anyone other than my physician or individuals responsible for designing and supervising my exercise program without my express written permission.

_____   _____

Signature of participant   Date

_____   _____

Signature of witness   Date

From E.T. Howley and D.L. Thompson, 2012, _Fitness professional's handbook, 6th ed._ (Champaign, IL: Human Kinetics).

Calibrating Equipment

To calibrate a measuring device is to check its accuracy by comparing it with a known standard and adjusting the device so that it provides an accurate reading. This section explains how to calibrate equipment used in exercise testing. These are suggestions only and should not be viewed as substitutes for the specific procedures recommended by the equipment manufacturers (29).

Treadmill Speed and Elevation Settings

The speed and grade settings on the treadmill must be calibrated because they determine physiological demand and are crucial in estimating CRF. These procedures should be used routinely to maintain test validity and reliability over time. A chart should be posted near each piece of equipment indicating when the calibration was done and by whom.

Calibrating Speed

An easy way to calibrate the speed on any treadmill is to measure the length of the belt and count the number of belt revolutions in a certain amount of time. To calibrate treadmill speed, follow these steps (29):

1. Measure the exact length of the belt in meters.
   a. Place a meter stick on the belt surface and mark a starting point.
   b. Advance the belt by hand, marking the belt 1 m at a time until you return to the starting point; record the value for belt length.
2. Place a small piece of tape near the edge of the belt surface.
3. Turn on the treadmill to a given speed by using the speed control.
4. Count 20 revolutions of the belt while tracking time with a stopwatch. Start your watch as the tape first moves past the fixed point, beginning the count with 0.
5. Convert the number of revolutions to revolutions per minute (rev · min^{-1}). For example, if the belt made 20 complete revolutions in 35 sec, then

$$35 \text{ sec} \div 60 \text{ sec} \cdot \text{min}^{-1} = 0.583 \text{ min},$$
$$20 \text{ rev} \div 0.583 \text{ min} = 34.3 \text{ rev} \cdot \text{min}^{-1}.$$

6. Multiply the calculated revolutions per minute (step 5) times the belt length (step 1). This gives the belt speed in meters per minute (m · min^{-1}). For example, if the belt length is 5.025 m, then

$$34.3 \text{ rev} \cdot \text{min}^{-1} \cdot 5.025 \text{ m} \cdot \text{rev}^{-1}$$
$$= 172.35 \text{ m} \cdot \text{min}^{-1}.$$

7. To convert meters per minute to miles per hour, divide the answer in step 6 by 26.8 (m · min^{-1}) · (mi · hr^{-1})$^{-1}$:

$$\frac{172.35 \text{ m} \cdot \text{min}^{-1}}{26.8 \, ([\text{m} \cdot \text{min}^{-1}] \cdot [\text{mi} \cdot \text{hr}^{-1}]^{-1})} = 6.43 \text{ mi} \cdot \text{hr}^{-1}$$

8. The value obtained in step 7 is the actual treadmill speed in miles per hour. If the speed indicator does not agree with this value, adjust the dial to the proper reading. Check the instruction manual for the location of the speed adjustment.
9. Repeat for a number of speeds to ensure accuracy across the speeds used in test protocols.

Calibrating Elevation

Treadmill manuals describe how to calibrate the grade using a simple carpenter's level and a square edge:

1. Use a carpenter's level to make sure that the treadmill is level, and check the zero setting on the grade meter under these conditions (with the treadmill electronics turned on). If the meter does not read zero, follow instructions to make the adjustment (usually by using the small screw on the face of the dial).
2. Elevate the treadmill so that the percentage grade dial reads approximately 20%. Measure the exact incline of the treadmill as shown in figure 7.7. When the bubble is exactly in the center of the tube in the level, the rise measurement is obtained.

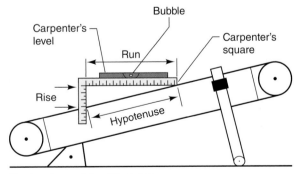

Grade = tangent θ = rise ÷ run
Grade = sine θ = rise ÷ hypotenuse

FIGURE 7.7 Calibrating grade using the tangent method (rise ÷ run) with a carpenter's square and level.

Reprinted, by permission, from E.T. Howley, 1988, The exercise testing laboratory. In *Resource manual for guidelines for exercise testing and prescription*, edited by S.N. Blair et al. (Philadelphia, PA: Lea & Febiger), 409.

3. Calculate the grade from the rise over the run and adjust the treadmill meter to read that exact grade. For example, if the rise is 4.5 in. (11.4 cm) and the run is 22.5 in. (57.2 cm), the fractional grade is calculated as follows:

$$\text{Grade} = \text{tangent } \theta = \text{rise} \div \text{run}$$
$$= 4.5 \text{ in.} \div 22.5 \text{ in.} = 0.20 = 20\%.$$

4. The rise-over-run method is a typical engineering method for calculating grade, giving the tangent of the angle (the opposite side divided by the adjacent side of the right triangle, as shown in figure 7.7). Although the sine of the angle (opposite side divided by the hypotenuse) provides the most accurate setting of grade, table 7.8 shows that the tangent value is a good approximation of the sine value for grades less than 20%, or 12°. The rise-over-run method can also be used to calibrate steep grades: Obtain the tangent value as described previously and simply look across table 7.8 to obtain the correct sine value to set on the treadmill dial. For example, if the rise-over-run method yielded 0.268, or 26.8% (tangent), the correct setting would be 25.9% (sine). The latter value is set on the grade dial of the treadmill.

TABLE 7.8 Natural Sines and Tangents

Degrees	Sine	Grade (%)	Tangent	Grade (%)
0	0.0000	0.0	0.0000	0.0
1	0.0175	1.7	0.075	1.7
2	0.0349	3.5	0.0349	3.5
3	0.0523	5.2	0.0524	5.2
4	0.0698	7.0	0.0699	7.0
5	0.0872	8.7	0.0875	8.7
6	0.1045	10.4	0.1051	10.5
7	0.1219	12.2	0.1228	12.3
8	0.1392	13.9	0.1405	14.0
9	0.1564	15.6	0.1584	15.8
10	0.1736	17.4	0.1763	17.6
11	0.1908	19.1	0.1944	19.4
12	0.2079	20.8	0.2126	21.3
13	0.2250	22.5	0.2309	23.1
14	0.2419	24.2	0.2493	24.9
15	0.2588	25.9	0.2679	26.8
20	0.3420	34.2	0.3640	36.4
25	0.4067	40.7	0.4452	44.5

Reprinted, by permission, from E.T. Howley, 1988, The exercise testing laboratory. In *Resource manual for guidelines for exercise testing and prescription*, edited by S.N. Blair et al. (Philadelphia, PA: Lea & Febiger), 409

KEY POINT

Calibrating the treadmill includes checking both speed and elevation.

Calibrating the Cycle Ergometer

The cycle ergometer must be calibrated routinely to ensure that the work rate is accurate. Altering either the pedal rate or the load on the wheel varies the work rate on the mechanically braked cycle ergometer. Work equals force times the distance through which the force acts: $w = f \cdot d$. The kilopond (kp), defined as the force acting on a mass of 1 kg at the normal acceleration of gravity, is the proper unit for force. However, the kilopond and the kilogram typically are used interchangeably in exercise testing.

On a mechanically braked cycle ergometer, the force (kilograms of weight on the wheel) is moved through a distance (in meters), so work is expressed in kilogram-meters (kgm). Because work is accomplished over time (e.g., minutes), the activity is referred to as a *work rate* or *power output* (kgm · min⁻¹), not a *workload*. On the Monark cycle ergometer, a point on the rim of the wheel travels 6 m per pedal revolution, so at 50 rev · min⁻¹, the wheel travels 300 m · min⁻¹. If a weight of 1 kg is hanging from that wheel, the work rate, or power output, is 300 kgm · min⁻¹. From these simple calculations you can see the importance of maintaining a correct pedal rate during the test—if the subject pedals at 60 rev · min⁻¹, the work rate is actually 20% higher (360 versus 300 kgm · min⁻¹) than it appears to be. The force setting (resistance on the wheel) also must be carefully set and checked because it tends to drift as the test progresses. It is crucial that the force (resistance) values on the scale are correct. The following four steps outline the procedure for calibrating the Monark cycle ergometer scale (5) (refer to figure 7.8).

1. Disconnect the belt at the spring.

2. Loosen the lock nut and use the adjusting screw on the front of the bike against which the force scale rests so that the vertical mark on the pendulum weight matches with 0 kp on the weight scale (see figure 7.8*a*). The pendulum must be swinging freely. Lock the adjustment screw with the lock nut. To keep the calibration weights from touching the flywheel, it may be easier to elevate the rear of the ergometer (with a 2×4 board on edge), set the zero as described previously, and proceed to the next step.

3. Suspend a 4.0 kg weight from the spring so that it's not in contact with the flywheel, and see if the pendulum moves to the 4.0 kp mark (see figure 7.8*b*). If it doesn't, alter the position or size of the adjusting weight in the pendulum (see figure 7.8*c*). By loosening the lock screw on the back of the pendulum weight, the adjusting weight can be lowered, raised, or replaced. Check the force scale again and calibrate the ergometer through the range of values used in your tests. If you used the 2×4

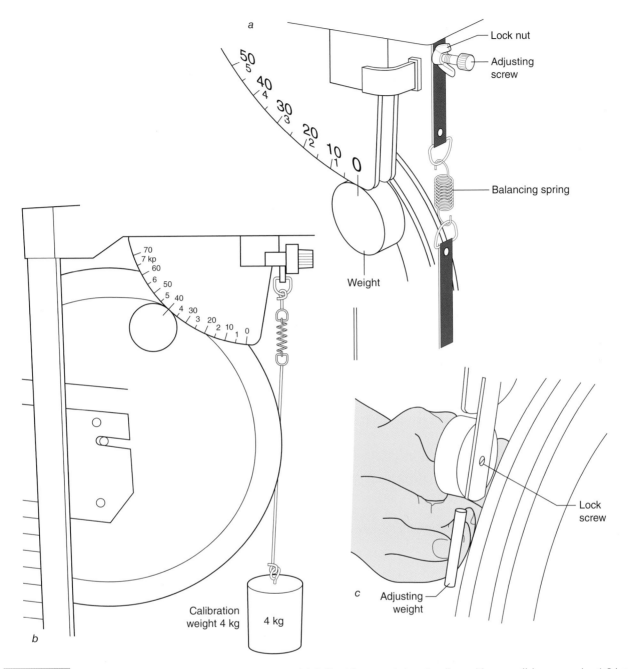

FIGURE 7.8 Calibrating the Monark cycle ergometer. *(a)* Adjust the pendulum to align with zero, *(b)* suspend a 4.0 kg weight from the spring, and *(c)* adjust the position or size of the weight in the pendulum.

Adapted, by permission, from Monark Sports and Medical, *Instruction manual, Monark model 818E* (Varberg, Sweden: Monark Exercise AB), 18.

to elevate the rear of the ergometer, remove it and reset the zero as described in step 2.

4. Reassemble the cycle ergometer.

KEY POINT

Calibrating the cycle ergometer involves establishing a true zero, hanging standard weights from the spring, and verifying that they line up with the readings on the scale.

Calibrating the Sphygmomanometer

A **sphygmomanometer** is a BP measurement system composed of an inflatable rubber bladder, an instrument that indicates the applied pressure, an inflation bulb that creates pressure, and an adjustable valve that deflates the system. The cuff and the measuring instrument are the most important for measurement accuracy. The cuff should be about 20% wider than the diameter of the limb to which it is applied, and when inflated, the bladder should not cause a bulging or displacement. If the bladder is too wide, BP will be underestimated; if it is too narrow, BP will be overestimated. Consequently, it is important to match cuff size to the subject being measured.

The device measuring the pressure, the manometer, can be a mercury or an aneroid type. The mercury type is the standard, and its calibration is easily maintained. The mercury column should rise and fall smoothly, form a clear meniscus, and read zero when the bladder is deflated. If the mercury sticks in the tube, remove the cap and swab out the inside. If it is very dirty, the tube should be removed and cleaned (with detergent, a water rinse, and alcohol for drying). If the mercury column falls below zero, add mercury to bring the meniscus exactly to the zero mark (12, 24, 29). Special care must be taken when handling toxic materials such as mercury; follow your institution's guidelines.

The aneroid gauge uses a metal bellows assembly that expands when pressure is applied, and the expansion moves the pointer on the indicator dial. A spring attached to the pointer moves the pointer downscale to zero when the bladder is deflated. This gauge should be calibrated at least once every 6 mo in a variety of settings using the mercury column just described. A simple Y tube (from the stethoscope) is used to connect the two systems (see figure 7.9). Readings should be taken with pressure falling to simulate the readings taken during an actual measurement (29).

KEY POINT

Using the correct size cuff is important when measuring BP. The mercury sphygmomanometer is the standard, and the aneroid gauge should be calibrated against the mercury column every 6 mo.

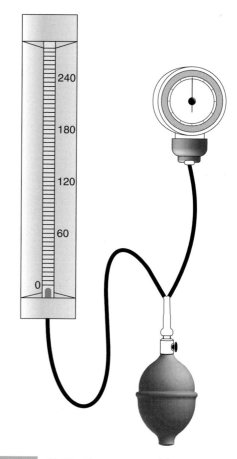

FIGURE 7.9 Calibrating an aneroid manometer with a mercury manometer.

Assessment of Body Composition

OBJECTIVES

The reader will be able to do the following:

1. Discuss how body composition affects health and describe the health implications of various patterns of body-fat distribution.

2. Compare and contrast hydrostatic weighing, air displacement plethysmography, bioelectrical impedance analysis (BIA), and skinfold measurement as means for estimating body composition.

3. Identify common measurement sites for skinfolds and girths.

4. Calculate and interpret BMI.

5. Assess body composition using a variety of techniques and describe the advantages and disadvantages of these techniques.

American media are filled with advertisements for programs designed to help people improve their health and fitness. Often the primary focus of these programs is weight loss. A healthy body weight and an appropriate amount of body fat are important aspects of physical fitness, and fitness professionals need to understand the importance of appropriate body composition, become aware of the various means for assessing body fat, and become proficient at estimating body fat through skinfold and girth measurements. As with other aspects of fitness assessment, paying attention to detail and gaining experience with the techniques are necessary to become proficient at estimating body fatness. This chapter is meant to assist fitness professionals in acquiring these skills.

Health and Body Composition

Body composition describes the component tissues of the body and is most often used to refer to the relative percentages of fat and fat-free tissues. **Fat-free mass (FFM)**, **fat mass (FM)**, and **percent body fat (%BF)** are the most frequently reported values in a body composition assessment. *Percent body fat* refers to the percentage of the total body mass that is composed of fat: %BF = (fat mass ÷ body mass) · 100%. *Fat-free mass* refers to the mass of the fat-free tissues of the body and often is used synonymously with the term **lean body mass**. Table 8.1 lists suggested age-based %BFs (30). Body composition is a vital aspect of overall fitness because of the ill effects related to excessively low or high body fatness. Various techniques are used to assess body composition, and fitness professionals should be skilled in their use.

Obesity is a condition in which a person has excess **adipose tissue**, or fat tissue. It may be classified either by %BF or by the relationship of height and weight (see section on BMI). Although there are no uniform standards for body-fat percentages, a %BF of >38% for females and >25% for males generally is considered in the obese range (21, 30). According to BMI standards, obesity is a value ≥ 30 kg · m^{-2} (26). **Overweight** is the condition in which a person is above the recommended weight range but is not yet in the obese category. A BMI of 25 to 29.9 kg · m^{-2} is considered in the overweight range. The **prevalence** of obesity and overweight among American adults and children has increased dramatically in the past 20 yr (5, 6, 10). Estimates from 2007 and 2008 show that nearly 34% of American adults are obese and another 34% are overweight (5). Thus, 68% of adults have a BMI of 25 kg · m^{-2} or higher. This is in sharp contrast with statistics from 1988 to 1994, when 22.9% of adults were obese and 55.9% had a BMI of 25 kg · m^{-2} or higher (6).

Obesity has been causally linked with numerous negative health consequences, including coronary artery disease (CAD), hypertension, stroke, type 2 diabetes, increased risk of various cancers, osteoarthritis, degenerative joint disease, abnormal blood lipid profile, and menstrual irregularities (26). Although precise estimates of the number of deaths that can be attributed to obesity vary considerably (7, 23, 25), hundreds of thousands of Americans die each year because of conditions either directly or indirectly linked to obesity. Because of the link between obesity and poor health, fitness professionals must provide clients with an accurate assessment of this important fitness component.

When people gain excess fat, genetics determines where the adipose tissue accumulates. Researchers are quite interested in learning how **body-fat distribution**, or **fat patterning**, affects health. **Android-type obesity** (i.e., male-pattern obesity, apple shape) refers to the excessive storage of fat in the trunk and abdominal areas. Excessive fat in the hips and thighs is labeled **gynoid-type obesity** (i.e., female-pattern obesity, pear shape). In terms of negative health consequences, android-type obesity appears to be the most dangerous, and it is closely linked with disease (8, 17). **Waist-to-hip ratio (WHR)** can be a useful tool for differentiating gynoid-type and android-type obesity. Waist circumference also is used to classify excessive trunk fat. Descriptions of how to take these measurements are presented later in this chapter.

Just as excessive body fat can be unhealthy, too little body fat also can compromise health. Among the many important roles of fat in human health are providing energy, helping with temperature regulation, and cushioning the joints. The minimum level of body fat needed to maintain health varies among individuals and depends on sex and genetics. The %BF thought to be necessary for good health, also known as **essential fat**, is 8% to 12% for women and 3% to 5% for men (30). Infertility, depression, impaired temperature regulation, and early death are among the outcomes of excessive weight loss. Extreme fat loss results from starvation imposed by internal or external forces. Eating disorders that result in self-starvation are discussed

TABLE 8.1   Age-Based Body Fat Percentage Standards for Adults

Men	Recommended range[a]
18-34 yr	8-22
35-55 yr	10-25
56 yr or older	10-25
Women	
18-34 yr	20-35
35-55 yr	23-38
56 yr or older	25-38

[a]Values are %BF levels considered generally healthy.

Based on Ratamess 2010.

KEY POINT

The prevalence of obesity and overweight is approximately 68% among U.S. adults. Significant health consequences (e.g., CVD, type 2 diabetes) may result from obesity. Disease risk is linked more closely with android-type obesity (apple shape) than with gynoid-type obesity (pear shape). Too little body fat also can lead to negative health outcomes.

in chapter 12. Because of the important link between health and body composition, a client's body fat should be analyzed during physical fitness assessments.

Methods for Assessing Body Composition

Numerous techniques have been used to estimate body composition. None of the methods currently used actually measure %BF; the only way to truly measure the volume of fat in the body would be to dissect and chemically analyze tissues in the body. The techniques routinely used to estimate %BF are based on the relationship between %BF and other factors that can be accurately measured, such as skinfold thicknesses or underwater weight. Because of the predictable relationship between the measured value and body composition, %BF can be estimated through these indirect methods.

Each of the techniques described in the following sections has advantages and disadvantages. Knowing these characteristics will help you decide wisely when choosing the method for body composition assessment. A comparison of important considerations can be found in table 8.2. For fitness professionals, ease of measurement, relative accuracy, and cost are the primary considerations when choosing a technique. In other situations (for research or clinical applications), the accuracy of the measurement may outweigh other considerations.

Anthropometric Methods: Body Mass Index

A widely used clinical assessment of the appropriateness of a person's weight is the **body mass index (BMI),** or Quetelet index. This value is calculated by dividing the weight in kilograms by height in meters squared.

BMI is a quick and easy method for determining if body weight is appropriate for body height. Table 8.3 lists the adult BMI categories. In the past, height–weight charts were used for this purpose, but BMI is currently the accepted method for interpreting the height–weight relationship. BMI does not differentiate between fat and fat-free weight, which is problematic when testing athletic individuals with a large lean mass. For example, a football linebacker who is 6 ft 2 in. (1.9 m) and weighs 220 lb (100 kg) is considered overweight according to BMI standards (BMI = 28.3 kg · m^{-2}), when in fact he may have a very low %BF. On the other hand, an inactive person with a similar height and weight is probably carrying excess adipose tissue.

Even with its limitations, for most adults there is a clear correlation between elevated BMI and negative health consequences (26). The recommended BMI range is 18.5 to 24.9 kg · m^{-2}. Overweight is classified as a BMI of 25 to 29.9 kg · m^{-2}, and a BMI of 30 kg · m^{-2} or higher is considered obese (1, 26). In screening situations where estimating body fat is impossible or impractical, BMI can be useful for providing feedback to people about the appropriateness of their body weight. It is important to note that BMI standards for children are age and sex specific (28, 29). Children at the 95th percentile or greater for their age and sex are considered obese. Consult the CDC growth charts for BMI standards for children (29).

TABLE 8.2 Comparison of Common Body Composition Techniques

	Equipment cost	Time required	Technician expertise	Day-to-day variation	Accuracy
Skinfolds	*	**	**	*	**
HW[1]	***	***	***	*	***
BIA[2]	* to **	*	*	**	**
DXA[3]	***	*	***	*	***
ADP[4]	***	*	*	*	***

* = low; ** = moderate; *** = high.

[1]Hydrostatic weighing

[2]Bioelectrial impedance analysis

[3]Dual-energy X-ray absorptiometry

[4]Air displacement plethysmography

TABLE 8.3 Body Mass Index Classification

Classification	BMI (kg · m⁻²)
Underweight	<18.5
Normal	18.5-24.9
Overweight	25.0-29.9
Obesity	
Class I	30.0-34.9
Class II	35.0-39.9
Class III (extreme obesity)	≥40.0

Based on NHLBI 1998.

Girth Measurements

Several girth measurements (body and limb circumferences) are used to either estimate body composition or describe body proportions. Girth measurements provide quick and reliable information. They are sometimes used in equations to predict body composition and may also be used to track changes in body shape and size during weight loss. The major disadvantage is that they provide little information about the fat and fat-free components of the body. For example, a bodybuilder's thigh can have a larger circumference yet less fat than that of an individual who is obese. A list of several commonly measured girths follows; refer to the *Anthropometric Standardization Reference Manual* (22) for additional circumference sites.

- Waist—narrowest part of the torso between the xiphoid process and the umbilicus
- Abdomen—circumference of the torso at the level of the umbilicus
- Hips—maximal circumference of the buttocks above the gluteal fold
- Thigh—largest circumference of the right thigh below the gluteal fold

WHR is a frequently used clinical application of girth measurements. This value is often used to reflect the degree of abdominal, or android-type, obesity. A WHR greater than 0.95 for young men or 0.86 for young women is associated with elevated health risks, while for men and women 60 to 69 yr old, a WHR of >1.03 and >0.9, respectively, is linked with disease risk (30).

Waist circumference (WC) alone can also provide valuable information about disease risk (13, 17, 26). A WC of greater than 102 cm (40 in.) in men or 88 cm (35 in.) in women significantly increases the risk of obesity-related disease (1). ACSM now uses BMI and WC as the techniques for classifying obesity for risk stratification (1).

When assessing girths, use the following procedures to standardize the measurements:

- Make sure the measuring tape is horizontal when measuring trunk circumference and is perpendicular to the long axis of the limb when measuring limbs. Use either a mirror or an assistant to help ensure that the tape is placed properly.
- Apply constant pressure to the tape without pinching the skin. Use a tape measure fitted with a handle that indicates the amount of tension exerted.
- When measuring limbs, measure on the right side of the body. Alternatively, measure on both sides and record the values for both right and left.
- Ensure that the person stands erect, relaxed, and with feet together.
- When measuring girths of the trunk, take the measurement after the person exhales and before the next breath begins.

Skinfold Measurements

Measuring skinfold thickness is one of the most frequently performed tests to estimate %BF. This quick, noninvasive, inexpensive method can provide a fairly accurate assessment of %BF. The value obtained by skinfold measurement is typically within 3.5% of the value measured with underwater weighing (30). Skinfold measurement is based on the assumption that, as a person gains adipose tissue, the increase in skinfold thickness is proportional to the additional fat weight.

Because of the widespread use of skinfold measurement, fitness professionals should master the skills involved. Accurately assessing skinfold thickness requires the correct performance of several steps: locating the skinfold site, pinching the skinfold away from the underlying tissue, measuring with the caliper, and choosing the proper equation. The following sections address each of these concerns.

Locating the Skinfold Site

It is critical to accurately determine the site of the skinfold measurement. To increase the accuracy of the measurement, especially for the inexperienced technician, the site should be located and then marked with a washable marker. This helps ensure that the calipers are placed in the correct position each time the skinfold is measured. All skinfold measurements should be taken on the right side of the body unless otherwise specified. Refer to table 8.4 and figure 8.1 for some of the most commonly used measurement sites. For a more complete description of determining skinfold sites, refer to the *Anthropometric Standardization Reference Manual* (22). Measuring skinfolds immediately after exercise should be avoided because exercise can shift fluid volume, leading to inaccurate results.

TABLE 8.4 Commonly Used Skinfold Sites

Skinfold site	Description
Abdomen	Measure the vertical fold 2 cm to the right of and level with the umbilicus. Make sure the head of the caliper is not in the umbilicus.
Triceps	Measure the vertical fold over the belly of the triceps muscle. The arm should be relaxed. The specific site is the posterior midline of the upper arm, half the distance between the acromion and olecranon processes.
Chest	Measure a diagonal fold along the natural line of the skin one-half (men) or one-third (women) the distance between the anterior axillary line and the nipple.
Midaxillary	Measure the vertical fold at the level of the xiphoid process on the midaxillary line.
Subscapular	Measure 2 cm below the inferior angle of the scapula along the diagonal fold at a 45° angle.
Suprailiac	Measure the diagonal fold in line with the natural angle of the iliac crest. Measure along the anterior axillary line just above the iliac crest.
Thigh	Measure the vertical fold over the quadriceps muscle on the midline of the thigh. Measure half the distance between the top of the patella and the inguinal crease. The leg should be relaxed.

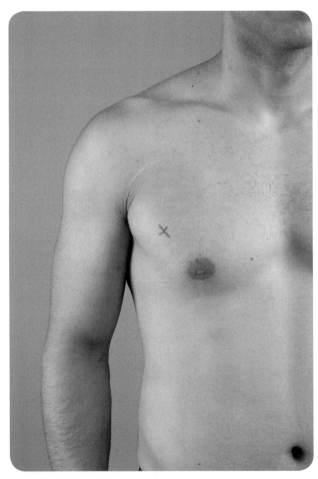 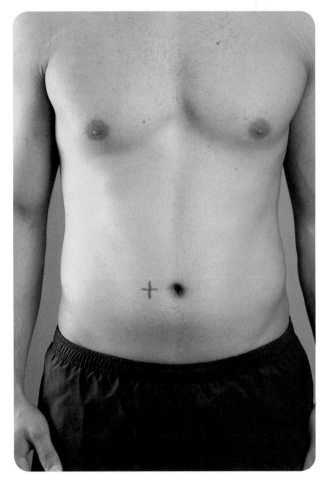

FIGURE 8.1 Skinfold testing sites.

Pinching the Skinfold

Once the correct location for the skinfold measurement is determined, the tester gently but firmly pinches and lifts the skinfold away from the underlying muscle in order to measure it. The following are guidelines for measuring skinfolds correctly:

1. Place the fingers perpendicular to the skinfold approximately 1 cm from the site to be measured.

2. Gently yet firmly pinch the skinfold between the thumb and the first two fingers and lift away from the underlying tissues. Place the jaws of the caliper perpendicular to the skinfold at the measurement site. The jaws of the caliper should be halfway between the bottom and top of the fold. Maintain the pinch while taking the measurement.

3. Read the measurement on the caliper 1 to 2 sec after the jaws contact the skin.

4. Wait at least 15 sec before taking a subsequent measurement. To allow time for the fold to return to normal, take one measurement at each site and then repeat measurements. If the second measurement varies by more than 1 to 2 mm, repeat the measurement a third time.

Measuring the skinfolds of individuals who are obese can be difficult, if not impossible. If the jaws of the caliper will not open wide enough to measure the skinfold, use an alternative method for assessing body composition. Girth measurements for predicting %BF (33, 34) along with BMI, WC, and WHR may be used instead.

Measuring With the Caliper

Skinfold thickness is measured with a skinfold caliper. The numerous commercially available calipers vary in price and accuracy. Lange and Harpenden calipers are the ones most often used in research settings because of their precision and reliability; however, other calipers may also be used effectively (2). Obviously, if the calipers do not measure skinfolds accurately, they will compromise the estimate of body fat. Measure with calipers that closely match those used in the development of the equation you are using.

Choosing the Proper Equation

Most skinfold equations were developed using underwater weighing as the criterion method and actually are designed to estimate body density. To develop skinfold equations, the body density of many people was measured (typically using hydrostatic weighing), and these values were compared with skinfold thickness through a statistical method called *regression analysis*. This statistical technique results in the development of an equation that reflects the relationship between skinfolds and body density. Inserting a client's skinfold measurements (and sometimes other information such as age) into these equations produces an estimate of the client's body density. Body density then is converted to %BF by using a two-compartment model equation such as the Siri equation, described later in this chapter.

Equations for Estimating Body Density From Skinfold Thicknesses

Women

3 sites $D_b = 1.0994921 - 0.0009929\,(X1) + 0.0000023\,(X1)^2 - 0.0001392\,(X2)$.

3 sites $D_b = 1.089733 - 0.0009245\,(X3) + 0.0000025\,(X3)^2 - 0.0000979\,(X2)$.

7 sites $D_b = 1.097 - 0.00046971\,(X4) + 0.00000056\,(X4)^2 - 0.00012828\,(X2)$.

    X1 = sum of triceps, suprailiac, and thigh skinfolds.

    X2 = age in years.

    X3 = sum of triceps, suprailiac, and abdominal skinfolds.

    X4 = sum of triceps, abdominal, suprailiac, thigh, chest, subscapular, and midaxillary skinfolds.

Men

3 sites $D_b = 1.10938 - 0.0008267\,(X1) + 0.0000016\,(X1)^2 - 0.0002574\,(X2)$.

3 sites $D_b = 1.1125025 - 0.0013125\,(X3) + 0.0000055\,(X3)^2 - 0.0002440\,(X2)$.

7 sites $D_b = 1.112 - 0.00043499\,(X4) + 0.00000055\,(X4)^2 - 0.00028826\,(X2)$.

    X1 = sum of chest, abdomen, and thigh skinfolds.

    X2 = age in years.

    X3 = sum of chest, triceps, and subscapular skinfolds.

    X4 = sum of triceps, abdominal, suprailiac, thigh, chest, subscapular, and midaxillary skinfolds.

From Jackson and Pollock, 1978; Jackson and Pollock, 1985; Jackson, Pollock, and Ward 1980.

Both generalized and population-specific skinfold equations have been developed (15, 30). Generalized equations estimate body composition in groups of people who vary greatly in age, body composition, and fitness. An advantage of these equations is that they can be used to estimate body composition in most people; however, the equations lose accuracy when testing individuals who are dissimilar to those used to develop the equations. These equations are also less accurate for people at either end of the fatness continuum.

Population-specific equations predict body composition in a particular subgroup of the population, such as female runners. The advantage of using population-specific equations is that they tend to have higher accuracy when testing people who fit the physical profile of those in the subgroup of interest.

Because sex influences the areas where fat is stored, separate skinfold equations for men and women have been developed. The Jackson and Pollock (14) equations for men and the Jackson, Pollock, and Ward (16) equations for women are generalized equations that are used widely. Note that the client's age is used in these equations. This is because the relationship between total body fat and subcutaneous fat changes with age; as a person ages, proportionally less fat is stored subcutaneously. Equations from these authors that require three or seven skinfold sites are listed in the sidebar Equations for Estimating Body Density From Skinfold Thicknesses. In addition, tables 8.5 and 8.6 provide quick references for estimating body fatness from skinfold thicknesses for men and women. To use these tables, total the sum of your client's skinfolds (chest, abdominal, and thigh sites for men; triceps, suprailiac, and thigh sites for women) and locate the corresponding value in the far left column. Then, locate the client's age in the top row. The intersection of the row and column is the client's estimated %BF.

KEY POINT

Skinfold measurements are a quick and relatively accurate method for estimating %BF; however, care must be taken in making these measurements if the values are to be reliable. Girth measurements, particularly WHR and WC, can be useful in assessing risk of obesity-related disease, and BMI is useful for classifying individuals into overweight and obese categories. The recommended BMI range is 18.5 to 24.9 kg · m^{-2}.

Densitometry

The density of an object is defined as the ratio of its weight to its volume (Density = weight ÷ volume). Two common procedures that estimate body composition based on densitometry are hydrostatic weighing and air displacement plethysmography. The foundation of these techniques is that various types of tissues in the body have different and consistent densities. Fat tissue has a density far less than either muscle or bone. Each of these techniques results in the assessment of total body volume and subsequently the calculation of body density.

Once the body density is calculated, it must be converted into %BF. To make this conversion, a **two-compartment model** is used. In a two-compartment model, all body tissues are classified as either fat or fat free. One of the most commonly used equations for this procedure is the Siri (32) equation: %BF = $(495 \div D_b) - 450$. In this model, the fat-free portion of the body is composed of all tissues except lipids and is assumed to have a density of 1.1 kg · L^{-1}. Fat is assumed to have a density of 0.9 kg · L^{-1}. It has been suggested that the inherent error (caused by variations in hydration or bone density) of this method is 2% to 2.8% in young Caucasian adults (20).

Fat density is fairly consistent among individuals; however, there are situations in which the density of the fat-free body is different from the assumed 1.1 kg · L^{-1}. For example, if a person's bone density is different from the standard used by Siri, then the assumption that the fat-free body density equals 1.1 kg · L^{-1} becomes invalid. This is the case for African Americans, who typically have a higher bone density than their Caucasian counterparts, and Schutte and colleagues (31) proposed that a different equation be used to calculate %BF for African American men. Many equations have been proposed to convert body density into %BF. Some of these are listed in table 8.7. For more equations and information on converting body density into %BF, see *ACSM's Guidelines for Exercise Testing and Prescription* (1) and Heyward and Wagner (12). Researchers sometimes use techniques more advanced than two-compartment models. Although these techniques are currently impractical for nonresearch settings, they are briefly described in the sidebar Body Composition Techniques in Research Settings: Multicompartment Models.

Hydrostatic Weighing

Hydrostatic (underwater) **weighing** is one of the most common means for estimating body composition in research settings and is often used as the **criterion method** for assessing %BF. A criterion method provides the standard against which other methodologies are compared. In this procedure, the participant is submerged in a tank of warm water and then exhales fully while technicians record the body mass (figure 8.2). The body mass while submerged and the body mass on land are used to calculate %BF.

Hydrostatic weighing is based on Archimedes' principle, which states that a submerged object is buoyed up by a force equal to the volume of water it displaces. This

TABLE 8.5 Estimating Percentage Body Fat for Men Using Age and the Sum of Chest, Abdominal, and Thigh Skinfolds

SUM OF SKIN-FOLDS (mm)	AGE TO THE LAST YEAR								
	Under 22	23-27	28-32	33-37	38-42	43-47	48-52	53-57	Over 57
8-10	1.3	1.8	2.3	2.9	3.4	3.9	4.5	5.0	5.5
11-13	2.2	2.8	3.3	3.9	4.4	4.9	5.5	6.0	6.5
14-16	3.2	3.8	4.3	4.8	5.4	5.9	6.4	7.0	7.5
17-19	4.2	4.7	5.3	5.8	6.3	6.9	7.4	8.0	8.5
20-22	5.1	5.7	6.2	6.8	7.3	7.9	8.4	8.9	9.5
23-25	6.1	6.6	7.2	7.7	8.3	8.8	9.4	9.9	10.5
26-28	7.0	7.6	8.1	8.7	9.2	9.8	10.3	10.9	11.4
29-31	8.0	8.5	9.1	9.6	10.2	10.7	11.3	11.8	12.4
32-34	8.9	9.4	10.0	10.5	11.1	11.6	12.2	12.8	13.3
35-37	9.8	10.4	10.9	11.5	12.0	12.6	13.1	13.7	14.3
38-40	10.7	11.3	11.8	12.4	12.9	13.5	14.1	14.6	15.2
41-43	11.6	12.2	12.7	13.3	13.8	14.4	15.0	15.5	16.1
44-46	12.5	13.1	13.6	14.2	14.7	15.3	15.9	16.4	17.0
47-49	13.4	13.9	14.5	15.1	15.6	16.2	16.8	17.3	17.9
50-52	14.3	14.8	15.4	15.9	16.5	17.1	17.6	18.2	18.8
53-55	15.1	15.7	16.2	16.8	17.4	17.9	18.5	19.1	19.7
56-58	16.0	16.5	17.1	17.7	18.2	18.8	19.4	20.0	20.5
59-61	16.9	17.4	17.9	18.5	19.1	19.7	20.2	20.8	21.4
62-64	17.6	18.2	18.8	19.4	19.9	20.5	21.1	21.7	22.2
65-67	18.5	19.0	19.6	20.2	20.8	21.3	21.9	22.5	23.1
68-70	19.3	19.9	20.4	21.0	21.6	22.2	22.7	23.3	23.9
71-73	20.1	20.7	21.2	21.8	22.4	23.0	23.6	24.1	24.7
74-76	20.9	21.5	22.0	22.6	23.2	23.8	24.4	25.0	25.5
77-79	21.7	22.2	22.8	23.4	24.0	24.6	25.2	25.8	26.3
80-82	22.4	23.0	23.6	24.2	24.8	25.4	25.9	26.5	27.1
83-85	23.2	23.8	24.4	25.0	25.5	26.1	26.7	27.3	27.9
86-88	24.0	24.5	25.1	25.7	26.3	26.9	27.5	28.1	28.7
89-91	24.7	25.3	25.9	26.5	27.1	27.6	28.2	28.8	29.4
92-94	25.4	26.0	26.6	27.2	27.8	28.4	29.0	29.6	30.2
95-97	26.1	26.7	27.3	27.9	28.5	29.1	29.7	30.3	30.9
98-100	26.9	27.4	28.0	28.6	29.2	29.8	30.4	31.0	31.6
101-103	27.5	28.1	28.7	29.3	29.9	30.5	31.1	31.7	32.3
104-106	28.2	28.8	29.4	30.0	30.6	31.2	31.8	32.4	33.0
107-109	28.9	29.5	30.1	30.7	31.3	31.9	32.5	33.1	33.7
110-112	29.6	30.2	30.8	31.4	32.0	32.6	33.2	33.8	34.4
113-115	30.2	30.8	31.4	32.0	32.6	33.2	33.8	34.5	35.1
116-118	30.9	31.5	32.1	32.7	33.3	33.9	34.5	35.1	35.7
119-121	31.5	32.1	32.7	33.3	33.9	34.5	35.1	35.7	36.4
122-124	32.1	32.7	33.3	33.9	34.5	35.1	35.8	36.4	37.0
125-127	32.7	33.3	33.9	34.5	35.1	35.8	36.4	37.0	37.6

Percentage of fat is calculated by the formula of Siri: %BF = $[(4.95 \div D_b) - 4.5] \cdot 100$, where D_b = body density.

Adapted, by permission, from M.L. Pollock, D.H. Schmidt and A.S. Jackson, 1980, "Measurement of cardiorespiratory fitness and body composition in a clinical setting," *Comprehensive Therapy* 6(9): 12-27.

TABLE 8.6 Estimating Percentage Body Fat for Women Using Age and Sum of Triceps, Suprailiac, and Thigh Skinfolds

SUM OF SKIN-FOLDS (mm)	AGE TO LAST YEAR								
	Under 22	23-27	28-32	33-37	38-42	43-47	48-52	53-57	Over 57
23-25	10.8	11.1	11.4	11.7	12.0	12.3	12.6	12.9	13.2
26-28	11.9	12.2	12.5	12.8	13.1	13.4	13.7	14.0	14.3
29-31	13.1	13.4	13.7	14.0	14.3	14.6	14.9	15.2	15.5
32-34	14.2	14.5	14.8	15.1	15.4	15.7	16.0	16.3	16.6
35-37	15.2	15.6	15.9	16.2	16.5	16.8	17.1	17.4	17.7
38-40	16.3	16.6	16.9	17.2	17.6	17.9	18.2	18.5	18.8
41-43	17.4	17.7	18.0	18.3	18.6	18.9	19.2	19.6	19.9
44-46	18.4	18.8	19.1	19.4	19.7	20.0	20.3	20.6	20.9
47-49	19.5	19.8	20.1	20.4	20.7	21.0	21.4	21.7	22.0
50-52	20.5	20.8	21.1	21.4	21.8	22.1	22.4	22.7	23.0
53-55	21.5	21.8	22.1	22.5	22.8	23.1	23.4	23.7	24.0
56-58	22.5	22.8	23.1	23.5	23.8	24.1	24.4	24.7	25.0
59-61	23.5	23.8	24.1	24.4	24.8	25.1	25.4	25.7	26.0
62-64	24.5	24.8	25.1	25.4	25.7	26.1	26.4	26.7	27.0
65-67	25.4	25.7	26.1	26.4	26.7	27.0	27.3	27.7	28.0
68-70	26.4	26.7	27.0	27.3	27.6	28.0	28.3	28.6	28.9
71-73	27.3	27.6	27.9	28.2	28.6	28.9	29.2	29.5	29.8
74-76	28.2	28.5	28.8	29.1	29.5	29.8	30.1	30.4	30.8
77-79	29.1	29.4	29.7	30.0	30.4	30.7	31.0	31.3	31.7
80-82	29.9	30.3	30.6	30.9	31.2	31.6	31.9	32.2	32.5
83-85	30.8	31.1	31.5	31.8	32.1	32.4	32.8	33.1	33.4
86-88	31.6	32.0	32.3	32.6	33.0	33.3	33.6	33.9	34.3
89-91	32.5	32.8	33.1	33.5	33.8	34.1	34.4	34.8	35.1
92-94	33.3	33.6	33.9	34.3	34.6	34.9	35.3	35.6	35.9
95-97	34.1	34.4	34.7	35.1	35.4	35.7	36.1	36.4	36.7
98-100	34.8	35.2	35.5	35.8	36.2	36.5	36.8	37.2	37.5
101-103	35.6	35.9	36.3	36.6	36.9	37.3	37.6	37.9	38.3
104-106	36.3	36.7	37.0	37.3	37.7	38.0	38.3	38.7	39.0
107-109	37.1	37.4	37.7	38.1	38.4	38.7	39.1	39.4	39.7
110-112	37.8	38.1	38.4	38.8	39.1	39.4	39.8	40.1	40.5
113-115	38.5	38.8	39.1	39.5	39.8	40.1	40.5	40.8	41.1
116-118	39.1	39.5	39.8	40.1	40.5	40.8	41.1	41.5	41.8
119-121	39.8	40.1	40.4	40.8	41.1	41.5	41.8	42.1	42.5
122-124	40.4	40.7	41.1	41.4	41.8	42.1	42.4	42.8	43.1
125-127	41.0	41.4	41.7	42.0	42.4	42.7	43.1	43.4	43.7
128-130	41.6	41.9	42.3	42.6	43.0	43.3	43.7	44.0	44.3

Percentage calculated using Jackson, Pollock, and Ward (15) and Siri (29) equations.

Adapted, by permission, from M.L. Pollock, D.H. Schmidt and A.S. Jackson, 1980, "Measurement of cardiorespiratory fitness and body composition in a clinical setting," *Comprehensive Therapy* 6(9): 12-27.

TABLE 8.7 Equations Used to Convert Body Density Into Body-Fat Percentage

Group	Sex	Equation
African American		
	Male	%BF = (437 ÷ D_b) − 393
	Female	%BF = (485 ÷ D_b) − 439
Caucasian		
	Male	%BF = (495 ÷ D_b) − 450
	Female	%BF = (501 ÷ D_b) − 457

%BF = body-fat percentage; D_b = body density.

Based on Heymsfield et al. 1990.

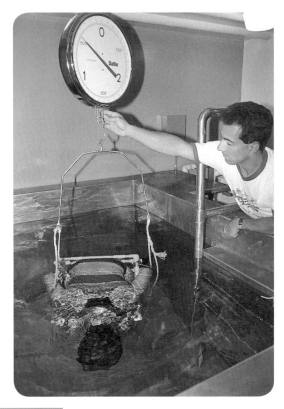

FIGURE 8.2 Hydrostatic weighing.

Reprinted, by permission, from V.H. Heyward and D.R. Wagner, 2004, *Advanced fitness assessment and exercise prescription*, 6th ed. (Champaign, IL: Human Kinetics), 193.

buoyant force causes the object to weigh less underwater than it does on land. The difference between land mass and underwater mass is used to calculate the volume of the object. Because the density of an object is calculated by dividing mass by volume, body density (D_b) can be calculated using the following formula.

$$D_b = \frac{M}{\dfrac{(M - M_{UW})}{D_{H_2O}} - RV - GV}$$

In addition to body mass (M) and mass underwater (M_{UW}), the density of the water (D_{H_2O}) in the hydrostatic

tank, the residual lung volume (RV), and the gastrointestinal air volume (GV) are needed for this calculation. Water density depends on water temperature and is necessary to convert mass into volume; therefore, accurate measurement of the water temperature is essential. Also, this equation corrects for the residual lung volume because any air in the lungs creates an additional buoyant effect that reduces underwater mass. The oxygen dilution technique described by Wilmore (35) is one of the most frequently used methods for assessing residual lung volume. Estimating instead of measuring residual lung volume dramatically decreases the accuracy of hydrostatic weighing. Because sex, age, and height correlate with residual lung volume, it can be estimated with a formula that incorporates the client's age and height (9). Formulas for males and females are shown in the sidebar Formulas to Calculate Residual Lung Volume From Height and Age. Since the volume of air trapped in the gastrointestinal tract cannot be measured, an estimate of 0.1 L is typically used.

Hydrostatic weighing accurately estimates body composition for most adults, and it remains a standard of comparison for other methods. Major disadvantages to this procedure are the time, expense, and technical expertise required. Also, many individuals are unable to undergo this procedure because of their discomfort with being underwater. Following are guidelines that will help ensure accurate assessment of body composition with hydrostatic weighing:

- The participant should not eat within 4 hr of testing.
- The participant should urinate and defecate before testing.
- The participant should wear as little clothing as possible. Remove any trapped air bubbles from clothing before weighing.
- Instruct the participant to exhale completely while submerged. (This will take practice for most individuals.)
- The participant should remain as motionless as possible while submerged.
- Perform several (5-10) trials to obtain consistent measurements.
- Measure, rather than estimate, residual volume.

Air Displacement Plethysmography

Another technique for determining %BF that uses the concept of density as the ratio of body mass to body volume is **air displacement plethysmography**. The Bod Pod is a commercially available air displacement plethysmograph (see figure 8.3). In this method, body volume is estimated while the subject sits in a sealed chamber. During testing, a computer-controlled diaphragm moves, changing the volume of the chamber. Pressure changes in the chamber

Formulas to Calculate Residual Lung Volume From Height and Age

Females

$$(0.009 \cdot \text{age in yr}) + (0.08128 \cdot \text{height in in.}) - 3.9 = \text{RV in L.}$$

Males

$$(0.017 \cdot \text{age in yr}) + (0.06858 \cdot \text{height in in.}) - 3.447 = \text{RV in L.}$$

From Goldman and Becklake 1959.

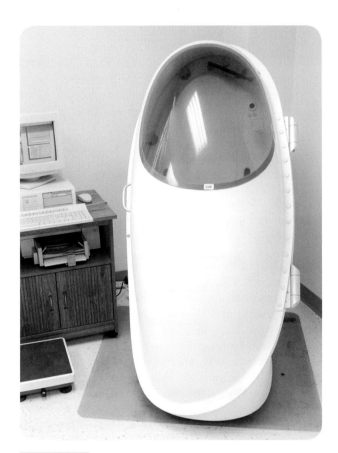

FIGURE 8.3 Bod pod.

Photo courtesy of COSMED USA, Inc.

are related to the size of the person being measured. By examining the pressure–volume relationship, body volume and, subsequently, body density are calculated (3, 24). Once body density is known, the two-compartment equations listed in table 8.7 can be used to estimate %BF.

The primary advantage of air displacement plethysmography compared with hydrostatic weighing is that it is quicker and is less anxiety-inducing for many individuals. Researchers continue to gather data on this device in an attempt to determine if it can be routinely substituted for hydrostatic weighing (4). The standard error of estimate for this technique varies among studies but is typically between 2% and 4% (30). The major disadvantage is the cost of the highly technical equipment needed to make the measurements. A major consideration for obtaining accurate measurements with the Bod Pod is that subjects must dress according to the manufacturer's specifications (i.e., in a tight-fitting swimsuit and swim cap).

Other Body Composition Techniques

In addition to the body composition techniques already discussed, a wide variety of others have been developed for use by clinicians, researchers, and fitness professionals. In the following paragraphs, you will learn about some of the most common techniques.

Dual-Energy X-Ray Absorptiometry

A technique that has gained wide acceptance in clinical settings is dual-energy X-ray absorptiometry (DXA). DXA was developed for measuring the density of bones. Although bone density measurement remains the primary use of this methodology, software has been developed that can estimate %BF from DXA scans. To estimate %BF from DXA, a total-body X-ray is performed with extremely low-dosage energy beams. As the X-rays pass through the subject, the density of all parts of the body is determined. Because fat, bone, and nonbone lean tissue have different densities, these three compartments can be identified (18).

Although DXA requires a full-body X-ray, the radiation exposure is minimal and is only a small fraction of the radiation exposure of a chest X-ray. Some researchers claim DXA as the new criterion method for body composition assessment; however, there are still unresolved issues for this technology. For example, differences in DXA software packages may result in varied body fat outcomes. Also, variations in body-segment thicknesses tend to alter DXA results (18). Studies investigating the error associated with this technique have reported errors ranging from 1.2% to 4.8% (20). This procedure is relatively quick (approximately 15 min) and has the potential for accurate results regardless of the age, sex, or race of the subject. The major prohibitive factors for using this procedure are cost and access to the equipment. Because of the radiation

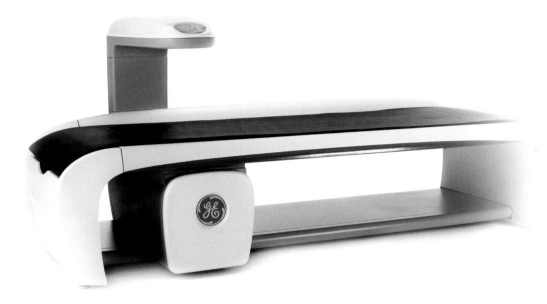

FIGURE 8.4 Dual energy X-ray absorptionmeter.

Reprinted, by permission, from V.H. Heyward and D.R. Wagner, 2004, *Advanced fitness assessment and exercise prescription*, 6th ed. (Champaign, IL: Human Kinetics), 201.

exposure involved, DXA equipment is housed in hospitals or clinically-oriented research centers. At present, DXA is used most frequently as a research tool and in the clinical assessment of body composition.

Magnetic resonance imaging (MRI) and computed tomography (CT) are also imaging techniques that provide important information to clinicians and researchers. One of the common uses of these techniques is to determine the amount of fat, particularly deep fat, found in the trunk. Because deep fat (visceral fat) is highly associated with disease, researchers use these techniques to quantify its distribution pattern. CT scans use X-rays to produce images of the fat and nonfat tissues, whereas MRI uses a strong magnetic field. The equipment necessary for this type of imaging is expensive and is found in clinical settings.

Bioelectrical Impedance Analysis

Bioelectrical impedance analysis (BIA) is a simple, quick, noninvasive method that can be used to estimate %BF. This technique is based on the assumption that tissues high in water content conduct electrical currents with less resistance than those with little water (27). Because adipose tissue contains little water, fat impedes the flow of electrical current.

BIA requires that a small electrical current be sent through the body. This current is undetectable to the person being tested (27). There are several types of commercially available BIA devices. Some place electrodes on the hand and foot, some are handheld, and others have contact points for the bottom of the feet and look similar to bathroom scales. Whatever the design of the machine, as the introduced current passes through the body, voltage decreases. This voltage drop (impedance) is used to calculate %BF.

Typically, other information such as sex, height, and age are used in conjunction with impedance to predict %BF.

BIA has gained wide acceptance in the fitness industry because it is easy, inexpensive, and noninvasive, and there are versions of these devices designed for in-home use by consumers. The accuracy of this technique depends on the type of equipment and equations used; however, a standard error of 2.7% to 6.3% commonly is reported (30). An issue that complicates the application of BIA is that the relationship between impedance and %BF varies among populations. In other words, for an accurate estimate of %BF, one must take into account age, gender, and other factors. Most commercially available devices have programmed equations to account for many of these factors. For more detailed information on choosing an appro-

> **KEY POINT**
>
> Two-compartment models divide the body into fat and fat-free components. Although the Siri two-compartment model is often used, other models are available. Both hydrostatic weighing and air displacement plethysmography use a two-compartment model. BIA is based on the principle that electrical currents flow more easily through more hydrated tissues (muscle) than through less hydrated tissues (fat). Although BIA is useful in body composition screening, steps should be taken to ensure that the client's hydration is normal at the time of testing. Multicompartment modeling and imaging techniques are used in research to assess body composition.

priate BIA equation, refer to *Applied Body Composition Assessment* by Heyward and Wagner (12). BIA does not produce accurate results for individuals with amputations, significant muscular atrophy, severe obesity, or diseases that alter the state of hydration. In addition, it is recommended that people with implanted defibrillators avoid BIA assessment until the safety of BIA for these individuals has been determined (27).

A person's state of hydration can greatly alter BIA results; therefore, it is essential to follow standardized guidelines with this assessment technique (27). Following is a list of these guidelines.

- Remove oil and lotions from the skin with alcohol before placing electrodes.

- Place electrodes precisely as directed by the manufacturer of the impedance device. Incorrect electrode placement greatly reduces the accuracy of BIA.

- If required to measure height, mass, or both, measure height to the nearest 0.5 cm and body mass to the nearest 0.1 kg.

- Ask clients to avoid any substance that alters the body's hydration state, such as alcohol or diuretics, for at least 48 hr before BIA. (Diuretics being taken under a doctor's direction should not be stopped.)

- Inform clients that during the 4 hr before assessment, they should avoid eating and should drink only enough water to maintain normal hydration.

- Instruct clients to avoid exercise for 12 hr preceding BIA.

- Note the phase of the menstrual cycle because of its ability to alter hydration levels.

Calculating Target Body Weight

As shown in table 8.1, healthy %BF ranges are quite different for females and males and cover a wide range. One of the important tasks of fitness professionals is helping clients determine an appropriate weight goal. Once an estimate of %BF has been obtained and %BF goals have been determined, the fitness professional can calculate an appropriate target weight. As discussed in chapter 12, setting reasonable goals for weight loss is a major factor in maintaining compliance. To calculate target body weight, you must know body weight, %BF, and the desired level of body fatness. An example of a calculation for target body weight is shown in the sidebar Calculating Target Body Weight.

KEY POINT

Target body weight can be calculated if current weight and body composition are known.

Body Composition Techniques in Research Settings: Multicompartment Models

A disadvantage to using two-compartment models in calculating body composition is the need to make broad generalizations about the composition and density of various body tissues. To avoid this problem, researchers sometimes use models that combine measurements to estimate body composition. Although these techniques must still rely on some basic assumptions about the body's makeup, fewer broad generalizations about its component parts are made. Therefore, these multicompartment models more accurately assess body composition.

An example of a multicompartment model is Siri's three-compartment model, in which the body is divided into fat, water, and solids (protein and mineral) (32). This model requires measuring total body density and total body water. Measurements of total body water are typically determined by having the participant ingest an isotope of hydrogen such as deuterium or tritium. After the ingested isotope spreads through the body's water, a fluid sample (e.g., urine, blood) can be used to calculate total body water. This model is particularly useful in clinical situations when patients have significantly altered body water. In cases where the bone mineral varies from what is assumed in a two-compartment model (e.g., in an osteoporotic patient), a technique requiring bone measurement is needed. Lohman (19) presented a model that divides the body into fat, protein and water, and mineral components. Both body density and bone mineral measurement (obtained via X-ray imaging) are needed for this technique. Sometimes bone and water measurements are added separately to body density to provide a four-compartment model (i.e., protein, mineral, fat, and water) (11).

Multicompartment models provide important criterion measures of body composition for researchers. Data from these methodologies are used to develop better field methods for assessing body composition in diverse populations. However, the cost, time, and technical expertise required for these processes make them impractical in nonresearch settings.

Calculating Target Body Weight

Total body mass, fat mass, fat-free mass, and the desired %BF must be known in order to calculate target body weight. The following equations are needed for these calculations.

$$\text{Fat mass (FM)} = \text{body mass} \cdot (\%BF \div 100\%).$$

$$\text{Fat-free mass (FFM)} = \text{body mass} - \text{FM}.$$

$$\text{Target body weight} = \frac{\text{FFM}}{1 - \left(\dfrac{\text{desired \% BF}}{(100)}\right)}$$

Example: A 40-yr-old woman weighs 155 lb (70 kg) and has a %BF of 30. Her goal is to reach 23% body fat. What is her target weight?

$$\text{FM} = 155 \text{ lb} \cdot (30 \div 100) = 46.5 \text{ lb.}$$

$$\text{FFM} = 155 \text{ lb} - 46.5 \text{ lb} = 108.5 \text{ lb.}$$

$$\text{Target body weight} = \frac{108.5}{1 - \left(\dfrac{23}{(100)}\right)} = 140.9 \text{ lb, or } 63.9 \text{ kg.}$$

STUDY QUESTIONS

1. What is the recommended BMI range? What is the BMI range for overweight? For obesity?

2. What are other names for the android-type obesity pattern? What conditions are linked to this obesity pattern?

3. Hydrostatic weighing and air displacement plethysmography use a two-compartment model for body composition. What are the two compartments assumed by this model?

4. Which technique applies a small electrical current to estimate %BF? What are ways that you can improve the accuracy of this technique?

5. What are important considerations when using skinfold measurements to estimate %BF that will help reduce measurement errors?

6. What are some advantages to using air displacement plethysmography?

7. What body composition technique is also used to measure bone density?

8. Why are multicompartment models of body composition assessment generally limited to research settings?

CASE STUDIES

You can check your answers by referring to appendix A.

1. Ms. Anderson is a 30-yr-old female who comes into your fitness facility wanting to lose weight. What are appropriate measurements and calculations for a fitness professional to make to assist Ms. Anderson with her goal?

2. Mr. Johnson is a 48-yr-old male who recently joined your fitness facility. At his initial evaluation you take the following measurements:

Height: 70 in. (178 cm)

Weight: 215 lb (97.5 kg)

Hip circumference: 39 in. (99 cm)

WC: 41 in. (104 cm)

Skinfolds: chest 35 mm, abdomen 49 mm, thigh 20 mm

Calculate and interpret Mr. Johnson's BMI, waist circumference, WHR, and %BF.

3. Mr. Johnson sets his initial %BF goal at 28%. Calculate the target body weight that will allow Mr. Johnson to achieve this goal.

REFERENCES

1. American College of Sports Medicine (ACSM). 2010. *ACSM's guidelines for exercise testing and prescription.* 8th ed. Baltimore: Lippincott Williams & Wilkins.

2. Cataldo, D., and V.H. Heyward. 2000. Pinch an inch: A comparison of several high-quality and plastic skinfold calipers. *ACSM's Health and Fitness Journal* 4:12-16.

3. Dempster, P., and S. Aitkens. 1995. A new air displacement method for the determination of human body composition. *Medicine and Science in Sports and Exercise* 27:1692-1697.

4. Fields, D., M. Goran, and M. McCrory. 2002. Body composition assessment via air-displacement plethysmography in adults and children: A review. *American Journal of Clinical Nutrition* 75:453-467.

5. Flegal, K.M., M.D. Carroll, C.L. Ogden, and L.R. Curtin. 2010. Prevalence and trends in obesity among U.S. adults, 1999-2008. *Journal of the American Medical Association* 303(3): 235-241.

6. Flegal, K.M., M.D. Carroll, C.L. Ogden, and C.L. Johnson. 2002. Prevalence and trends in obesity among U.S. adults, 1999-2000. *Journal of the American Medical Association* 288:1723-1727.

7. Flegal, K.M., B.I. Graubard, D.F. Williamson, and M.H. Gail. 2005. Excess deaths associated with underweight, overweight, and obesity. *Journal of the American Medical Association* 293:1861-1867.

8. Folsom, A., L. Kushi, K. Anderson, P. Mink, J. Olson, C.-P. Hong, T. Sellers, D. Lazovich, and R. Prineas. 2000. Associations of general and abdominal obesity with multiple health outcomes in older women. *Archives of Internal Medicine* 160:2117-2128.

9. Goldman, H.I., and M.R. Becklake. 1959. Respiratory function tests. *American Review of Tuberculosis and Pulmonary Disease* 79:457-467.

10. Hedley, A.A., C.L. Ogden, C.L. Johnson, M.D. Carroll, L.R. Curtin, and K.M. Flegal. 2004. Prevalence of overweight and obesity among U.S. children, adolescents, and adults, 1999-2002. *Journal of the American Medical Association* 291:2847-2850.

11. Heymsfield, S.B., S. Lichtman, R.N. Baumgartner, J. Wang, Y. Kamen, A. Aliprantis, N. Richard, and J. Pierson. 1990. Body composition of humans: Comparison of two improved four-compartment models that differ in expense, technical complexity, and radiation exposure. *American Journal of Clinical Nutrition* 52:52-58.

12. Heyward, V.H., and D.R. Wagner. 2004. *Applied body composition assessment.* 2nd ed. Champaign, IL: Human Kinetics.

13. Hu, G., J. Tuomilehto, K. Silventoinen, N. Barengo, and P. Jousilahti. 2004. Joint effects of physical activity, body mass index, waist circumference and waist-to-hip ratio with the risk of cardiovascular disease among Finnish men and women. *European Heart Journal* 25:2212-2219.

14. Jackson, A.S., and M.L. Pollock. 1978. Generalized equations for predicting body density of men. *British Journal of Nutrition* 40:497-504.

15. Jackson, A.S., and M.L. Pollock. 1985. Practical assessment of body composition. *Physician and Sportsmedicine* 13:76-90.

16. Jackson, A.S., M.L. Pollock, and A. Ward. 1980. Generalized equations for predicting body density of women. *Medicine and Science in Sports and Exercise* 12:175-182.

17. Janssen, I., P.T. Katzmarzyk, and R. Ross. 2004. Waist circumference and not body mass index explains obesity-related health risk. *American Journal of Clinical Nutrition* 79:379-384.

18. Kohrt, W.M. 1995. Body composition by DXA: Tried and true? *Medicine and Science in Sports and Exercise* 27:1349-1353.

19. Lohman, T.G. 1986. Applicability of body composition techniques and constants for children and youth. In *Exercise and Sports Science Reviews*, ed. K.B. Pandolf, 325-357. New York: Macmillan.

20. Lohman, T.G. 1992. *Advances in body composition assessment.* Champaign, IL: Human Kinetics.

21. Lohman, T.G., L. Houtkooper, and S.B. Going. 1997. Body fat measurement goes high-tech: Not all are created equal. *ACSM's Health and Fitness Journal* 1:30-35.

22. Lohman, T.G., A.F. Roche, and R. Martorell. 1988. *Anthropometric standardization reference manual.* Champaign, IL: Human Kinetics.

23. Mark, D.H. 2005. Deaths attributable to obesity. *Journal of the American Medical Association* 293:1918-1919.

24. McCrory, M.A., T.D. Gomez, E.M. Bernauer, and P.A. Mole. 1995. Evaluation of a new air displacement plethysmograph for measuring human body composition. *Medicine and Science in Sports and Exercise* 27:1686-1691.

25. Mokdad, A.H., J.S. Marks, D.F. Stroup, and J.L. Gerberding. 2004. Actual causes of death in the United States, 2000 [published correction appears in *JAMA* 2005; 293:298]. *Journal of the American Medical Association* 291:1238-1245.

26. National Heart, Lung, and Blood Institute. 1998. *Clinical guidelines on the identification, evaluation, and treatment of overweight and obesity in adults* (NIH Publication No. 98-4083). Bethesda, MD: National Institutes of Health—National Heart, Lung, and Blood Institute.

27. National Institutes of Health (NIH). 1994. *Bioelectrical impedance analysis in body composition measurement: NIH Technology Assessment Conference statement.* Bethesda, MD: National Institutes of Health.

28. Ogden, C.L., and K.M. Flegal. 2010. Changes in terminology for childhood overweight and obesity. *National Health Statistics Reports* 25:1-5.

29. Ogden, C.L., R.J. Kuczmarski, K.M. Flegal, Z. Mei, S. Guo, R. Wei, L.M. Gummer-Strawn, L.R. Curtin, A.F. Roche, and C.L. Johnson. 2002. Centers for Disease Control and Prevention 2000 growth charts for the United States: Improvements to the 1977 National Center for Health Statistics version. *Pediatrics* 109:45-60.

30. Ratamess, N. 2010. Body composition status and assessment. In *ACSM's resource manual for guidelines for exercise testing and prescription*, 6th edition, ed. J.K. Ehrman, 264-281. Baltimore: Lippincott Williams & Wilkins.

31. Schutte, J.E., E.M. Townsend, J. Hugg, R.F. Shoup, R.M. Malina, and C.G. Blomqvist. 1984. Density of lean body mass is greater in blacks than in whites. *Journal of Applied Physiology: Respiratory, Environmental, and Exercise Physiology* 56:1647-1649.

32. Siri, W.E. 1961. Body composition from fluid spaces and density: Analysis of methods. In *Techniques for measuring body composition*, ed. J. Brozek and A. Henschel, 223-244. Washington, DC: National Academy of Sciences.

33. Weltman, A., S. Levine, R.L. Seip, and Z.V. Tran. 1988. Accurate assessment of body composition in obese females. *American Journal of Clinical Nutrition* 48:1179-1183.

34. Weltman, A., R.L. Seip, and Z.V. Tran. 1987. Practical assessment of body composition in obese males. *Human Biology* 59:523-536.

35. Wilmore, J. 1969. A simplified method for determination of residual volume. *Journal of Applied Physiology* 27:96-100.

Assessment of Muscular Fitness

Kyle McInnis and Avery Faigenbaum

OBJECTIVES

The reader will be able to do the following:

1. Define terminology used to describe muscular fitness.

2. Discuss precautions that enhance participant safety during muscular fitness assessments.

3. Describe various methods of assessing muscular fitness, including repetition maximum tests, push-up and abdominal curl-up tests, the YMCA bench press test, and others.

4. Identify methods for standardizing testing protocols to increase accuracy and reproducibility of test results.

5. Describe how to interpret the results from various muscular fitness tests.

6. Describe how to assess muscular strength and endurance in older adults .

7. Describe the benefits, safety, and precautions for assessing muscular fitness in clients who are at elevated risk for adverse cardiovascular responses such as those with high BP or CHD.

8. Describe the benefits, safety, and precautions for assessing muscular fitness in children and adolescents.

Muscular fitness

Muscular fitness refers to the integrated status of **muscular strength** (maximal force a muscle can generate) and **muscular endurance** (ability of a muscle to make repeated contractions or to resist muscular fatigue) (4, 18, 24). Muscular fitness is important in both promoting and maintaining health and enhancing athletic performance (3). Accordingly, in its position stand on the recommended quantity and quality of exercise to achieve and maintain fitness (3) and its public health recommendations (21), ACSM promotes routine resistance and strengthening exercise. In general, ACSM recommends that resistance training of a moderate to high intensity, sufficient to develop and maintain muscle mass, be performed at least twice per week as part of a well-rounded fitness program (see chapter 13). This chapter describes tests commonly used in the health and fitness setting to assess muscular strength and endurance. Particular emphasis is given to strength tests that can be performed safely in the fitness setting, especially those that do not require specialized equipment or sophisticated procedures. Assessing muscular fitness and functional capabilities in special populations such as older adults, people at increased cardiovascular risk, and children or adolescents is described.

Preliminary Considerations

Muscular fitness often is assessed by the number of repetitions a person can perform with a given weight. This may be viewed as a continuum with strength at one end of the assessment scale and endurance at the other (figure 9.1) (4). According to ACSM (4), tests allowing few repetitions (<5) before momentary muscle fatigue measure muscular strength, whereas those that require high numbers of repetitions (>15) measure muscular endurance. However, the performance of a maximal repetition range (e.g., 4, 6, or 8 repetitions) also can assess strength. Performing fitness tests to assess muscular strength and endurance before commencing exercise training or as part of a fitness screening can provide valuable information about a client's baseline fitness. For example, results from a muscular fitness test can be compared with established standards and can help identify weaknesses in certain muscle groups or muscle imbalances that could be targeted in exercise training programs. The information obtained during baseline muscular fitness assessments also can serve as a basis for designing individualized exercise training programs. An equally useful application of fitness testing is to show a client's progress over time as a result of the training program.

For safety purposes, all participants who undergo fitness testing should first complete a medical history questionnaire and, if necessary, seek consultation from a qualified health care provider to obtain advice on modifying exercise participation. This may include people with known cardiovascular or orthopedic conditions. The ACSM procedures for administering a careful health risk assessment have

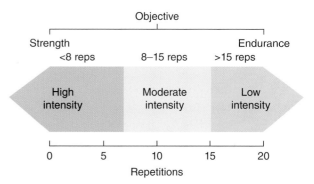

FIGURE 9.1 Classification of intensity of resistance exercise for training and assessment. Weight loads allowing few reps (<15) test for muscular strength, and weight loads that can be repeatedly lifted (>15 reps) assess muscular endurance.

Adapted from American College of Sports Medicine 2006.

been described in detail in this textbook (see chapter 2) and elsewhere (4).

• Standardization of testing protocols. According to ACSM (4), people should participate in familiarization (practice) sessions, adhere to one test protocol, and perform a proper warm-up in order to obtain a reliable score that can be used to track true physiologic adaptations over time. Other standardized conditions that promote safe muscular fitness tests that yield valid and reproducible results include ensuring that the participant uses a strict posture, a predetermined speed of contractions, and a full ROM on all lifts. Safety measures should be reviewed. Additionally, the muscular fitness tests should be specific to the training program.

• Familiarization. To obtain a reliable test score that can be used to track physiological adaptations over time, people should become familiar with the testing equipment and protocol by participating in one or more practice sessions with qualified instruction.

• Warm-up. A 5 to 10 min general warm-up including brief cardiorespiratory exercise, calisthenics, and several light repetitions of the specific testing exercise should precede muscular fitness testing. This increases muscle temperature and localized blood flow and promotes appropriate cardiovascular responses to exercise (3, 4). Warm-up procedures that involve the performance of moderate- to high-intensity dynamic movements for the upper and lower body may be of particular value when testing people who have resistance training experience (4, 10).

• Specificity. Muscular strength and endurance are specific to the muscle or muscle group, the type of muscular action (static or dynamic, concentric or eccentric), the speed of muscular action (slow or fast), and the joint angle being tested (18, 24). Accordingly, muscular fitness tests should be similar to the exercises used during the training program.

- Safety. Safety measures related to the testing equipment and providing proper instruction should be employed before testing.

- Interpretation of results. The availability of health criteria or population-specific norms should be considered when choosing a test, particularly when classifying a participant's test data, such as when performing a fitness screening. However, availability of norms is less of a concern when the test is used primarily to detect improvements in muscular fitness, where the absolute strength values (e.g., kilograms lifted) or relative scores (e.g., kilograms lifted per kilogram of body weight) can be compared during repeated testing.

Muscular Strength

Muscular strength refers to the maximal force that can be generated by a specific muscle or muscle group. Isometric or static strength (constant muscle length during muscle activation) can be measured conveniently with a variety of devices, including cable tensiometers and handgrip dynamometers, which measure strength at one specific point in the ROM. The peak force achieved in such tests is called the **maximum voluntary contraction (MVC)**. These tests and devices occasionally are used in research and academic settings but are not used routinely by most health and fitness practitioners. Thus, the procedures for these tests are described in detail elsewhere (5, 18).

Isokinetic testing involves the assessment of maximal muscle tension throughout a range of joint motion at a constant angular velocity (e.g., $60° \cdot sec^{-1}$). Isokinetic testing devices measure peak rotational force, or torque, and data are obtained with specialized equipment that allows the tester to control the speed of rotation (degrees per second) around various joints (e.g., knee, hip, shoulder, elbow). Although the data collected from isokinetic strength assessments may be useful to health and fitness professionals, the necessary computerized equipment is expensive and therefore limits isokinetic testing almost entirely to rehabilitation and research settings. Consequently, isokinetic strength evaluations may not be a practical consideration for most health and fitness practitioners.

The most common type of strength assessment performed by fitness professionals is **dynamic testing**, which involves movement of the body (e.g., push-up) or an external load (e.g., bench press). Dynamic testing is typically inexpensive because it does not require specialized equipment. Moreover, dynamic assessments can be performed with a variety of equipment, such as free weights (barbells and dumbbells) or weight-stack machines, and they can test any major muscle or muscle group through a variety of exercises. Exercises typically used for dynamic strength testing in fitness centers include the bench press, lat pull-down, and leg press.

Components of Muscular Fitness Related to Promoting or Maintaining Good Health, Fitness, and Athletic Performance

Health Aspects of Muscular Fitness

- Preservation or enhancement of fat-free mass and resting metabolic rate
- Preservation or enhancement of bone mass with aging
- Improved glucose tolerance and insulin sensitivity
- Reduced HR and BP response while lifting any submaximal load (which reduces myocardial oxygen demand during activities requiring muscular force)
- Lowered risk of musculoskeletal injury, including low-back pain
- Improved ability to carry out ADLs in older age
- Improved balance and decreased risk of falls in older age
- Improved self-esteem

Performance Aspects of Muscular Fitness

- Enhanced muscular strength and muscular endurance
- Enhanced speed, power, agility, and balance
- Reduced risk for musculoskeletal injuries
- Improved body composition for various events and activities
- Improved confidence for performing certain athletic events and activities involving high levels of muscular fitness
- Enhanced performance in most athletic activities

Adapted from American College of Sports Medicine 2009.

KEY POINT

Muscular strength is best assessed by using a resistance that requires maximum or near-maximum resistance with few repetitions, whereas muscular endurance is assessed by using lighter loads with a greater number of repetitions. In either case, muscular fitness can be assessed safely in the health and fitness setting and provides important information for individualized exercise prescription. An ideal application of these tests is to evaluate changes in muscular fitness over time using standardized testing procedures that ensure valid and reproducible results.

Repetition Maximum Testing

The gold standard of dynamic strength testing is the **1-repetition maximum (1RM)**, the heaviest weight that can be lifted only once using good form (4). In general, 1RM tests are good indicators of strength and can be performed safely in the health and fitness setting with qualified supervision, for example, by fitness professionals who adhere to current guidelines of exercise leadership such as those described in this chapter and by ACSM (3,4). The fitness professional should ensure proper positioning of the client (e.g., grip position and foot stance) and must be readily available to assist in case of a failed repetition. Also, beginners must learn how to exert maximal effort by participating in several familiarization sessions with each strength testing protocol prior to testing. Untrained clients tend to misinterpret submaximal effort for maximal effort due to lack of training experience. Proper familiarization and the presence of experienced spotters who can recognize potentially hazardous situations (e.g., poor exercise technique) will enhance the safety and reliability of strength testing procedures. Maximal or near-maximal strength tests have been shown to be safe for most people, including those with known or latent CHD and risk factors (12). Nonetheless, caution should be used when testing older adults, people at heightened cardiac risk, pregnant women, and people with certain orthopedic concerns (4). In some cases, it may be prudent to delay or even avoid testing until a qualified health care provider has determined the person to be clinically stable.

Multiple **repetition maximum (RM)** tests that involve 8 to 12 repetitions can also safely and effectively assess strength in healthy adults as well as people with stable chronic health conditions, such as high BP or diabetes, that are under control (29). Moreover, when the purpose of testing is to define an initial training load, multiple RM testing minimizes the potential error compared with extrapolating the exercise intensity as a percentage of 1RM. For example, the maximum weight a person can lift 10 times during testing can be used to identify an appropriate weight load for this number of repetitions performed during training and provides an index of strength changes over time, independent of the true 1RM.

The procedures used to assess 1RM can be modified to test any given number of repetitions (e.g., 10RM). Moreover, it is possible to estimate the 1RM when multiple RM tests are used. For instance, the 10RM weight has been shown to be approximately 75% of the 1RM weight (21). Although a fair amount of individual variability can be expected when extrapolating 1RM from 10RM, this may be desirable in some cases. Regardless of the RM testing protocol, fitness professionals must communicate with the client to determine a progression pattern of loading that is consistent with the client's capacity. Asking questions (e.g., "Can you lift five more pounds?" or "Are you close to your max?"), offering encouragement, and showing concern for the client during the testing session can help to ensure maximal performance.

Interpreting Results

It is best to express strength as a ratio of weight lifted during a single or multiple RM test relative to body weight when comparing strength assessments of people who differ in body mass, such as when comparing men and women. The following procedure describes how to determine a strength ratio from a 10RM test (21):

1. Determine the heaviest weight the client can lift for 10 good repetitions (10RM weight load).
2. Convert the 10RM weight load to a 1RM estimation by dividing the weight load by 0.75.
3. Divide the estimated 1RM by the client's body weight to obtain the strength ratio.

For example, a client who weighs 140 lb (63.5 kg) and completes 10 leg presses with 120 lb (54.4 kg) has an estimated 1RM of 120 ÷ 0.75, or 160 lb (72.6 kg). Her leg press weight ratio is 1.14 (160 ÷ 140).

Normative Data

Normative strength scores such as lower- or upper-body strength ratios for various age and sex categories have been published in *ACSM's Guidelines for Exercise Testing and Prescription* (4). However, most normative data have been derived from a relatively homogeneous sample of subjects (mostly middle- to upper-class Caucasians) using only certain types of resistance training equipment, which limits interpretation of test scores. For example, because equipment design can vary significantly from one manufacturer to another and because of inherent differences in using free weights versus machine weights, strength scores can vary widely using different testing equipment. Thus, client scores can only be compared with norms generated from tests performed with the same type of equipment.

Procedures for 1RM Testing

1. The subject performs a light warm-up set of 5 to 10 repetitions at 40% to 60% of perceived maximum (e.g., light to moderate exertion).

2. After a 1 min rest, the subject performs 3 to 5 repetitions at 60% to 80% of perceived maximum (e.g., moderate to hard exertion).

3. The subject attempts a 1RM lift. If the lift is successful, the subject rests 3 min and repeats the test with a heavier load. This process is continued until a failed attempt occurs. The goal is to find the 1RM within 3 to 5 attempts to avoid excessive fatigue.

4. The 1RM is reported as the weight of the last successfully completed lift with proper exercise technique.

Adapted, by permission, from W. Kraemer et al., 2006, Strength Training: Development and evaluation of methodology. In *Physiological assessment of human fitness*, edited by P.J. Maud and C. Foster (Champaign, IL: Human Kinetics), 119-150.

Future research is needed to provide norms for a variety of resistance training equipment as well as norms for diverse races, ethnicities, and age groups.

Comparing Pretraining and Posttraining

Often, the primary purpose of a muscular fitness test is to evaluate changes in strength over the course of a fitness program. Periodic muscle fitness testing is particularly appealing because it eliminates the need to compare individual data with data provided in normative tables. The frequency of follow-up testing depends on the quality and quantity of exercise training by the client as well as the client's desire and the availability of staff. When multiple tests are performed over time, useful feedback to the client should include the *percentage improvement of strength or endurance* (i.e., percentage change between tests). This is obtained by dividing the pretraining score by posttraining score and multiplying by 100. For example, if Mrs. Smith performs a 10RM baseline of 40 lb (18.1 kg) on the chest press and improves to 60 lb (27.2 kg) during follow-up testing, she has demonstrated a 50% strength gain ([60 − 40 ÷ 40] · 100%) on that lift. This information can provide positive reinforcement about the efficacy of the training program. In cases when the client does not improve, recommendations for altering the exercise program can be made based on the client's goals.

Muscular Endurance

Muscular endurance is the ability of a muscle group to repeatedly contract over a time long enough to cause muscular fatigue or to maintain a specific percentage of the MVC for a prolonged time (4). Equipment (e.g., free weights or machines) for measuring strength can be used to assess **local muscular endurance**. In addition, simple field tests such as an abdominal curl-up (crunch) test (11, 14) or the maximum number of push-ups that can be performed

without rest (8) can be used to evaluate the endurance of the abdominal or upper-body muscles, respectively. These field tests can be used either independently or in combination with other methods of strength or endurance assessment, such as RM testing. Tests such as the abdominal curl-up or the push-up can screen for muscle weaknesses related to various health indicators. For example, scientific data suggest that poor abdominal strength or endurance predisposes muscular low-back pain and that the curl-up test can help identify people who have abdominal strength or endurance weakness that may contribute to low-back pain (4, 22). Moreover, the muscles of the upper body, such as those tested by the push-up, are used in many daily activities such as raking or gardening, carrying luggage, or painting. Thus, these tests are a practical way to evaluate a client's muscular fitness and to provide useful feedback to the client about how muscular conditioning affects many common activities.

Push-Up and Curl-Up Tests

The procedures used to perform the push-up and curl-up (abdominal crunch) tests as described by ACSM (4) are presented and shown in figures 9.2 and 9.3 (push-up test) and 9.4 (curl-up test). The push-up test evaluates muscular endurance of the upper body, including the triceps, deltoid, and pectoral muscles. There are two standard push-up positions: one with the hands and toes in contact with the floor and the other with the hands and knees in contact with the floor (the modified push-up position). The procedures for administering the test are similar and either position may be used for men or women since the position should be based on strength, not gender. However, the norms for the standard push-up are for men and the norms for the modified push-up are for women. When women perform the standard push-up and men perform the modified push-up, pre- and posttraining scores can be compared to evaluate improvement over time; however, the table of norms should not be used in these circumstances. As with RM testing, the push-up and curl-up tests should be used with caution when testing older adults and people at heightened cardiac risk. The curl-up test should not be used for pregnant women after the first trimester or for other people with certain orthopedic or musculoskeletal concerns such as low-back pain (4).

The bent-knee curl-up test evaluates abdominal muscle endurance. Full sit-up tests are unsatisfactory because hip flexor involvement during the sit-up motion may harm

the low back (see chapter 10). Even though the traditional sit-up has been modified, as it is in the bent-knee position, the low back is still stressed during the motion. Consequently, the bent-knee curl-up test has been modified to reduce the potential for low-back injury and to better assess abdominal muscle function (11).

Both the push-up and curl-up tests are relatively simple, inexpensive methods for assessing muscular endurance,

Push-Up and Abdominal Curl-Up (Crunch) Test Procedures

Push-Up

1. Explain the purpose of the test to the client (to determine how many push-ups can be completed in order to reflect upper-body muscular strength and endurance).

2. Inform clients of proper breathing technique (to exhale with the effort, which occurs when pushing away from the floor).

3. The push-up test usually is administered with male subjects in the up position with hands shoulder-width apart, back straight, and head up, using the toes as the pivotal point. For female subjects, the modified knee push-up position often is used, with legs together, lower legs in contact with mat, ankles plantar flexed, back straight, hands shoulder-width apart, and head up. (Note: Some males will need to use the modified position, and some females can use the full-body position).

4. The subject must lower the body until the chin touches the mat. The stomach should not touch the mat.

5. For both men and women, the back must be straight at all times and the subject must push up to a straight-arm position.

6. Demonstrate the test and allow the client to practice if desired.

7. Remind the client that the maximal number of push-ups performed consecutively without rest is counted as the score.

8. Begin the test when the client is ready. Stop the test when the client strains forcibly or is unable to maintain the appropriate exercise technique for two consecutive repetitions.

Curl-Up (Crunch)

1. Explain the purpose of the test to the client (to determine how many curl-ups can be completed in order to reflect the strength and endurance of the abdominal muscles).

2. Explain proper breathing technique (to exhale with the effort, which occurs when curling up from the floor).

3. Have the client assume a supine position on a mat, with the knees at 90°. The arms are at the sides, with the tips of the fingers touching a piece of masking tape. A second piece of masking tape is placed 10 cm beyond the first. Clients slide the arms along the floor as they curl up, and they stop the curl-up when their fingers reach the second piece of tape.*

4. Set a metronome to 50 beats · min^{-1}. Instruct the client to perform slow, controlled curl-ups to lift the shoulder blades off the mat (the trunk makes a 30° angle with the mat) in time with the metronome (25 curl-ups · min^{-1}). The low back should be flattened before curling up.

5. Demonstrate the test and allow the client to practice if desired.

6. Have the client perform as many curl-ups as possible without pausing, up to a maximum of 25.**

*Alternatives include (a) holding the hands across the chest and counting when the trunk reaches a 30° position and (b) placing the hands on the thighs and curling up until the hands reach the kneecaps. Elevating the trunk to 30° is the important part of the movement.

**An alternative includes doing as many curl-ups as possible in 1 min.

Adapted from American College of Sports Medicine 2010.

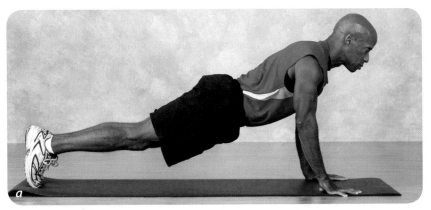

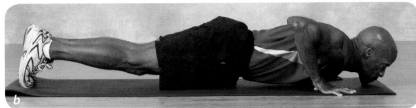

FIGURE 9.2 Proper form for the (a) starting position and (b) finishing position of the standard push-up test, as described by ACSM (4).

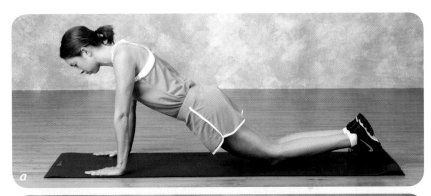

FIGURE 9.3 Proper form for the (a) starting position and (b) finishing position of the modified push-up test, as described by ACSM (4).

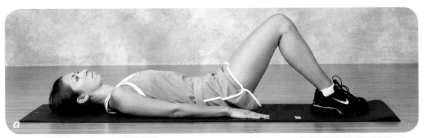

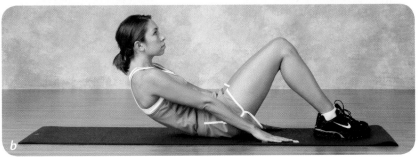

FIGURE 9.4 Proper form for the (a) starting position and (b) finishing position of the abdominal curl-up test, as described by ACSM (4).

and both can be used for men and women of various ages. Results of the standard push-up test for men and modified push-up test for women and curl-up tests for men and women can be compared with the standards in tables 9.1 and 9.2. As with RM testing, the push-up and curl-up tests can be performed on multiple occasions over time to reliably assess changes in muscular endurance that occur with training. Finally, very deconditioned people, especially those who are overweight or obese, may find these tests difficult, and poor results obtained during testing may discourage them from exercise participation. Thus, for each participant, the fitness professional must carefully consider whether these tests are appropriate and likely to yield useful information. In such circumstances where relatively low strength prohibits performance of extended repetitions (i.e., <15), the curl-up and push-up tests are not adequate to assess muscular endurance.

YMCA Bench Press Test

There are alternatives to the push-up and curl-up tests. The fitness professional can adapt resistance training equipment to measure muscular endurance by selecting an appropriate submaximal level of resistance and measuring the number of repetitions or the duration of static contraction before fatigue. For example, the YMCA bench press test involves performing standardized repetitions at a rate of 30 lifts · min^{-1} to test muscular endurance of the upper body (17). Men use an 80 lb (36.3 kg) barbell and women use a 35 lb (15.9 kg) barbell, and subjects are scored by the number of successful repetitions completed. The main disadvantage of the test is that it uses a fixed weight, which favors heavier clients over lighter clients. Also, the fixed weight may be too heavy for deconditioned or older clients to lift repeatedly. On the other hand, the load may be too light for very fit subjects, who may perform significantly more repetitions than typically used during training.

Despite these limitations, this test can be used independently or in combination with other tests in the overall assessment of muscular fitness in clients who have experience using free weights. The procedures for this test are summarized next, and norms are shown in tables 9.3 and 9.4.

1. Use a 35 lb (15.9 kg) straight barbell for women or an 80 lb (36.3 kg) straight barbell for men. A spotter should be present during the test.

2. Set a metronome to 60 beats · min^{-1}.

TABLE 9.1 Fitness Categories by Age and Gender for Push-Up Test Using Number Completed

Fitness	20-29 YR M	20-29 YR F	30-39 YR M	30-39 YR F	40-49 YR M	40-49 YR F	50-59 YR M	50-59 YR F	60-69 YR M	60-69 YR F
Excellent	≥36	≥30	≥30	≥27	≥25	≥24	≥21	≥21	≥18	≥17
Very good	29-35	21-29	22-29	20-26	17-24	15-23	13-20	11-20	11-17	12-16
Good	22-28	15-20	17-21	13-19	13-16	11-14	10-12	7-10	8-10	5-11
Fair	17-21	10-14	12-16	8-12	10-12	5-10	7-9	2-6	5-7	1-4
Needs improvement	≤16	≤9	≤11	≤7	≤9	≤4	≤6	≤1	≤4	≤1

Canadian Standardized Test of Fitness Operations Manual, 3rd ed., Health Canada, 2003. Reproduced with permission from the Minister of Public Works and Government Services Canada, 2011.

TABLE 9.2 Fitness Categories by Age and Gender for Curl-Up Test Using Number Completed in 1 Minute

Fitness	20-29 YR M	20-29 YR F	30-39 YR M	30-39 YR F	40-49 YR M	40-49 YR F	50-59 YR M	50-59 YR F	60-69 YR M	60-69 YR F
Excellent	25	25	25	25	25	25	25	25	25	25
Very good	21-24	18-24	18-24	19-24	18-24	19-24	17-24	19-24	16-24	17-24
Good	16-20	14-17	15-17	10-18	13-17	11-18	11-16	10-18	11-15	8-16
Fair	11-15	5-13	11-14	6-9	6-12	4-10	8-10	6-9	6-10	3-7
Needs improvement	≤10	≤4	≤10	≤5	≤5	≤3	≤7	≤5	≤5	≤2

Canadian Standardized Test of Fitness Operations Manual, 3rd ed., Health Canada, 2003. Reproduced with permission from the Minister of Public Works and Government Services Canada, 2011.

3. Have the subject begin with the bar in the down position touching the chest, with the elbows flexed and hands shoulder-width apart.

4. Count 1 repetition when the elbows fully extend. After each extension, the participant should lower the bar to touch the chest.

5. Instruct the client to complete up or down movements in time to the 60 beats $\cdot$ min^{-1} rhythm, which should be 30 lifts $\cdot$ min^{-1}.

6. Count the total number of repetitions completed in good form.

KEY POINT

The most common type of muscle fitness assessment in the fitness setting is dynamic strength testing with a single or multiple RM protocol. Although lack of adequate normative data often limits the evaluation of individual test data, such tests are valuable for tracking strength and muscular endurance improvement. Field tests such as the push-up and abdominal curl-up tests provide a practical approach for evaluating muscular fitness, either alone or together with other types of muscular fitness evaluations.

RESEARCH INSIGHT

The purpose of a study by Curry et al. (10) was to compare three warm-up protocols including static stretching, dynamic stretching (i.e., dynamic warm-up such as walking lunges or quick sprints), and light aerobic activity on selected measures of ROM and power in untrained females. A total of 24 healthy females (aged 23-29 yr) attended one familiarization session and three test sessions on nonconsecutive days within 2 wk. A within-subject design protocol with the testing investigators blinded to the subjects' warm-up was followed. Each session started with 5 min of light aerobic cycling followed by pretest baseline measures. Another 5 min of light aerobic cycling was completed, followed by one of the three randomly selected warm-up interventions (static stretching, dynamic stretching, or light aerobic activity). Analysis of the data revealed that warm-ups with an active component tended to have beneficial effects. The data suggest that dynamic stretching has greater ability than static stretching to enhance performance on strength and power tests.

TABLE 9.3 YMCA Bench Press Norms for Number of Repetitions Completed for Men Using 80 lb (36.3 kg)

	AGE (YR)					
Fitness	18-25	26-35	36-45	46-55	56-65	66+
Excellent	44-64	41-61	36-55	28-47	24-41	20-36
Good	34-41	30-37	26-32	21-25	17-21	12-16
Above average	29-33	26-29	22-25	16-20	12-14	9-10
Average	24-28	21-24	18-21	12-14	9-11	7-8
Below average	20-22	17-20	17-14	9-11	5-8	4-6
Poor	13-17	12-16	9-12	5-8	2-4	2-3
Very poor	<10	≤9	≤6	≤2	≤1	≤1

Adapted from Golding 2000.

TABLE 9.4 YMCA Bench Press Norms for Number of Repetitions Completed for Women Using 35 lb (15.9 kg)

	AGE (YR)					
Fitness	16-25	26-35	36-45	46-55	56-65	65+
Excellent	42-66	40-62	33-57	29-50	24-42	18-30
Good	30-38	29-34	26-30	20-24	17-21	12-16
Above average	25-28	24-28	21-24	14-18	12-14	8-10
Average	20-22	18-22	16-20	10-13	8-10	5-7
Below average	16-18	14-17	12-14	7-9	5-6	3-4
Poor	9-13	9-13	6-10	2-6	2-4	0-2
Very poor	≤6	≤6	≤4	≤1	≤1	0

Adapted from Golding 2000.

Testing Older Adults

The number of older adults in the United States is expected to increase exponentially over the next several decades. For instance, in 1990 there were 31.2 million U.S. adults (13%) aged 65 or older, but this number is expected to more than double to 70.3 million (20%) by the year 2030 (27). Because people are living longer, it is becoming increasingly important to find ways to extend active, healthy lifestyles and to reduce physical frailty in later years (2, 25). Assessing muscular strength and local muscular endurance as well as other aspects of physical fitness in older adults can reveal physical weaknesses and be used to design exercise programs that improve strength before serious functional limitations occur.

Senior Fitness Test

In response to the need for improved assessment for older adults, Rikli and Jones (31) developed a functional fitness test battery, the Senior Fitness Test (SFT). This test evaluates the key physiological parameters (i.e., strength, endurance, agility, and balance) needed to perform everyday physical activities that are often difficult in later years. One aspect of the SFT is the 30 sec chair stand test (see Research Insight). This test, as well as others of the SFT, meets scientific standards for reliability and validity, is simple and easy to administer in the field setting, and has performance norms for men and women aged 60 to 94 based on a study of more than 7,000 older Americans (30). This test also has been shown to correlate well with other strength tests such as the 1RM. The fitness professional can use the SFT to safely and effectively assess muscular strength and endurance in most older adults.

Assessing Muscular Fitness With the Senior Fitness Test

Before testing, all participants should warm up and follow other preliminary procedures as described earlier. In addition, the following instruction is recommended as a standardization procedure for administering the chair stand test and the arm curl test to all clients:

> Do the best you can on each test item but never push yourself to a point of overexertion or beyond what you think is safe for you.

30 Sec Chair Stand Test

The 30 sec chair stand test, which reflects lower-body strength, involves counting the number of times within 30 sec that the subject can rise to a full stand from a seated position without pushing off with the arms (figure 9.5). Studies have shown that chair stand performance, a common method of assessing lower-body strength in older adults, correlates well with major criterion indicators of lower-body strength (e.g., isokinetic-measured knee extensor and knee flexor strength), stair-climbing ability, walking speed, and risk of falling (6), and it has been found to detect normal age-related declines in strength (9). Further, the chair stand has been found to be safe and sensitive in detecting the effects of physical training in older adults (19, 26). Table 9.5 summarizes the normal range of scores of participants aged 60 to 94. The normal range is defined as the middle 50% of the population tested for each age group, with the lower limits being equivalent to the 25th percentile rank and the upper limits equivalent to the 75th percentile rank within each 5 yr age group.

Arm Curl Test

Upper-body function, including arm strength and local muscular endurance, is important in executing many everyday activities such as carrying groceries, lifting a suitcase, and picking up grandchildren (27). The 30 sec single-arm curl test, a measure of upper-body strength and endurance, determines the number of times a dumbbell (5 lb, or 2.3 kg, for women and 8 lb, or 3.6 kg, for men) can be curled through a full ROM in 30 sec. The prescribed protocol includes holding the weight in a handshake grip at full extension (to the side of the chair) and then supinating during flexion so that the palm of the hand faces the biceps at full flexion (figure 9.6). Results of studies indicate that the 30 sec arm curl test is a good predictor of both biceps strength and overall upper-body strength (30). Most participants, including those with arthritis, are able to perform the arm curl test without much discomfort and are less bothered performing the arm curl test described here than the maximum grip strength protocol commonly used as a strength measure in other studies (30). Results obtained from the 30 sec arm curl test can be compared with the norms presented in table 9.4.

Testing Clients With Cardiovascular Disease

Moderate resistance training performed just twice a week improves muscular fitness, prevents and manages a variety of chronic medical conditions, modifies coronary risk factors, and enhances psychosocial well-being for people with CVD, including high BP (hypertension), diabetes, and CHD (16). Resistance training could benefit most adults living with heart disease and its associated risk factors such as high BP and type 1 or type 2 diabetes. This is because many people with and without cardiovascular conditions do not regularly participate in muscular strengthening exercises and lack the physical strength and self-confidence to perform common daily activities that require muscular effort (29). Consequently, authoritative professional health

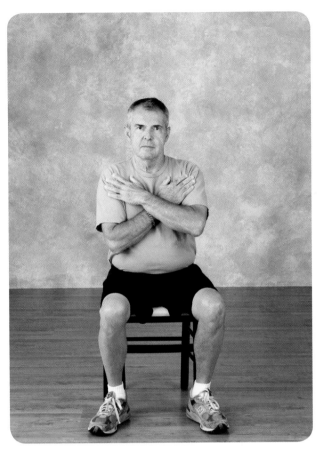 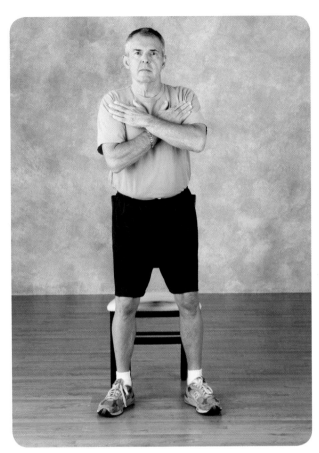

FIGURE 9.5 The 30 sec chair stand test (31).

TABLE 9.5 Normal Range of Scores on the 30 Sec Chair Stand and 30 Sec Arm Curl Tests for Older Adults

	AGE (YR)						
	60-64	**65-69**	**70-74**	**75-79**	**80-84**	**85-89**	**90-94**
CHAIR STAND (# OF STANDS)							
Women	12-17	11-16	10-15	10-15	9-14	8-13	4-11
Men	14-19	12-18	12-17	11-17	10-15	8-14	7-12
ARM CURL (# OF REPS)							
Women	13-19	12-18	12-17	11-17	10-16	10-15	8-13
Men	16-22	15-21	14-21	13-19	13-19	11-17	10-17

Normal is defined as the middle 50% of the population. Participants scoring above or below these ranges would be considered above normal or below normal for their age.

Reprinted, by permission, from R.E. Rikli and C.J. Jones, 2001, *Senior fitness test manual* (Champaign, IL: Human Kinetics), 143.

organizations, including the AHA (29), ACSM (4), and American Association of Cardiovascular and Pulmonary Rehabilitation (AACVPR) (1), support resistance training as an adjunct to endurance exercise in their current recommendations and guidelines on exercise for people with CVD. Resistance training is also recommended in the evidence-based clinical practice guidelines on cardiac rehabilitation (32).

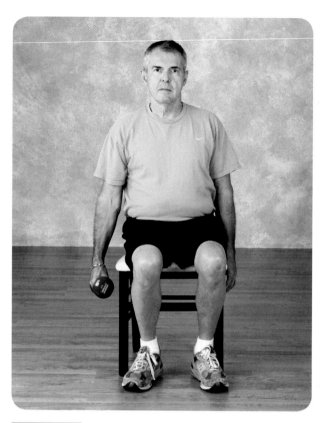 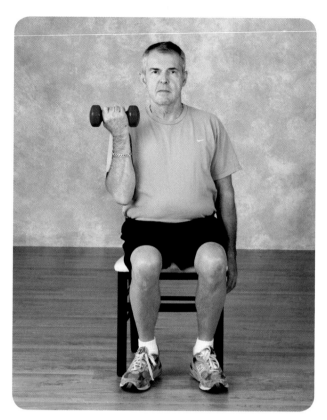

FIGURE 9.6 The 30 sec arm curl test (31).

Both moderate- and high-intensity (40%-80% 1RM) resistance testing and training can be performed safely by cardiac patients deemed low risk (e.g., patients with absence of angina or serious ventricular arrhythmias during normal activities, with good left ventricular function, and with good exercise capacity) (29). Moreover, despite concerns that resistance exercise elicits abnormal cardiovascular pressor responses such as severely elevated BP in patients with CHD or controlled hypertension, studies have found that strength tests and resistance training in these individuals typically elicit clinically acceptable HR and BP responses (12, 28). Specific data on the benefits and safety of resistance training in women with CHD and patients with poor left ventricular function, such as those with CHF, are limited, and these areas require additional investigation. Current exercise guidelines suggest that patients with uncontrolled hypertension (>160/90 mmHg), unstable angina pectoris, uncompensated CHF, poor left ventricular function (ejection fraction < 30%), abnormal hemodynamic responses during a clinical exercise test, severe orthopedic limitations, or uncontrolled metabolic diseases (e.g., uncontrolled diabetes or thyroid disease) should not undergo strength testing or training until their clinical status improves or stabilizes and until they receive appropriate medical clearance (29).

As with GXT, the risk of a serious cardiac event during strength testing can be minimized by proper preparticipation screening and close supervision by fitness professionals, particularly those with specialized training and certification regarding people who have special health concerns. When testing patients with known or suspected CHD or hypertension, the fitness professional should do preliminary work to establish appropriate weight loads and instruct the participant on proper lifting techniques. This should include demonstrating proper ROM and speed of movement for each exercise as well as correct breathing patterns to avoid the Valsalva maneuver. The monitoring of resting and recovery BP (e.g., every few min) and identification and evaluation of abnormal signs and symptoms should be standard protocol during the initial evaluation of the cardiovascular response during testing. Exaggerated BP responses, clinical signs or symptoms of CHD, or any other abnormal findings as previously described by ACSM that occur during resistance testing or training indicate termination of the activity until further evaluation by a qualified health care provider (4). Because BP measured immediately after exercise tends to underestimate values during contractions, the fitness professional should act conservatively when evaluating cardiovascular responses to testing in this population (15, 20).

RESEARCH INSIGHT

Measuring lower-body strength is critical in evaluating the functional performance of older adults. Jones, Rikli, and Beam's 1999 study (23) assessed the test–retest reliability and validity of a 30 sec chair stand as a measure of lower-body strength in adults over the age of 60. Seventy-six community-dwelling older adults (mean age = 70.5 yr) volunteered to participate in the study, which involved performing two 30 sec chair stand tests and two maximum leg press tests, each conducted on separate days 2 to 5 days apart. Test–retest interclass correlations of .84 for men and .92 for women, together with a nonsignificant change in scores from day 1 to day 2, indicated that the 30 sec chair stand has good stability reliability. A moderately high correlation between chair stand performance and maximum weight-adjusted leg press performance for both men and women ($r = .78$ and $.71$, respectively) supported the criterion-related validity of the chair stand as a measure of lower-body strength. Construct (or discriminant) validity of the chair stand was demonstrated by the ability of the test to detect differences among groups of various ages and physical activity levels. As expected, chair stand performance decreased significantly across age groups in decades—from the 60s to the 70s to the 80s ($p < .01$)—and was significantly lower for participants who were less active than for participants who were highly active ($p < .0001$). It was concluded that the 30 sec chair stand provides a reliable and valid indicator of lower-body strength in generally active, community-dwelling older adults.

Studies thus far have shown no adverse hemodynamic responses in low-risk cardiac patients who perform 1RM or multiple RM testing for upper- and lower-body exercises (12, 15). Moreover, there is no scientific evidence suggesting that 1RM testing is riskier than 10RM testing for low-risk cardiac patients. However, multiple RM testing (e.g., 5RM or 10RM) is a more conservative and, therefore, sensible approach to testing clients with a history of CVD. Thus, multiple RM testing that includes higher repetitions (i.e., 10-15) rather than single or low repetitions is a recommended practice for the fitness professional to assess strength and endurance in people with stable CHD. Regardless of the number of repetitions used during testing, the initial resistance or weight should be moderate to allow the participant to achieve the proper repetition range by work-

ing at a level that is somewhat hard (i.e., 13-15 on Borg's original RPE scale; see chapter 5) (7). Furthermore, the procedures for strength assessment previously described in this chapter can be applied safely to clients with a history of known or occult CHD who are clinically stable and to clients with controlled hypertension, diabetes, or other cardiovascular high risk factors. Careful screening and astute monitoring of abnormal signs or symptoms, such as angina, dizziness, or light-headedness, are paramount to minimize any potential risks while simultaneously maximizing the benefits of resistance testing or training for people with and without known CVD.

Testing Children and Adolescents

Along with CRF, flexibility, and body composition, muscular strength is an important component of health-related fitness in children and adolescents (13). Enhancing muscular strength helps young people develop proper posture, reduce the risk of injury, improve body composition, and enhance motor skills such as sprinting and jumping (4, 13). Assessing muscular strength and endurance with the push-up and abdominal curl-up is common in most physical education programs and YMCA recreation programs, whereas maximal load lifting (e.g., 1RM and 10RM) is often used to evaluate training-induced changes in performance in youth sport centers and pediatric research facilities (13). Standardized testing procedures have been developed for young people, and normative data for children and teenagers are available in most physical education textbooks. When properly administered, a variety of fitness measures can be used to assess a child's strength, develop a personalized fitness program, track progress, and motivate participants.

Unsupervised or poorly administered strength assessments may not only discourage young people from participating in fitness activities but also result in injury. Qualified fitness professionals should demonstrate how to properly perform each exercise, allow the child to practice a few repetitions of each exercise, and offer guidance when necessary. This is particularly important when testing untrained youth who may not be aware of the inherent risks associated with resistance training equipment. In addition, it is important to obtain informed consent from the parent or legal guardian before initiating muscular fitness testing or a formal exercise program for children. The informed consent explains potential benefits and risks of resistance testing or training, the right to withdraw at any time, and issues regarding confidentiality.

When assessing fitness in young people, avoid the pass–fail mentality that may discourage some boys and girls from participating. Instead, refer to the assessment as a *challenge* in which all participants can feel good about their performance and get excited about monitoring their progress (4). Fitness professionals should also understand that children are not simply miniature adults. Since children are physically and psychologically less mature than adults, evaluating any measure of physical fitness requires special considerations. Fitness professionals should develop a friendly rapport with each child, and the exercise area should be nonthreatening. Because most children have limited experience performing at maximum exertion, fitness professionals should reassure children that they can safely perform exercise at a high exertion. Moreover, positive encouragement can motivate children to help ensure a valid test outcome. Following the strength assessment, cool down afterward with gentle calisthenics and stretching exercises.

KEY POINT

Muscular fitness testing is useful for a variety of special populations, including older adults, people at increased cardiovascular risk, and children and adolescents. Although strength tests, particularly those involving maximal exertion, were once thought to evoke unsafe physiological responses in these populations, scientific evidence shows that such tests are safe and can provide valuable information for the resistance training prescription if properly administered and performed. For older adults and people at elevated cardiovascular risk, proper screening by a physician or other qualified health care professional is warranted to promote safe and effective muscular fitness evaluations.

STUDY QUESTIONS

1. Define *muscular fitness*.
2. What would you include in a standardization procedure to improve the reliability of a strength test?
3. Describe the procedures for measuring a 1RM.
4. Describe two tests for measuring muscular endurance, one using weights and one using body weight as the resistance.
5. How you would compare the strength of two people who differ markedly in body weight?
6. Describe a lower-body and an upper-body muscular endurance test for seniors.
7. What is the more conservative approach to measuring strength in cardiac patients with regard to RM testing?
8. Describe two muscular endurance tests used with schoolchildren as part of a fitness testing battery.

CASE STUDIES

You can check your answers by referring to appendix A.

1. A middle-aged female who recently joined your fitness facility would like to participate in an initial fitness assessment and receive advice about beginning an overall fitness program. She has not participated in a structured exercise program for several years, although she reports that she leads an active lifestyle and often achieves moderate amounts of physical activity throughout the day. Her preparticipation health history questionnaire reveals that she is without signs, symptoms, or diagnosis of any cardiovascular, metabolic, or musculoskeletal conditions. With a classmate playing the role of this client, practice the following procedures presented in this chapter:

   a. Explain, demonstrate, and perform the procedures for the push-up test.
   b. Using the client information just described, explain, demonstrate, and perform the procedures for the curl-up test.
   c. Using the client information just described, explain, demonstrate, and perform the procedures for the 1RM bench press test.

REFERENCES

1. American Association of Cardiovascular and Pulmonary Rehabilitation (AACVPR). 2006. *AACVPR cardiac rehabilitation resource manual.* Champaign, IL: Human Kinetics.

2. American College of Sports Medicine (ACSM). 2009. Exercise and physical activity for older adults. *Medicine and Science in Sports and Exercise* 41:1510-1530.

3. American College of Sports Medicine (ACSM). 2009. Progression models in resistance training for healthy adults. *Medicine and Science in Sports and Exercise* 41:687-708.

4. American College of Sports Medicine (ACSM). 2010. *ACSM's guidelines for exercise testing and prescription.* 8th ed. Baltimore: Lippincott Williams & Wilkins.

5. Bohannon, R.W. 1990. Muscle strength testing with hand-held dynamometers. In *Muscle strength testing: Instrumented and non-instrumented systems,* ed. L.R. Amundsen, 69-112. New York: Churchill Livingstone.

6. Bohannon, R.W. 1995. Sit-to-stand test for measuring performance of lower extremity muscles. *Perceptual and Motor Skills* 80:163-166.

7. Borg, G. 1982. Psychophysical bases of perceived exertion. *Medicine and Science in Sports and Exercise* 14:377-381.

8. Government of Canada, Fitness and Amateur Sport. 1986. *Canadian Standardized Test of Fitness operations manual.* 3rd ed. Ottawa: Author.

9. Csuka, M., and D.J. McCarty. 1985. Simple method for measurement of lower extremity muscle strength. *Journal of the American Medical Association* 78:77-81.

10. Curry, B.S., D. Chengkalath, G.J. Crouch, M. Romance, and P.J. Manns.2009. Acute effects of dynamic stretching, static stretching, and light aerobic activity on muscular performance in women. *Journal of Strength and Conditioning Research* 23:1811-1819.

11. Diener, M.H., L.A. Golding, and D. Diener. 1995. Validity and reliability of a one-minute half sit-up test of abdominal muscle strength and endurance. *Sports Medicine Training and Rehabilitation* 6:105-119.

12. Faigenbaum, A., G. Skrinar, W. Cesare, W. Kraemer, and H. Thomas. 1990. Physiologic and symptomatic responses of cardiac patients to resistance exercise. *Archives of Physical Medicine and Rehabilitation* 71:395-398.

13. Faigenbaum, A.D., W.J. Kraemer, C.J. Blimke, I. Jeffreys, L.J. Micheli, M. Nitka, and T.W. Rowland. 2009. Youth resistance training: Updated position statement paper from the National Strength and Conditioning Association. *Journal of Strength and Conditioning Research* 23(5 Suppl): S60-S79.

14. Faulkner, R.A., E.S. Springings, A. McQuarrie, and R.D. Bell. 1989. A partial curl-up protocol for adults based on an analysis of two procedures. *Canadian Journal of Sports Science* 14:135-141.

15. Featherstone, J.F., R. Holly, and E. Amsterdam. 1993. Physiologic responses to weightlifting in coronary artery disease. *American Journal of Cardiology* 71:287-292.

16. Fletcher, G.F., G. Balady, V.F. Froelicher, L.H. Hartley, W.L. Haskell, and M.L. Pollock. 1995. Exercise standards: A statement for healthcare professionals from the American Heart Association. *Circulation* 91:580-615.

17. Golding, L.A., ed. 2000. *YMCA fitness testing and assessment manual.* 4th ed. Champaign, IL: Human Kinetics.

18. Graves, J.E., M.L. Pollock, and C.X. Bryant. 2001. Assessment of muscular strength and endurance. In *ACSM's resource manual for guidelines for exercise testing and prescription.* 4th ed. Ed. J.L. Roitman, 376-380. Baltimore: Williams & Wilkins.

19. Guralnik, J.M., E.M. Simosick, L. Ferrucci, R.J. Glynn, L.F. Berkman, D.G. Blazer, P.A. Scherr, and R.B. Wallace. 1994. A short physical performance battery assessing lower extremity function: Association with self-reported disability and prediction of mortality and nursing home admission. *Journal of Gerontology* 49:M85-M94.

20. Haslam, K.A., S.N. McCartney, R.S. McKelvie, and J.D. MacDougall. 1988. Direct measurements of arterial blood pressure during formal weightlifting in cardiac patients. *Journal of Cardiopulmonary Rehabilitation* 8:213-225.

21. Haskell, W.L., I.M. Lee, R.R. Pate, K.E. Powell, S.N. Blair, B.A. Franklin, C.A. Macera, G.W. Heath, P.D. Thompson, and A. Bauman. 2007. Physical activity and public health: Updated recommendation for adults from the American College of Sports Medicine and the American Heart Association. *Medicine and Science in Sports and Exercise* 39:1423-1434.

22. Jackson, A.W., J.R. Morrow, P.A. Brill, and H.W. Kohl. 1998. Relations of sit-up and sit-and-reach to low back pain in adults. *Journal of Orthopaedic and Sports Physical Therapy* 27:22-26.

23. Jones, C.J., R.E. Rikli, and B.C. Beam. 1999. A 30 s chair-stand test as a measure of lower body strength in community residing older adults. *Research Quarterly for Exercise and Sports* 70:113-119.

24. Kraemer, W., N. Ratamess, A. Fry, and D. French. 2006. Strength training: Development and evaluation of methodology. In *Physiological assessment of human fitness,* ed. P. Maud and C. Foster, 119-150. Champaign, IL: Human Kinetics.

25. Lawrence, R., and A.M. Jette. 1996. Disentangling the disablement process. *Journals of Gerontology, YES Series B, Psychological Sciences and Social Sciences* 51b:5173-5182.

26. McMurdo, M., and L. Rennie. 1993. A controlled trial of exercise by residents of old people's homes. *Age and Aging* 22:11-15.

27. Federal Interagency Forum on Aging Related Statistics. 2000. *Older Americans 2000: Key indicators of well-being.* Hyattsville, MD: Author.

28. Pollock, M., and W. Evans. 1999. Resistance training for health and disease. *Medicine and Science in Sports and Exercise* 31:10-11.

29. Pollock, M.L., B.A. Franklin, G.J. Balady, L. Bernard, M.D. Chaitman, J.L. Fleg, B. Fletcher, M. Limacher, I.L. Pina, R.A. Stein, M. Williams, and T. Bazzarre. 2000. Resistance exercise in individuals with and without cardiovascular disease benefits, rationale, safety, and prescription. *Circulation* 101:828-833.

30. Rikli, R.E., and C.J. Jones. 1999. Development and validation of a functional fitness test for community residing older adults. *Journal of Aging and Physical Activity* 7:129-161.

31. Rikli, R.E., and C.J. Jones. 2001. *Senior fitness test manual.* Champaign, IL: Human Kinetics.

32. Wenger, N.K., E.S. Froelicher, L.K. Smith, P.A. Ades, K. Berra, J.A. Blumenthal, C.M. Cerro, A.M. Dattilo, D. Davis, R.F. DeBusk, J.P. Drozda, B.J. Fletcher, B.A. Franklin, H. Gaston, P. Greenland, P.E. McBride, C.G.A. McGregor, N.B. Oldridge, J.C. Piscarella, and F.J. Rogers. 1995. *Cardiac rehabilitation as secondary prevention: Clinical practice guideline* (AHCPR publication no. 96-0672). Rockville, MD: U.S. Department of Health and Human Services, Public Health Service, Agency for Health Care Policy and Research and the National Heart, Lung, and Blood Institute.

Assessment of Flexibility and Low-Back Function

Wendell Liemohn

OBJECTIVES

The reader will be able to do the following:

1. Describe the relationship between flexibility or ROM and low-back function.

2. List five factors that can affect flexibility or ROM.

3. Describe the amount of flexion that can occur between the rib cage and the sacrum and state a general rule for performing lumbar extension exercises.

4. Explain why having good ROM at the hip joint is important to having a healthy back.

5. Describe the pros and cons of the sit-and-reach test.

Flexibility relates to the ability to bend without breaking; **flexion** is the act of bending or being bent. In applied anatomy, *flexion* denotes a bending movement that occurs in the sagittal plane as two body segments are brought together (see chapter 3). When you bend over and touch your toes from the standing position, you demonstrate flexion at both iliofemoral (hip) joints and limited flexion in the lower intervertebral joints of the spine (2). When you return to the standing position, the movement is called *extension;* moving the trunk backward beyond your normal standing posture is called *hyperextension* (see chapter 3). Individuals may be considered flexible if they can show great mobility in either forward bending (flexion) or backward bending (hyperextension), because both movements meet the criteria for the definition of flexion. Because there is potential confusion in describing the ability to hyperextend as flexibility, the term *range of motion (ROM)* frequently is used in place of *flexibility.* The two terms, however, often are interchanged.

Having functional ROM at all joints of the musculoskeletal system ensures efficient body movement, which is one reason why flexibility is a key component of physical fitness. Although some people might be considered to have very good ROM because they perform well in a flexibility test, flexibility is a joint-specific characteristic. In other words, having good ROM in trunk flexion does not guarantee having good ROM in trunk extension. Moreover, sometimes ROM relates to a person's genotype (i.e., is hereditary), and in other cases it relates more to the person's activities. For example, many years of ballet or gymnastics training should make a person more flexible than someone of the same age, same sex, and comparable genotype who did not participate in such training. Natural selection can also be a factor; a person without good innate flexibility might not strive to do well in ballet or gymnastics.

If the body is viewed as a kinetic chain, any asymmetrical tightness or looseness in the joints of the lower extremities could affect the spine. Good ROM is also considered desirable for low-back function. ROM at the hip joint is of particular concern because the position of the sacrum (and contiguous pelvis) is the foundation for the spine, and this position is controlled by muscles originating on the pelvis

or spine and inserting on the femur. ROM of the spine itself is typically not viewed as problematic; however, too much mobility can contribute to instability. For example, if a disc and its supporting ligaments were damaged and the person's ability to control the supporting muscles were insufficient, further injury to the spine could occur. (Motor control of the spine is discussed further in chapter 14.)

Factors Affecting Range of Motion

Many factors affect ROM. Although age, sex, and genotype may be good predictors, there are always exceptions.

Age and Sex

ROM depends on several demographic variables. For example, ROM typically decreases in adulthood; however, it is unknown how much of this diminution is attributable to aging or to the reduction in physical activity related to aging. Females are generally considered to be more flexible than males; commonly cited examples include elbow hyperextension (because of shorter olecranon processes) and flexibility in the pelvic area (because of shallower pelvises) (1). However, the opposite has been found in extension of the spine (26). It is difficult to discriminate between the effects of one's genotype and one's lifestyle when ROM is the topic of discussion (3).

Nature and Nurture

Individuals may increase ROM by participating in flexibility training programs, although, as mentioned previously, a person's genotype can limit flexibility. Some people have relatively poor flexibility; no matter how hard they train, their flexibility improves nominally. Some research suggests that improving ROM may relate more to the ability to tolerate pain than to actual changes in connective-tissue length (17, 20). Moreover, McGill (19) makes a strong argument that tight hamstrings can enhance performance in sports such as basketball. Obviously this issue is extremely complex.

Posture

If individuals do not use their full ROM at a joint, tendinous tissue may compensate by shortening. It then becomes difficult to make some of the movements needed in ADLs. For example, a person sitting at a computer desk several hours each day might develop a greater thoracic curve (i.e., dorsal kyphosis) and rounded shoulders (see figure 10.1*a*). If this posture becomes habitual and no countermeasures are taken to change it, tendinous tissue that previously permitted good movement can shorten and correction of this posture may become difficult, if not impossible, to correct. A much better posture to assume at a desk is seen

KEY POINT

Flexibility and ROM are joint specific. Having good ROM at the hip joint can decrease the chances of having low-back problems. Once a low-back problem has occurred, increasing ROM at the hip joint may be a goal in a therapeutic exercise program. However, in some cases a damaged motion segment may enable too much ROM and cause instability.

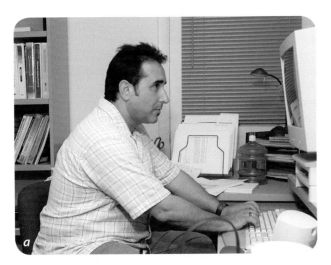
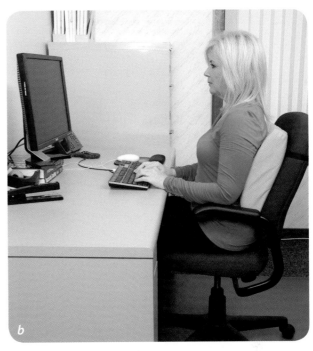

FIGURE 10.1 Connective-tissue structures (e.g., ligaments and tendons) adapt to habitual poor sitting posture (e.g., rounding of the upper back or less lordotic curve in the lumbar region) by lengthening in response to stress (*a*); this adaptation is called *ligamentous creep* and *disc creep*. Without an attempt to remove these stresses or to develop counterbalancing ones, poor sitting postures can transfer to poor standing postures. The person in (*b*) demonstrates a properly balanced sitting posture.

in figure 10.1*b*. In the spine, injuries typically occur near the end of ROM, which should be remembered especially when the spine moves while under load.

Disease

Disease can negatively affect ROM. Arthritis and osteoporosis and their effect on ROM are discussed next.

Arthritis

Arthritis can have a debilitating effect on ROM because it affects articular cartilage. Articular cartilage, also called *hyaline cartilage,* is **avascular** (i.e., it does not have a blood supply), which means its healing capability is poor. Thus, if one or more joints are injured or diseased, the body's compensatory adaptations may work for a while but often become deficient with aging. Because articular cartilage does not repair itself well, fibrocartilage and bony spicules may replace the cartilage, further diminishing joint movement. Two common types of arthritis are **rheumatoid arthritis** and **osteoarthritis**. Rheumatoid arthritis affects females more than males and can occur anytime in life but most often occurs between the ages of 25 and 60. It appears to be an autoimmune disease in some cases, but the exact cause is unknown; it can affect a few joints (pauciarticular) or many joints (polyarticular). Osteoarthritis is much more prevalent and accounts for 90% to 95% of arthritis cases.

It can be considered a disease of aging, because after age 70 it affects about 85% of the population. Its cause is usually some injury or mechanical derangement; however, in some cases the cause is unknown.

Lack of mobility attributable to arthritis often occurs in joints such as the fingers or the knee; however, arthritis also can decrease mobility in the spine if the site is a facet joint (see figure 10.2). Because articular cartilage is avascular, it depends on the diffusion of nutrients from tissue fluid, and so further deterioration can result from lack of movement. Thus, it is desirable for people with arthritis to maintain as much movement and ROM as possible. (See also chapter 14.)

Osteoporosis

Osteoporosis is characterized by a loss in BMD or bone mass. Although it is seen particularly in women after menopause, it can also affect men and may be genetically influenced. Common osteoporotic sites include the hip, wrist, and vertebrae; a common characteristic of these sites is that cancellous bone predominates (see chapter 3). In the spine, osteoporosis can cause buckling and compression of vertebrae. A person with this condition may show extreme curves in the spine as well as loss of ROM. Fortunately, cancellous bone can become denser through weight-bearing activities and resistance training. (See also chapter 17.)

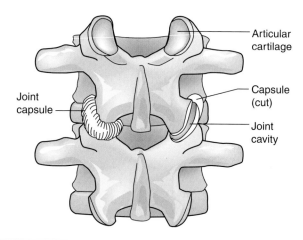

FIGURE10.2 Posterior junctions between two vertebrae often are referred to as *facet joints*. Facet joints are synovial joints and have articular cartilage; if articular cartilage is damaged, arthritis can occur.

Adapted, by permission, from W. Liemohn, 2001, *Exercise prescription and the back* (New York, NY: McGraw-Hill), 11. © The McGraw-Hill Companies.

KEY POINT

Factors relating to ROM include age, sex, heredity, posture, and disease. If joint ROM is not used, it may be lost. Although declines in ROM relate to increased age, some result from a decline in physical activity or from injury. ROM relates to both nature and nurture, meaning that a person's genotype and activities can affect it. Habitual poor posture also can decrease ROM. Arthritis is a disease of the joints and thus tends to decrease joint ROM. Osteoporosis can reduce spine ROM because of its destructive effect on vertebral bodies.

Range of Motion and Low-Back Function

Spinal carriage is functionally integrated with most movements because many movements emanate from the spine. An argument has been made that the spine and its associated tissues are the primary engine of locomotion in humans (7). Accepting this view demands an appreciation of the importance of maintaining good spinal mobility; however, this mobility must also be under muscle control.

Spinal Range of Motion

If one were to bend forward at the waist from an upright standing position (with the movement occurring primarily in the lumbar spine), the nuclei of lumbar intervertebral discs would drift in the direction of the spinous processes of the lumbar vertebrae. If this person were to resume an upright posture and then hyperextend at the lumbar spine, the nuclei of the lumbar discs would drift anteriorly.

As noted in figure 10.3, the flexion movement between the rib cage and the sacrum is, in essence, a straightening of the normal lumbar **lordotic curve**. Although spinal mobility may progressively decline in all planes with aging, McKenzie (21) contends that greater decline occurs in extension because this movement is used less as a person ages. Unfortunately, spine extension is often ignored or misinterpreted in exercise programs (see chapter 14). Although ballistic extension movements (and ballistic rotation movements) of the spine are inappropriate, slow and controlled extension to maintain ROM and strengthen the erector spinae is appropriate in exercise programs. Nevertheless, if the back is actively extended, the person should not exceed the upper limit of the normal lumbar lordosis as seen in standing (25).

Scoliosis is an extreme lateral curvature of the thoracic spine. Although it typically cannot be corrected by exercise, potentially inappropriate exercise could exacerbate the condition (23). If the fitness professional thinks that a client might have a scoliosis, the professional can use the Adam's test to get a better perception of its presence (figure 10.4). Although there are many causes for scoliosis, usually the cause is unknown. A length discrepancy between the legs leading to a lateral tilt of the pelvis is associated

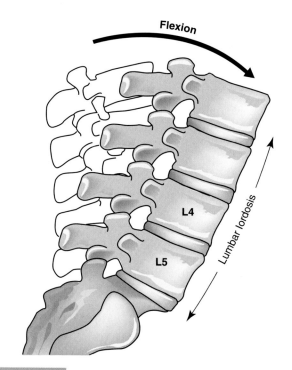

FIGURE10.3 In forward movement of the trunk, lumbar flexion per se does not occur. What some may view as lumbar flexion is in essence a removal of the lordotic curve.

Adapted, by permission, from W. Liemohn, 2001, *Exercise prescription and the back* (New York, NY: McGraw-Hill), 40. © The McGraw-Hill Companies.

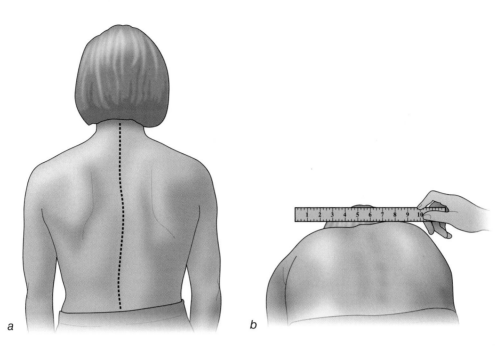

a   b

FIGURE 10.4 Adam's test. Viewing the spinous processes as the subject stands does not always clearly reveal a scoliotic curve. However, if you watch from behind as the subject bends forward, a rib hump may be noted (placing a straight edge on the latter magnifies its presence).

Adapted, by permission, from C.A. Oatis, 2004. *Kinesiology: The mechanics and pathomechanics of human movement* (Philadelphia: Lippincott Williams & Wilkins), 844.

with scoliosis and low-back pain; however, the evidence that scoliosis causes low-back pain is not conclusive. Depending on the degree of scoliosis, a person with this condition may present with a different posturing of the rib cage during abdominal strengthening exercises because of the spinal rotation that scoliosis may cause.

The fitness professional should obtain advice from an appropriate medical professional before prescribing trunk exercises for any client with suspected scoliosis.

Iliofemoral Range of Motion

The muscles crossing the hip joint sometimes are viewed as guy-wires because they can limit movement of the pelvis by bracing it (see figure 10.5). If any of these guy-wires are too tight, the trunk musculature, regardless of how well it is developed, may have difficulty controlling pelvic position. Because the sacrum (in the pelvis) is the foundation of the 24 vertebrae stacked on it, pelvic positioning plays an important role in the integrity of the spine. For example, tightness in the hip flexors such as the psoas can produce an anterior or forward pelvic tilt, and tightness in the hip extensors such as the hamstrings can produce a backward or posterior pelvic tilt (see figure 10.5). Thus, if either of these muscle groups is tight, the ability of the abdominal muscles to control pelvic positioning is adversely affected. Individuals who cannot control their pelvic positioning with their abdominal muscles are predisposed to low-back pain, which is one of the reasons why ROM at the iliofemoral joint is important.

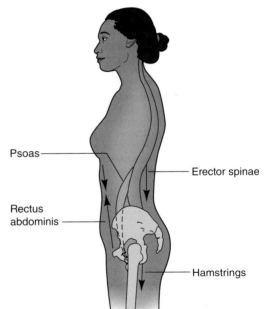

Psoas

Rectus abdominis

Erector spinae

Hamstrings

FIGURE 10.5 The muscles crossing the hip joint can be viewed as guy-wires. If, for example, the hamstring guy-wires are too tight, they will tend to posteriorly rotate the pelvis, making it difficult for the rectus abdominis to control pelvic positioning. Inability to control pelvic positioning with the abdominal musculature predisposes a person to low-back problems.

There also may be tightness in the iliotibial (IT) band, which can limit adduction of the thigh. Tightness in the piriformis muscle can limit movement in the transverse plane; this is a little more complex because such tightness can limit outward or inward rotation of the femur depending on the angle between hip and thigh (25).

KEY POINT

Spinal flexion between the rib cage and the sacrum is limited to the straightening of the normal lordotic curve. Although maintaining spine extension ROM is important, ballistic back extension movements should be avoided, and back extension should not exceed the exerciser's normal lumbar lordosis. IT band and piriformis tightness also have a deleterious effect on the biomechanics of the iliofemoral joint (24).

Measuring Spinal and Hip Range of Motion

Some techniques used to measure ROM as it relates to low-back function are specific to the spine or to the hip joint. Others concurrently measure ROM of the spine and the hip joint.

Trunk Extension Range of Motion

In Imrie and Barbuto's (10) test for back extension, the back musculature is not actively used. This test is considered a passive test of back ROM because the hyperextension movement in the spine results from arm and shoulder muscle contraction (see figure 10.6). An active test of spine extension ROM, called the *trunk lift*, was developed by the Cooper Institute for Aerobics Research (6). It is an active test because muscles of the spine (i.e., erector

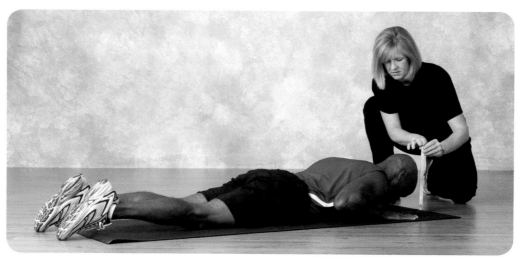

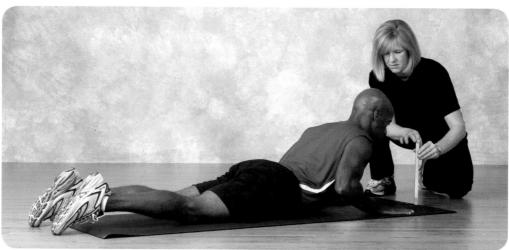

FIGURE 10.6 Passive back ROM test (10). While keeping the anterior part of the pelvis (i.e., anterior superior iliac spines) in contact with the floor, the subject elevates the torso with arm and shoulder muscles; the muscles of the back are not used in this movement. The score is the perpendicular distance from the suprasternal notch to the floor. People with longer trunks tend to have better scores, which should be considered when interpreting test scores. Scoring: 30 cm (12 in.) or more is excellent, 20 cm (8 in.) is good, and 10 cm (4 in.) is fair.

spinae and multifidus) hyperextend the spine (see figure 10.7). Because both trunk extensor strength and ROM contribute to performance in the trunk lift and only ROM contributes to performance in the passive test, we used multiple regression analyses to further study performance on these tests by university students. Somewhat to our surprise, we found that the two tests in essence measured the same construct (14); thus, this area could benefit from further research. However, because the passive test is purer in that it only measures ROM and strength is not a factor, there are advantages to its use.

Hip Range of Motion

The Thomas test typically is used to measure tightness in the hip flexors (see figure 10.8). Two of the more popular tests used to measure tightness of the hamstrings are the relatively new knee extension test, which is active (see figure 10.9), and the often-used straight leg raise test, which is passive (see figure 10.10). In some instances it may be desirable to check for tightness in the IT bands and in the piriformis muscles; however, these tests are more difficult to administer (see figures 10.11 and 10.12; 28).

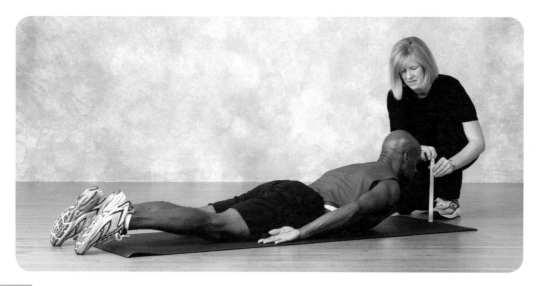

FIGURE 10.7 Active back ROM and strength test. In this test, the subject slowly lifts the torso by contracting the erector spinae and multifidus muscle groups until the chin is a maximum of 30 cm (12 in.) from the mat. This test is from the Cooper Institute for Aerobics Research (6); although norms were not presented, most individuals tested should be able to raise the chin at least 15 cm (6 in.). People with longer trunks tend to have better scores, which should be considered when interpreting test scores.

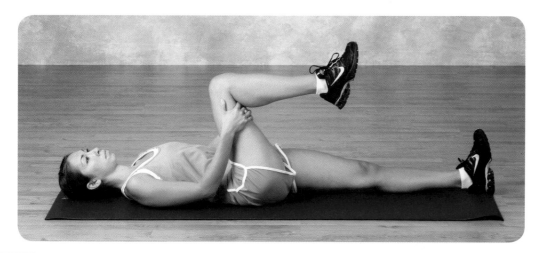

FIGURE 10.8 Thomas test. The subject pulls the contralateral leg toward the chest until the low back touches the testing surface. The thigh should remain in contact with the testing table or floor (11). If it does not, the degree of elevation indicates the tightness of the hip flexors. The tester must ensure that there is not too much posterior rotation of the pelvis. Some subjects may be able to posteriorly rotate the pelvis beyond the point where the low back touches the testing surface, which could result in a false positive (i.e., with too much posterior rotation of the pelvis, anyone's hip flexors might look tight).

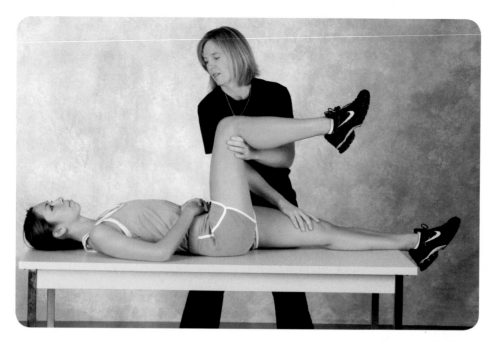

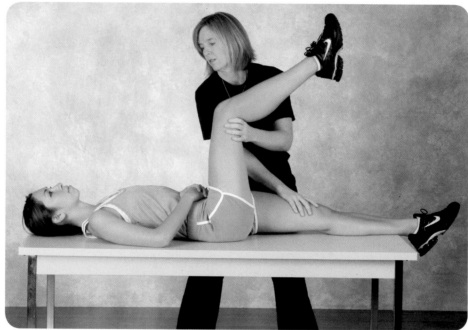

FIGURE 10.9 Active knee extension test. In this test, sometimes referred to as the *90/90 test*, the thigh of one leg is raised perpendicular (i.e., 90° to the testing surface) with the lower leg 90° to the thigh (the tester will have to hold the thigh in this position). The subject then actively extends the lower leg. A score of zero indicates that the leg was moved 90° (i.e., perpendicular to the table and in line with the thigh); a score of 10 indicates that the leg was moved 80°. A score of 5 to 15 is desirable. Many therapists like this test because the subject controls the amount of movement.

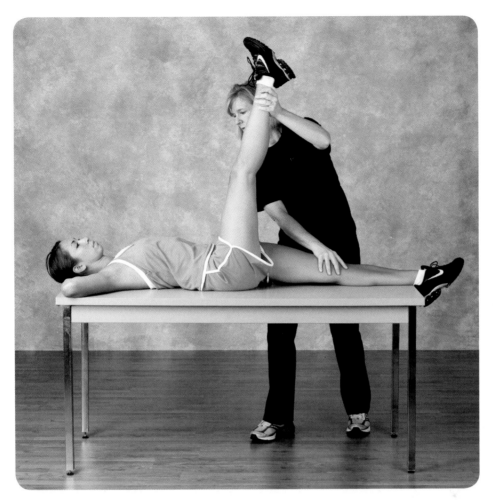

FIGURE 10.10 Passive straight leg raise test. In the test that is recommended, the pelvis is first posteriorly rotated until the low back is snug against the table; one leg is then raised by the tester while ensuring that the other one remains extended and flat on the testing surface. ROM in flexion can be determined with a goniometer placed on its axis on the greater trochanter or an inclinometer placed just below the tibial tubercle. A minimum of 80° is desirable on the passive straight leg raise. If many subjects are being tested, a protractor-type device can be contrived (e.g., marked on wall) to speed up the testing process; however, the measurement will not be as precise.

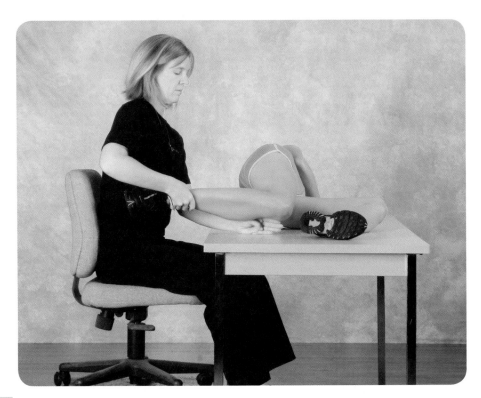

FIGURE 10.11 Ober test (IT band tightness). The pelvis is in the neutral position with the hips stacked. The score is the number of finger-breadths that the medial femoral condyle remains elevated from the testing surface (27). This test can be helpful in determining the effect of exercise programming on IT band tightness, a problem seen in runner's knee (also referred to as *patellofemoral syndrome* or *chondromalacia patella*).

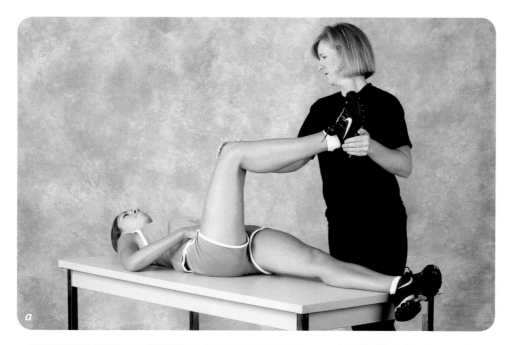

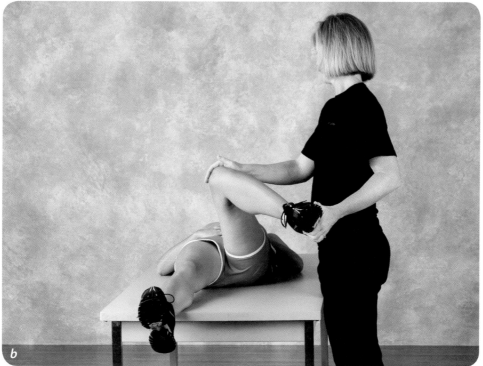

FIGURE 10.12 Piriformis test. Examining piriformis ROM is difficult and thus should be done *only* by those with appropriate experience. It includes (*a*) assessment below 90° of hip flexion (in this position it is an external rotator and abductor) and (*b*) assessment above 90° of hip flexion (in this position it is an internal rotator and adductor) (27). This test can help determine the effect of exercise programming on piriformis tightness.

Combined Tests of Range of Motion in Trunk and Hip Flexion

The fingertips-to-floor and sit-and-reach tests have often been used under the pretense that they measure flexibility in the low back as well as at the hip joint. It has been shown, however, that although both can be used to measure hip joint flexibility (e.g., hamstring length), in their conventional use neither effectively measures low-back ROM (18). Because the sit-and-reach is used more than the fingertips-to-floor test as a field test, it is examined here in greater detail. Most of the following comments apply to its use either as an exercise or as a test.

Using the sit-and-reach test as an exercise has been questioned. For example, if the hamstrings are tight and the sitting stretch is performed ballistically, the spine may be obligated to absorb these stresses, and over time these repetitive motions may have serious consequences for low-back function. Moreover, even if the sit-and-reach is done slowly, the static postures resulting during the stretching phase can place high compressive forces on the intervertebral discs (19, 22). Cailliet (5) cautioned that this exercise might damage ligaments of the spine, particularly if the hamstrings are tight.

To reduce the stress on the spine in the sit-and-reach test, Cailliet (5) recommended what he called a *protective hamstring stretch* (see figure 10.13). In this exercise, the hamstrings of each leg are alternately stretched while the nonstretched limb is bent at the knee joint with its foot flat on the floor next to the contralateral knee. Cailliet contended that lumbosacral stress is less in this hamstring stretch than in the more typical sit-and-reach test with both legs extended; if this is true, the same reasoning would warrant administering the sit-and-reach test with only one leg extended. However, we examined lumbosacral movement in university students tested with both legs extended as well as with just one leg extended and found that less flexion (which would imply less stress) was not seen in Cailliet's version of the sit and reach (15). Nevertheless, Cailliet's protective hamstring stretch has other advantages (e.g., permits checking for symmetry), and it is preferred because it is deemed safer for the spine than the sit-and-reach test with both legs extended.

The sit-and-reach test has also been questioned because it does not allow for proportional differences between arm, trunk, and leg length. In response, Hopkins and Hoeger (8) developed a protocol that purportedly controls for some of this variance (see figure 10.14). More recent research by others suggests that the adjustment for limb length did not improve validity (9).

We noted that performance on the sit-and-reach test was significantly better with the ankle of the tested leg in passive plantar flexion as opposed to the fixed dorsiflexion posture usually required when the test is administered (13).

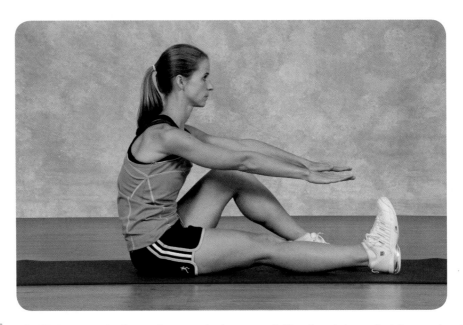

FIGURE 10.13 In Cailliet's protective hamstring stretch, the extensibility of each lower limb is examined. By placing the foot of the nonexamined leg adjacent to the knee of the straightened leg, the posterior rotation of the pelvis decreases the turning moment of inertia of the torso and there is less chance of hyperflexion and disc compression in the lumbar area.

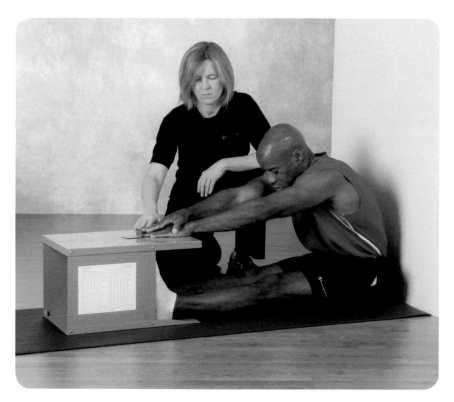

FIGURE 10.14 In the Hopkins and Hoeger sit-and-reach, the tester notes how far the subject can reach with the back against the wall. After this number is recorded, the subject then slowly bends forward to determine how far he can reach beyond the first number recorded.

Our research suggests that factors such as tightness in the connective-tissue structures located behind the knee and tension on the **sciatic nerve** can affect performance on the sit-and-reach. (We used a sit-and-reach box that restrained only the heel of the tested leg and permitted the foot to plantar flex into the box.) More recently Hui and Yuen (9) reported on a test that also permits plantar flexion of the foot of the tested leg and does not require a sit-and-reach box (see figure 10.15).

Even though the sit-and-reach has medical contraindications and a host of factors can affect performance on it, it still has value as a field test provided that test users are aware of its shortcomings. Following are suggestions that can make the sit-and-reach a better test.

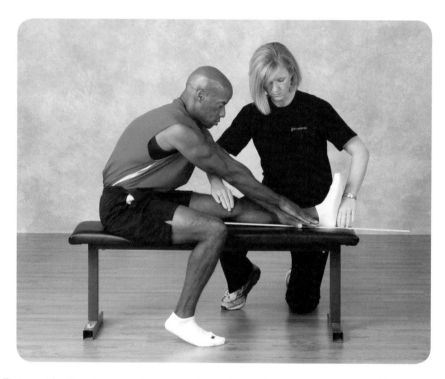

FIGURE 10.15 The modified back-saver sit-and-reach (9). The only equipment required is a meter stick and a bench. Because the ankle is permitted to passively plantar flex, connective-tissue tightness behind the knee, as well as other factors such as sciatic nerve tension, does not affect performance.

Modification Considerations for the Sit-and-Reach

- It is argued that the number of centimeters reached is not the most valid indicator of performance. The test administrator is better advised to examine the subject's quality of movement. Look for the angle of the sacrum (see figure 10.16) and the smoothness of the spinal curve. These relatively simple determinations can make the sit-and-reach a measure of low-back mobility as well as of hamstring length. These and other quality points are delineated in figure 10.16.

- It is recommended that the subject extend only one leg during the sit-and-reach test. Although this technique doubles the number of measurements required, the tester will also be able to evaluate symmetry. As stated previously, lower-extremity symmetry is desirable with respect to strength and flexibility, because imbalance may have an untoward effect on the spine.

- If a sit-and-reach box is used to make measurements, it is recommended that it be altered to permit passive plantar flexion at the ankle joint; however, normative data are not available for this modification. To alter the standard sit-and-reach box, simply replace the vertical surface under the cantilever extension with a 4 cm rod, which permits plantar flexion into the box but restrains the heel. This adjustment is not necessary if the protocol of Hui and Yuen (9) is followed.

Considerations for Spinal Range of Motion

Although it may be desirable in some instances, measuring ROM of the spine presents complexities that are probably not in the province of most readers of this chapter. The complexities relate to the ability to find bony landmarks and using special equipment such as an inclinometer. If the fitness professional is interested in reading about techniques of measuring spinal ROM, refer to the chapter references (2, 12, 16).

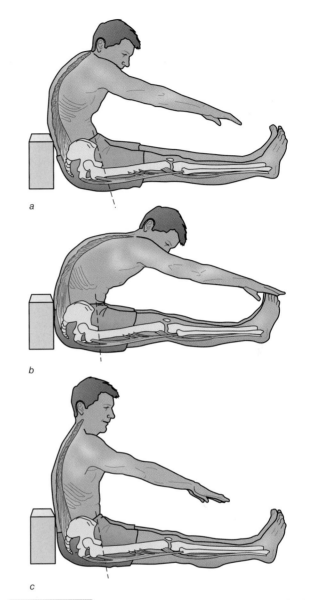

FIGURE 10.16 Sit-and-reach test. Quality points to look for include *(a)* tight hamstrings (note tilt of pelvis), tight low back, and stretched upper back; *(b)* normal length of hamstrings and low back; and *(c)* tight hamstrings (note tilt of pelvis) and tight low back.

KEY POINT

If a person with tight hamstrings practices the sit-and-reach maneuver with both legs extended, the soft-tissue structures of the spine can be damaged. In administering the sit-and-reach test, the fitness professional should consider the quality of the movement; it can be more important than the number of centimeters reached.

STUDY QUESTIONS

1. Why are sitting postures often deemed more detrimental to low-back function than standing postures?

2. Some of the tests that were presented in this chapter require an extremely good understanding of the nuances of human movement capability. Why could it be a mistake to administer one of these tests if you do not have a good understanding of these nuances?

3. Differentiate between rheumatoid arthritis and osteoarthritis. One could make an argument that at times either one could be more delimiting than the other. Discuss what factors appear to have an impact on ROM.

4. Movement capability in the lumbar spine is often misunderstood. Describe the movements and the factors that limit each.

5. Why is hip ROM important to a healthy back?

6. A prime reason for administering the sit-and-reach test is that it is easy to administer. Discuss why it would be a mistake to put too much stock in a client's performance on such a test.

7. Why is the guy-wire concept relevant to people who lead exercise activities?

8. Define and differentiate between active and passive ROM.

CASE STUDIES

You can check your answers by referring to appendix A.

1. After learning that one of the participants in your physical fitness program was told that his hamstrings were tight, you administer the sit-and-reach test to get some baseline data. Somewhat to your surprise, you find that he can reach beyond his toes. What quality factors (other than centimeters reached) in his sit-and-reach performance might you further examine to explain this disparity? What other hamstring length test might you administer?

2. Another client's record indicates that previous results from the Thomas test show she has very tight hip flexors. However, when you administer the Thomas test, you do not find evidence of tightness in the hip flexors. Assume that this person has done nothing to increase her ROM and that you are confident that you administered the Thomas test correctly. Explain how the previous administrator of the test might have erred.

3. Assume that you note a definite scoliosis in a client with whom you are planning exercise activities. Why is it important that you obtain good advice before prescribing exercises of the axial skeleton for this individual? Whom might you ask for this advice?

REFERENCES

1. Alter, M.J. 2004. *Science of flexibility.* Champaign, IL: Human Kinetics.

2. Beattie, P.F. 2004. Structure and function of the bones and joints of the lumbar spine. In *Kinesiology—The mechanics and pathomechanics of human movement,* ed. C.A. Oatis, 539-562. Philadelphia: Lippincott Williams & Wilkins.

3. Biering-Sorensen, F. 1984. Physical measurements as risk indicators for low-back trouble over a one-year period. *Spine* 9(2): 106-119.

4. Cady, L.D., D.P. Bischoff, E.R. O'Connell, P.C. Thomas, and J.H. Allan. 1979. Strength and fitness and subsequent back injuries in firefighters. *Journal of Occupational Medicine* 21(4): 269-272.

5. Cailliet, R. 1988. *Low back pain syndrome.* Philadelphia: Davis.

6. Cooper Institute for Aerobics Research. 1992. *The prudential Fitnessgram.* Dallas: Author.

7. Gracovetsky, S. 1988. *The spinal engine.* New York: Springer-Verlag.

8. Hopkins, D.R., and W.W.K. Hoeger. 1992. A comparison of the sit-and-reach test and the modified sit-and-reach test in the measurement of flexibility for males. *Journal of Applied Sport Science Research* 6:7-10.

9. Hui, S.S., and P.Y. Yuen. 2000. Validity of the modified backsaver sit-and-reach test: A comparison with other protocols. *Medicine and Science in Sports and Exercise* 32(9): 1655-1659.

10. Imrie, D., and L. Barbuto. 1988. *The back power program.* Toronto: Stoddart.

11. Kendall, F.P., E.K. McCreary, and P.G. Provance. 1993. *Muscles: Testing and function.* 4th ed. Baltimore: Williams & Wilkins.

12. Lee, R. 2002. Measurement of movements of the lumbar spine. *Physiotherapy Theory and Practice* 18:159-164.

13. Liemohn, W., S.B. Martin, and G. Pariser. 1997. The effect of ankle posture on sit-and-reach test performance in young adults. *Journal of Strength and Conditioning Research* 11:239-241.

14. Liemohn, W., M. Miller, T. Haydu, S. Ostrowski, S. Miles, and S. Riggs. 2000. An examination of a passive and an active back extension range of motion (ROM) tests. *Medicine and Science in Sports and Exercise* 32(5): S307.

15. Liemohn, W., G.L. Sharpe, and J.F. Wasserman. 1994. Lumbosacral movement in the sit-and-reach and in Cailliet's protective-hamstring stretch. *Spine* 19:2127-2130.

16. Liemohn, W., and G. Pariser, 2001. Flexibility, range of motion, and low back function. In *Exercise prescription and the back*, ed. W. Liemohn, 37-64. New York: McGraw-Hill Medical.

17. Magnusson, S.P., E.B. Simonsen, P. Aagaard, G.W. Gleim, M.P. McHugh, and M. Kjaer. 1995. Viscoelastic response to repeated static stretching in the human hamstring muscle. *Scandinavian Journal of Medicine and Science in Sports* 5:342-347.

18. Martin, S.B., A.W. Jackson, J.R. Morrow, and W. Liemohn. 1998. The rationale for the sit-and-reach test revisited. *Measurement in Physical Education and Exercise Science* 2(2): 85-92.

19. McGill, S. 2004. *Ultimate back fitness and performance.* Waterloo, ON: Wabuno.

20. McHugh, M.P., I.J. Kremenic, M.B. Fox, and G.W. Gleim. 1998. The role of mechanical and neural restraints to joint range of motion during passive stretch. *Medicine and Science in Sports and Exercise* 30(6): 928-932.

21. McKenzie, R. 1981. *The lumbar spine—Mechanical diagnosis and therapy.* Waikanae, New Zealand: Spinal.

22. Nachemson, A. 1975. Towards a better understanding of low-back pain: A review of the mechanics of the lumbar disc. *Rheumatology Rehabilitation* 14:129-143.

23. Oatis, C.A. 2004. *Kinesiology: The mechanics and pathomechanics of human movement.* Baltimore: Lippincott Williams & Wilkins.

24. Pope, M.H., T. Bevins, D.G. Wilder, and J.W. Frymoyer. 1985. The relationship between anthropometric, postural, muscular, and mobility characteristics of males ages 18-55. *Spine* 10:644-648.

25. Saal, J.S., and J.A. Saal. 1991. Strength training and flexibility. In *Conservative care of low back pain,* ed. A.H. White and R. Anderson, 65-77. Baltimore: Williams & Wilkins.

26. White, A.A., and M.M. Panjabi. 1990. *Clinical biomechanics of the spine.* Philadelphia: Willliams & Wilkins.

27. Williams, R., J. Binkley, R. Bloch, C.H. Goldsmith, and T. Minuk. 1993. Reliability of the modified-modified Schober and double inclinometer methods for measuring lumbar flexion and extension. *Physical Therapy* 73:26-37.

28. Zuhosky, J.P., and J.L. Young. 2001. Functional physical assessment for low back injuries in the athlete. In *Exercise prescription and the back, ed.* W. Liemohn, 67-88. New York: McGraw-Hill Medical.

Exercise Prescription for Health and Fitness

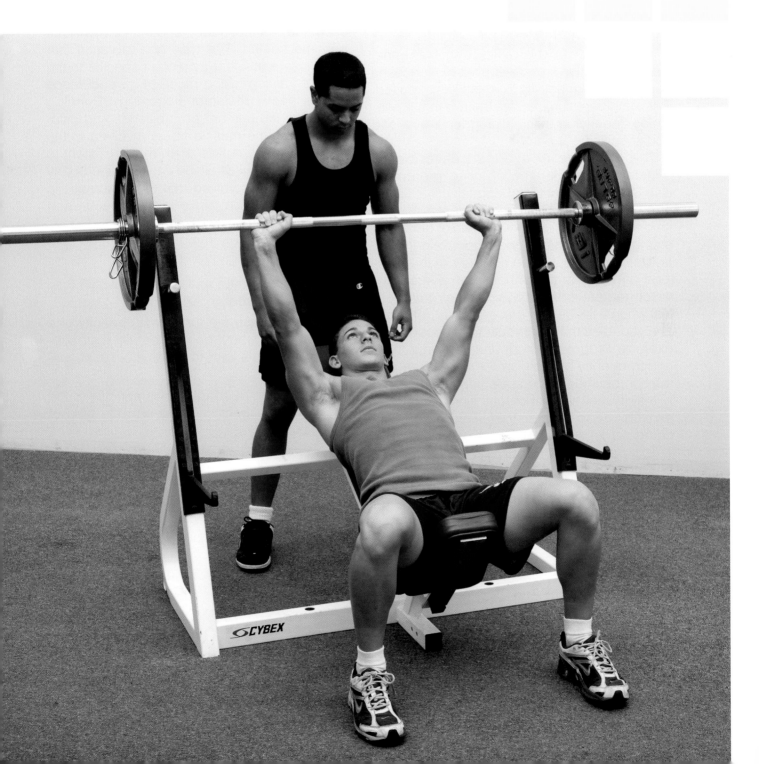

PART IV

In part IV we provide guidelines for exercise programming for each of the fitness components: cardiorespiratory fitness (CRF) (chapter 11), weight management (chapter 12), muscular strength and endurance (chapter 13), and flexibility and low-back function (chapter 14). The degree to which a tissue such as bone, skeletal muscle, or cardiac muscle functions depends on the activity to which it is exposed. This statement summarizes the two major principles underlying training programs: overload and specificity.

The principle of overload describes a dynamic characteristic of living creatures: Use increases functional capacity. If a tissue or organ system is required to work against a load to which it is not accustomed, it becomes stronger. The common adage for this principle is "Use it or lose it." The corollary of the overload principle is the principle of reversibility, which indicates that physiological gains are lost when a tissue or organ system is not used. The variables that contribute to overload in an exercise program include intensity, duration, and frequency of exercise. As we will see, it is the combination of these elements that results in a sufficient amount of total work, or energy expenditure, to increase the functional capacity of the cardiorespiratory system.

The principle of specificity states that the training effects derived from an exercise program are specific to the exercise performed and the muscles involved. For example, a person who runs for exercise shows little change in the arm muscles. A person who exercises at a low intensity that recruits only slow-twitch muscle fibers will see little or no training effect in the fast-twitch fibers. If muscle fibers are not used, they cannot adapt, and thus they will not become trained. The type of adaptation that occurs as a result of training is specific to the type of training taking place (e.g., endurance versus heavy resistance training). Running increases the number of capillaries and mitochondria in the muscle fibers involved in the exercise, which makes them more resistant to fatigue. Resistance training causes hypertrophy of the muscles involved due to an increase in the amount of contractile proteins, actin and myosin, in the muscle.

Following is a summary of overload and specificity:

- Tissues adapt to the load to which they are exposed.

- To increase the functional capacity of a tissue, it must be overloaded (i.e., subjected to a load to which it is not accustomed).

- The type of adaptation is specific to the muscle fibers involved and the type of exercise.

- Endurance exercise increases mitochondria and capillary numbers.

- Resistance training increases the contractile proteins and the size of the muscle.

Exercise Prescription for Cardiorespiratory Fitness

OBJECTIVES

The reader will be able to do the following:

1. Characterize the dose of exercise in an exercise prescription and identify means by which a health-related effect might occur.

2. Describe the public health recommendation for physical activity.

3. Explain the concepts of overload and specificity as they relate to training programs.

4. Describe general guidelines related to CRF programs, including those related to warm-up and cool-down.

5. Develop an exercise prescription with the exercise intensity, duration, and frequency needed to achieve and maintain CRF goals.

6. Express exercise intensity in terms of energy production, HR, and RPE.

7. Contrast the approaches used for developing exercise prescriptions for the general public, for the fit population, and for people whose complete GXT results are available.

8. Describe the differences between a supervised and an unsupervised program.

9. Describe how temperature and humidity, altitude, and pollution affect exercise prescriptions.

There is no question that higher levels of physical activity, exercise, and CRF are linked to reduced risk of many chronic diseases and death from all causes (13, 25, 41, 62, 64, 65). Of the hundreds of health objectives for the United States, *Healthy People 2020* (63) selected physical activity as one of the top 10 health indicators. Figure 11.1 from Myers et al. (40) shows that as CRF increases, the risk of death decreases. There are two important takeaway messages from this figure. First, the greatest decrease in risk occurs when moving from the lowest 20% (quintile) of CRF to the next level, and second, the risk continues to decrease with increases in fitness (more is better). The results from this study were consistent with those in the classic study of Blair et al. (5), which found that risk levels off at a CRF level of only 9 METs for women and 10 METs for men.

As we move through this chapter it will become clear that it is not difficult to achieve levels of physical activity and CRF consistent with a lower risk of chronic disease. This knowledge forms the basis for the public health physical activity recommendations. Consequently, the primary purpose of this chapter is to show how to prescribe physical activity and exercise to improve CRF in adults. Later chapters present additional information on prescribing physical activity and exercise for children, older adults, and those with known diseases.

Prescribing Exercise

There is a close parallel between the fitness professional's desire to know the proper **dose** of exercise needed to bring about a desired **effect** (response) and the physician's need to know the type and quantity of a drug needed to cure a disease. In fact, the ACSM–AMA program called *Exercise is Medicine* speaks to that connection, and materials are available to help fitness professionals interact with medical personnel (http://exerciseismedicine.org/fitpros.htm). If we think about prescriptions from a medical perspective, there is a difference between what is needed to cure a headache and what is needed to cure tuberculosis. In the same way, there is no question that the dose of physical activity required to achieve a high level of performance is different from that required to improve a health-related outcome (e.g., lower BP, lower risk of CHD). Similarities can be drawn between the dose–response relationship for medications and that for exercise, which is shown in figure 11.2 (18).

• Potency. The potency of a drug is a relatively unimportant characteristic in that it makes little difference whether the effective dose is 1 mg or 100 mg as long as the drug can be administered in an appropriate dosage (18). Likewise in exercise prescriptions, walking 4 mi (6.4 km)

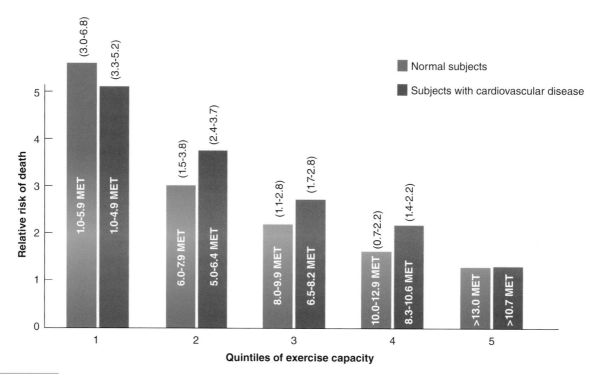

FIGURE 11.1 Relative risk of all-cause mortality to quintiles of exercise capacity (METs) among normal subjects and those with CVD.

Reprinted, by permission, from J.M. Myers et al., 2002, "Exercise capacity and mortality among men referred for exercise testing," *New England Journal of Medicine* 346: 793-801. ©Massachusetts Medical Society.

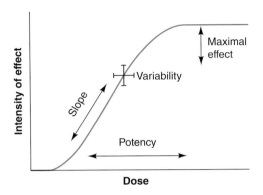

FIGURE 11.2 Representative dose–effect curve with four characterizing parameters.

Reprinted, by permission, from A. Goodman, 1975, *Pharmacological basis of therapeutics* (New York, NY: McGraw-Hill), 25. ©The McGraw-Hill Companies.

at a moderate pace is as effective in expending calories as running 2 mi (3.2 km).

- Slope. The slope of the curve describes how much of an effect comes from a change in dose (18). Some physiological measures such as HR and lactate response to a fixed exercise task change quickly (in days) for a dose of exercise, whereas some health-related effects (e.g., changes in serum cholesterol) are realized only after many months of exercise.

- Maximal effect. The maximal effect (efficacy) of a drug varies with the type of drug. For example, morphine can relieve pain of all intensities, whereas aspirin is effective against only mild to moderate pain (18). Similarly, strenuous exercise can increase $\dot{V}O_2max$ and modify risk factors, whereas light to moderate exercise can improve risk factors but only minimally affect $\dot{V}O_2max$.

- Variability. The effect of a drug varies among and within individuals depending on the circumstances (18). In terms of exercise, gains in $\dot{V}O_2max$ attributable to endurance training show considerable variation, even when the initial $\dot{V}O_2max$ value is controlled for (11).

- Side effect. No drug produces a single effect (18), and the effects might include adverse (side) effects that limit the usefulness of the drug. For exercise, the side effects might include an increased risk of injury.

KEY POINT

An exercise dose reflects the interaction of the intensity, frequency, duration, and type of exercise. Many health-related benefits are derived from participation in physical activity and exercise, and within limits, more is better. These benefits are not dependent on an increase in CRF, but there is no question that a higher level of CRF is related to a lower risk of chronic disease.

Unlike most drugs, which people stop taking when a disease is cured, physical activity is needed throughout life to promote its health-related and fitness effects. The exercise dose usually is characterized by the intensity, frequency, duration, and type of activity; we discuss each of these in detail later in this chapter. Over the past two decades, we have learned much more about how much physical activity is needed to achieve a variety of health outcomes. The recent detailed review carried out before the development of the first edition of the *U.S. Physical Activity Guidelines* (64) supported and added to the findings of earlier reports (13). The following Research Insight provides current information on the health benefits associated with regular physical activity in adults and older adults.

RESEARCH INSIGHT

The following information provides the level of evidence (strong, moderate, weak) that supports the connection between physical activity and various health outcomes in adults and older adults. An impressive amount of research has been done over the past 40 years to allow us to make such statements (64, 65).

Strong evidence
- Lower risk of early death
- Lower risk of CHD
- Lower risk of stroke
- Lower risk of high BP
- Lower risk of adverse blood lipid profile
- Lower risk of type 2 diabetes
- Lower risk of metabolic syndrome
- Lower risk of colon and breast cancer
- Prevention of weight gain
- Weight loss, particularly when combined with a reduced caloric intake
- Improved CRF and muscular strength
- Prevention of falls
- Reduced depression
- Better cognitive function (for older adults)

Moderate to strong evidence
- Better functional health (older adults)
- Reduced abdominal obesity

Moderate evidence
- Lower risk of hip fracture
- Lower risk of lung and endometrial cancer
- Weight maintenance after weight loss
- Increased bone density
- Improved sleep quality

As mentioned in chapter 1, the health-related benefits of physical activity are not dependent on an increase in CRF. That said, there is no question that an increase in $\dot{V}O_2$max is associated with a decrease in the risk of many chronic diseases and death from all causes. The purpose of this chapter is to show fitness professionals how to help people accomplish that goal.

Short- and Long-Term Responses to Exercise

Haskell has indicated that in addition to understanding the cause-and-effect connection between physical activity and specific outcomes, we need to distinguish between short-term (acute) and long-term (training) responses (23, 24). The responses in the days and weeks following the initiation of a dose of exercise can vary substantially, depending on the variable being measured:

- Acute responses—Responses occur with one or several exercise bouts but do not improve further.

- Rapid responses—Benefits occur early and plateau.

- Linear responses—Gains are made continuously over time.

- Delayed responses—Responses occur only after weeks of training.

The need for such distinctions can be seen in figure 11.3 (34), which shows proposed dose–response relationships between physical activity, defined as minutes of exercise per week at 60% to 70% of maximal work capacity, and a variety of physiological responses:

- BP and insulin sensitivity are most responsive to exercise.

- Changes in $\dot{V}O_2$max and resting HR are intermediate.

- Serum lipid changes such as increases in HDL are delayed.

The dose–response relationship of exercise has important implications when exercise is used alone or in concert with medication to control disease; we discuss this further in chapter 25.

Public Health Recommendations for Physical Activity

Given the previous discussion, it should be no surprise that it is difficult to provide a single exercise prescription that addresses all the issues related to preventing and treating various diseases. Despite this, there has been a great need

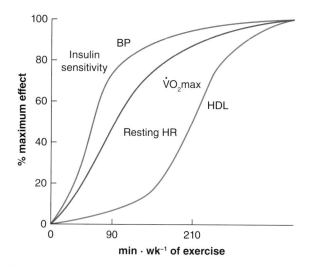

FIGURE 11.3 Proposed dose–response relationships between amount of exercise performed per week at 60% to 70% maximum work capacity and changes in BP and insulin sensitivity (curve on left), which appear most sensitive to exercise; maximum oxygen consumption ($\dot{V}O_2$max) and resting HR, which are parameters of physical fitness (middle curve); and lipid changes, such as increases in HDL (curve on right).

Reprinted from G.L. Jennings et al., 1991, "What is the dose-response relationship between exercise training and blood pressure?," *Annals of Medicine* 23: 313-318, by permission of Taylor & Francis, Ltd. www.tandfco.uk/journals.

to provide a general exercise recommendation to improve the health status of all adults in the United States. ACSM and the CDC responded to this need by publishing public health guidelines for physical activity in 1995 (42): Every U.S. adult should accumulate 30 min or more of moderate-intensity physical activity on most, preferably all, days of the week.

In 2007, ACSM and the AHA released an update to this 1995 public health guideline for physical activity (42), and in 2008 the first U.S. Physical Activity Guidelines were released (64). Both guidelines supported the original statement but attempted to provide more clarity about the roles of moderate versus strenuous (vigorous) exercise in meeting the recommendation (25, 64). Because of the similarity between the two, we will present only the U.S. Physical Activity Guidelines.

- People can realize the health-related benefits of physical activity by doing 150 to 300 min of moderate-intensity activity per week, or 75 to 150 min of vigorous-intensity activity per week, or some combination of the two (e.g., walking briskly for 30 min on 3 days · wk^{-1} and jogging for 30 min on 2 days · wk^{-1} would meet the minimum goal).

- The 150 min of moderate-intensity activity or 75 min of vigorous-intensity activity is the minimum goal.

- The range of physical activity is given because more health-related benefits can be realized by doing additional activity (i.e., more is better).
- Doing the activity in multiple intermittent bouts (e.g., 10 min each) is an alternative way of meeting the goals.

In addition, the new guidelines recommend resistance training on at least 2 days · wk^{-1} to improve or maintain muscular strength and endurance (25, 64). Note that these new guidelines spell out the number of minutes per week but not the number of days per week to exercise. That does not mean that one should do the 150 min of moderate-intensity activity in 1 day and rest for 6 days. For reasons that will be discussed later, spreading out exercise over the course of the week makes it easier to schedule and reduces the risk of injury (64).

The health-related gains associated with physical activity are realized when the volume of physical activity is between 500 and 1,000 MET-min · wk^{-1} (64). Moderate-intensity activity is defined as absolute intensities of 3.0 to 5.9 METs, and vigorous-intensity activity is defined as intensities of 6.0 METs or more.

- For example, walking at 3 mi · hr^{-1} (4.8 km · hr^{-1}) requires 3.3 METs, an activity at the low end of the moderate-intensity range. If the person walks at this speed for 30 min, an energy expenditure of 99 MET-min (3.3 METs times 30 min) is achieved. If done 5 days · wk^{-1}, the weekly volume of activity is 495 MET-min.
- If a person were to jog at 5 mi · hr^{-1} or 8 km · hr^{-1} (8 METs) for 25 min, the volume would be 200 MET-min. If done 3 days · wk^{-1}, the weekly energy expenditure would be 600 MET-min.
- The fact that it takes about twice the time when doing moderate-intensity activity to achieve the same energy expenditure as when doing vigorous-intensity activity leads to the 2:1 ratio when comparing the time it takes to meet the guidelines for these intensities (150 versus 75 min).

Those who meet the upper end of the activity guidelines (1,000 MET-min · wk^{-1}) have a greater chance of achieving and maintaining a normal body weight (see chapters 12 and 19). How do we convert MET-min to kcal of energy expended? If a person is 75 kg and walks at 3.0 mi · hr^{-1} (4.8 km · hr^{-1} or 3.3 METs) for 150 min · wk^{-1}, for example, the number of kcal expended can be computed as described in chapter 6:

$$75 \text{ kg} \cdot 3.3 \text{ kcal} \cdot \text{kg}^{-1} \cdot \text{hr}^{-1} =$$
$$248 \text{ kcal} \cdot \text{hr}^{-1} \cdot 2.5 \text{ hr} = 620 \text{ kcal} \cdot \text{wk}^{-1}.$$

Table 11.1 shows the number of MET-min and kcal expended at various exercise intensities for those meeting

TABLE 11.1 Walk, Jog, and Run Speeds; METs and MET-Minutes; and Estimated Kilocalories Expended by a 75 kg (165 lb) Adult for 150 min and 300 min of Weekly Physical Activity

Speed mi · hr^{-1} (km · hr^{-1})	METs	150 min · wk^{-1} MET-min †	150 min · wk^{-1} kcal †	300 min · wk^{-1} MET-min †	300 min · wk^{-1} kcal †
Rest	1.0	150	190	300	380
2.5 (4.0)	3.0	450	565	900	1,130
3.0 (4.8)	3.3	495	620	990	1,240
4.0 (6.4)	5.0	750	940	1,500	1,880
4.3 (6.9)	6.0	900	1,125	1,800	2,250
5.0 (8.0)	8.0	1,200	1,500	2,400	3,000
6.0 (9.7)	10.0	1,500	1,875	3,000	3,750
7.0 (11.3)	11.5	1,725	2,155	3,450	4,310
8.0 (12.9)	13.5	2,025	2,530	4,050	5,060
10.0 (16.1)	16.0	2,400	3,000	4,800	6,000

2.5 to 4.3 mi · hr^{-1} (4.0-6.9 km · hr^{-1}) = walk; 5 to 10 mi · hr^{-1} (8.0-16.0 km · hr^{-1}) = jog/run

† kilocalories for 75 kg adult when exercising at the given intensity for either 150 or 300 min. These are gross energy expenditure values during exercise; thus, they include the energy expenditure at rest and not just the additional energy expenditure due to the activity. Kilocalories calculated using 1 MET = 1 kilocalorie per kilogram per hour and rounded to nearest 5 kilocalories.

U.S. Department of Health and Human Services. 2008.

the 150 and 300 min goals. Obviously, someone who is fit has a greater capacity to work at a higher intensity and meet the goal in a shorter time. Consequently, benefits are gained not only when a sedentary person becomes active but also when a moderately active person engages in more vigorous exercise that increases energy expenditure and functional capacity ($\dot{V}O_2$max). This chapter provides the steps for developing an exercise prescription to improve CRF in apparently healthy people.

KEY POINT

To achieve the physical activity energy expenditure associated with substantial health benefits, either moderate-intensity or vigorous-intensity physical activity can be used. The goal is to achieve between 500 and 1,000 MET-min · wk^{-1} of physical activity energy expenditure.

General Guidelines for Cardiorespiratory Fitness Programs

To apply the principles of overload and specificity in exercise programs (see the introduction to part IV), activities that overload the heart and respiratory system need to be used. Activities that involve the large muscle groups contracting in a rhythmic and continuous manner can overload the cardiorespiratory system. Activities involving a small muscle mass and resistance training exercises are less appropriate because they tend to generate high cardiovascular loads relative to energy expenditure (see chapter 4). Activities that improve CRF are high in caloric cost and therefore help to achieve a goal of relative leanness. So, how does a fitness professional get someone started in a CRF program?

Screen Participants

If the person has not already done so, have her fill out a health status form. Chapter 2 provides guidelines for who should and should not seek medical clearance before exercising.

Encourage Regular Participation

Exercise must become a valuable part of a person's lifestyle. It is not something that can be done sporadically, nor will doing it for only a few months or years build up a fitness reserve. Dramatic gains accomplished through fitness activities are lost quickly with inactivity (see chapter 4). Only people who continue activity as a way of life enjoy its long-term benefits.

Provide a Variety of Activities

A fitness program starts with easily quantified activities, such as walking or cycling, so that the proper exercise intensity can be achieved. After a minimum level of fitness is achieved, a variety of activities are included in the program. Chapter 22 outlines three phases of physical activity: Work up to walking briskly each day, gradually begin jogging and work up to jogging continuously for 2 to 3 mi (3.2-4.8 km), and introduce a variety of activities, including group exercise.

Program for Progression

Given the importance of helping sedentary people become active, the emphasis in any health-related fitness program that includes such participants should be to start slowly and, when in doubt, do too little rather than too much. A 10% increase in the number of minutes done per week is a reasonable increase in the quantity of activity to minimize injury risk. One should gradually increase the number of minutes per session and the number of days per week before increasing the intensity (64). For example, sedentary participants who are interested in jogging should begin a training program by walking a distance that they can complete without feeling fatigued or sore. With time, the participants will be able to walk farther and faster without discomfort. After they can walk several miles briskly without stopping, they can gradually work up to jogging continuously during each workout. When the participants are first ready to begin jogging, introduce the interval workout (walking, jogging, walking, jogging). As they adapt to the interval workouts, they will be able to gradually increase the amount of jogging while decreasing the distance walked (see the walking and jogging programs in chapter 22). The importance of progression cannot be overemphasized, whether the client is a child, adult, or older adult (64).

Adhere to Format for a Fitness Workout

The main body of the fitness workout consists of dynamic activities using large muscle groups at an intensity high enough and a duration long enough to accomplish enough total work to specifically overload the cardiorespiratory system. Stretching and light endurance activities are included before the workout (warm-up) and after the workout (cool-down) for safety and for improving low-back function.

There are physiological, psychological, and safety reasons for including the warm-up and cool-down. In general, the warm-up and cool-down should consist of the following:

- Activities similar to those in the main body of the workout but at a lower intensity (e.g., walking, jogging, or cycling below THR)
- Stretching exercises for the muscles involved in the activity as well as for those in the midtrunk area (see chapter 14)
- Muscular endurance exercises, especially for the muscles in the abdominal region (see chapter 14)

These activities help participants ease into and out of a workout and promote a healthy low back. If a workout is going to be shorter than usual, the main body of the workout is the part that should be adjusted so that 5 to 10 min are retained for the warm-up and cool-down.

Conduct Periodic Fitness Tests

Routine health-related fitness testing to determine a participant's progress can be motivational and may help alter programs that are not achieving desired results. The fitness professional can help by setting realistic goals for the next testing session when discussing test results. A general rule would be a 10% improvement in 3 mo in the test scores that need to change. Once the person has reached a desirable fitness level, the goal is to maintain that level.

KEY POINT

People interested in a fitness program should be screened for risk factors and encouraged to exercise regularly. The program should provide a variety of activities that use large muscle groups and overload the heart and respiratory system, and the participant should start slowly and progress gradually to higher levels of work. The workout should have a warm-up and a cool-down, including stretching and muscular endurance exercises for the midtrunk. Periodic CRF tests can be used to alter the exercise prescription.

Formulating the Exercise Prescription

The CRF training effect depends on the degree to which the systems are overloaded; that is, it depends on the intensity, duration, and frequency of training. **Intensity** generally is expressed as a percentage of some maximal physiological response, usually oxygen uptake ($\%\dot{V}O_2$max), HR ($\%$HRmax), or derivatives of these—oxygen uptake reserve ($\dot{V}O_2$R) or HR reserve (HRR). These are described in detail in the next section. The interaction of intensity (low to high), duration (short to long), and frequency (seldom to

often) should result in an energy expenditure (total work) of 500 to 1,000 MET-min $\cdot$ wk^{-1} (64).

Intensity

How hard does a person have to work to sufficiently overload the cardiovascular and respiratory systems to increase CRF? To answer this question, we must first define the various expressions of exercise intensity and show how they relate to each other.

- Percentage of maximal oxygen uptake ($\%\dot{V}O_2$max). Across a broad range of CRF levels, many physiological responses are normalized (i.e., made similar between individuals) when the intensity of exercise is expressed as a percentage of $\dot{V}O_2$max ($\%\dot{V}O_2$max). A person who is working at 24.5 ml $\cdot$ kg^{-1} $\cdot$ min^{-1} and has a $\dot{V}O_2$max of 35 ml $\cdot$ kg^{-1} $\cdot$ min^{-1} is working at 70% $\dot{V}O_2$max. This approach has been used extensively to develop exercise guidelines, as can be seen in the *ACSM's Guidelines for Exercise Testing and Prescription* and ACSM position stands. However, in recent updates of these documents, the relative intensity is expressed as the percentage of oxygen uptake reserve ($\%\dot{V}O_2$R) (3, 4).

- Percentage of oxygen uptake reserve ($\%\dot{V}O_2$R). $\dot{V}O_2$R is calculated by subtracting 1 MET (3.5 ml $\cdot$ kg^{-1} $\cdot$ min^{-1}) from the subject's $\dot{V}O_2$max. For example, if a subject's $\dot{V}O_2$max is 35 ml $\cdot$ kg^{-1} $\cdot$ min^{-1}, the $\dot{V}O_2$R is 35 − 3.5 ml $\cdot$ kg^{-1} $\cdot$ min^{-1} = 31.5 ml $\cdot$ kg^{-1} $\cdot$ min^{-1}. The $\%\dot{V}O_2$R is calculated by subtracting 1 MET from the exercise oxygen uptake, dividing by the subject's $\dot{V}O_2$R, and multiplying by 100%. For instance, if this person is exercising at 24.5 ml $\cdot$ kg^{-1} $\cdot$ min^{-1}, the exercise intensity is 67% $\dot{V}O_2$R: (24.5 − 3.5 ml $\cdot$ kg^{-1} $\cdot$ min^{-1}) ÷ (35 − 3.5 ml $\cdot$ kg^{-1} $\cdot$ min^{-1}) $\cdot$ 100% = 67% $\dot{V}O_2$R. The $\%\dot{V}O_2$R equals the HR response when HR is expressed as a percentage of the HRR (58, 59).

- Percentage of HRR ($\%$HRR). The HRR is calculated by subtracting resting HR from maximal HR. The $\%$HRR is a percentage of the difference between resting and maximal HR and is calculated by subtracting resting HR from exercise HR, dividing by HRR, and multiplying by 100%.

1. A 20-year old man is exercising at 160 beats $\cdot$ min^{-1}.
2. He has a maximal HR of 200 beats $\cdot$ min^{-1} and a resting HR of 60 beats $\cdot$ min^{-1}.
3. Consequently, he is working at 71% of the HRR: (160 − 60 beats $\cdot$ min^{-1}) ÷ (200 − 60 beats $\cdot$ min^{-1}) $\cdot$ 100%.

For many years, $\%$HRR was believed to be linked to $\%\dot{V}O_2$max on a one-to-one basis; that is, 70% HRR = 70% $\dot{V}O_2$max. However, Swain and colleagues (58, 59) pointed out that although this is the case when fit people exercise vigorously, it is not the case for low intensities of exercise, especially when they are performed by people with low fitness levels. For example, a 3 MET activity for someone with a 5 MET maximal aerobic power is 60% $\dot{V}O_2$max but only 50% $\dot{V}O_2$R: $(3 - 1\ MET) \div (5\ METs - 1\ MET) \cdot 100\%$. An advantage of expressing exercise intensity as %HHR is that %$\dot{V}O_2$R is numerically identical to %HRR across the fitness continuum.

- Percentage of maximal HR (%HRmax). Because of the linear relationship between HR (above 110 beats · min^{-1}) and $\dot{V}O_2$ during dynamic exercise, investigators and clinicians have long used a simple percentage of maximal HR (%HRmax) to estimate %$\dot{V}O_2$max in setting exercise intensity. This method of expressing exercise intensity is easier to teach than is %HRR.

- Rating of perceived exertion (RPE). The RPE is not viewed as a substitute for prescribing exercise intensity by HR, but once the relationship between the HR and RPE has been established, RPE can be used in its place (3). However, the RPE may not consistently translate to the same intensity for different modes of exercise, so do not expect the RPE to exactly match a %HRmax or %HRR (4).

Table 11.2 shows the categories of exercise intensity as described in the 2008 report of the U.S. Physical Activity Guidelines Advisory Committee (65) and the 2010 edition of *ACSM's Guidelines for Exercise Testing and Prescription*, with %$\dot{V}O_2$R and %HRR used to set the standard for the other expressions of exercise intensity (4). These are shown on the left side of the table, with intensities ranging from very light to maximal. It must be noted that in the 2011 ACSM Position Stand on the quantity and quality of exercise for developing and maintaining cardiorespiratory fitness, (3) the number of categories was reduced from six to five, shrinking the light-exercise classification to 30-39% HRR and stretching out the vigorous-intensity classification to 60-89% HRR. Because we believe these new classifications have little impact on developing an exercise prescription, we have chosen to use the classification cut points from the 2010 edition of the ACSM Guidelines.

The RPE values are based on the Borg RPE scale (6). The values in table 11.2 for %HRmax and %$\dot{V}O_2$max accurately reflect the relationship between them and %$\dot{V}O_2$R (%HRR) (32). Further, table 11.2 provides the absolute exercise intensities (in METs) for each of the intensity classifications for four groups that vary in $\dot{V}O_2$max. Looking across the table from the 12 MET to the 5 MET column, there is little difference between %$\dot{V}O_2$max and %$\dot{V}O_2$R at higher $\dot{V}O_2$max values, especially at higher exercise intensities; however, the differences are more obvious for the very light to moderate intensities and lower $\dot{V}O_2$max values.

For people with $\dot{V}O_2$max values of 12 METs, %$\dot{V}O_2$max is similar to %$\dot{V}O_2$R:

TABLE 11.2 Classification of Physical Activity Intensity

	RELATIVE INTENSITY			ENDURANCE ACTIVITY — INTENSITY (METS AND %$\dot{V}O_2$MAX) IN HEALTHY ADULTS DIFFERING IN $\dot{V}O_2$							
				$\dot{V}O_2$MAX = 12 METS		$\dot{V}O_2$MAX = 10 METS		$\dot{V}O_2$MAX = 8 METS		$\dot{V}O_2$MAX = 5 METS	
Intensity	%HRR %$\dot{V}O_2$R*	%HR$_{max}$^{y}	RPE‡	METs	%$\dot{V}O_2$max	METs	%$\dot{V}O_2$max	METs	%$\dot{V}O_2$max	METs	%$\dot{V}O_2$max
Very light	<20	<50	<10	<3.2	<27	<2.8	<28	<2.4	<30	<1.8	<36
Light	20-39	50-63	10-11	2.3-5.3	27-44	2.8-4.5	28-45	2.4-3.7	30-47	1.8-2.5	36-51
Moderate	40-59	64-76	12-13	5.4-7.5	45-62	4.6-6.3	46-63	3.8-5.1	48-64	2.6-3.3	52-67
Hard/vigorous	60-84	77-93	14-16	7.4-10.2	63-85	6.4-8.6	64-86	5.2-6.9	65-86	3.4-4.3	68-87
Very hard	≥85	≥94	≥17-19	≥10.3	≥86	≥8.7	≥87	≥7.0	≥87	≥4.4	≥88
Maximal	100	100	20	12	100	10	100	8	100	5	100

*%$\dot{V}O_2$R = percentage of oxygen uptake reserve; %HRR = percentage of heart rate reserve.

^{y}%HRmax = 0.7305 (%$\dot{V}O_2$max) + 29.95 (Londeree and Ames 1976); values based on 10 MET group.

‡Borg rating of perceived exertion 6-20 scale (Borg 1988).

%$\dot{V}O_2$max = [(100% − 90% $\dot{V}O_2$ R) MET max^{-1}] + % $\dot{V}O_2$ R (personal communication, Dave Swain, 2000).

Adapted from American College of Sports Medicine 1998; Howley 2001.

- Moderate intensity equals 40 to 59 %$\dot{V}O_2R$ and 45 to 62 %$\dot{V}O_2$max.

- Hard (vigorous) intensity equals 60 to 84 %$\dot{V}O_2R$ and 63 to 85 %$\dot{V}O_2$max.

For people with $\dot{V}O_2$max values of 5 METs, %$\dot{V}O_2$max is higher than %$\dot{V}O_2R$:

- Moderate intensity equals 40 to 59 %$\dot{V}O_2R$ and 52 to 67 %$\dot{V}O_2$max.

- Hard (vigorous) intensity equals 60 to 84 %$\dot{V}O_2R$ and 68 to 87 %$\dot{V}O_2$max.

- Consequently, for people of average or higher CRF, the difference between %$\dot{V}O_2$max and %$\dot{V}O_2R$ is small, and these expressions will be used interchangeably except where noted otherwise.

The %HRmax values listed in table 11.1 were derived from an equation by Londeree and Ames (36).

$$\%HRmax = 0.7305 \ (\%\dot{V}O_2max) + 29.95.$$

This equation is similar to those of Swain and colleagues (57) and of Hellerstein and Franklin (27). There was little difference in the %HRmax values across the four fitness groups for each of the intensity classifications, so the %$\dot{V}O_2$max values for the 10 MET fitness group were used to provide the %HRmax values for table 11.2. Table 11.2 allows the fitness professional to consistently classify data on exercise intensity, whether they are expressed in oxygen uptake (METs), HR, or RPE.

The 1998 ACSM position stand recommended a range of exercise intensities from 40% to 84% of HRR to achieve CRF goals. However, the position stand also indicated that the lower end of this continuum of intensities (i.e., 40%-49% HRR) is appropriate for people who are quite unfit (3). That is consistent with the need of this group to focus on moderate-intensity physical activity that can be carried out long enough to achieve health-related benefits and perhaps gains in CRF.

- For the average sedentary person, the appropriate range of exercise intensities for achieving CRF goals is 50% to 84% HRR.

- For older, deconditioned adults, 40% to 59% HRR is a good place to start.

- For adults who are physically active and at the high end of the fitness scale, intensities greater than 80% HRR are appropriate.

- However, for most people who are cleared to participate in a structured exercise program, 60% to 80% HRR seems to be the optimal range of exercise intensities.

Figure 11.5 shows that exercise at the high end of the scale has been associated with more cardiac complications (10, 27). Exercise intensity must be balanced against the duration so that the person can exercise long enough to expend 500 to 1,000 MET-min $\cdot$ wk^{-1}, the higher volume being consistent with greater improvements in CRF and greater reductions in chronic disease risk factors (64, 65). If the exercise intensity is too high, the person may not be able to exercise long enough to achieve the desired energy expenditure.

Duration

How many minutes of exercise should a person do per session? Figure 11.5 shows that improvements in $\dot{V}O_2$max increase with the **duration** of the exercise session. However, the optimal duration of an exercise session depends on the intensity. The **total work** accomplished in a session is the most important variable determining CRF gains, once the minimal intensity **threshold** is achieved (4). If the goal were to accomplish 300 kcal of total work in an exercise session in which the participant works at 10 kcal $\cdot$ min^{-1} (2 L of oxygen per min), the duration of the session would have to be 30 min. If the person were working at half that intensity, 5 kcal $\cdot$ min^{-1}, the duration would have to be twice as long. A half hour of exercise can be taken as one 30 min session, two 15 min sessions, or three 10 min sessions. Figure 11.5 also shows that when the duration of hard exercise (75% $\dot{V}O_2$max) exceeds 30 min, the risk of orthopedic injury increases (43).

Frequency

Why recommend that a person do 3 to 5 workouts each week if 2 would suffice? Figure 11.4 shows that gains in

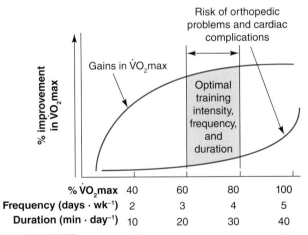

% $\dot{V}O_2$max	40	60	80	100
Frequency (days $\cdot$ wk^{-1})	2	3	4	5
Duration (min $\cdot$ day^{-1})	10	20	30	40

FIGURE 11.4 Effects of increased frequency, duration, and intensity of exercise on $\dot{V}O_2$max. This figure demonstrates the increasing risk of orthopedic problems attributable to exercise sessions that are too long or conducted too many times per week. The probability of cardiac complications increases with exercise intensity beyond that recommended for improving CRF.

KEY POINT

CRF improves with exercise intensities of 40% to 84% HRR. The intensity threshold for a training effect is lower (40%-59% HRR) for people who are sedentary, and it is higher (>80% HRR) for people who are physically active and have high CRF. The optimal training intensity for the average person is approximately 60% to 80% HRR. The duration of an exercise session should balance the exercise intensity to result in an energy expenditure of 500 to 1,000 MET-min · wk⁻¹, the higher volume being consistent with greater improvements in health benefits and CRF. The optimal frequency of training, based on improvement in CRF and a low risk of injuries, is 3 to 4 times · wk⁻¹ for exercise intensities rated as *hard*.

CRF increase with the frequency of exercise but begin to level off at 4 days · wk⁻¹. People who start a fitness program and are doing vigorous-intensity exercise should plan to exercise 3 or 4 days · wk⁻¹. The long-recommended work-a-day then rest-a-day routine has been validated by improvements in CRF, low incidence of injuries, and achievement of weight-loss goals. Although exercising for fewer than 3 days · wk⁻¹ can improve CRF, the participant would have to exercise at a higher intensity, and weight-loss goals might be difficult to achieve (43). Exercising for more than 4 days · wk⁻¹ at a vigorous intensity for previously sedentary people seems to be too much and results in more dropouts and injuries and less psychological adjustment to the exercise (10, 43).

Determining Intensity

How is exercise intensity set for a particular client? This section reviews direct and indirect methods to determine appropriate exercise intensity, with a focus on the typically sedentary individual. The approach would be the same for people with very low or very high levels of physical activity and CRF, but different intensity guidelines would be used.

Metabolic Load

The most direct way to determine the appropriate exercise intensity is to use a percentage of the measured maximal oxygen consumption. Remember, the optimal range of exercise intensities associated with improved CRF in typically sedentary individuals is 60% to 80% $\dot{V}O_2$max. The advantage of measuring oxygen consumption to determine exercise intensity is that the method is based on the criterion test for CRF—maximal oxygen consumption. The major disadvantages are the expense and difficulty of measuring oxygen consumption for each person and trying to suit specific fitness activities to meet the specific metabolic demand for each person.

QUESTION: A 75 kg man completes a maximal GXT, and his $\dot{V}O_2$max is 3.0 L · min⁻¹. This equals 15 kcal · min⁻¹ (5 kcal · L⁻¹ · 3 L · min⁻¹), 40 ml · kg⁻¹ · min⁻¹, and 11.4 METs. At what exercise intensities should he work to be at 60% to 80% $\dot{V}O_2$max?

1. 60% of 3.0 L · min⁻¹ = 1.8 L · min⁻¹;
   80% of 3.0 L · min⁻¹ = 2.4 L · min⁻¹.
2. 60% of 15 kcal · min⁻¹ = 9 kcal · min⁻¹;
   80% of 15 kcal · min⁻¹ = 12 kcal · min⁻¹.
3. 60% of 40 ml · kg⁻¹ · min⁻¹ = 24 ml · kg⁻¹ · min⁻¹;
   80% of 40 ml · kg⁻¹ · min⁻¹ = 32 ml · kg⁻¹ · min⁻¹.
4. 60% of 11.4 METs = 6.8 METs;
   80% of 11.4 METs = 9.1 METs.

ANSWER:

He should use activities that require the following:

1.8 to 2.4 L · min⁻¹

9 to 12 kcal · min⁻¹

24 to 32 ml · kg⁻¹ · min⁻¹

6.8 to 9.1 METs

At what exercise intensities does he work to be at 60% and 80% $\dot{V}O_2$R? Using the preceding data, we find that $\dot{V}O_2$R = 40 ml · kg⁻¹ · min⁻¹ − 3.5 ml · kg⁻¹ · min⁻¹ = 36.6 ml · kg⁻¹ · min⁻¹.

For 60% $\dot{V}O_2$R:

Target $\dot{V}O_2$ = 0.6 (36.5 ml · kg⁻¹ · min⁻¹) + 3.5 ml · kg⁻¹ · min⁻¹,

Target $\dot{V}O_2$ = 21.9 + 3.5 = 25.4 ml · kg⁻¹ · min⁻¹ = 7.3 METs

For 80% $\dot{V}O_2$R:

Target $\dot{V}O_2$ = 0.8 (36.5 ml · kg⁻¹ · min⁻¹) + 3.5 ml · kg⁻¹ · min⁻¹,

Target $\dot{V}O_2$ = 29.2 + 3.5 = 32.7 ml · kg⁻¹ · min⁻¹ = 9.3 METs

Answer: He should use activities that require the following:

25.4 to 32.7 ml · kg⁻¹ · min⁻¹

7.3 to 9.3 METs

When these exercise intensity values are known, appropriate exercises can be selected from tables listing the energy costs of various activities. However, this is a very cumbersome method for prescribing exercise. Prescribing on the basis of the caloric cost of the activity does not take into consideration the effect that environmental (e.g., heat, humidity, altitude, cold, pollution), dietary (e.g., hydration state), and other variables have on a person's response to some absolute exercise intensity. The ability of participants to complete a workout depends on their physiological responses and perception of effort rather than the metabolic cost of the activity itself. Fortunately, by using specific HR values that are approximately equal to 60% to 80% $\dot{V}O_2$max, it is possible to formulate an exercise prescription that takes many of these factors into consideration. These HR values form the **target heart rate (THR)** range. How is the THR range determined?

Target Heart Rate: Direct Method

As described in chapters 4 and 7, HR increases linearly with the metabolic load. In the direct method for determining THR, HR is monitored at each stage of a maximal GXT. HR is then plotted on a graph against the $\dot{V}O_2$ (or MET) equivalents of each stage of the test. The fitness professional determines the THR range by taking the percentages of $\dot{V}O_2$max (%$\dot{V}O_2$max) at which the person should train and finding what the HR responses were at those points. Figure 11.5 shows this method being used for a subject with a functional capacity of 10.5 METs. Work rates of 60% to 80% of maximal METs demanded HR responses of 132 to 156 beats · min⁻¹. The HR values become the intensity guide for the subject and represent the THR range (3).

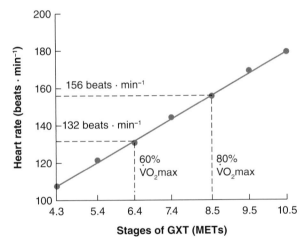

FIGURE 11.5 Direct method of determining the THR zone when maximal aerobic power (functional capacity) is measured during a GXT.

Target Heart Rate: Indirect Methods

In contrast to the direct method, which requires the participant to complete a maximal GXT, two indirect methods have been developed to estimate an appropriate THR. These are the HRR method and the %HRmax method.

Heart Rate Reserve Method

HRR is the difference between resting and maximal HR. For a maximal HR of 200 beats · min⁻¹ and a resting HR of 60 beats · min⁻¹, the HRR is 140 beats · min⁻¹. As shown in figure 11.6, the percentage of the HRR equals the percentage of $\dot{V}O_2$R across the range of exercise intensities (58,

59). For participants with average to high levels of CRF, %HRR approximately equals %$\dot{V}O_2$max.

The HRR method of determining the THR range, made popular by Karvonen, requires a few simple calculations (35):

1. Subtract the resting HR from the maximal HR to obtain the HRR.

2. Calculate 60% and 80% of the HRR.

3. Add each value to the resting HR to obtain the THR range.

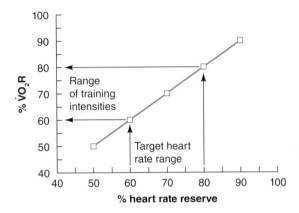

FIGURE 11.6 Relationship of %HRR and %$\dot{V}O_2$R.
Adapted from Swain et al. 1998.

QUESTION: A 40-yr-old male participant has a measured maximal HR of 175 beats · min⁻¹ and a resting HR of 75 beats · min⁻¹. What is his THR range as calculated by the Karvonen (HRR) method?

ANSWER:

1. HRR = 175 beats · min⁻¹ − 75 beats · min⁻¹ = 100 beats · min⁻¹.

2. 60% of 100 beats · min⁻¹ = 60 beats · min⁻¹, and 80% of 100 beats · min⁻¹ = 80 beats · min⁻¹.

3. 60 beats · min⁻¹ + 75 beats · min⁻¹ = 135 beats · min⁻¹ for 60% $\dot{V}O_2$max.

   80 beats · min⁻¹ + 75 beats · min⁻¹ = 155 beats · min⁻¹ for 80% $\dot{V}O_2$max.

The advantages of using this procedure to determine exercise intensity are that the recommended THR is always between the person's resting and maximal HRs and the %HRR equals the %$\dot{V}O_2$R across the entire range of CRF. Although the resting HR varies and can be influenced by factors such as caffeine, lack of sleep, dehydration, emotional state, and training, this variation does not introduce serious errors into calculating the THR by the Karvonen method (22). Consider the following example.

QUESTION: The 40-yr-old subject mentioned previously participates in an endurance training program, and his resting HR decreases by 10 beats · min⁻¹. Because maximal HR (175 beats · min⁻¹) is not affected by training, what happens to his THR range?

ANSWER:

1. The HRR now equals 175 beats · min⁻¹ − 65 beats · min⁻¹ = 110 beats · min⁻¹.

2. 60% of 110 beats · min⁻¹ = 66 beats · min⁻¹ + 65 beats · min⁻¹ = 131 beats · min⁻¹.

3. 80% of 110 beats · min⁻¹ = 88 beats · min⁻¹ + 65 beats · min⁻¹ = 153 beats · min⁻¹.

Consequently, the change in resting HR had only a minimal effect on the THR range.

Percentage of Maximal Heart Rate Method

Another method of determining THR range is to use a fixed percentage of the maximal HR (%HRmax). The advantage of this method is its simplicity and the fact that it has been validated across many populations (27, 37, 57). Figure 11.7 shows the relationship between %HRmax and %V̇O₂max.

It is clear that %HRmax and %V̇O₂max are linearly related and that %HRmax can be used to estimate the metabolic load in training programs. The usual guideline to estimate reasonable exercise intensity for the typically sedentary person is 70% to 85% HRmax. This THR range equals approximately 55% to 75% V̇O₂max and results in an intensity prescription that is slightly more conservative than that generated by the HRR method when 60% to 80% of HRR is used. The range of 75% to 90% HRmax is more similar to 60% to 80% V̇O₂max and HRR. The following example shows how to use the %HRmax method to calculate the THR range.

QUESTION: How can you calculate a THR range if you don't know what the resting HR is? Use the data from the 40-yr-old subject mentioned previously, who had a measured maximal HR of 175 beats · min⁻¹.

ANSWER:

Take 75% and 90% of the maximal HR:

75% of 175 beats · min⁻¹ = 131 beats · min⁻¹, and

90% of 175 beats · min⁻¹ = 158 beats · min⁻¹.

These values are similar to those calculated using the HRR method described earlier. Table 11.3 shows the relationship between %V̇O₂max and %HRmax across the range of exercise intensities from 50% to 85% V̇O₂max. Using this table simplifies the process of making specific intensity recommendations by using the %HRmax method.

Threshold

As mentioned earlier, the intensity of exercise that provides an adequate stimulus for cardiorespiratory improvement varies with activity level and age and spans the range of 40% to 84% V̇O₂R and V̇O₂max. In a systematic review of the literature, Swain and Franklin verified the low end of the threshold range. They found that the threshold for improvement in V̇O₂max was only 30% HRR for people with V̇O₂max values less than 40 ml · kg⁻¹ · min⁻¹ and only 46% HRR for people with higher V̇O₂max values; however, higher intensities more effectively increased V̇O₂max (60). Consequently, for most of the population, the optimal intensity threshold is in the following ranges:

- 60% to 80% of V̇O₂max, HRR, and V̇O₂R
- 75% to 90% of HRmax

As we discussed at the beginning of this section, the threshold is toward the lower part of the range (50%-60% HRR) for older, sedentary populations and toward the upper part of the range (>80% HRR) for younger, more fit populations. The middle of the range (70% HRR, 70% V̇O₂max, or 80% HRmax) is an *average* training intensity and is appropriate for the typical apparently healthy person who wishes to be involved in a regular fitness program. Participating in activities at these intensities constitutes

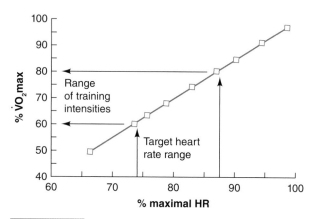

FIGURE 11.7 Relationship of %HRmax and %V̇O₂max.

Adapted from Londeree and Ames 1976.

TABLE 11.3 Relationship of %HRmax and %V̇O₂max

%V̇O₂max	%HRmax
50	66
55	70
60	74
65	77
70	81
75	85
80	88
85	92

From Londeree and Ames 1976.

RESEARCH INSIGHT

Tanaka, Monahan, and Seals (61) evaluated the validity of the classic formula of 220 − age for estimating HRmax. They analyzed 351 published studies and cross-validated these findings with a well-controlled laboratory study. They found almost identical results for both approaches: HRmax = 208 − 0.7 · age. This new formula yields HRmax values that are 6 beats · min^{-1} lower for 20-yr-olds and 6 beats · min^{-1} higher for 60-yr-olds. Although the new formula yields better estimates of HRmax on average, the investigators emphasize that the estimated HRmax for a given individual is still associated with a standard deviation of 10 beats · min^{-1}.

RESEARCH INSIGHT

The two indirect HR methods for estimating exercise intensity are simply guidelines to use in an exercise program, and small differences between methods are not important. Both approaches must be used as guidelines because, as for any prediction equation, an error is involved in estimating the %$\dot{V}O_2$max value. For example, even though we estimate that a person is at 70% $\dot{V}O_2$max when the HR is 81% HRmax (see table 11.3), in reality, 68% (1 SD) of the true values are between 64% and 76% $\dot{V}O_2$max for that HR value, and we don't know exactly where in that range any individual is (36). Because of this uncertainty, the calculated THR values should be used as guidelines in helping clients increase or maintain CRF. The fitness professional needs other indicators of exercise intensity to compensate for some of the inherent uncertainty in the THR prescription (see later in this chapter).

an overload on the cardiorespiratory system, resulting in adaptation over time.

Maximal Heart Rate

The indirect methods for determining exercise intensity use HRmax, and it is recommended that the HRmax be measured directly (by maximal GXT) when possible. If HRmax cannot be measured, then any estimation must consider the effect of age on it. Previously, HRmax had been estimated by subtracting age from 220. However, this formula underestimates HRmax for older adults (see Research Insight).

Any estimate of HRmax is a potential source of error for both the HRR and the %HRmax methods of calculating a THR. For example, given that 1 standard deviation (SD) of this estimate of HRmax is about 10 beats · min^{-1}, a 45-yr-old's true HRmax may be anywhere between 145 and 205 beats · min^{-1} (3 SD) rather than the estimated 175. However, 68% (1 SD) of the population would be between 165 and 185 beats · min^{-1}. If the HRmax is known (e.g., from a GXT), the fitness professional should use this measured HRmax to determine THR rather than using the estimate with its potential error (37). Estimating HRmax is another reason for using caution when relying solely on the THR range as an indicator of exercise intensity. The potential for error exists both in the estimate of HRmax and in the equations in which various percentages of HRmax are used to predict %$\dot{V}O_2$max. The intensity levels should only be considered as guidelines (see Research Insight).

Use of Target Heart Rate

The concept of an intensity threshold provides the basis for regular fitness workouts. Low-intensity activity around the house, yard, and office should be encouraged, but specific workouts above the intensity threshold are necessary to

achieve optimum CRF results. At the other extreme, people who push themselves near their maximum do not have a fitness advantage because similar results can be obtained at a lower intensity that is above the threshold.

The THR can be used as an intensity guide for large-muscle-group, continuous, whole-body activities such as walking, running, swimming, rowing, cycling, skiing, and dancing. However, the same training results may not occur from activities using small muscle groups or resistance exercises, because these exercises elevate the HR much higher for the same metabolic load.

The THR range associated with improvements in CRF and health-related outcomes is 50 to 84 %HRR, however, people who are less active and have more risk factors should use the lower end of the THR range. For example, moderate-intensity activity, equal to only 40 to 59 %HHR, is well within the capabilities of most people and carries a low risk of injury or complications (64). That is why it is the best starting place for most sedentary deconditioned people. Further, many clients may wish to continue doing moderate-intensity activity and not move to vigorous-intensity activity, because it suits them and they can work it into their schedule. More active people with fewer risk factors can use the upper end of the THR range. The THR can be divided by 6 to provide the desired 10 sec THR. If the person's HRmax is unknown, the estimated THR for 10 sec, by age and activity level, can be found in table 11.4. People can learn to exercise at their THRs by walking or jogging for several minutes and then stopping and immediately taking a 10 sec HR. If their HR is not within the target range, they should adjust the intensity by going slower or faster for a few minutes and then taking another 10 sec count. Using the THR to set exercise intensity has many advantages:

- It has a built-in individualized progression (i.e., as people increase their fitness, they have to work harder to achieve the THR).
- It accounts for environmental conditions (e.g., a person decreases the intensity while working in very hot temperatures).
- It is easily determined, learned, and monitored.

These recommendations are appropriate for most people, but individuals differ in terms of the threshold needed for a training effect, the rate of adaptation to the training, and how exercise feels to them. The fitness professional must use subjective judgment, based on observations of the person exercising, to determine whether the intensity should be higher or lower. If the work is so easy that the person experiences little or no increase in ventilation and is able to work without effort, then the intensity should be increased. At the other extreme, if a person shows signs of working very hard and is still unable to reach THR, then a lower intensity should be chosen. In this case, the top part of the THR range might be above the person's true HRmax because the 220 − age formula only roughly estimates the true value. The fitness professional should not rely on the THR as the only method of judging whether the participant is exercising at the correct intensity; attention should be paid to other signs and symptoms of overexertion. The Borg RPE scale might be useful in this regard.

Rating of Perceived Exertion

The Borg RPE scale that is used to indicate the subjective sensation of effort experienced during a GXT (see chapter 7) can be used in prescribing exercise for the apparently healthy person (6). Exercise perceived as just below somewhat hard to just above hard, a rating of 12 to 16 on the original RPE scale, approximates 40% or 50% to 84% of HRR or 60% or 65% to 90% of HRmax (3, 4). As mentioned earlier, the RPE is not a substitute for prescribing exercise intensity by HR (3). However, if the HRmax is not known and the THR range is perceived as too low or too high, an RPE rating can estimate the overall effort experienced by the person, and the exercise intensity can then be adjusted accordingly. Further, as a participant becomes accustomed to the physical sensations experienced when exercising at the THR range, there will be less need for frequently measuring the pulse rate. In the *2008 U.S. Physical Activity Guidelines*, a 10-point relative intensity (level-of-effort) scale was recommended, with 5 to 6 being moderate intensity and 7 to 8 being vigorous intensity (64).

KEY POINT

The exercise intensity for a CRF training effect can be described in a variety of ways: 40% or 50% to 84% $\dot{V}O_2R$ (HRR), 60% or 65% to 90% HRmax, and 12 to 16 on the original RPE scale.

Exercise Recommendations for the Untested Masses

Certain general recommendations can be made for anyone wanting to begin a fitness program. Although the fitness professional might wish to have each client undergo a complete testing protocol before beginning exercise, that simply is not realistic. In addition, people without known health problems who follow these general guidelines can begin to exercise at low risk. In fact, the CHD risks of continuing not to exercise are greater than those of begin-

TABLE 11.4 Estimated 10 Sec Target Heart Rate for People Whose Maximal Heart Rate Is Unknown

Population	INTENSITY %$\dot{V}O_2$max	AGE (YR) 20	30	40	50	60	70	80
Inactive with several risk factors	50	22	21	20	18	17	16	15
	55	23	22	21	19	18	17	16
Normal activity with few risk factors	60	24	23	22	20	19	18	17
	65	25	24	23	21	20	19	18
	70	26	25	24	22	21	20	18
	75	28	26	25	24	22	21	19
	80	29	28	26	25	23	22	20
Very active with low risk	85	30	29	27	26	24	23	21
	90	31	30	28	27	25	24	22

Data from Londeree and Ames 1976.

When Moderate-Intensity Exercise May Be Hard

The U.S. Physical Activity Guidelines (64) recommend 150 min · wk⁻¹ or more of moderate-intensity (3-5.9 METs) physical activity. The fitness professional must recognize that the range of 3 to 5.9 METs may be moderate exercise for some but hard exercise for others. Figure 11.8 shows that the relative intensity for a fixed exercise varies considerably across the range of $\dot{V}O_2$max values (32, 65). Consequently, some people with low $\dot{V}O_2$max values would function in the intensity range consistent with achieving gains in $\dot{V}O_2$max, whereas those with higher CRF values would not. This example emphasizes the need to consider the THR range and RPE when following recommendations that specify absolute exercise intensities (e.g., METs).

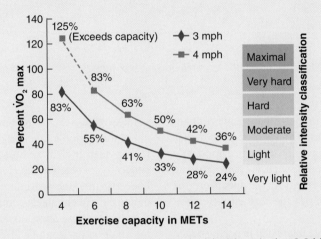

FIGURE 11.8   Relative exercise intensity for walking at 3.0 mi · hr⁻¹ (4.8 km · hr⁻¹ or 3.3 METs) and 4.0 mi · hr⁻¹ (6.4 km · hr⁻¹ or 5.0 METs) expressed as a percent of $\dot{V}O_2$max for adults with an exercise capacity ranging from 4 to 14 METs.

From: U.S. Department of Health and Human Services (DHHS), 2008, Physical Activity Guidelines Advisory Committee report 2008, Fig. D.1, page D-7. www.health.gov/paguidelines/committeereport.aspx.

ning a moderate-intensity exercise program. Figure 11.9 summarizes the recommendations for achieving health, fitness, and performance goals. On the left side we see the U.S. Physical Activity Guidelines for adults, the starting place for most sedentary deconditioned individuals (64). We want to emphasize that there is no structural barrier between what is needed for health and what is needed for fitness. The high end of moderate intensity (59% HRR) is clearly not different from the low end of vigorous intensity (60% HRR); think of the two categories as a continuum to realize much of the same benefits that we have discussed throughout the text. The fitness professional's challenge is to match the starting point to the client's status and progress the client through a program in a manner that is safe and consistent with the client's goals, which may change as fitness improves.

Exercise Programming for the Fit Population

Exercise recommendations for people who are regularly active and have achieved a reasonable level of physical fitness tend to be associated with less risk, and these participants require less supervision. People who become fit

can simply continue their program using the guidelines in the middle box of figure 11.9. As fitness improves, higher absolute intensities of exercise (e.g., faster jogging speeds) will be needed for the HR to stay in the THR range. Some people in this group may want to focus on performance, in contrast to health and fitness, as the primary goal. A wide variety of programs, activities, races, and competitions are available to address the needs of this group.

The THR range will be calculated as described before, but very fit individuals can work at the top part of the range (≥85% of $\dot{V}O_2$max or >90% of HRmax). As mentioned earlier, individuals who are less fit can start working out at the low end of the range and still experience a training effect. Those who are more fit need to work at the top end of the range to maintain a high level of fitness.

Training for competition demands more than the training intensity needed for CRF. Individuals who do interval-type training programs have peak HRs close to maximum during the intervals. The recovery period between the intervals should include some work at a lower intensity (near 40%-50% $\dot{V}O_2$max) to help metabolize the lactate produced during the interval (12) and to reduce the chance of cardiovascular complications that can occur when a person comes to a complete rest at the end of a strenuous exercise bout (44).

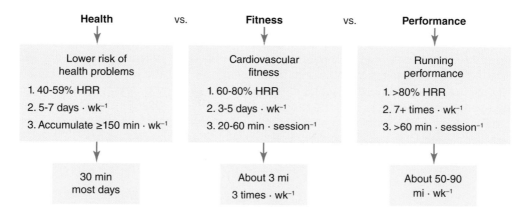

FIGURE 11.9 Contrasting recommendations for achieving health, fitness, and performance goals.

For people who participate in sports that are intermittent in nature but that still require high levels of aerobic fitness for success, a running and jogging program is a good way to maintain general conditioning when not participating in the primary sport. However, given the specificity of training, there is no substitute for the real activity when conditioning for a sport.

As figure 11.9 shows, people interested in performance who work at the top end of the THR range, exercise 5 to 7 or more times each week, and exercise for longer than 60 min each exercise session are doing much more than those interested in fitness, and it should be no surprise that they tend to experience more injuries (64). When the risk of injury during exercise is coupled with the inherent risks associated with competitive activities, it is clear that alternative activities should be planned that can be done when participation in the primary activity is not possible. This planning reduces the chance of becoming detrained when injuries do occur. Further, the alternative activities can be used as a part of the regular activity program to reduce the chance of an injury in the first place.

Exercise Prescriptions Using Complete Graded Exercise Test Results

In the previous sections, the exercise recommendations were based on little or no specific information about the people involved. In many adult fitness programs, potential participants have had a general medical exam or a maximal GXT with appropriate monitoring of HR, BP, and possibly ECG responses. Unfortunately, this information is not always used in designing the exercise program; instead, the measured HRmax is used in the THR formulas and the rest of the data are ignored. This section outlines the steps that should be followed when the fitness professional assists in making the exercise recommendation using information about the person's functional capacity and cardiovascular responses to graded exercise. The fitness professional is not generally involved in the clinical evaluation of a GXT, but understanding the procedures used to make clinical judgments clearly enhances communication with the program director, exercise specialist, and physician. The following information on using GXTs for exercise prescription and programming was written with this intent.

Program Selection

Exercise program options include exercising alone, in small groups, in fitness clubs, and in clinically oriented settings. The fitness professional must consider a variety of factors before recommending participation in a supervised or an unsupervised program.

Supervised Program

The risk factors, the response to the GXT, the health and activity history, and personal preference influence the type of program in which a client should participate. Generally, the higher the risk, the more important it is that the person participate in a supervised program. People at high risk for CHD and those who have diseases such as diabetes, hypertension, asthma, and CHD should be encouraged to participate under supervision, at least at the beginning of an exercise program. The personnel in the supervised program are trained to provide the necessary instruction in the appropriate activities, to help monitor the participant's response to the activity, and to administer appropriate first aid or emergency care.

Supervised programs run the gamut from those conducted within a hospital for patients with CHD and other diseases to programs conducted in fitness clubs for people at low risk for CHD. In general, as a person moves along the continuum from inpatient to outpatient, less formal

Using Graded Exercise Tests for Exercise Prescription and Programming

Analyzing Graded Exercise Test for Exercise Prescription

1. Analyze the person's history and list the known risk factors for CHD; also, identify those factors that might have a direct bearing on the exercise program, such as orthopedic problems, previous physical activity, and current interests.
2. Determine if the functional capacity is a true maximum or if it is limited by a sign or symptom. Express the functional capacity in METs, and record the highest HR and RPE achieved without significant signs or symptoms.
3. If ECG was monitored, itemize the person's ECG changes as indicated by the physician.
4. Examine the HR and BP responses to see if they are normal.
5. List the symptoms reported at each stage.
6. List the reasons why the test was stopped (e.g., ECG changes, falling SBP, dizziness).

Designing an Exercise Program From a Graded Exercise Test

1. Given the overall response to the GXT, decide to either refer for additional medical care or initiate an exercise program.
2. Identify the THR range and approximate MET intensities of selected activities needed to be within that THR range.
3. Specify the frequency and duration of activity needed to meet the goals of increased CRF and weight loss.
4. Recommend that the person (a) participate in either a supervised or an unsupervised program, (b) be monitored or unmonitored, and (c) do group or individual activities.
5. Select a variety of activities at the appropriate MET level that allow the person to achieve THR. Consider environmental factors, medication, and any physical limitations of the participant when making this recommendation.

monitoring is required. In addition, the background and training of the personnel tend to vary. Exercise programs aimed at maintaining the fitness level of CHD patients who have gone through a hospital-based program have medical personnel and emergency equipment appropriate for the population being served. Supervised fitness programs for the apparently healthy have a fitness professional who can focus more on the appropriate exercise, diet, and other lifestyle behaviors needed to improve health.

The supervised program offers a socially supportive environment for people to become and stay active. This is important, given the difficulty of changing lifestyle behaviors (see chapter 23). The group program allows for more variety in activities (e.g., group games) and reduces the chance of boredom. For the program to be effective in the long run, the program leader should try to wean the participants from the group in a way that encourages them to maintain their activity patterns when they are no longer in the program. See the following Research Insight for information about how pedometers were effective in increasing the physical level of patients in a cardiac rehabilitation program.

Unsupervised Program

Despite the risks just described, the vast majority of people at risk for or already having CHD participate in unsupervised exercise programs. Reasons for this include the limited number of supervised programs, the level of interest of the participant and physician in such programs, and the financial resources required to participate in such programs.

Participation in an unsupervised exercise program requires the fitness professional or physician to clearly communicate how to begin and maintain the exercise program. The emphasis in beginning an unsupervised exercise program is on low to moderate intensity (i.e., 40%-50% $\dot{V}O_2R$, 50% $\dot{V}O_2$max, or 65% HRmax), because the threshold for a training effect is lower in deconditioned people. The goal is to increase the duration of the activity, with exercise frequency approaching every day. This reduces the chance of muscular, skeletal, or cardiovascular problems caused by the exercise intensity and increases muscle function with the expenditure of a relatively large number of calories. In addition, the regularity of the exercise program

RESEARCH INSIGHT

Shipe (55) assessed whether the provision of a pedometer and exercise diary could increase the activity levels of phase II cardiac rehabilitation program (CRP) patients on the days they did not attend the 12 wk program (Tuesday, Thursday, Saturday, and Sunday). Members of the control group were given a blinded pedometer, and the physical activity information stored on the pedometer was downloaded at regular weekly intervals when they came to class. Members of the experimental group received a pedometer that they could view as well as an exercise diary to record their daily step counts (the information on their pedometers also was downloaded each week). Control patients wore the pedometer during all of their waking hours and were encouraged to increase their overall activity levels in accordance with the standard level of care. Patients in the experimental group were encouraged to gradually increase their step counts on the days they did not attend phase II CRP (i.e., non-CRP days) until they were accumulating 2,000 steps a day above their baseline levels for those days. Over the 12 wk program, the experimental group increased its daily step count on non-CRP days from 3,763 at week 1 to 5,772 at week 5 and maintained that level (i.e., 6,400 steps each day at wk 12); the control group remained virtually unchanged (3,175 at wk 1 versus 3,364 at wk 12). Clearly, the use of pedometers and an exercise diary helped these phase II CRP patients to be more active.

KEY POINT

Exercise recommendations for the general public emphasize moderate intensity (40%-59% HRR) and regular participation. Exercise performed at 60% to 80% HRR for 20 to 40 min 3 or 4 days $\cdot$ wk^{-1} increases and maintains CRF. Exercise recommendations for very fit individuals emphasize the top end of the training intensity (>80% $\dot{V}O_2R$) and frequent (almost daily) participation. The potential for injury is greater for such performance-driven workouts. For people who undergo a comprehensive diagnostic GXT with ECG monitoring, all test results are used to select an optimal and safe exercise prescription. Participants with multiple risk factors for CHD and those with existing diseases benefit from participating in a supervised program. However, most of these individuals will participate in an unsupervised program, necessitating clear communication about the exercise prescription and safety concerns.

encourages a positive habit. The outcome of such programs results in participants being able to conduct their daily affairs with more comfort and sets the stage for people who would like to exercise at higher levels.

In an unsupervised exercise program, the client should be provided explicit information about the intensity (THR), duration, and frequency of exercise so that no doubt remains about what should be done. For example, the exercise recommendation might read, "Walk 1 mi (1.6 km) in 30 min each day for 2 wk. Monitor and record your heart rate." The person must be told how to take the pulse rate and be encouraged to follow through on the recording. (See chapter 22 for more details.)

Updating the Exercise Program

During participation in an endurance training program, the capacity for work increases. The best sign of this is that the recommended exercise is no longer sufficient to reach THR; clearly the person is adapting to the exercise. Taking the HR during a regular activity session provides a sound basis for upgrading the intensity or duration of the exercise session.

The exercise program, including the THR, should be updated periodically. The need to update is greater for those with a lower initial level of fitness and a greater number of risk factors. A person who has a low functional capacity because of heart disease, orthopedic limitations, or chronic inactivity (which might include prolonged bed rest) has difficulty reaching a true maximum on a first treadmill test. Further, he experiences the greatest improvements in the shortest time during the fitness program. This person benefits from frequent retesting because the test allows progress (or the lack thereof) to be monitored, and it may give new information that influences the exercise prescription.

If the client has had a change in medication that influences the HR response to exercise, the exercise program must be reevaluated, especially if the exercise prescription was originally based on the initial HR response. These issues are found more in clinical rehabilitation programs, but as Exercise is Medicine initiatives come into place, fitness professionals will have to become more aware of how to help patients make a transition to fitness facilities.

For people who reach a true maximum in the first test, actual THR will change little during a fitness program because the HRmax is affected very little by regular endurance exercise. However, these people still benefit from regular evaluation of the overall exercise program because their activity interests may change or they may develop orthopedic problems that did not exist before. The reevaluation allows fitness professionals to probe for information that may enable them to refer the person for treatment at a time when treatment will do the most good. Such contact increases the chance that the person will stay involved in an activity program—the most important factor in maintaining aerobic fitness.

Environmental Concerns

THR is used to indicate the proper exercise intensity in health-related fitness programs. However, environmental factors such as heat, humidity, pollution, and altitude can elevate HR and RPE during an exercise session, which may shorten the session and reduce the participant's chance of expending sufficient calories to meet energy balance goals. Fortunately, by decreasing the exercise intensity, the fitness professional can work around these environmental problems to provide a safe and effective exercise prescription. This section discusses the effects of various environmental factors on the exercise prescription and what the fitness professional can do about them.

Environmental Heat and Humidity

Chapter 4 describes the increases in body temperature that occur with exercise, the mechanisms of heat loss called into play, and the benefits of becoming acclimatized to the heat. Our core temperature (37 °C, or 98.6 °F) is within a few degrees of a value that could lead to death by heat injury. As described in chapter 26, to prevent a progression from the least to the most serious heat injury, people should recognize and attend to a series of stages from heat cramps to heatstroke. Preventing the problem in the first place is a better approach than treating the problem after it has occurred.

Each of the following factors influences susceptibility to heat injury and can alter the HR and metabolic responses to exercise:

- Fitness. Fit people have a lower risk of heat injury (1, 17), can tolerate more work in the heat (14), and acclimatize to heat faster (8).

- Acclimatization. Exercising for 7 to 14 days in the heat increases the capacity to sweat, initiates sweating at a lower body temperature, and reduces salt loss. Body temperature and HR responses are lower during exercise, and the chance of salt depletion is reduced (1, 4, 8).

- Hydration. Inadequate hydration reduces sweat rate and increases the chance of heat injury (1, 8, 51, 52). In general, during exercise the focus should be on replacing water, not salt or carbohydrate stores.

- Environmental temperature. Exercising in temperatures greater than skin temperature results in a heat gain by convection and radiation. Evaporation of sweat must compensate for this gain if body temperature is to remain at a safe level.

- Clothing. As much skin surface as possible should be exposed to encourage evaporation, although the skin should be protected from the sun by using sunblock. Materials should be chosen that wick sweat to the surface for evaporation; materials impermeable to water increase the risk of heat injury and should be avoided.

- Humidity (water vapor pressure). Evaporation of sweat depends on the water vapor pressure gradient between skin and environment. In warm and hot environments, relative humidity is a good index of the water vapor pressure, with a lower relative humidity facilitating the evaporation of sweat.

- Metabolic rate. During times of high heat and humidity, decreasing the exercise intensity decreases the heat load as well as the strain on the physiological systems that must deal with it.

- Wind. Wind places more air molecules in contact with the skin and can influence heat loss in two ways: If there is a temperature gradient for heat loss between the skin and the air, wind will increase the rate of heat loss by convection. In a similar manner, wind increases the rate of evaporation, assuming the air can accept moisture.

Recommendations for Fitness

Members of a fitness program should be educated about all of the heat-related factors just mentioned. The fitness professional might suggest the following:

- Learning about the symptoms of heat illness (e.g., cramps, lightheadedness) and how to deal with them (see chapter 26)

- Exercising in the cooler parts of the day to avoid heat gain from the sun or from building or road surfaces heated by the sun

- Gradually increasing exposure to high heat and humidity over 7 to 14 days to safely acclimatize to these environmental conditions

- Drinking water before, during, and after exercise and weighing in each day to monitor hydration

- Wearing only shorts and a tank top in order to expose as much skin as possible, but being careful to use sunblock to reduce the chance of skin cancer

- Taking HR measurements several times during the activity and reducing exercise intensity to stay in the THR zone

The last recommendation is most important: HR is a sensitive indicator of dehydration, environmental heat load, and acclimatization, and variation in any of these factors will modify the HR response to any fixed submaximal exercise. It is therefore important for fitness participants to monitor HR regularly and slow down to stay within the THR zone. RPE also can be used in extreme heat to provide an index of the overall physiological strain that the participant is experiencing.

Implications for Performance

Any athlete performing in an environment that is not conducive to heat loss is at an increased risk of heat injury. This has been a major problem for football, where clothing and equipment prevent heat loss, but the increased number of people participating in 10K races, marathons, and triathlons has shifted our focus to them (1, 20, 33). In the latter cases, the athlete has a high metabolic rate while exercising in direct exposure to the sun. In response to this problem and on the basis of sound research, ACSM developed position stands on exercise-related thermal injuries (1). The elements in this position stand are consistent with the information presented at the beginning of this section.

Environmental Heat Stress

The preceding discussion mentioned high temperature and relative humidity as factors increasing the risk of heat injuries. To quantify the overall heat stress associated with an environment, a **wet-bulb globe temperature (WBGT)** guide has been developed (1). This overall heat stress index is composed of the following measurements:

- **Dry-bulb temperature (T_{db})**—Ordinary measure of air temperature taken in the shade.

- **Black-globe temperature (T_g)**—Measure of the radiant heat load in direct sunlight; temperature is measured inside a copper globe (15 cm diameter) painted flat black.

- **Wet-bulb temperature (T_{wb})**—Measurement of air temperature with a thermometer whose mercury bulb is covered with a wet cotton wick, which makes it sensitive to the relative humidity (water

vapor pressure) and provides an index of the ability to evaporate sweat.

The formula used to calculate the WBGT temperature shows the importance of the wet-bulb temperature, which makes up 70% (0.7) of the WBGT index, in determining heat stress (1). This is related to the role the wet-bulb temperature plays in estimating the ability to evaporate sweat, the most important heat-loss mechanism in most situations. The formula is as follows:

$$WBGT = 0.7\, T_{wb} + 0.2\, T_g + 0.1\, T_{db}.$$

The risk of **hyperthermia** (heat illness), including **exertional heat stroke (EHS)**, attributable to environmental stress while wearing shorts, socks, shoes, and a T-shirt is rated on the following scale (1, 50):

WBGT exceeds 27.9 °C (>82.1 °F).
Extreme risk of hyperthermia; cancel or postpone.

WBGT = 25.7 to 27.8 °C (78.1-82 °F).
Extreme caution; high risk for unfit, nonacclimatized.

WBGT = 22.3 to 25.6 °C (72.1-78 °F).
Extreme caution; risk of hyperthermia increased for all.

WBGT = 18.4 to 22.2 °C (65.1-72 °F).
Caution: moderate risk of hyperthermia; high-risk people monitored or not compete.

WBGT 10 to 18.3 °C (50-65 °F).
Low risk of hypothermia and hypothermia, but EHS can occur.

The risk of **hypothermia** while wearing shorts, socks, shoes, and a T-shirt also must be considered in distance running. A WBGT index of <10 °C (<50 °F) is associated with an increased risk of hypothermia, especially in wet and windy conditions, but EHS can still occur (1).

Table 11.5 provides an estimate of the WBGT using just air temperature and relative humidity. Because this table

TABLE 11.5 Estimate of Wet-Bulb Globe Temperature From Air Temperature and Relative Humidity

	WBGT (°F)										
RH%	60	65	70	75	80	85	90	95	100	105	110
90	60	64	69	74	79	85	90	95	100	105	110
80	59	63	68	72	77	82	88	93	99	105	110
70	58	62	66	71	76	80	85	90	96	102	108
60	57	60	66	69	73	78	83	87	93	98	103
50	55	59	63	67	71	75	80	84	89	94	99
40	54	58	62	65	69	73	77	82	88	90	95
30	53	57	60	64	67	71	76	79	83	87	91
20	52	55	58	62	65	69	72	76	79	83	87
10	51	54	57	60	63	68	69	73	76	79	82

For inside or outside, WBGT can be estimated from air temperature at the time and place of exercise. Relative humidity is very sensitive to air temperature. If the exercise occurs in direct sunlight, add 4 °F to the estimated WBGT. To convert °F to °C, subtract 32 and divide by 1.8.

Adapted, by permission, from American College of Sports Medicine, 2001, *ACSM's resource manual for guidelines for exercise testing and prescription*, 4th ed. (Philadelphia, PA: Lippincott, Williams & Wilkins), 213.

does not include radiant heat load (globe temperature), 4 °F should be added to the estimated WBGT if exercise is conducted in direct sunlight (4).

Exercise and Cold Exposure

Exercising in the cold can create problems if certain precautions are not taken. As mentioned previously, a WBGT of less than 10 °C (50 °F) is associated with hypothermia. Hypothermia is a decrease in body temperature that occurs when heat loss exceeds heat production, and it is clinically defined as a core temperature below 35 °C (95 °F). In cold air, there is a larger gradient for convective heat loss from the skin; cold air also is dryer (has a low water vapor pressure) and facilitates the evaporation of moisture from the skin to further cool the body. The combined effects can be deadly, as shown in Pugh's report of three deaths during a walking competition of 45 mi (72 km) that was performed in very cold temperatures (46).

Factors related to hypothermia include environmental variables, such as temperature, water vapor pressure, wind, and whether air or water are involved; personal characteristics, such as age and gender; insulating factors, such as clothing and subcutaneous fat; and the capacity for sustained energy production. Each of these factors is discussed in the following paragraphs.

Environmental Factors

Conduction, convection, and radiation depend on a temperature gradient between the skin and the environment; the larger the gradient, the greater the rate of heat loss.

What surprises many is that the environmental temperature does not have to be below freezing to cause hypothermia. Other environmental factors interact with temperature to facilitate heat loss, namely, wind and water (2).

Windchill Index

The rate of heat loss at any given temperature is influenced directly by wind speed. Wind increases the number of cold air molecules coming into contact with the skin, increasing the rate of heat loss. The **windchill index** indicates the temperature equivalent (under calm air conditions) for any combination of temperature and wind speed (see figure 11.10). This index allows the fitness professional to properly gauge the cold stress associated with a variety of wind velocities and temperatures. Keep in mind that for activities such as running, riding, or cross-country skiing into the wind, the speed of the activity must be added to the wind speed to evaluate the full impact of the windchill. For example, cycling at 20 mi · hr^{-1} (32 km · hr^{-1}) into calm air at 0 °F (−17.8 °C) has a windchill value of −22 °F (−30.0 °C)! However, wind is not the only factor that can increase the rate of heat loss at any given temperature.

Water

Heat is lost 25 times faster in water than in air of the same temperature. Unlike air, water offers little or no insulation where it meets the skin, so heat is lost rapidly from the body. Movement in cold water increases heat loss from the arms and legs (29), so it is better to stay as still as possible in long-term unplanned immersions or to wear a wetsuit for anticipated activities in cold water.

Temperature (°F)

Calm	40	35	30	25	20	15	10	5	0	−5	−10	−15	−20	−25	−30	−35	−40	−45
5	36	31	25	19	13	7	1	−5	−11	−16	−22	−28	−34	−40	−46	−52	−57	−63
10	34	27	21	15	9	3	−4	−10	−16	−22	−28	−35	−41	−47	−53	−59	−66	−72
15	32	25	19	13	6	0	−7	−13	−19	−26	−32	−39	−45	−51	−58	−64	−71	−77
20	30	24	17	11	4	−2	−9	−15	−22	−29	−35	−42	−48	−55	−61	−68	−74	−81
25	29	23	16	9	3	−4	−11	−17	−24	−31	−37	−44	−51	−58	−64	−71	−78	−84
30	28	22	15	8	1	−5	−12	−19	−26	−33	−39	−46	−53	−60	−67	−73	−80	−87
35	28	21	14	7	0	−7	−14	−21	−27	−34	−41	−48	−55	−62	−69	−76	−82	−89
40	27	20	13	6	−1	−8	−15	−22	−29	−36	−43	−50	−57	−64	−71	−78	−84	−91
45	26	19	12	5	−2	−9	−16	−23	−30	−37	−44	−51	−58	−65	−72	−79	−86	−93
50	26	19	12	4	−3	−10	−17	−24	−31	−38	−45	−52	−60	−67	−74	−81	−88	−95
55	25	18	11	4	−3	−11	−18	−25	−32	−39	−46	−54	−61	−68	−75	−82	−89	−97
60	25	17	10	3	−4	−11	−19	−26	−33	−40	−48	−55	−62	−69	−76	−84	−91	−98

Wind (mph)

Frostbite occurs in: 30 min · 10 min · 5 min

Windchill (°F) = 35.74 + 0.6215T − 35.75($V^{0.16}$) + 0.4275T($V^{0.16}$)

T = air temperature (°F)   V = wind speed (mph)

FIGURE 11.10 Windchill index.

Courtesy of the NOAA National Weather Service www.nws.noaa.gov

237

Personal Characteristics

Both age and sex influence the ability to respond to a cold environment. The fitness professional should give special attention to those at greater risk of hypothermia.

Age

Adults older than 60 yr may be less responsive to cold stress due to a reduced capacity to vasoconstrict the skin blood vessels and conserve body heat. In addition, from a behavioral standpoint, they respond later to a drop in environmental temperature than younger people. Because of their higher body surface area-to-mass ratios and lower body fat, children may experience a greater drop in body temperature when exposed to the same cold environment as adults (2).

Sex

Sex differences exist in the ability to respond to a cold-water challenge. These are primarily related to sex differences in body fatness, subcutaneous fat, and muscle mass (2).

Insulating Factors

The rate at which heat is lost from the body is related inversely to the insulation between the body and the environment. The insulating quality is related to the thickness of subcutaneous fat, the ability of clothing to trap air, and whether the clothing is wet or dry.

Body Fat

Subcutaneous fat thickness is an excellent indicator of total body insulation per unit surface area through which heat is lost (26). For example, in one report an obese man was able to swim for 7 hr in 16 °C water with no change in body temperature, but a thinner man had to leave the water in 30 min with a core temperature of 34.5 °C (47). For this reason, long-distance swimmers tend to have more body fat than short-distance swimmers; the higher body fatness provides more buoyancy, requiring less energy to swim at any set speed (28).

Clothing

Clothing can extend our natural subcutaneous fat insulation, allowing us to endure very cold environments. The insulation quality of clothing is given in clo units, where 1 clo unit is the insulation needed at rest (1 MET) to maintain core temperature when the environmental temperature is 21 °C (70 °F), the relative humidity is 50%, and the air movement is 6 mi · hr⁻¹ (9.7 km · hr⁻¹) (7). As the air temperature falls, clothing with a higher clo value must be worn to maintain core temperature because the gradient between skin and environment is increasing. Figure 11.11 shows the insulation needed at various energy expenditures across a broad range of environmental temperatures, from −60 to 80 °F (−51.1 to 26.7 °C) (7). As energy production increases, insulation must decrease to maintain core temperature. When clothing is worn in layers, insulation can be removed as needed to maintain core temperature. By following these steps, the sweat rate will be reduced and the clothing will retain more of its insulating value.

If the clothing becomes wet, its insulating quality decreases because the water can now conduct heat away from the body about 25 times better than air can (29). A primary goal, then, is to avoid wetness caused by either sweat or weather. This problem is exacerbated by the very dry air of the cold environment, which causes a greater evaporation of moisture. When this problem of cold, dry air and wet clothing is coupled with windy conditions, the risk is even greater. The wind not only provides for greater convective heat loss, as described in the windchill section, but it also accelerates evaporation (21).

Energy Production

Energy production can modify the amount of insulation needed to maintain core temperature and prevent hypothermia (see figure 11.11). When thin (>16.8% body fat) male subjects were immersed in cold water, the drop in body temperature that occurred at rest was prevented when they exercised at an energy expenditure of about 8.5 kcal · min⁻¹ (38, 39). Although being physically fit does not affect the thermoregulatory responses to cold, a fit person can exercise for a longer time at a higher metabolic rate, which can help maintain core temperature (2).

Table 11.6 shows the progression of signs and symptoms of hypothermia that occur as body temperature decreases (56). It is important to deal with these problems on-site rather than wait until the person can be taken to an emer-

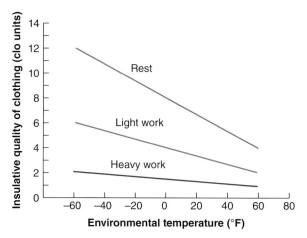

FIGURE 11.11 As work intensity increases, less insulation is needed to maintain core temperature.

Data from Burton and Edholm 1955.

TABLE 11.6 Clinical Symptoms of Hypothermia

Core temperature (°C)	Symptoms and signs
35	Maximal shivering
34	Amnesia, poor judgment
33	Ataxia, apathy
30	Cardiac arrhythmias
26	No response to pain
23	No corneal reflexes
18-19	EEG silence, asystole

Adapted from American College of Sports Medicine 2006.

gency room. According to Sharkey (54), do the following to help a person with hypothermia:

- Get the person out of the cold, wind, and rain.
- Remove all wet clothing.
- Provide warm drinks, dry clothing, and a warm, dry sleeping bag for a mildly impaired person.
- Keep the person awake; if semiconscious, undress the person and put him in a sleeping bag with another person.
- Find a heat source, such as a campfire.

Effect of Air Pollution

Air pollution includes gases and particulates that are products of the combustion of fossil fuels. The smog that results when these pollutants are highly concentrated can have detrimental effects on health and performance. The gases can affect performance by decreasing the capacity to transport oxygen, increasing airway resistance, and altering the perception of effort required when the eyes burn and the chest hurts.

Physiological responses to these pollutants are related to the amount, or dose, received. Several factors determine the dose:

- Concentration of the pollutant
- Duration of exposure to the pollutant
- Volume of air inhaled

The volume of air inhaled is large during exercise, and this is one reason why physical activity should be curtailed during times of peak pollution (15). The following discussion focuses on the major air pollutants: particulate matter, ozone, sulfur dioxide, and carbon monoxide.

Particulate Matter

The air is full of microscopic and submicroscopic particles, many of which can be tied to motor vehicles (especially diesel vehicles) and industrial sources. Over the past several years, more attention has been directed on the very small particles because of their potential to promote pulmonary infection and to actually cross the epithelium to enter the blood circulation (16). Fine-particle pollution elevates BP in people with preexisting CVD and may contribute to an increased risk of cardiac mortality and morbidity (53, 66).

Ozone

The **ozone** in the air we breathe is generated by the reaction between ultraviolet (UV) light and emissions from internal combustion engines. There is evidence that a single 2 hr exposure to a high ozone concentration, 0.75 parts per million (PPM), decreases $\dot{V}O_2$max; further, recent studies show that a 6 to 12 hr exposure to a concentration of only 0.12 PPM (the U.S. air quality standard) decreases lung function and increases respiratory symptoms. Interestingly, people can adapt to ozone exposure, showing diminished responses to subsequent exposures during the ozone season. Concern about long-term lung health suggests, however, that it would be prudent to avoid heavy exercise during the time of day when ozone and other pollutants are highest (15).

Sulfur Dioxide

Sulfur dioxide (SO$_2$) is produced by smelters, refineries, and electrical utilities that use fossil fuel for energy generation. SO$_2$ does not affect lung function in most people, but it causes bronchoconstriction in people who have asthma—a response influenced by the temperature and humidity of the inspired air. Nose breathing is encouraged to scrub the SO$_2$, and drugs such as cromolyn sodium and beta-agonists can partially block the response to SO$_2$ (15).

Carbon Monoxide

Carbon monoxide (CO) is derived from the burning of fossil fuel (coal, oil, gasoline) and wood as well as from cigarette smoke. CO can bind to hemoglobin (HbCO) and decrease the capacity for oxygen transport. The CO concentration in blood is generally less than 1% in nonsmokers but may be as high as 10% in smokers (49). As mentioned in chapter 4, beyond an HbCO concentration of 4.3%, there is a 1% reduction in $\dot{V}O_2$max for each 1% increase in the HbCO concentration. In contrast, when one exercises at about 40% $\dot{V}O_2$max, the HbCO concentration can be as high as 15% before endurance is affected. The cardiovascular system simply has a greater capacity to respond with a larger cardiac output when the oxygen concentration of the blood is reduced during submaximal work (30, 48, 49). This, of course, requires a higher HR for the same work rate, and participants need to reduce the intensity of exercise during exposure to CO to stay in the THR range. Because it takes about 2 to 4 hr to remove half the CO from the blood once the exposure has been removed, CO can have a lasting effect on performance (15). Unfortunately, it is difficult to predict what the actual CO concentration will be in any given environment. Because we must consider the previous exposure to the pollutant, as well as the length of time and rate of ventilation associated with the current exposure, the following guidelines are provided for exercising in an area with air pollution (49):

- Reduce exposure to the pollutant before exercise because the physiological effects are time and dose dependent.
- Stay away from areas where you might receive a high dose of CO: smoking areas, high-traffic areas, and urban environments.
- Do not schedule activities during the times when pollutants are at their highest levels because of traffic: 7 to 10 a.m. and 4 to 7 p.m.

Air Quality Index

The air quality index (AQI) is a measure of air quality for five major air pollutants regulated by the U.S. Clean Air Act: ground-level ozone, particulate matter, carbon monoxide, sulfur dioxide, and nitrogen dioxide. The AQI is shown in figure 11.12 as a color-coded chart with interpretations of

what the numerical values mean. This information is generally provided in a local community's weather forecast. The fitness professional should interpret the AQI information to suit the individual—some people experience symptoms at lower levels of pollution than others do (9).

Effect of Altitude

An increase in altitude decreases the partial pressure of oxygen and reduces the amount of oxygen bound to hemoglobin. As a result, the volume of oxygen carried in each liter of blood decreases. As mentioned in chapter 4, maximal aerobic power steadily decreases with increasing altitude, so by 2,300 m (7,500 ft) the value is only 88% of that measured at sea level. This means that an activity that demanded 88% of $\dot{V}O_2$max at sea level now requires 100% of the new $\dot{V}O_2$max.

More than maximal aerobic power is affected by altitude exposure. Any submaximal work rate is going to demand a higher HR at altitude compared with sea level (shown in figure 11.13). This is because each liter of blood has less oxygen at altitude, and thus more blood is required to deliver the same quantity of oxygen to the tissues. Consequently, the HR response is elevated at any given submaximal work rate. To stay within the THR range, a person must decrease the intensity of the exercise when at altitude. As with exercising in high heat and humidity, monitoring the THR allows the exerciser to modify the intensity of the activity relative to any additional environmental demand (31).

Levels of health concern	Numerical value	Meaning
Good	0–50	Air quality is considered satisfactory, and air pollution poses little or no risk
Moderate	51–100	Air quality is acceptable; however, for some pollutants there may be a moderate health concern for a very small number of people who are unusually sensitive to air pollution.
Unhealthy for sensitive groups	101–150	Members of sensitive groups may experience health effects. The general public is not likely to be affected.
Unhealthy	151–200	Everyone may begin to experience health effects; members of sensitive groups may experience more serious health effects.
Very unhealthy	201–300	Health alert: everyone may experience more serious health effects
Hazardous	301–500	Health warnings of emergency conditions. The entire population is more likely to be affected.

FIGURE 11.12 Color-coded AQI chart.

From: http://www.airnow.gov/index.cfm?action=aqibasics.aqi\

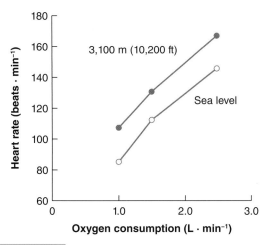

FIGURE 11.13 The effect of altitude on the HR response to submaximal exercise.

Based on Grover et al. 1967.

KEY POINT

In conditions of high heat and humidity, the exerciser should decrease the work rate to stay in the THR zone. Exercisers should acclimatize to heat over 7 to 14 days to reduce the risk of heat injury. Advise participants to drink water before, during, and after exercise and to exercise in the early morning to reduce environmental heat load. When exercising in cold weather, participants should wear clothing in layers and remove layers to minimize sweating and to stay dry. Participants should become aware of the AQI readings in their communities and avoid exercising at times and in places in which air pollution is a problem. When exercising at altitude, participants should decrease work intensity to stay in the THR zone.

STUDY QUESTIONS

1. What do the terms *intensity*, *frequency*, and *duration* mean in describing the dose of physical activity?

2. How might you calculate the volume or amount of physical activity done in a week?

3. Explain the principle of overload.

4. What is the public health recommendation for physical activity for both moderate and vigorous intensities?

5. What is the range of exercise intensities, in %HRR, associated with increasing CRF? Where does moderate-intensity physical activity fit in that range?

6. What is the optimal range of exercise intensities associated with increasing CRF for most people who are cleared to participate in a structured exercise program?

7. What %HRmax values would you use to match the intensities in question 6?

8. What does *progression* mean when it comes to helping a person become physically active?

9. What should clients learn to check to help maintain the optimal relative intensity when the environmental temperature and relative humidity are elevated?

10. What is the air quality index (AQI), and how could you obtain information about air quality in your own community?

CASE STUDIES

You can check your answers by referring to appendix A.

In the first two case studies you are given general information about a client, data on risk factors, and the results of an exercise test. Analyze each case, delineate the risk factors, and react to the person's responses to the test (whether normal or not). Then, on the basis of your analysis, make some recommendations for the client regarding an exercise program and risk-factor reduction program.

1. Paul, a Caucasian male, is 36 yr old, weighs 88 kg, is 178 cm tall, and has 28% body fat. Blood chemistry values indicate that his total cholesterol is 270 mg · dl⁻¹ and HDL-C is 38 mg · dl⁻¹. His mother died of a heart attack at the age of 63, and his father had a heart attack at the age of 68. He is sedentary and has engaged in no endurance training since college. The following are the results of a maximal GXT conducted by his physician.

TEST: Balke, 3 mi · hr⁻¹ (4.8 km · hr⁻¹); 2.5% every 2 min

% Grade	METs	SBP (mmHg)	DBP (mmHg)	HR (beats · min⁻¹)	ECG	Symptoms
2.5	Rest	126	88	70	Normal	—
5	4.3	142	86	142	Normal	—
7.5	5.4	184	88	150	Normal	—
10	6.4	162	86	160	Normal	—
12.5	7.4	174	84	168	Normal	—
15	8.5	186	84	176	Normal	—
17.5	9.5	194	84	190	Normal	Calf tight
	10.5	198	84	198	Normal	Fatigue

2. Mary is a 38-yr-old Hispanic American female and is 170 cm tall, weighs 61.4 kg, and has 30% body fat. Blood chemistry values indicate a total cholesterol of 188 mg · dl⁻¹ and an HDL-C of 59 mg · dl⁻¹. Her resting BP is 124/80 mmHg. Family history indicates that her father had a nonfatal heart attack at the age of 67. She has smoked one pack of cigarettes per day for the past 13 yr, and her lifestyle is sedentary. The table to the right is the result of her submaximal cycle ergometer test.

TEST: YMCA cycle test

Work rate (kpm · min⁻¹)	HR (min 2)	HR (min 3)
150	118	120
300	134	136

Pedal rate = 50 rev · min⁻¹; predicted HRmax = 182 beats · min⁻¹; seat height = 6; and 85% HRmax = 155 beats · min⁻¹.

3. You are asked to make a presentation to a group of sedentary faculty members at your school on how to begin a physical activity program to accrue the health-related benefits discussed in this chapter. What guidance would you provide to help them each achieve their goals? Discuss the kind of general screening that you would recommend (that they could do at the meeting) and how you would instruct them to begin the program (specify the frequency, intensity, and time) that ultimately leads to the goal of 150 min of moderate-intensity physical activity per week. You may assume that everyone can walk without pain.

REFERENCES

1. American College of Sports Medicine (ACSM). 2007. Exertional heat illness during training and competition. *Medicine and Science in Sports and Exercise* 39:556-572.

2. American College of Sports Medicine (ACSM). 2006. Prevention of cold injuries during exercise. *Medicine and Science in Sports and Exercise* 38:2012-2029.

3. American College of Sports Medicine (ACSM). 2011. The recommended quantity and quality of exercise for developing and maintaining cardiorespiratory, musculoskeletal, and neuromotor fitness in apparently healthy adults: guidance for prescribing exercise. *Medicine and Science of Sports and Exercise* 43(7): 1334-1359.

4. American College of Sports Medicine (ACSM). 2010. *ACSM's guidelines for exercise testing and prescription.* 8th ed. Philadelphia: Lippincott Williams & Wilkins.

5. Blair, S.N., H.W. Kohl III, R.S. Paffenbarger, Jr., D.G. Clark, K.H. Cooper, and L.W. Gibbons. 1989. Physical fitness and all-cause mortality. *Journal of the American Medical Association* 262:2395-2401.

6. Borg, G. 1998. *Borg's perceived exertion and pain scales.* Champaign, IL: Human Kinetics.

7. Burton, A.C., and O.G. Edholm. 1955. *Man in a cold environment.* London: Edward Arnold.

8. Buskirk, E.R., and D.E. Bass. 1974. Climate and exercise. In *Science and medicine of exercise and sport,* ed. W.R. Johnson and E.R. Buskirk, 190-205. New York: Harper & Row.

9. Campbell, M.E., Q. Li, S.E. Gingrich, R.G. Macfarlane, and S. Cheng. 2005. Should people be physically active outdoors on smog alert days? *Canadian Journal of Public Health* 96:24-28.

10. Dehn, M.M., and C.B. Mullins. 1977. Physiologic effects and importance of exercise in patients with coronary artery disease. *Cardiovascular Medicine* 2:365.

11. Dionne, F.T., L. Turcotte, M.-C. Thibault, M.R. Boulay, J.S. Skinner, and C. Bouchard. 1991. Mitochondrial DNA sequence polymorphism, V̇O₂max, and response to endurance training. *Medicine and Science in Sports and Exercise* 23:177-185.

12. Dodd, S., S.K. Powers, T. Callender, and E. Brooks. 1984. Blood lactate disappearance at various intensities of recovery exercise. *Journal of Applied Physiology* 57:1462-1465.

13. Dose–response issues concerning physical activity and health: An evidence-based symposium (Suppl.). 2001. *Medicine and Science in Sports and Exercise* 33(6).

14. Drinkwater, B.L., J.E. Denton, I.C. Kupprat, T.S. Talag, and S.M. Horvath. 1976. Aerobic power as a factor in women's response to work within hot environments. *Journal of Applied Physiology* 41:815-821.

15. Folinsbee, L.J. 1990. Discussion: Exercise and the environment. In *Exercise, fitness, and health,* ed. C. Bouchard, R.J. Shephard, T. Stephens, J.R. Sutton, and B.D. McPherson, 179-183. Champaign, IL: Human Kinetics.

16. Frampton, M.W., M.J. Utell, W. Zareba, G. Oberdorster, C. Cox, L.S. Huang, P.E. Morrow, F.E. Lee, D. Chalupa, L.M. Frasier, D.M. Speers, and J. Stewart. 2004. Effects of exposure to ultrafine carbon particles in healthy subjects and subjects with asthma. *Research Report—Health Effects Institute* 126:1-63.

17. Gisolfi, G.V., and J. Cohen. 1979. Relationships among training, heat acclimation, and heat tolerance in men and women: The controversy revisited. *Medicine and Science in Sports and Exercise* 11:56-59.

18. Goodman, L.S., and A. Gilman, eds. 1975. *The pharmacological basis of therapeutics.* New York: Macmillan.

19. Grover, R., J. Reeves, E. Grover, and J. Leathers. 1967. Muscular exercise in young men native to 3,100 m altitude. *Journal of Applied Physiology* 22:555-564.

20. Hanson, P.G., and S.W. Zimmerman. 1979. Exertional heatstroke in novice runners. *Journal of the American Medical Association* 242:154-157.

21. Hardy, J.D., and P. Bard. 1974. Body temperature regulation. In vol. 2 of *Medical physiology.* 13th ed. Ed. V.B. Mountcastle, 1305-1342. St. Louis: Mosby.

22. Haskell, W.L. 1978. Design and implementation of cardiac conditioning programs. In *Rehabilitation of the coronary patient,* ed. N.K. Wenger and H.K. Hellerstein, 203-241. New York: Wiley.

23. Haskell, W.L. 1984. The influence of exercise on the concentrations of triglyceride and cholesterol in human plasma. *Exercise and Sport Sciences Reviews* 12:205-244.

24. Haskell, W.L. 2001. What to look for in assessing responsiveness to exercise in a health context. *Medicine and Science in Sports and Exercise* 33:S454-S458.

25. Haskell, W.L., I.-M. Lee, R.R. Pate, K.E. Powell, S.N. Blair, B.A. Franklin, C.A. Macera, G.W. Heath, P.D. Thompson, and A. Bauman. 2007. Physical activity and public health: Updated recommendations for adults from the American College of Sports Medicine and the American Heart Association. *Medicine and Science in Sports and Exercise* 39:1423-1434.

26. Hayward, M.G., and W.R. Keatinge. 1981. Roles of subcutaneous fat and thermoregulatory reflexes in determining ability to stabilize body temperature in water. *Journal of Physiology* (London) 320:229-251.

27. Hellerstein, H.K., and B.A. Franklin. 1984. Exercise testing and prescription. In *Rehabilitation of the coronary patient.* 2nd ed. Ed. N.K. Wenger and H.K. Hellerstein, 197-284. New York: Wiley.

28. Holmer, I. 1979. Physiology of swimming man. *Exercise and Sport Sciences Reviews* 7:87-123.

29. Horvath, S.M. 1981. Exercise in a cold environment. *Exercise and Sport Sciences Reviews* 9:221-263.

30. Horvath, S.M., P.R. Raven, T.E. Dahms, and D.J. Gray. 1975. Maximal aerobic capacity of different levels of carboxyhemoglobin. *Journal of Applied Physiology* 38:300-303.

31. Howley, E.T. 1980. Effect of altitude on physical performance. In *Encyclopedia of physical education, fitness, and sports: Training, environment, nutrition, and fitness,* ed. G.A. Stull and T.K. Cureton, 177-187. Salt Lake City: Brighton.

32. Howley, E.T. 2001. Type of activity: Resistance, aerobic and leisure versus occupational physical activity. *Medicine and Science in Sports and Exercise* 33:S364-S369.

33. Hughson, R.L., H.J. Green, M.E. Houston, J.A. Thompson, D.R. MacLean, and J.R. Sutton. 1980. Heat injuries in Canadian mass-participation runs. *Canadian Medical Association Journal* 122:1141-1144.

34. Jennings, G.L., G. Deakin, P. Korner, I. Meredith, B. Kingwell, and L. Nelson. 1991. What is the dose–response relationship between exercise training and blood pressure? *Annals of Medicine* 23:313-318.

35. Karvonen, M.J., E. Kentala, and O. Mustala. 1957. The effects of training heart rate: A longitudinal study. *Annales Medicinae Experimentalis et Biologiae Fenniae* 35:307-315.

36. Londeree, B.R., and S.A. Ames. 1976. Trend analysis of the %$\dot{V}O_2$max-HR regression. *Medicine and Science in Sports* 8:122-125.

37. Londeree, B.R., and M.L. Moeschberger. 1982. Effect of age and other factors on maximal heart rate. *Research Quarterly for Exercise and Sport* 53:297-304.

38. McArdle, W.D., J.R. Magel, T.J. Gergley, R.J. Spina, and M.M. Toner. 1984. Thermal adjustment to cold-water exposure in resting men and women. *Journal of Physiology: Respiratory, Environmental and Exercise Physiology* 56:1565-1571.

39. McArdle, W.D., J.R. Magel, R.J. Spina, T.J. Gergley, and M.M. Toner. 1984. Thermal adjustments to cold-water exposure in exercising men and women. *Journal of Applied Physiology* 56:1572-1577.

40. Myers, J., M. Prakash, V. Froelicher, D. Do, S. Partington, and J.E. Atwood. 2002. Exercise capacity and mortality among men referred for exercise testing. *New England Journal of Medicine* 346:793-801.

41. Paffenbarger, R.S., R.T. Hyde, and A.L. Wing. 1986. Physical activity, all-cause mortality, and longevity of college alumni. *New England Journal of Medicine* 314:605-613.

42. Pate, R.R., M. Pratt, S.N. Blair, W.L. Haskell, C.A. Macera, and C. Bouchard. 1995. Physical activity and public health: A recommendation from the Centers for Disease Control and Prevention and the American College of Sports Medicine. *Journal of the American Medical Association* 273:402-407.

43. Pollock, M.L., L.R. Gettman, C.A. Mileses, M.D. Bah, J.L. Durstine, and R.B. Johnson. 1977. Effects of frequency and

duration of training on attrition and incidence of injury. *Medicine and Science in Sports* 9:31-36.

44. Pollock, M.L., and J.H. Wilmore. 1990. *Exercise in health and disease.* 2nd ed. Philadelphia: Saunders.

45. Powers, S.K., and E.T. Howley. 1997. *Exercise physiology.* Madison, WI: Brown & Benchmark.

46. Pugh, L.G.C. 1964. Deaths from exposure in Four Inns Walking Competition, March 14-15, 1964. *Lancet* 1:1210-1212.

47. Pugh, L.G.C., and O.G. Edholm. 1955. The physiology of Channel swimmers. *Lancet* 2:761-768.

48. Raven, P.B. 1980. Effects of air pollution on physical performance. In vol. 2 of *Encyclopedia of physical education: Physical fitness, training, environment and nutrition related to performance,* ed. G.A. Stull and T.K. Cureton, 201-216. Salt Lake City: Brighton.

49. Raven, P.B., B.L. Drinkwater, R.O. Ruhling, N. Bolduan, S. Taguchi, J. Gliner, and S.M. Horvath. 1974. Effect of carbon monoxide and peroxyacetylnitrate on man's maximal aerobic capacity. *Journal of Applied Physiology* 36:288-293.

50. Roberts, W.O. 2007. Heat and cold: What does the environment do to marathon injury? *Sports Medicine* 37:400-403.

51. Sawka, M.N., R.P. Francesconi, A.J. Young, and K.B. Pandolf. 1984. Influence of hydration level and body fluids on exercise performance in the heat. *Journal of the American Medical Association* 252(9): 1165-1169.

52. Sawka, M.N., A.J. Young, R.P. Francesconi, S.R. Muza, and K.B. Pandolf. 1985. Thermoregulatory and blood responses during exercise at graded hypohydration levels. *Journal of Applied Physiology* 59:1394-1401.

53. Sharman, J.E., J.R. Cockcroft, and J.S. Coombes. 2004. Cardiovascular implications of exposure to traffic air pollution during exercise. *QJM* 97:637-643.

54. Sharkey, B.J. 1990. *Physiology of fitness.* 3rd ed. Champaign, IL: Human Kinetics.

55. Shipe, M. 2009. The effects of a pedometer intervention on the physical activity patterns of cardiac rehabilitation participants. Unpublished PhD dissertation, University of Tennessee.

56. Sutton, J.R. 1990. Exercise and the environment. In *Exercise, fitness, and health,* ed. C. Bouchard, R.J. Shephard, T. Stephens, J.R. Sutton, and B.D. McPherson, 165-178. Champaign, IL: Human Kinetics.

57. Swain, D.P., K.S. Abernathy, C.S. Smith, S.J. Lee, and S.A. Bunn. 1994. Target heart rates for the development of cardiorespiratory fitness. *Medicine and Science in Sports and Exercise* 26:112-116.

58. Swain, D.P., and B.C. Leutholtz. 1997. Heart rate reserve is equivalent to %$\dot{V}O_2$reserve, not to %$\dot{V}O_2$max. *Medicine and Science in Sports and Exercise* 29:410-414.

59. Swain, D.P., B.C. Leutholtz, M.E. King, L.A. Haas, and J.D. Branch. 1998. Relationship between % heart rate reserve and % $\dot{V}O_2$reserve in treadmill exercise. *Medicine and Science in Sports and Exercise* 30:318-321.

60. Swain, D.P., and B.A. Franklin. 2002. $\dot{V}O_2$ reserve and the minimal intensity for improving cardiorespiratory fitness. *Medicine and Science in Sports and Exercise* 34:152-157.

61. Tanaka, H., K.D. Monahan, and D.R. Seals. 2001. Age-predicted maximal heart rate revisited. *Journal of the American College of Cardiology* 37:153-156.

62. U.S. Department of Health and Human Services (DHHS). 1996. *Surgeon General's report on physical activity and health.* Washington, DC: Author.

63. U.S. Department of Health and Human Services (DHHS). 2010. *Healthy people 2020.* www.healthypeople.gov/2020/topicsobjectives2020/default.aspx.

64. U.S. Department of Health and Human Services (DHHS). 2008. *2008 physcial activity guidelines for Americans.* www.health.gov/paguidelines/guidelines/default.aspx.

65. U.S. Department of Health and Human Services (DHHS). 2008. Physical Activity Guidelines Advisory Committee report 2008. www.health.gov/paguidelines/committeereport.aspx.

66. Zanobetti, A., M.J. Canner, P.H. Stone, J. Schwartz, D. Sher, E. Eagan-Bengston, K.A. Gates, L.H. Hartley, H. Suh, and D.R. Gold. 2004. Ambient pollution and blood pressure in cardiac rehabilitation patients. *Circulation* 110:2184-2189.

Exercise Prescription for Weight Management

OBJECTIVES

The reader will be able to do the following:

1. Identify factors that contribute to obesity.

2. Describe the role that energy balance plays in weight loss and weight maintenance.

3. Provide guidelines for caloric intake to facilitate appropriate weight loss.

4. Discuss the role of exercise in weight loss and weight maintenance.

5. Prescribe safe and effective exercise programs for weight management.

6. Describe strategies for behavioral change for weight control.

7. List reasons to avoid quick-fix weight-loss techniques.

8. Recognize signs of eating disorders.

9. Provide healthy guidelines for gaining weight.

Americans spend billions of dollars each year on weight loss. The weight-loss industry provides a broad spectrum of goods and services, including over-the-counter and prescription drugs, motivational and educational books, weight-loss clinics, and online support for weight loss. Weight-loss support groups have sprung up in many environments, including schools, health clinics, and churches. Despite this multibillion-dollar industry, U.S. obesity prevalence is at an all-time high. Recent evidence shows that 68% of American adults are classified as either overweight or obese (11). Unfortunately, this same trend is found among U.S. children (13, 17, 32). Although many Americans lose the fight against obesity, many successfully lose excess weight, and some manage to maintain a healthy weight throughout their lives. The lessons from these people provide a road map for successful weight control (18, 44).

Increasing Prevalence of Obesity in the United States

In the early 1960s, 13.4% of American adults were obese (i.e., had a BMI ≥ 30 kg · m⁻²) (10). Recent national statistics (from 2007-2008) revealed that obesity has soared to 33.8% (11). Figure 12.1 shows the increasing prevalence of obesity during the past four decades for both men and women. Some segments of the population have even more dramatic values. For example, obesity prevalence for non-Hispanic black women is currently approximately 50%, an 11.5% increase since the early 1990s (11, 12). Because of the rapid changes in obesity prevalence in the past few decades, this trend does not appear to be causally linked to genetics. As discussed later, lifestyle changes seem to be the major culprit.

Adults commonly accumulate additional adipose tissue as they age. This gradual accumulation of fat is sometimes called **creeping obesity**. Part of this change in body composition is attributable to a natural loss of muscle caused by aging. A decreasing metabolic rate, a more sedentary lifestyle, and unadjusted eating patterns, however, appear to be the most important factors in this increased body fat (8). Although some fat accumulation is acceptable (see chapter 8, table 8.1), when BMI climbs to obese levels, negative health consequences follow (30, 31).

KEY POINT

Although Americans spend billions of dollars each year on weight loss, the prevalence of obesity is increasing. Over two-thirds of adults are overweight or obese. People tend to accumulate fat as they age, but excessive fat accumulation is unhealthy.

Etiology of Obesity

The cause of obesity cannot be described simply, because many factors contribute to its development. Ultimately, **positive caloric balance** (i.e., taking in more calories than are expended) leads to obesity. Factors contributing to obesity can be discussed under two broad categories: genetics and lifestyle.

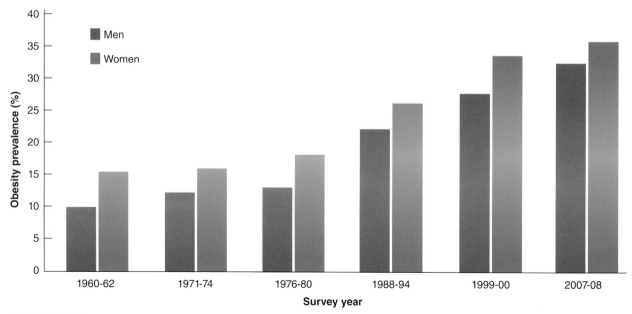

FIGURE 12.1 Prevalence of obesity among American adults.
Data from Flegal et al. 2010; Flegal et al. 2002.

Genetics

Although estimates vary based on study design, evidence generally suggests that inheritance contributes 30% to 70% of the interindividual variation in obesity (27). In evaluating the genetic influence on obesity, researchers have attempted to differentiate among factors that are genetic and sociocultural. Bouchard and colleagues (7) estimate that approximately 25% of the variance in percent body fat is attributable to genetics. Interestingly, these authors found that inheritance has a larger effect on total fat and deep deposits of adipose tissue than on subcutaneous fat. Additional evidence on the importance of genetics comes from data demonstrating that the BMI of adopted children is more similar to that of their biological parents than to that of their adoptive parents (35). The recent discoveries of genes linked with obesity provide additional evidence that genetic factors help determine the likelihood of being obese and developing diseases that accompany obesity (e.g., type 2 diabetes) (38). Research continues in an attempt to understand the link between genetics and obesity.

Many genes are linked with obesity (26, 37), and recently 18 new loci were shown to be associated with BMI (34). The expression of each gene depends on environmental factors (e.g., availability of fatty foods, social influences); therefore, the genetics of obesity is complex and much is yet to be learned (6, 27). A negative consequence of our growing knowledge of the genetic link to obesity is that people with many overweight family members may become discouraged and believe that they can do nothing about their weight status. Although genetics can contribute to the development of obesity, a primary reason that people become obese is lifestyle. Loos and Bouchard (27) suggest that only a small percentage of individuals have true genetic obesity that would be present regardless of the environment. These authors suggest that the majority of people who develop obesity in modern Western societies (an environment where high-density food is abundant and physical activity is not a part of everyday life) might be normal weight or at worst overweight in a less obesogenic environment (27). Fitness professionals must emphasize to clients that genetics may predispose certain people to obesity, but those people still have a great capacity to affect their body weight.

Lifestyle

The choices people make about energy expenditure and caloric intake predominantly influence the development of obesity. The number of calories consumed, the types of foods eaten, and the amount of daily activity all affect body weight. If more calories are consumed than are expended, the positive caloric balance results in weight (fat) gain. To lose fat weight, a **negative caloric balance** must be established. This balance can be achieved by decreasing caloric intake, increasing caloric expenditure, or both. National data comparing 1971 with 2000 show that the American daily calorie intake increased by 168 kcal · day^{-1} for men and 335 kcal · day^{-1} for women (45), and daily physical activity rates during these same years did not increase to offset the change in energy intake. Thus the typical American today weighs just over 24 lb (18 kg) more than the typical American of 40 years ago (33). During the early part of the 21st century, caloric intake has remained steady (46). Likewise, obesity prevalence appears to have leveled off at around 34% (11).

Food Intake

When excess calories (particularly fat calories) are consumed, the energy is stored as fat. From an evolutionary standpoint, fat storage is a positive adaptation to variations in food availability. In other words, fat accumulation occurs during times of plenty, and this stored energy is used when food supplies are low. In populations that have a constant abundance of food with high caloric density, this mechanism often results in excessive fat accumulation.

Health professionals sometimes question whether individuals who are obese typically consume more calories than their counterparts who are average weight. Dietary-recall studies provide little clear information about this issue because people tend to underreport dietary intake and overestimate physical activity (25). Some research suggests that subjects who are obese particularly underreport consumption of high-fat and snack foods (42). Highly advanced research procedures in which people ingest isotopes of oxygen and hydrogen (doubly labeled water) indicate that individuals who are overweight expend and consume more calories than people of normal weight (41). The higher energy expenditure is caused by the metabolic cost of supporting excess body weight. The reason extra calories are consumed is not known and is likely related to a variety of complex factors.

Types of Food Eaten and Obesity

When fat is consumed, it is stored as adipose tissue more readily than either protein or carbohydrate is. From a theoretical perspective, the low thermic effect of fat (i.e., the energy needed to digest, absorb, transport, and store fat), the ease with which fat is stored as adipose tissue, and the high caloric density of high-fat foods make fat a likely culprit in the development of obesity. National data indicate that during the past 30 years, the percentage of calories from fat in the typical American diet has gone down (45). However, since the total energy intake has increased, the actual number of calories from fat intake has changed very little.

Several studies indicate that people who are obese and overweight tend to consume a higher percentage of calories from fat than people of normal weight consume (42). It appears that the availability of foods high in fat and simple sugars puts individuals at higher risk for obesity. In cultures where the majority of calories consumed are complex carbohydrate, the rates of obesity are lower than those in the United States.

Daily Energy Expenditure

Researchers have found a relationship between low physical activity and an increased likelihood of obesity (2). Amish adults who live an active life that is similar to what was typical in the late 19th century have much lower rates of obesity compared with the average American (5). Additionally, women who walk more daily have a lower BMI, WC, and body-fat percentage compared with women who are less active (20, 23, 36). Because these are cross-sectional studies, it is impossible to say whether low physical activity leads to obesity or obesity causes people to reduce their activity levels. The longitudinal CARDIA study has shown that adults who maintain active lifestyles over a 20-year period gain significantly less weight and add fewer inches to their waists (16).

The role of regular exercise in weight loss is complex and has been reviewed by several authors (2, 15, 31). Increased physical activity helps create a negative caloric balance, and in combination with dietary restriction, it can lead to weight loss (2). Some studies support the role of exercise in maintaining fat-free mass and metabolic rate during weight loss. Although exercise without dietary restriction typically does not lead to major weight reduction, the long-term positive consequences of physical activity on weight maintenance are clear (2). Exercise is a strong predictor of long-term weight maintenance (2, 24, 43, 44). Additionally, regular physical activity attenuates age-related weight gain (10, 16).

KEY POINT

Both genetics and lifestyle contribute to obesity. Caloric intake, food choices, and daily physical activity are all aspects of lifestyle that affect fat accumulation. A positive caloric balance results in weight gain; a negative caloric balance results in weight loss.

Maintaining a Healthy Weight

Numerous methods can be used to maintain a healthy weight or to lose weight when necessary. Fitness professionals should encourage clients to choose weight maintenance or weight-loss techniques that are effective yet pose little threat to overall health. The following sections outline practices that most adults can implement safely.

Assessing Daily Caloric Need

Whether planning individualized programs for weight loss or weight maintenance, it is helpful to know the number of calories the client needs to sustain her current body weight. You can gain this knowledge by estimating daily caloric need. **Daily caloric need** is the number of calories a person needs to sustain current body weight, assuming that activity levels remain constant. The resting metabolic rate, **thermic effect of food**, and energy consumed by daily activities determine the daily caloric need (figure 12.2).

Resting metabolic rate (RMR) is the number of calories expended to maintain the body during resting conditions. For most people, RMR is 60% to 70% of their daily caloric need. For people who engage in regular, vigorous exercise, the RMR may account for a smaller proportion of daily caloric need because the energy requirements of exercise account for a larger percentage. RMR can be measured in a laboratory using indirect calorimetry. To accurately measure RMR, assess the client when he has not eaten for several hours, has not exercised vigorously for the past 12 hr, and has been in a resting, reclined position for 30 min (28). Because of the cost of indirect calorimetry and the strict control needed to obtain accurate results, measuring RMR is not always practical; therefore, a number of equations have been developed to predict RMR. These RMR equations are based on the following principles:

- RMR is proportional to body size.
- RMR decreases with age.
- Muscle is more metabolically active than fat.

The larger the body, the more calories needed to sustain it. This relationship is reflected in all RMR equations. In addition to body size, age significantly affects RMR. As a person ages, RMR decreases, meaning that the daily caloric need decreases with age. Generally RMR equations are sex-specific because males often have more fat-free mass than females have and fat-free mass requires more energy compared with fat tissue.

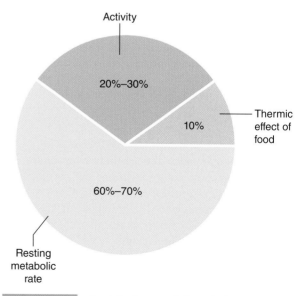

FIGURE 12.2 Contributors to daily caloric need.

If a client's fat-free mass is known, the following equation can be used to predict RMR (9). There is no need for sex-specific equations when fat-free mass is known, because a gram of muscle has the same metabolic need whether it resides in a male or female body.

$$\text{RMR (kcal} \cdot \text{day}^{-1}) = 370 + (21.6 \cdot \text{fat-free mass in kg}).$$

When determining daily caloric need, an estimate of the calories burned in physical activity is needed. This assessment requires information about work and leisure activity. Although there are numerous ways to gather information about daily activity, one typical method is an activity log in which the client records work and leisure activity. Once the activity pattern is established, the caloric cost of various activities can be calculated (see chapter 6) and used to estimate the energy burned in activity. Estimating this energy is especially important if working with a client who trains extensively. Alternatively, you can estimate daily caloric need by using the methods outlined in Calculating Daily Energy Needs.

The smallest part of the daily caloric need comes from the thermic effect of food. This is the energy needed to digest, absorb, transport, and store the food that is eaten. Although this value may vary slightly depending on the food eaten, the thermic effect of food typically accounts for 10% of the daily caloric need (29).

Changing Lifestyle to Promote a Healthy Weight

Although each individual must assess which areas of her lifestyle contribute to excessive weight accumulation, common steps that benefit the majority of people who are attempting to lose weight include the following:

- Reduce total calories.
- Reduce fat intake.
- Increase physical activity.
- Change eating behaviors.

As previously mentioned, a negative caloric balance must be established for weight loss. The number of calories consumed while attempting to lose weight should be determined by the client's health, caloric need, and ultimate weight-loss goals. Most healthy adults who need to lose weight can institute a short-term low-calorie diet (LCD) consisting of 800 to 1,500 kcal $\cdot$ day^{-1} without major adverse consequences. Very low-calorie diets (VLCDs) are sometimes used in specialized settings to treat individuals with extreme obesity. In these cases, physicians and dietitians provide patient oversight. VLCDs can lead to substantial weight loss, and years of study with this approach has yielded protocols with few negative side effects (39).

ACSM recommends that weekly weight-loss goals should target a loss of 1 to 2 lb or 0.5 to 0.9 kg (1). A general guideline is to establish a caloric deficit of 3,500 to 7,000 kcal $\cdot$ wk^{-1} (500-1,000 kcal $\cdot$ day^{-1}), which theoretically results in a 1 to 2 lb loss (0.5 to 0.9 kg) of fat each week (1 lb of fat = 3,500 kcal). ACSM also recommends that people restricting their caloric intake limit their fat intake to less than 30% of total calories (1). These are general recommendations, and people with special needs (e.g., athletes, older adults, people with metabolic disorders) may require

Calculating Daily Energy Needs

The Institute of Medicine (14) recommends the following equations for calculating a person's daily caloric need, or estimated energy requirement (EER). These formulas require the client's age in years, height in meters, weight in kilograms, and level of physical activity.

Adult Man

$$\text{EER} = 662 - 9.53(\text{age}) + \text{PA} [15.91(\text{weight}) + 539.6(\text{height})].$$

Adult Woman

$$\text{EER} = 354 - 6.91(\text{age}) + \text{PA} [9.36(\text{weight}) + 726(\text{height})].$$

PA reflects a person's level of daily physical activity. Use the following table to choose the appropriate PA value.

Activity level	PA value (men)	PA value (women)
Sedentary—extremely limited activity	1.0	1.0
Low active—typical activities of daily living only	1.11	1.12
Active—regular moderate physical activity	1.25	1.27
Very active—regular vigorous exercise	1.45	1.45

a different approach to weight loss. Caloric restriction can lead to decreased RMR and fat-free mass. The decrease in RMR and loss of fat-free mass will be greater in dieters with large daily caloric deficits (31).

Exercise Prescription for Weight Management

ACSM recommends a combined approach of exercise and moderate caloric restriction for people attempting weight loss (1, 2). Although debate continues over the precise contribution of exercise to weight management, a combination of exercise and moderate calorie restriction appears to be most effective in maintaining lean mass and avoiding excessive decreases in RMR. Existing data clearly demonstrate that people who are successful in maintaining weight loss engage in regular aerobic activity (44). Studies also show that regular exercise helps prevent weight gain (10, 16, 21). From a theoretical perspective, adding exercise to everyday life can significantly alter body weight. For example, expending just 100 kcal · day⁻¹ beyond daily caloric need for a year creates a caloric deficit of 36,500 kcal. ACSM recommends that individuals engage in a minimum of 150 min of moderate-intensity exercise per week and further states that additional exercise (200-300 min · wk⁻¹) is more likely to be associated with successful weight control (1, 2). The following are specific recommendations for weight loss with exercise (1):

- Frequency: 5 to 7 days · wk⁻¹.
- Intensity: initially moderate (40%-60% HRR), then progressing to higher intensity (50%-75% HRR).
- Duration: progress from short, easily tolerated bouts to 45 to 60 min daily. Multiple daily bouts can be used with bout duration of 10 min or longer.
- Type: aerobic exercise targeting large muscle groups. Resistance exercise is recommended as a supplement to aerobic activity.

In addition to the physical benefits, psychological variables improve with exercise. Improvements in self-

KEY POINT

Daily caloric need is determined by RMR, the thermic effect of food, and activity levels. Reducing total calories, decreasing fat intake, increasing physical activity, and changing eating behaviors are some common steps that will benefit many people who are attempting to lose weight. The exercise prescription for weight management should involve weekly aerobic activity of at least 150 min. When weight reduction is needed, most healthy adults can safely initiate weight-loss goals of 1 to 2 lb (0.5 to 0.9 kg) per week.

esteem and self-efficacy are commonly reported outcomes of regular exercise. The empowerment that comes from becoming more fit can add to the resolve to live a healthy lifestyle and maintain a healthy weight.

Behavior Modification for Weight Loss and Maintenance

The majority of attempts to lose weight and maintain weight loss are unsuccessful. Behavior modification (changes in lifestyle habits) is an important component of successful weight-loss and maintenance programs (31). For additional information on behavior modification, see chapter 23.

When people are committed to changing eating and activity patterns, a number of strategies can improve the chances of long-term success. During the initial phase of weight loss (the action stage; see chapter 23), implementing these strategies requires a great deal of effort and there is a significant chance of failure (i.e., relapse). After 6 mo or more of using these strategies (the maintenance stage; see chapter 23), changes in diet and lifestyle become more natural. Some strategies effective for losing weight and maintaining weight loss are discussed next. Not every person responds well to the same techniques, so clients should be considered separately and an individualized plan developed for each.

Keeping Records

Before implementing a weight-loss or maintenance program, it is wise to examine current eating patterns. This is most easily done with an eating diary or food log. A sample food log is provided in chapter 5. Remember, it is important to gather information about the types and quantities of food eaten as well as the social and emotional circumstances surrounding eating.

Careful record keeping accomplishes several objectives. First, food logs document the problem areas of food intake. Many people are unaware of the total calories or the amount of fat they consume daily. Second, eating diaries document the social and emotional cues to eating. After keeping records for a while, individuals begin to recognize the factors other than hunger that lead to eating (e.g., socializing with friends, watching television, feeling stressed). To combat these cues to eating, the social and emotional situations that trigger overeating must be recognized and strategies developed to overcome them. Third, recording food intake makes eating a cognitive process. For many people, eating is a habit, and they automatically choose how much and what to eat without conscious consideration. As discussed next, planning appropriate meals and snacks is an important component of successful weight loss.

Planning Meals and Snacks

Weight loss does not occur by accident; it takes a concerted effort. Purchasing appropriate foods and planning meals are imperative for success. One of the most helpful practices in controlling food intake is not purchasing high-fat and calorie-dense food. Substituting low-calorie and low-fat foods for high-calorie and high-fat foods also can substantially affect weight loss. For example, substituting a cup (8 fl oz, or 237 ml) of 1% milk for a cup of whole milk decreases caloric intake by approximately 50 kcal. If a person drinks 2 cups of milk per day, this substitution will reduce caloric intake by 36,500 kcal in 1 yr!

Meal planning is also essential. In busy households, planning healthy meals often becomes a low priority, and this can lead to meals that are easy to prepare but do not promote health or weight control. One technique for overcoming time constraints is buying breakfast foods that are quick to prepare yet are nutritious and relatively low in calories (e.g., fresh fruit, low-fat yogurt, whole-grain cereals). These foods provide a morning meal that offsets hunger and includes important nutrients.

Because many Americans are not at home for the noon meal, they often eat at restaurants that are convenient, affordable, and quick, including fast-food restaurants. Although several fast-food chains have added healthier items to their menus, the majority of fast food is high in both fat and calories. Individuals who choose to eat fast food are less successful at maintaining weight loss compared with those who avoid these food choices (19). Planning ahead might allow some people to carry their lunch to work and ensure that they can choose from a variety of healthy foods for this important meal.

The evening meal contributes a significant percentage of the daily caloric intake of many Americans. It is not uncommon for people who have limited their food intake during the day to overindulge at night. Because of the effort required to cook a meal, many people eat at restaurants or purchase packaged meals that tend to be high in fat and calories. The effort necessary for cooking nutritious meals can be reduced by doing the following:

- Cook and store meals ahead of time.
- Find a variety of low-calorie meals that are quick and easy to prepare.
- Purchase food ahead of time to avoid unnecessary shopping.
- Keep a variety of fresh vegetables on hand.

It is also important to consider the foods available for snacks. Although avoiding food between meals may be ideal for some, there are times when snacks are necessary. Foods that are nutritious and also low in calories are the best choices (e.g., fresh fruit, raw vegetables, low-fat yogurt).

Establishing a Support System

Studies have shown the benefit of having a support system when trying to lose weight (31). The source of the support, however, will vary depending on the client. A support system may be a friend, significant other, parent, coworker, therapist, or support group. Fitness professionals should encourage clients in a weight-loss or maintenance program to seek out other people to encourage them in their efforts. For some people, the reasons for overeating are emotional and deeply rooted. In these cases, a trained therapist may be needed.

A lot of people are encouraged by supporting others who also are attempting to lose weight. Many commercial weight-loss centers provide support groups, which serve several functions: They provide a group to whom participants are accountable, a setting in which helpful hints and success stories can be shared, and a nonthreatening environment where all of the participants are pursuing the same objective. In addition, Internet support groups are gaining popularity. Some of these services are free and others charge a membership fee. Consumers should seek out Internet services that meet their needs.

Committing to Behavioral and Outcome-Oriented Goals

Clients must develop goals that encourage healthy eating. Goal setting is important to help individuals remain focused on weight loss or weight maintenance. It should be a mutual exchange between the fitness professional and the client. The fitness professional provides information about healthy weight-loss or management practices, and the client identifies the behavioral goals to which she is willing to commit.

Typically, weight loss is outcome oriented (i.e., the end result is the measure of success). Weight-loss goals should be reasonable for the client and should follow the guidelines listed previously in this chapter. In contrast to outcome goals, behavioral goals focus on the process of weight loss, not the final outcome. Behavioral goals can help the client make behavior and lifestyle changes that will affect weight loss or maintenance. These goals may target altering eating patterns, making wise food choices, and increasing daily energy expenditure. An example of a behavioral goal is, "I will walk the stairs to my office daily rather than riding the elevator." More specific information on goal setting can be found in chapter 23.

Designing a Reward System

Part of human nature is the desire to be rewarded for accomplishing goals. When designing a weight-loss or maintenance program, it is wise to provide motivation by rewarding success. As with goal setting, it is vital that the client be involved in developing the rewards that will be used. One rule that fitness professionals should encourage, however, is to avoid using food as a reward. The reward program should recognize the achievement of both outcome-oriented and behavioral goals. This is important because attaining an outcome goal may take much longer than it may take to change certain behaviors. Also, there will be times when a person's weight plateaus; behavioral goals should be rewarded during these times. Here are some examples of rewards:

- Purchasing new clothes
- Purchasing hobby items (e.g., books, music, tools)
- Taking a trip
- Attending special events (e.g., movies, concerts, lectures)

Avoiding Self-Defeating Behaviors

Certain situations increase the likelihood of overeating. A client trying to lose weight needs to acknowledge these situations and institute measures to minimize the chance of succumbing to self-defeating behaviors. For example, a person who snacks on high-calorie foods late at night might avoid purchasing such foods and also implement a behavioral objective of not eating after 7:00 p.m. A person who loves pizza but tends to overindulge when going out to a restaurant might make pizza at home using low-fat ingredients and vegetables as toppings.

There are special times (e.g., birthdays, holiday dinners) when people will want to eat foods that are not a part of their weight management plan. Fitness professionals should emphasize to clients that a lapse in eating (or activity) should not mean an end to the weight management plan. Clients should be encouraged to immediately return to their healthy eating and exercise plan after the lapse. Fitness professionals might help clients who feel guilty by suggesting they view the lapse not as a failure but as an opportunity for renewing the commitment to weight loss or maintenance.

Combining Moderate Caloric Restriction and Aerobic Exercise

Regular exercise is an important facet of successful weight loss and weight maintenance. As mentioned, ACSM (1, 2) and the National Institutes of Health (31) support the use of exercise for weight loss and maintenance. The majority of weight-loss studies that compare diet with diet plus exercise show that the combined approach leads to greater weight loss (31). The standard aerobic activity recommendation of at least 150 min · wk^{-1} should be considered a minimum for people attempting to lose or maintain weight (1, 2). Progressing to 200 to 300 min · wk^{-1} is likely to provide additional assistance with weight control. See previous comments in this chapter and also chapter 19 for more information on exercise prescription for weight loss or weight maintenance.

Changing Unhealthy Eating Patterns

Specific eating patterns have been linked with excessive weight gain (8). Being aware of these behaviors and implementing plans to avoid them increases the likelihood of successful weight management. These four changes in eating patterns are recommended:

- Slow down.
- Make wise substitutions.
- Consume a variety of nutritious foods.
- Eat smaller and fewer portions.

People often eat rapidly and then feel uncomfortably full for several minutes after they finish eating. When food is eaten rapidly, inadequate time is allowed for the satiety mechanisms to help curb hunger. This results in people overeating before they realize that they are no longer hungry. To help slow their eating, people can put down eating utensils between bites, pause at least 30 sec between bites, and chew food completely and swallow before taking another bite (8).

Substituting foods that contain less fat and calories for foods that are high in fat and calories can significantly reduce caloric intake. For example, a person who eats a roasted chicken breast without the skin instead of a fried chicken breast with the skin will save approximately 160 kcal. The wise consumer looks closely at the total calories in a food as well as the calories that are contributed by fat. Reducing fat intake not only helps with weight control but also may help improve the blood lipid profile.

One problem that people face when trying to manage weight is diet burnout. It is not uncommon to find dieters who consume only certain foods. To avoid becoming bored and frustrated with a diet, it is important to consume a variety of healthy, low-calorie, and tasty foods. This objective is linked to the planning process. Maintaining variety in the diet not only helps avoid boredom but also provides nutritional balance.

When attempting to lose weight, one of the most helpful changes is to decrease the portion size as well as the number of portions consumed. Many people habitually fill their plates and eat everything on the plate. Also, social norms can contribute to the struggle to control weight. For example, Americans may demonstrate to their hosts that they enjoy the provided food by eating extra portions. Taking smaller portions of foods as well as avoiding second helpings can contribute significantly to caloric restriction.

Committing to Lifelong Maintenance

Weight loss is only temporary unless a plan is in place to maintain the loss. In examining the variables that predict success in maintaining weight loss, Lavery and Loewy (24) concluded, "There are no quick-fix, easy solutions to obesity. The solution is the harsh realization of the need for permanent lifestyle changes to maintain a desired weight status." Fitness professionals should help clients understand the need to commit to long-term lifestyle changes rather than focus solely on short-term weight-loss goals. It is encouraging, however, to learn that long-term maintenance of weight loss is much more likely once people have kept the weight off for 2 to 5 yr (44).

KEY POINT

Some strategies for successful weight management are keeping records, planning meals and snacks, developing a support system, designing a reward system, committing to both outcome-oriented and behavioral goals, avoiding self-defeating behaviors, combining moderate caloric restriction with aerobic exercise, changing unhealthy eating patterns, and committing to lifelong weight maintenance.

Gimmicks and Gadgets for Weight Loss

Over the years numerous devices have been marketed for weight loss. The majority of these devices are ineffective, and, unfortunately, some are potentially harmful.

Saunas and sweat suits have sometimes been recommended to help weight loss by burning off or melting away fat, but this is a false claim. These devices may induce short-term (i.e., a few hours) loss of weight by dehydration. They do not burn fat but can cause people to sweat profusely. Overusing saunas and sweat suits can lead to severe dehydration. Further, the warmer core temperature that is caused by these devices could harm fetuses during the first trimester of pregnancy.

Other devices such as vibrating belts, body wraps, and electrical stimulators have been used in attempted weight loss. Although these devices may not be harmful, the scientific evidence does not support their weight-loss claims. The money spent on these devices would be better spent on proven techniques. Additionally, people who put faith and effort into these unproven techniques may delay making lifestyle changes that lead to long-term weight loss and maintenance.

A widely held myth is that exercise emphasizing a particular body part will cause that area to lose fat faster than the rest of the body uses it. This false theory is called **spot reduction**. People commonly perform sit-ups or curl-ups in an attempt to decrease their waistlines. Although these are terrific exercises for increasing the strength and endurance of the abdominal muscles, they are not very effective for burning fat. As a person establishes a caloric deficit through regular aerobic exercise, fat loss occurs all over the body, not just at the parts he would like to see decrease.

Programs that advertise rapid, large weight losses are typically deceptive. The rapid weight losses at the beginning of such programs primarily result from lost water weight. Also, dietary plans that establish extremely large caloric deficits substantially reduce RMR and lean body mass and do not establish healthy, lifelong eating habits. As stated earlier, diets consisting of fewer than 800 kcal $\cdot$ day^{-1} are not generally recommended (31). Information about fad diets is highlighted in the sidebar Focus on Fad Diets.

KEY POINT

A number of quick fixes for weight loss are marketed, but these products are often ineffective and sometimes dangerous.

Focus on Fad Diets

Diet plans that promise incredible results can be found easily on bookshelves, in advertisements, and on the Internet. Many people are looking for quick, easy ways to lose weight, and entrepreneurs are eager to supply them. No one description summarizes all fad diets. Many focus on eating one food or food group, whereas others emphasize avoiding certain foods. Most of these plans are low in calories and may result in weight loss. However, these diets often do not emphasize a balanced diet with an adequate supply of essential nutrients. Over time, these nutritional deficiencies have the potential to lead to serious health consequences. Because of this potential for negative health consequences, the AHA has declared war on fad diets.

Another problem with these diets is that they do not lead to lifestyle changes that result in permanent weight loss. Many people follow these diets for a brief time and then regain their excess weight when they return to their previous pattern of overconsuming calories. These diets typically focus on food rather than on behavior change (e.g., increasing physical activity, using food substitution). For more information on making healthy diet choices, see the websites of the American Dietetic Association (www.eatright.org), U.S. Department of Agriculture (www.choosemyplate.gov), and National Institute of Diabetes and Digestive and Kidney Diseases (www.niddk.nih.gov).

Disordered Eating Patterns

Certain conditions exist in which an eating pattern can have a serious negative effect on health. **Eating disorders** are clinically diagnosed conditions in which the unhealthy eating patterns may lead to severe declines in health and even to death. **Anorexia nervosa**, **bulimia nervosa**, and **binge-eating disorder** are three of the eating disorders recognized by the American Psychiatric Association (APA) (4). **Disordered eating** refers to subclinical, unhealthy eating patterns that are often the precursors of eating disorders.

In the United States, anorexia nervosa occurs at a rate of 0.5% to 1% and bulimia nervosa occurs at a rate of 2% to 4% (22). No single mechanism has been identified as the primary cause of disordered eating or eating disorders. It appears that genetic, psychological, and sociocultural factors may predispose a person to these conditions. In the United States, these conditions are most common in young women from middle and high socioeconomic environments and in female athletes in sports that emphasize extreme leanness. It is hypothesized that the social pressure to be thin as well as discomfort with sexual development contribute to unhealthy eating patterns in young women. For female athletes, the pressure to perform in some sports is linked with extremely low body weights. For example, it has been reported that more than 60% of female gymnasts exhibit disordered eating patterns (22).

In anorexia nervosa, a preoccupation with body weight leads to self-starvation. People with anorexia nervosa typically view themselves as overweight even when their weight is substantially below normal. The APA lists the following criteria for diagnosis of anorexia nervosa (4):

- Purposefully maintaining weight at less than 85% of expected weight for age and height
- Extreme fear of gaining weight or fat
- Unhealthy body image in which the person feels overweight even when underweight; often associated with a severe intertwining of body image and self-esteem and a disregard for the seriousness of maintaining an extremely low body weight
- Absence of at least three consecutive menstrual cycles in postmenarchal women

Bulimia nervosa is characterized by consuming large amounts of food followed by food purging (4). Misuse of laxatives, self-induced vomiting, and excessive exercise are among the methods that may be used to purge. To meet the diagnostic criteria established by the APA, a person must engage in this behavior at least twice a week for 3 mo. Patients with bulimia nervosa, similar to those with anorexia nervosa, have an impaired body image and fear losing control over their body weight. Both anorexia nervosa and bulimia nervosa should be considered life-threatening disorders.

Binge-eating disorder is characterized by consuming large amounts of food in a short time (4). Unlike bulimia nervosa, binge eating is not associated with purging. Binge episodes are often initiated by emotional or psychological cues (e.g., loneliness, anxiety) rather than by physical hunger. These binges typically occur when the person is alone and may be followed by shame, guilt, and depression. To be clinically diagnosed with binge-eating disorder, a person must engage in at least two binges per week for 6 mo (4). The prevalence of binge-eating disorder in the general population has been estimated at 2%. In contrast, 25% to 70% of obese individuals seeking treatment for weight loss may have this disorder (40).

Recognizing the signs of disordered eating is necessary for successful intervention. Some common signs of disordered eating are listed in the sidebar Signs of Disordered Eating. Fitness professionals who observe these signs should discuss the issue in a nonconfrontational manner with the client. However, when approached, many people will deny the existence of a problem. Asking gentle questions about the client's health (e.g., "How are you feeling?" or "Are you a little tired?") is one way to attempt to break the ice on this delicate subject. Successful intervention for eating disorders requires a multidisciplinary approach combining medical, nutritional, and psychological professionals (3). Knowledge of local support groups or professionals who work with patients who have eating disorders will allow fitness professionals to recommend places for clients to receive help. For additional information and support for dealing with eating disorders, refer to the National Eating Disorders Association (www.nationaleatingdisorders.org) and the National Institute of Mental Health (www.nimh.nih.gov).

KEY POINT

Eating disorders can significantly impair health and may even result in death. Anorexia nervosa, bulimia nervosa, and binge-eating disorder are three eating disorders recognized by the APA. Intervention for eating disorders should be multidisciplinary and should include psychological counseling.

Strategies for Gaining Weight

Before concluding this chapter, we must mention that some individuals struggle to increase their body weight.

Signs of Disordered Eating

- A preoccupation with food, calories, and weight
- Repeatedly expressed concerns about being or feeling fat, even when weight is average or below average
- Increasing self-criticism about the body
- Secretly eating or stealing food
- Eating large meals, then disappearing or making trips to the bathroom
- Consuming large amounts of food not consistent with current body weight
- Bloodshot eyes, especially after trips to the bathroom
- Swollen parotid glands at the angle of the jaw, giving a chipmunk-like appearance
- Vomitus or odor of vomitus in the bathroom
- Wide fluctuations in weight over a short time
- Bouts of severe caloric restriction
- Excessive laxative use
- Compulsive, excessive exercise that is not part of the planned training regimen
- Unwillingness to eat in front of others
- Expression of self-deprecating thoughts after eating
- Wearing baggy or layered clothing
- Mood swings
- Appearing preoccupied with the eating behavior of others
- Continual drinking of diet soda or water

Based on Johnson 1994.

Fitness professionals should encourage these individuals to accumulate fat-free mass rather than all-fat weight. This will necessitate adding resistance training to the exercise routine. Various nutritional supplements are touted as supposedly guaranteed ways to increase muscle mass. However, as mentioned in chapter 5, even those who are training intensely need only about 1.5 g of protein per kilogram of body weight. Supplements such as creatine monohydrate may contribute somewhat to weight gain, but much of the change comes from greater water retention in the muscle.

The following are tips for increasing weight over time. When individuals continually lose weight or struggle to gain weight, a physician should be consulted about the possibility of underlying conditions.

- Increase caloric intake by 200 to 1,000 kcal · day^{-1} by increasing the meal size, number of meals, or number of between-meal snacks.
- Increase the number of healthy snacks consumed. Choose bread, fruit, granola, and other nutritious foods.
- Consume complex carbohydrate (e.g., whole-wheat pasta, whole-grain bread, brown rice, potatoes) to get the majority of additional calories.
- Add resistance training to the daily routine. Weight training is an effective means for increasing fat-free mass.
- When training intensely, make sure each day to consume 1.5 g of protein for each kilogram of body weight.
- Increase consumption of milk and fruit juices. These excellent choices not only provide additional calories but also essential nutrients.

KEY POINT

The additional calories needed to increase weight should come from increasing the number of healthy snacks or the size of meals. Adding resistance training to the exercise routine may help increase muscle mass.

STUDY QUESTIONS

1. What is the current obesity prevalence for U.S. adults?

2. Define *positive caloric balance*. Does it lead to weight loss or weight gain?

3. What roles do genetic factors play in development of obesity?

4. What three factors contribute to the daily caloric need?

5. What is the standard recommendation for daily caloric deficit when attempting weight loss?

6. Why is exercise important for those who are attempting weight loss or maintenance?

7. What are some behavioral strategies that can be useful for weight loss and maintenance?

8. List the signs of disordered eating.

CASE STUDIES

You can check your answers by referring to appendix A.

Ms. Kim is a 55-yr-old female who comes to your facility for an initial evaluation. She complains that she has gained 20 lb (9 kg) in the last 5 yr, and she wants to lose that extra weight. She is 5 ft 5 in. (1.65 m) and weighs 160 lb (72.6 kg). She currently does not exercise and has a sedentary job.

1. Calculate her estimated daily energy requirements.

2. In order for her to lose approximately 1 lb (0.5 kg) a week, what calorie intake would you recommend?

3. Assume Ms. Kim begins a weekly exercise program in which she will walk (3.5 mph or 5.6 kph) for 30 min on 5 days $\cdot$ wk^{-1}. How many additional calories will this expend each day? (Hint: See chapter 6.) Describe the effect this will have on weight loss.

REFERENCES

1. American College of Sports Medicine (ACSM). 2010. *ACSM's guidelines for exercise testing and prescription.* 8th ed. Baltimore: Lippincott Williams & Wilkins.

2. American College of Sports Medicine (ACSM). 2009. Appropriate physical activity intervention strategies for weight loss and prevention of weight regain for adults. *Medicine and Science in Sports and Exercise* 41(2): 459-471.

3. American College of Sports Medicine (ACSM). 2007. The female athlete triad. *Medicine and Science in Sports and Exercise* 39(10): 1867-1882.

4. American Psychiatric Association (APA). 1994. *Diagnostic and statistical manual of mental disorders.* Washington, DC: Author.

5. Bassett, D.R., P.L. Schneider, and G.E. Huntington. 2004. Physical activity in an Old Order Amish community. *Medicine and Science in Sports and Exercise* 36:79-85.

6. Beamer, B.A. 2003. Genetic influences on obesity. In *Obesity: Etiology, assessment, treatment and prevention,* ed. R.E. Anderson, 43-56. Champaign, IL: Human Kinetics.

7. Bouchard, C., L. Perusse, C. Leblanc, A. Tremblay, and G. Theriault. 1988. Inheritance of the amount and distribution of human body fat. *International Journal of Obesity* 12:205-215.

8. Cottrell, R.R. 1992. *Weight control.* Guilford, CT: Dushkin.

9. Cunningham, J.J. 1991. Body composition as a determinant of energy expenditure: A synthetic review and a proposed general prediction equation. *American Journal of Clinical Nutrition* 54:963-969.

10. DiPietro, L. 1999. Physical activity in the prevention of obesity: Current evidence and research issues. *Medicine and Science in Sports and Exercise* 31: S542-S546.

11. Flegal, K.M., M.D. Carroll, C.L. Ogden, and L.R. Curtin. 2010. Prevalence and trends in obesity among U.S. adults, 1999-2008. *Journal of the American Medical Association* 303(3): 235-241.

12. Flegal, K., M. Carroll, C. Ogden, and C. Johnson. 2002. Prevalence and trends in obesity among U.S. adults, 1999-2000. *Journal of the American Medical Association* 288:1723-1727.

13. Flegal, K.M. 1999. The obesity epidemic in children and adults: Current evidence and research issues. *Medicine and Science in Sports and Exercise* 31:S509-S514.

14. Food and Nutrition Board, Institute of Medicine. 2002. *Dietary reference intakes for energy, carbohydrate, fiber, fat, fatty acids, cholesterol, protein, and amino acids.* Washington, DC: National Academies Press.

15. Grundy, S.M., G. Blackburn, M. Higgins, R. Lauer, M.G. Perri, and D. Ryan. 1999. Physical activity in the prevention and treatment of obesity and its comorbidities: Roundtable consensus statement. *Medicine and Science in Sports and Exercise* 31:S502-S508.

16. Hankinson, A.L., M.L. Daviglus, C. Bouchard, M. Carnethon, C.E. Lewis, P.J. Schreiner, K. Liu, and S. Sidney.

2010. Maintaining a high physical activity level over 20 years and weight gain. *Journal of the American Medical Association* 304(23): 2603-2610.

17. Hedley, A.A., C.L. Ogden, C.L. Johnson, M.D. Carroll, L.R. Curtin, and K.M. Flegal. 2004. Prevalence of overweight and obesity among U.S. children, adolescents, and adults, 1999-2002. *Journal of the American Medical Association* 291:2847-2850.

18. Hill, J.O., and E.L. Melanson. 1999. Overview of the determinants of overweight and obesity: Current evidence and research issues. *Medicine and Science in Sports and Exercise* 31:S515-S521.

19. Holden, J.H., L.L. Darga, S.M. Olson, D.C. Stettner, E.A. Ardito, and C.P. Lucas. 1992. Long-term follow-up of patients attending a combination very-low calorie diet and behaviour therapy weight loss programme. *International Journal of Obesity* 16:605-613.

20. Hornbuckle, L.M., D.R. Bassett Jr., and D.L. Thompson. 2005. Pedometer-determined walking and body composition variables in African-American women. *Medicine and Science in Sports and Exercise* 37:1069-1074.

21. Jebb, S.A., and M.S. Moore. 1999. Contribution of a sedentary lifestyle and inactivity to the etiology of overweight and obesity: Current evidence and research issues. *Medicine and Science in Sports and Exercise* 31:S534-S541.

22. Johnson, M.D. 1994. Disordered eating. In *Medical and orthopedic issues of active and athletic women*, ed. R. Agostini, 141-151. Philadelphia: Hanley & Belfus.

23. Krumm, E.M., O.L. Dessieux, P. Andrews, and D.L. Thompson. 2006. The relationship between daily steps and body composition in postmenopausal women. *Journal of Women's Health* 15(2): 202-210.

24. Lavery, M.A., and J.W. Loewy. 1993. Identifying predictive variables for long-term weight change after participation in a weight loss program. *Journal of the American Dietetic Association* 93:1017-1024.

25. Lichtman, S.W., K. Pisarska, E.R. Berman, M. Pestone, H. Dowling, E. Offenbacher, H. Weisel, S. Heshka, D.E. Matthews, and S.B. Heymsfield. 1992. Discrepancy between self-reported and actual caloric intake and exercise in obese subjects. *New England Journal of Medicine* 327:1893-1898.

26. Loos, R.J.F. 2009. Recent progress in the genetics of common obesity. *British Journal of Clinical Pharmacology* 68(6): 811-829.

27. Loos, R.J.F., and C. Bouchard. 2003. Obesity—is it a genetic disorder? *Journal of Internal Medicine* 254:401-425.

28. Molé, P.A. 1990. Impact of energy intake and exercise on resting metabolic rate. *Sports Medicine* 10:72-87.

29. Montoye, H.J., H.C.G. Kemper, W.H.M. Saris, and R.A. Washburn. 1996. *Measuring physical activity and energy expenditure.* Champaign, IL: Human Kinetics.

30. Must, A., J. Spandano, E.H. Coakley, A.E. Field, G. Colditz, and W.H. Dietz. 1999. The disease burden associated with overweight and obesity. *Journal of the American Medical Association* 282:1523-1529.

31. National Heart, Lung and Blood Institute. 1998. *Clinical guidelines on the identification, evaluation, and treatment of overweight and obesity in adults* (NIH Publication No.

98-4083). Bethesda, MD: National Institutes of Health—National Heart, Lung, and Blood Institute.

32. Ogden, C.L., M.D. Carroll, L.R. Curtin, M.M. Lamb, and K.M. Flegal. 2010. Prevalence of high body mass index in U.S. children and adolescents, 2007-2008. *Journal of the American Medical Association* 303(3): 242-249.

33. Ogden, C.L., C.D. Fryar, M.D. Carroll, and K.M. Flegal. 2004. *Mean body weight, height, and body mass index, United States 1960-2002* (Advance data from vital and health statistics; No. 347). Hyattsville, MD: National Center for Health Statistics.

34. Speliotes, E.K, C.J. Willer, S.I. Berndt, et al. 2010. Association analyses of 249,796 individuals reveal 18 new loci associated with body mass index. *Nature Genetics* 42(11): 937-950.

35. Stunkard, A.J., T.I.A. Sørensen, C. Hanis, T.W. Teasdale, R. Charkraborty, W.J. Schull, and F. Schulsinger. 1986. An adoption study of human obesity. *New England Journal of Medicine* 314:193-198.

36. Thompson, D.L., J. Rakow, and S.M. Perdue. 2004. Relationship between accumulated walking and body composition in middle-aged women. *Medicine and Science in Sports and Exercise* 36:911-914.

37. Van Vliet-Ostaptchouk, J.V., M.H. Hofker, Y.T. van der Schouw, C. Wijmenga, and N.C. Onland-Moret. 2009. Genetic variation in the hypothalamic pathways and its role on obesity. *Obesity Reviews* 10:593-609.

38. Vimaleswaran, K.S., and R.J.F. Loos. 2010. Progress in the genetics of common obesity and type 2 diabetes. *Expert Reviews in Molecular Medicine* 12: e7. doi:10.1017/S1462399410001389.

39. Volpe, S.L. 2010. Weight management. In *ACSM's resource manual for guidelines for exercise testing and prescription.* 6th ed. Ed. J.K. Ehrman, 524-536. Baltimore: Lippincott Williams & Wilkins.

40. Wadden, T.A., and A.J. Stunkard. 1993. Psychosocial consequences of obesity and dieting: Research and clinical findings. In *Obesity: Theory and therapy*, ed. A.J. Stunkard and T.A. Wadden, 163-177. New York: Raven Press.

41. Welle, S., G.B. Forbes, M. Statt, R.R. Barnard, and J.M. Amatruda. 1992. Energy expenditure under free-living conditions in normal-weight and overweight women. *American Journal of Clinical Nutrition* 55:14-21.

42. Westerterp, K.R. 2000. The assessment of energy and nutrient intake in humans. In *Physical activity and obesity*, ed. C. Bouchard, 133-149. Champaign, IL: Human Kinetics.

43. Williamson, D.F., J. Madans, R.F. Anda, J.C. Kleinman, H.S. Kahn, and T. Byers. 1993. Recreational physical activity and ten-year weight change in a US national cohort. *International Journal of Obesity* 17:279-286.

44. Wing, R.R., and J.O. Hill. 2001. Successful weight loss maintenance. *Annual Review of Nutrition* 21:323-341.

45. Wright, J.D., J. Kennedy-Stephenson, C.Y. Wang, M.A. McDowell, and C.L. Johnson. 2004. Trends in intake of energy and macronutrients—United States, 1971-2000. *Morbidity and Mortality Weekly Report* 53:80-82.

46. Wright, J.D., and C.-Y. Wang. 2010. Trends in intake of energy and macronutrients in adults from 1999-2000 through 2007-2008. *NCHS Data Brief*, no. 49.

Exercise Prescription for Muscular Fitness

Avery Faigenbaum and Kyle McInnis

OBJECTIVES

The reader will be able to do the following:

1. Explain the physiological principles of overload, specificity, and progressive resistance and how they relate to exercise programming for developing muscular fitness.

2. Describe the following methods of resistance training: isometrics, dynamic constant external resistance training, variable resistance training, isokinetics, and plyometrics.

3. Describe the modes of resistance training.

4. Discuss the health and fitness benefits of resistance training and understand precautions that enhance participant safety.

5. Describe the variables that are used to design resistance training programs and discuss the relationship among the amount of resistance used, the training volume, the repetition velocity, and the rest intervals between sets and exercises.

6. Understand periodization and its application in the design of exercise programs, and differentiate between overreaching and overtraining.

7. Describe the following systems of resistance training: single set, multiple set, circuit training, preexhaustion, and assisted training.

8. Discuss the safety, benefits, and recommendations of resistance training for youth, older adults, pregnant women, and people considered to be at elevated cardiovascular or musculoskeletal risk.

Traditionally, **resistance training** was used primarily by adult athletes to enhance sport performance and increase muscle size. Today, resistance training is recognized as a method of enhancing the health and fitness of men and women of all ages and abilities (6, 7, 35, 94). Despite preconceived concerns associated with this type of training, resistance training has become a popular fitness trend in commercial, community, clinical, and corporate health and fitness facilities (91). Current public health guidelines aim to increase participation in muscle-strengthening activities to improve overall health and fitness (92).

Like aerobic training, regular resistance training provides a variety of health and fitness benefits that may enhance quality of life while reducing the risk of several chronic diseases (see table 13.1). Resistance training is recommended by national health organizations such as the AHA and ACSM and is performed by everyone from children to older adults, pregnant women, and patients with

chronic disease (6, 94). For fitness professionals, the ability to design safe and effective resistance training programs for people of all ages, fitness levels, and health conditions is a valuable asset. This chapter focuses on principles of resistance training that can be used in designing exercise programs for enhancing muscular fitness in untrained and trained people. Advanced resistance training programs for developing speed, strength, and power for elite athletes are available elsewhere (7, 17, 67, 73, 88).

In this chapter, the term *resistance training* refers to a method of conditioning designed to increase a person's ability to exert or resist force. This term encompasses a wide range of resistive loads (from light manual resistance to plyometric jumps) and a variety of training modalities, including free weights (barbells and dumbbells), weight machines, elastic tubing, medicine balls, stability balls, and body weight. Resistance training should be distinguished from the competitive sports of **weightlifting**, **powerlifting**, and **bodybuilding**. Weightlifting and powerlifting are

TABLE 13.1 Effects of Aerobic Endurance Training and Resistance Training on Health and Fitness Variables

Variable	Aerobic exercise	Resistance exercise
BMD	↑↑	↑↑
Body composition		
%BF	↓↓	↓
LBM	↔	↑↑
Strength	↔	↑↑↑
Glucose metabolism		
Insulin response to glucose challenge	↓↓	↓↓
Basal insulin levels	↓	↓
Insulin sensitivity	↑↑	↑↑
Serum lipids		
HDL-C	↑↔	↑↑↔
LDL-C	↓↔	↓↔
Resting HR	↓↓	↔
SV, resting and maximal	↑↑	↔
BP at rest		
Systolic	↓↔	↔
Diastolic	↓↔	↓↔
$\dot{V}O_2$max	↑↑↑	↑↑↔
Submaximal and maximal endurance time	↑↑↑	↑↑
Basal metabolism	↑	↑↑

↑ = values increase; ↓ = values decrease; ↔ = values remain unchanged; single arrow = small effect; double arrows = medium effect; triple arrows = large effect; %BF = percent body fat; LBM = lean body mass; HDL-C = high-density lipoprotein cholesterol; LDL-C = low-density lipoprotein cholesterol; HR = heart rate; SV = stroke volume; BP = blood pressure.

Adapted, by permission, from M.L. Pollock et al., 2000, "Resistance exercise in individuals with and without cardiovascular disease," *Circulation* 101: 828-833.

sports in which athletes attempt to lift maximal amounts of weight, and bodybuilding is a sport in which the goal is muscle size and symmetry.

Muscular endurance refers to the ability of a muscle or muscle group to perform repeated contractions against a submaximal resistance. **Strength** is defined as the maximal force that a muscle or muscle group can generate at a specified velocity, and **power** refers to the rate of performing work and is the product of strength and speed of movement. *Muscular fitness* is a general term that includes muscular endurance, strength, and power and is related to promoting and maintaining good health and fitness. For ease of discussion, the terms *children* and *youth* are broadly defined in this chapter to include the preadolescent and adolescent years, and the terms *older* and *senior* have been defined to include adults aged 65 and older.

Principles of Training

A key factor in any resistance training program is appropriate program design. Since the act of resistance training itself does not ensure gains in muscular performance, the resistance training program needs to be based on sound training principles and must be carefully prescribed in order to maximize training outcomes. Although factors such as initial fitness level, heredity, nutritional status (e.g., diet composition and hydration), health habits (e.g., sleep), and motivation influence the rate and magnitude of the adaptation that occurs, there are four principles that determine the effectiveness of all resistance training programs: progression, regularity, overload, and specificity. These principles of resistance training can be remembered as the PROS.

Principle of Progression

According to the principle of progression, the demands placed on the body must continually and progressively increase over time in order to result in long-term fitness gains. Although it is impossible to improve at the same rate over long-term periods, the systematic manipulation of program variables over time can limit training plateaus and optimize training adaptations (5). This does not mean that heavier weights should be used in every workout, but rather that over time exercise sessions should become more challenging in order to create a more effective exercise stimulus. Without a more challenging stimulus that is consistent with individual needs, goals, and abilities, the human body has no reason to adapt any further. This principle is particularly important after the first 2 or 3 mo of resistance training, when the threshold for training-induced adaptations in conditioned people is higher (5).

The training stimulus should increase at a rate that is compatible with the training-induced adaptations. Beginners can progress relatively fast whereas slower rates of improvement are appropriate for people with experience in resistance training. A reasonable guideline for a beginner is to increase the training weight about 5% to 10% and decrease the **repetitions** (the number of times a movement is completed) by 2 to 4 once a given load can be performed for the desired number of repetitions with proper exercise technique. For example, if an adult female can easily perform 12 repetitions of the chest press using 100 lb (45 kg), she should increase the weight to 110 lb (50 kg) and decrease the repetitions to 8 if she wants to continue to gain muscular strength. Alternatively, she could increase the number of **sets** (groups of repetitions), increase the number of repetitions, or add another chest exercise (e.g., dumbbell fly) to her routine. The decision on how this person will progress should be based on her training experience and personal goals.

Principle of Regularity

In order to make continual gains in muscular fitness, resistance training must be performed regularly several times per week. Inconsistent training will result in only modest training adaptations, and prolonged inactivity will result in a loss of muscular strength and size. The adage, "Use it or lose it," is appropriate for exercise programming because training-induced adaptations cannot be stored. Although adequate recovery is needed between training sessions, the principle of regularity states that long-term gains in muscle strength and performance will be realized only if the program is performed on a regular basis.

Principle of Overload

For more than a century, the **overload** principle has been a tenet of resistance training. The overload principle states that to enhance muscular performance, the body must exercise at a level beyond that at which it is normally stressed. For example, an adult male who can easily complete 10 repetitions with 20 lb (9 kg) while performing a barbell curl must increase the weight, the repetitions, or the number of sets if he wants to increase his arm strength. If the training stimulus is not increased beyond the level to which the muscles are accustomed, training adaptations will not occur. Overload is typically manipulated by changing the exercise intensity, total repetitions, repetition speed, rest periods, type of exercise, and training volume (5). This process is often referred to as *progressive overload* and is the basis for maximizing long-term training adaptations.

Principle of Specificity

The principle of **specificity** refers to the adaptations that take place as a result of a training program. The adaptations to resistance training are specific to the muscle actions, velocity of movement, exercise ROM, muscle groups, energy systems, and intensity and volume involved in training (5, 51). Specificity is often referred to as the *SAID principle*, which stands for **s**pecific **a**daptations to **i**mposed **d**emands. In essence, every muscle or muscle group must be trained to make gains in strength and local muscular endurance. For instance, exercises such as the squat and leg press can enhance lower-body strength, but they will not affect upper-body strength.

KEY POINT

Gains in strength and muscular endurance will occur only if the overload is greater than that to which the muscle or muscle group is normally accustomed. To make continual gains, training must progress gradually and be performed regularly. The program design will influence the training-induced adaptations that occur. The most beneficial resistance training programs are designed to meet individual needs, goals, and abilities.

The adaptations that take place in a muscle or muscle group will be as simple or as complex as the stress placed on them. For example, because basketball requires multijoint and multiplanar movements (i.e., in the frontal, sagittal, and transverse planes), basketball players should perform complex exercises that closely mimic the movements and energy demands of their sport. The specificity principle also can be applied to designing resistance training programs for people who want to enhance their ability to perform ADLs such as stair-climbing and house cleaning, which also require multijoint and multiplanar movements. The most effective resistance training programs target specific muscle groups and energy systems.

Program Design Considerations

As with exercise programs that enhance CRF, resistance training programs should be based on the participant's interests, current fitness level, health needs, clinical status, and personal goals as well as on the principles of resistance training. By assessing the individual needs of each participant and applying principles of training to the program design, safe and effective resistance training programs can be developed for each person. However, because the magnitude of adaptation to a given exercise stimulus varies from person to person, fitness professionals must be aware of interindividual differences and be prepared to alter the program to reduce the risk of injury and to optimize gains.

Health Status

The health status of each person should be assessed before the resistance training begins. As discussed in chapter 2, each participant should complete a health and medical questionnaire, and the fitness professional should review it to make decisions about further medical evaluation. Additional questions on the HSQ regarding past resistance training experiences, previous musculoskeletal injuries, presence of known cardiovascular conditions, and personal goals can also help with designing the resistance training program.

Fitness Level

An important factor to consider when designing resistance training programs is the participant's previous experience with resistance training, or training age. Those who are the least experienced in resistance training tend to have a greater capacity for improvement compared with those who have been resistance training for several years. Although any reasonable program can increase the strength of untrained people, more comprehensive programs are often needed to produce desirable adaptations in trained people. For example, a 32-yr-old person with 5 yr of resistance training experience (i.e., a training age of 5 yr) may not achieve the same strength gains in a given time as a 25-yr-old person who has no experience with resistance training (i.e., a training age of 0 yr). The potential for adaptation gradually decreases as training age increases. Thus, as people gain experience with resistance training, they need more advanced programs so that they may continue to gain muscular strength (5, 34).

Training Goals

After the preexercise screening, participants should establish realistic short- and long-term goals. The results of a muscular fitness evaluation (see chapter 9) along with the participant's interests can be used to help set realistic and measurable goals. To improve compliance, these goals ideally are set by the participant with guidance from a knowledgeable fitness professional. Typical goals are to increase muscle strength and decrease body fat. An effort to establish realistic goals and increase confidence to achieve those goals is important because it may help people avoid unrealistic expectations that ultimately can lead to discouragement and poor adherence. Testing fitness periodically and reviewing individualized workout logs can help the fitness professional assess training progress and modify the program. Understanding that resistance training programs designed to improve health and fitness are quite different from training programs designed to enhance sport performance will further promote the development of and adherence to programs suited to a participant's needs.

Types of Resistance Training

Several types of resistance training can be used to enhance muscular strength and muscular endurance. Although each method has advantages and disadvantages, there are several factors to consider when selecting one type of training over another or including multiple types of training within a given program. The most common types of resistance training include isometrics, dynamic constant external resistance training, variable resistance training, isokinetics, and plyometrics.

Isometrics

Isometric training, or static resistance training, refers to muscle actions in which muscle length does not change. This type of training is usually performed against an immovable object such as a wall or a weight machine loaded with a heavy weight. The concept of isometric training was popularized in the 1950s when Hettinger and Muller reported remarkable gains in muscle strength resulting from one daily 6 sec isometric contraction at two-thirds of maximal force (42). Although subsequent studies also reported gains in strength resulting from isometric training, the reported gains were substantially less than those reported earlier (35).

An advantage of isometric training is that specialized equipment is not required and the cost is minimal. Increases in strength and muscle **hypertrophy** (an increase in size or mass) can occur from this type of training; however, a major limitation is that the strength gains are specific to the joint angle at which the training occurred. For example, if isometric training of the elbow flexors is performed at a joint angle of 90°, muscle strength will increase at this joint angle but not necessarily at other angles. Even though there seems to be about 20° of carryover on either side of the joint angle, the same isometric exercise must be performed at varying joint angles in order to increase strength throughout the full ROM. Isometric training may help to maintain muscle strength and prevent muscle **atrophy** (a decrease in size or mass) when a limb is immobilized in a cast, but gains in functional strength (e.g., stair-climbing) and motor performance (e.g., sprinting and jumping) as a result of isometric training are unlikely to occur if isometric training takes place only at one joint angle.

Factors such as the number of repetitions performed, duration of contractions, intensity of contractions, and frequency of training can influence the strength gains resulting from isometric training. In general, isometric training characterized by maximal voluntary muscle actions performed for 3 to 5 sec for 15 to 20 repetitions at least 3 times · wk^{-1} tends to optimize strength gains (35). Because of the nature of isometric training, it is particularly important to avoid the breath-holding Valsalva maneuver, which reduces venous return to the heart and increases SBP and DBP. During all types of resistance training, regular breathing patterns (i.e., exhalation while lifting and inhalation while lowering) should be encouraged.

Dynamic Constant External Resistance (DCER) Training

Resistance training that involves a lifting and lowering phase is called *dynamic*. Exercises using free weights (e.g., barbells and dumbbells) and weight machines are dynamic because the weight is lifted and lowered through a predetermined ROM. Although the term *isotonic* traditionally was used to describe this type of training, it literally means "constant *(iso)* tension *(tonic)*." Because tension exerted by a muscle as it shortens varies with the mechanical advantage of the joint and the length of the muscle fibers at a particular joint angle, the term *isotonic* does not accurately describe this training method. As shown in figure 13.1, during a barbell curl, the elbow flexors are strongest at approximately 100° and weakest at 60° (elbows fully flexed) and at 180° (elbows fully extended). The same principle applies to other muscle groups. DCER better describes resistance training in which the weight does not

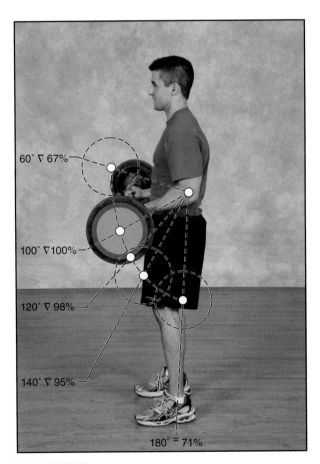

FIGURE 13.1 Variation in strength relative to the angle of the elbow flexors during the biceps curl.

change during the lifting, or **concentric**, and lowering, or **eccentric**, phase of an exercise.

DCER training is the most common method of resistance training for enhancing health and fitness. Endless combinations of sets and repetitions and a variety of training equipment can be used for DCER training. Although there is not enough scientific evidence to make any specific recommendations regarding the most effective speed for DCER training (e.g., 4 sec or 14 sec per repetition), it is likely that the performance of various training speeds within a program may provide the most effective training stimulus. Weight machines generally limit the user to fixed planes of motion. However, they are easy to use and are ideal for isolating muscle groups. Free weights are less expensive and can be used for a wide variety of exercises that require greater proprioception, balance, and coordination. Several free-weight exercises (e.g., barbell squat and bench press) require the use of a spotter who can assist the lifter in case of a failed repetition. In addition to improving health and fitness, DCER training is also used to enhance motor performance skills and sport performance.

During DCER training, the weight lifted does not change throughout the ROM. Because muscle tension can vary significantly during a DCER exercise, the heaviest weight that can be lifted throughout a full ROM is limited by the strength of a muscle at the weakest joint angle. As a result, DCER exercise provides enough resistance in some parts of the movement range but not enough resistance in others. For example, during the barbell bench press, more weight can be lifted during the last part of the exercise than in the first part of the movement when the barbell is being pressed off the chest. This is a limitation of DCER training that should be recognized when choosing starting weights for beginners.

In an attempt to overcome this limitation, mechanical devices that operate through a lever arm or cam have been designed to vary the resistance throughout the ROM of an exercise (see figure 13.2). These devices, called *variable resistance machines*, theoretically force the muscle to contract maximally throughout the ROM by varying the resistance to match the exercise strength curve. These machines can be used to train all the major muscle groups, and by automatically changing the resistive force throughout the movement range, they provide proportionally less resistance in weaker segments of the movement and more resistance in stronger segments of the movement. As with all weight machines, variable resistance machines provide a specific movement path. This makes the exercise easier to perform compared with free-weight exercises, which require balance, coordination, and the involvement of stabilizing muscle groups. These features make variable resistance machines a popular mode of resistance training for people who desire safe and simple exercise sessions.

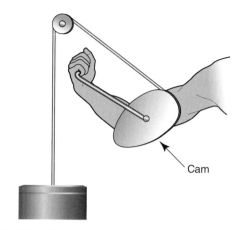

FIGURE 13.2 Variable resistance device for the biceps muscle in which a cam alters the resistance throughout the ROM.

Adapted, by permission, from D. Wathen and F. Roll, 1994, Training methods and modes. In *Essentials of strength training and conditioning*, by National Strength and Conditioning Association, edited by T.R. Baechle (Champaign, IL: Human Kinetics), 408.

Isokinetics

The term *isokinetics* refers to muscular actions performed at a constant angular limb velocity. Isokinetic training involves specialized and expensive equipment, and most isokinetic devices are designed to train only single-joint movements. Isokinetic machines generally are not used in fitness centers, but they are used by physical therapists and athletic trainers for injury rehabilitation. Unlike other types of resistance training, in isokinetics, the speed of movement rather than the resistance is controlled. During isokinetic training, any force applied to the isokinetic machine is met with an equal reaction force. Although it is theoretically possible for a muscle to contract maximally through the full ROM of an exercise, this seems unlikely during isokinetic training because of the acceleration at the beginning and deceleration at the end of the ROM.

Isokinetic training studies have generally found that strength gains are specific to the training velocity (18). Isokinetic training at a slow movement velocity (e.g., $60°\cdot\text{sec}^{-1}$) will increase strength at that velocity, but strength gains at faster velocities are unlikely to occur. If the purpose of the training program is to increase strength at higher velocities (e.g., for enhanced sport performance), high-speed isokinetic training appears prudent. Although further research is warranted, the best approach may be to perform isokinetic training at slow, intermediate, and fast velocities to develop strength and power at a variety of movement speeds.

Plyometrics

Plyometric training, first known simply as *jump training*, refers to a specialized method of conditioning designed to enable a muscle to reach maximal force in the shortest possible time (20). Unlike an exercise such as the bench press, plyometric training is characterized by quick, powerful movements that involve rapid stretching of a muscle (eccentric muscle action) immediately followed by rapid shortening (concentric muscle action). This type of muscle action, sometimes called *stretch–shortening cycle exercise*, provides a physiological advantage because the muscle force generated during the concentric muscle action is potentiated by the preceding eccentric muscle action (71). Although both muscle actions are important, the amount of time it takes to change direction from the eccentric to the concentric muscle action is a critical factor in plyometric training. This amount of time is the **amortization phase** and should be as short as possible (<0.1 sec) in order to maximize training adaptations. Both mechanical factors (i.e., increased stored elastic energy) and neurophysiological factors (i.e., change in the force–velocity relationship of the muscle) contribute to the increased force production resulting from plyometric training (71).

Exercises that involve explosive jumping, skipping, hopping, and throwing can be considered plyometric. Although plyometric exercises often are associated with high-intensity drills such as depth jumps (i.e., jumping from a box to the ground and then immediately jumping upward), common activities such as jumping jacks and hopscotch are also plyometric exercises because every time the feet hit the ground, the quadriceps go through a stretch–shortening cycle. Strength and power athletes in sports such as American football, volleyball, and track and field regularly perform plyometric exercises as part of their conditioning program. More recently, this type of training has become popular in group exercise classes and fitness programs.

Since plyometric exercises can greatly stress muscles, connective tissues, and joints, they need to be carefully prescribed to reduce the likelihood of musculoskeletal injury. In some cases, the risks of performing plyometric exercises may outweigh the potential benefits for untrained or overweight people who may lack the strength and coordination to perform the exercises properly. In other cases, plyometrics may be a worthwhile addition to the exercise program of a trained individual who wants to join a recreational basketball league. Clearly, the prescription of plyometric exercises needs to be individualized and based on a person's health history, training experience, and personal goals. It seems prudent to restrict plyometric training to people who have developed a foundation of muscle strength by first participating in a general resistance training program.

It is also reasonable to begin plyometric training with lower-intensity drills and gradually progress to higher-intensity drills as technique and performance improve. In one case report, a 12-yr-old boy developed exertional rhabdomyolysis after he was instructed to perform excessive repetitive squat jumps (>250) in a physical education class (22). Exertional rhabdomyolysis is a serious medical condition that can result in severe muscle soreness and renal failure. Clearly, there is the potential for injury or illness to occur if the intensity, volume, or frequency of resistance training exceed the ability of the participant.

Other considerations for plyometric training include proper footwear, adequate space, shock-absorbing landing surfaces (e.g., suspended floor or grass playing field), and training frequency (20). Although research has yet to determine the minimal training threshold for maximizing training adaptations from plyometric exercise, it is always better to undertrain than overtrain and risk an injury. It seems reasonable to begin plyometric training with 1 to 3 sets of 6 to 10 repetitions of several low-intensity exercises for the upper and lower body twice a week on nonconsecutive days. Fitness professionals who have experience with plyometric training should provide demonstrations and coaching cues in order to enhance learning, improve technique, and reduce the likelihood of injury. Additional training guidelines and examples of plyometric drills are available elsewhere (20, 70).

KEY POINT

Various types of resistance training can increase muscular strength, muscular endurance, and power. The effects of isometric training are generally limited to the joint angle at which the training occurs. DCER training refers to exercises performed throughout a ROM with free weights and weight machines. Isokinetic training occurs at a constant limb velocity with maximal force exerted throughout the ROM of the joint. Plyometric training exploits the muscle cycle of lengthening and shortening to increase speed of movement and muscle power.

Modes of Resistance Training

Various modes of resistance training can be used to accommodate the needs of young people, adults, and seniors. Provided that the principles of training are adhered to, almost any mode of resistance training can be used to enhance muscular fitness. Some types of equipment are relatively easy to use, while others require balance, coordination, and high levels of skill. The decision to use a certain mode of resistance training should be based on each client's needs, goals, and abilities. The major modes of resistance training are weight machines, free weights (barbells and dumbbells), body-weight exercises, and a broadly defined category of balls, bands, and elastic tubing.

Single-joint exercises such as the biceps curl target a specific muscle group and require less skill. Multijoint exercises such as the bench press involve more than one joint or major muscle group and require more balance and coordination. Although both single-joint and multijoint exercises enhance muscular fitness, multijoint exercises are considered to be more effective for increasing muscle strength because they involve a greater amount of muscle mass and therefore enable a heavier weight to be lifted (5, 51). Multijoint exercises have also been shown to have the greatest acute metabolic and anabolic hormonal (e.g., testosterone and growth hormone) response, which could favorably influence resistance training that targets improvements in muscle size and body composition (52). Table 13.2 summarizes the advantages and disadvantages of weight machines, free weights (barbells and dumbbells), body-weight exercises, and balls, bands, and elastic tubing.

Weight machines are designed to train all the major muscle groups and can be found in most fitness centers. Both single-joint (e.g., leg extension) and multijoint (e.g., leg press) exercises can be performed on weight machines, which are relatively easy to use because the exercise motion is controlled by the machine and typically occurs in only one anatomical plane. This may be particularly important when designing resistance training programs for sedentary or inexperienced participants. Also, several weight-machine exercises such as the lat pull-down and leg curl are difficult to mimic with free weights. Weight machines are designed to fit the average male or female, so smaller people may not be able to properly position themselves on the equipment. A seat pad or back pad can be used to adjust body position to allow for a better fit. Some companies now manufacture weight machines specifically for children. These machines are smaller versions of adult-sized machines and have weight increments that are appropriate for younger populations.

Free weights are also popular in fitness centers and come in a variety of shapes and sizes. Although it may take longer to master proper exercise technique when using free weights compared with weight machines, free weights have several advantages. For example, proper fit is not an issue with adjustable barbells and dumbbells because one size fits all. Free weights also offer a greater variety of exercises than weight machines because they can be moved in many directions. Another benefit of free weights is that they require the use of stabilizing and assisting muscles to hold the correct body position during an exercise. As such, free-weight training can occur in different planes. This is particularly true with dumbbells because they train each side of the body independently.

In general, free weights allow the participant to train functionally by encouraging different muscle groups to work together while performing exercises that are similar to the participant's chosen sport or activity. However, unlike weight machines, several free-weight exercises require the aid of a spotter who can assist the lifter in case of a failed repetition. Using a spotter is particularly important when performing the bench press. In an epidemiological evaluation of injuries related to resistance training, a large number of injuries occurred with free weights and the most common mechanism of injury was weights dropping on the person (49). Accidents such as these underscore the importance of close supervision and an appropriate progression of training loads when training with free weights.

Body-weight exercises such as push-ups, pull-ups, and curl-ups are some of the oldest modes of resistance training. An example of using body weight as a form of resistance is Pilates exercise and to some extent certain forms of yoga that particularly target stability and core strength (i.e., abdominal muscles, lower back, hips). Obviously, a major advantage of body-weight training is that equipment is not needed and a variety of exercises can be performed. Conversely, a limitation of body-weight training is the difficulty in adjusting the body weight to the individual's strength level. Sedentary or overweight participants may not be strong enough to perform even one push-up or pull-up. In such cases, body-weight exercises not only may be ineffective, they may have a negative effect on program compliance. Exercise machines that allow people to perform body-weight exercises such as pull-ups and dips by using a predetermined percentage of their body weight are available. These machines provide an opportunity for

TABLE 13.2 Comparison of Modes of Resistance Training

	Weight machines	Free weights	Body weight	Balls and cords[a]
Cost	High	Low	None	Very low
Portability	Limited	Variable	Excellent	Excellent
Ease of use	Excellent	Variable	Variable	Variable
Muscle isolation	Excellent	Variable	Variable	Variable
Functionality	Limited	Excellent	Excellent	Excellent
Exercise variety	Limited	Excellent	Excellent	Excellent
Space requirements	High	Variable	Low	Low

[a]Medicine balls, stability balls, and elastic cords.

participants of all abilities to incorporate body-weight exercises into their resistance training program.

Stability balls, medicine balls, and elastic tubing are safe and effective alternatives to weight machines and free weights. Medicine balls first became popular in the 1950s, and stability balls and elastic tubing have been used by therapists for many years. Now fitness professionals are using balls and bands for resistance training and conditioning. Not only are stability balls, medicine balls, and elastic tubing relatively inexpensive, they can also be used to enhance strength, muscular endurance, and power. In addition, exercises performed with balls and tubing can challenge proprioception, which carries added benefits, including gains in agility, balance, and coordination.

Stability balls are lightweight, inflatable balls about 45 to 75 cm in diameter that add the elements of balance and coordination to any exercise while targeting selected muscle groups. Although many exercises can be performed

with stability balls, they are often used to develop core (i.e., abdominal, hip, and low-back) strength and improve posture. When participants sit on a stability ball, their feet should be at a 90° angle. The firmer the ball, the more difficult the exercise will be. Since proper body alignment is crucial when performing an exercise on a stability ball, fitness professionals should know how to perform each exercise correctly and when to modify an exercise to meet individual needs and abilities. Many types of exercise programs using stability balls can be created to enhance strength, muscular endurance, and flexibility (40, 60). Figure 13.3 illustrates the performance of abdominal curls on a stability ball.

Medicine balls come in a variety of shapes and sizes (about 1 kg to more than 10 kg) and are a safe and effective alternative to free weights and weight machines. In addition to performing squats or chest presses with a medicine ball, participants can use the ball in throwing drills—such

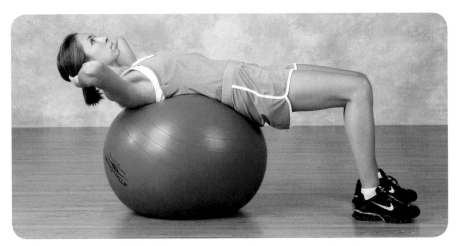

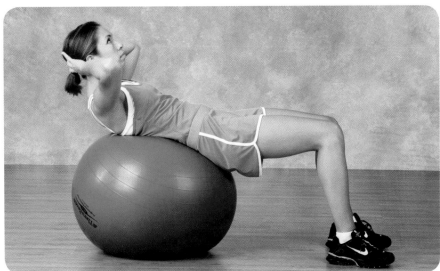

FIGURE 13.3 Abdominal curl on a stability ball.

as throwing from participant to instructor or against the wall—to enhance upper-body explosive power. High-speed training with medicine balls adds a new dimension to resistance training that can benefit men and women of all ages. Further, since medicine balls typically require the body to function as a unit instead of as separate parts, they are particularly effective for mimicking natural body positions and movement speeds that occur in daily life and game situations. Progressive medicine-ball training that can be used in one-on-one settings or group fitness classes is available (40, 60). Figure 13.4 illustrates the medicine-ball squat.

Resistance training with an elastic band involves performing an exercise against the force required to stretch the band and then return it to its unstretched state. A variety of exercises can be performed by holding the ends of the cord with both hands or attaching one end of the cord to a fixed object. For safety reasons, fitness professionals should ensure that the cord is secured under both feet or to a fixed object before performing any exercise. Incorporating exercises with stability balls, medicine balls, and elastic tubing into a workout session can be challenging, motivating, beneficial, and fun. Figure 13.5 illustrates a chest press with an elastic band.

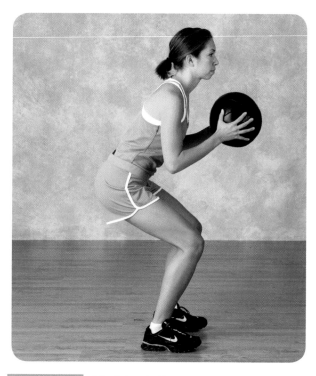

FIGURE 13.4 Medicine-ball squat.

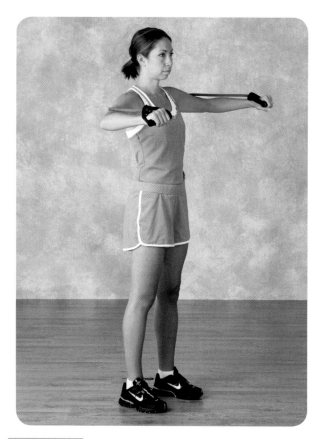

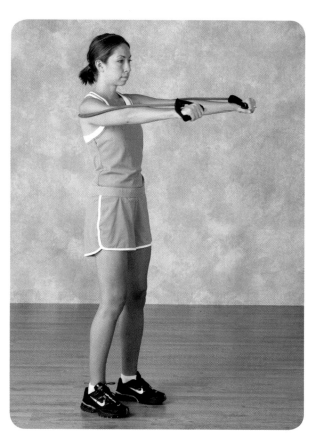

FIGURE 13.5 Chest press with elastic band.

KEY POINT

Weight machines, free weights, body-weight exercises, medicine balls, stability balls, and elastic bands can be used to enhance muscular fitness. When designing resistance training programs, fitness professionals should evaluate the advantages and disadvantages of each training mode to meet individual needs, goals, and abilities.

Safety Issues

Resistance training programs should be designed by fitness professionals who are knowledgeable about safe and effective training methods. Although all resistance training activities have some degree of medical risk, the chance of injury can be reduced by following established training guidelines and safety procedures. Without proper supervision and instruction, injuries that require medical attention may occur. An evaluation of resistance-training-related injuries presenting to U.S. emergency rooms revealed that 27% of all reported injuries in adults were considered accidental (e.g., dropped weights, improper use of equipment, tripping over equipment) and could have been prevented with strict adherence to safety guidelines (65). The mechanism of injury in the aforementioned study was considered nonaccidental if it resulted from exertion (sprain or strain), overuse, or equipment malfunction (65). Further, these researchers reported that men suffered more trunk injuries than women, whereas women had more foot and leg injuries than men (72), Figure 13.6 illustrates the percentage of resistance-training-related injuries at each body part for men and women who presented to U.S. emergency rooms (72). Clearly, people who resistance train should receive instruction on appropriate training guidelines and equipment use. General safety recommendations for designing and instructing resistance training programs are given next.

Supervision and Instruction

People who want to participate in resistance training should first receive guidance and instruction from qualified fitness professionals who understand principles of resistance training and appreciate individual differences. Fitness professionals should be able to correctly perform the exercises they prescribe and should be able to modify exercise form and technique if necessary. They should know which exercises require spotters and should be prepared to offer assistance in case of a failed repetition. When working in a health or fitness facility, the staff should be attentive and should try to position themselves with a clear view of the training center so that they can quickly access people who need assistance. In addition, the fitness staff is responsible for enforcing safety rules

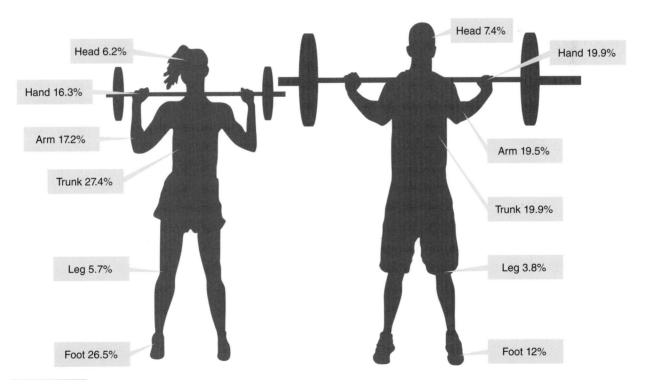

FIGURE 13.6 Percentage of injuries at each body location for men and women.

Reprinted, by permission, from C. Quatman, 2009, "Sex differences in "weightlifting" injuries presenting to United States emergency rooms" *Journal of Strength and Conditioning Research* 23: 2061-2067. Journal of strength and conditioning research by National Strength & Conditioning Association (U.S.) Reproduced with permission of LIPPINCOTT WILLIAMS & WILKINS INC in the format Journal via Copyright Clearance Center.

Safety Recommendations for Resistance Training

- Review participants' HSQs before they begin resistance training.
- Provide adequate supervision and instruction when necessary.
- Regularly practice emergency procedures.
- Encourage participation in warm-up and cool-down activities.
- Move carefully around the resistance training area, and don't back up without looking first.
- Fix broken or malfunctioning equipment immediately or put an out-of-order sign on it.
- Use collars on all plate-loaded barbells and dumbbells.
- Be aware of proper spotting procedures and offer assistance when needed.
- Model appropriate behavior and do not allow horseplay in the fitness center.
- Demonstrate correct exercise technique and do not allow participants to train improperly.
- Periodically check all resistance training equipment.
- Ensure the training environment is free of clutter and appropriately maintained.
- Stay up to date with current resistance training guidelines and safety procedures for special populations.

(e.g., wear proper footwear, store weights safely, no foolish play in the fitness center) and safe training procedures (e.g., emphasizing proper exercise technique rather than the amount of weight lifted). Not only can fitness professionals enhance the safety of resistance training, but they can help clients maximize strength gains (58) when they develop and supervise personalized programs.

Training Environment

If exercise is to take place in a public, community, worksite, or school-based fitness center, the training area should be well lit and large enough to handle the number of people exercising in the facility at any given time. The facility should be clean and the equipment should be well maintained. Equipment pads that come in contact with the skin should be cleaned daily, and cables, guide rods, and chains on machines should be checked weekly. Equipment should be spaced to allow easy access to each resistance training exercise, and equipment such as free weights and collars should be returned to the proper storage area after each use. Recommended temperature (68-72 °F, or 20.0-22.2 °C), humidity (60% or less), and air circulation (at least 8 air exchanges every hr) should be maintained in the resistance training area (3). Additional recommendations for fitness facility maintenance and risk management are available elsewhere (3).

Warm-Up and Cool-Down

Resistance training should be preceded by warm-up activities. A general warm-up increases body and muscle temperature, increases blood flow, and may enhance performance (6). This type of warm-up typically includes 5 to 10 min of moderate- to high-intensity aerobic exercise such as slow jogging or stationary cycling. More recently, dynamic warm-up protocols that include moderate- to high-intensity hops, skips, and jumps and various movement-based exercises for the upper and lower body have proven to be effective (89, 97). Although a general warm-up can elevate muscle temperature, a well-designed dynamic warm-up can also enhance motor unit excitability, improve kinesthetic awareness, and increase strength and power (16, 36). Although the exact mechanisms that explain how a dynamic warm-up might improve muscle performance are unclear, most factors seem to be related to a neuromuscular phenomenon known as *postactivation potentiation*, or PAP (78). In this phenomenon, muscular performance is acutely enhanced as a result of prior activity performed at a relatively high intensity.

A specific warm-up involves movements that are similar to the resistance training exercises that are about to be performed. For example, after a general or dynamic warm-up, a lifter could perform a light set of 10 repetitions on

KEY POINT

Qualified supervision and instruction, a safe training environment, and adherence to established training guidelines will help minimize the risk of injury during resistance training. Fitness professionals should educate participants about safe training procedures and design programs that are consistent with each person's needs and abilities. Warm-up and cool-down activities can enhance performance and reduce the likelihood of muscle soreness and injury.

the bench press before performing the training set with a heavier weight. It makes sense to physically and mentally prepare for the demands of resistance training by spending a few minutes warming up. After a resistance workout, it's a good idea to cool down with general calisthenics and static stretching exercises. A cool-down can help relax the body and possibly reduce muscle stiffness and soreness.

Resistance Training Guidelines

Guidelines for resistance training are not as universally accepted as recommendations for enhancing aerobic fitness. Although sports medicine organizations recognize the importance of resistance training for health and fitness, there has been considerable debate regarding training volume (i.e., sets · repetitions · weight lifted). In particular, the efficacy of performing either single or multiple sets has captured the interest of some exercise scientists (35, 53, 76). Yet, despite various claims about the best training approach, there does not appear to be one optimal combination of sets, repetitions, and exercises that promotes long-term adaptations in muscular fitness for all people. Rather, many program variables may be altered to achieve desirable outcomes provided that the tenets of resistance exercise are followed. Clearly, resistance training programs need to be individualized and based on a person's training history and personal goals.

There are many factors to consider when designing a resistance training program, including the following (35):

1. Choice of exercise
2. Order of exercise
3. Resistance used
4. Training volume (total number of sets and repetitions)
5. Rest intervals between sets and exercises
6. Repetition velocity
7. Training frequency

By varying one or more of these variables, endless resistance training programs can be designed. But since different people will respond differently to the same resistance training program, decisions must be based on an understanding of exercise science, individual needs, and personal goals. The ACSM's resistance training guidelines for apparently healthy adults are summarized in the sidebar Summary of the ACSM's Resistance Training Guidelines for Healthy Adults.

Choice of Exercise

A limitless number of exercises can be used to enhance muscular strength, power, and local muscular endurance (90). Selected exercises should be appropriate for a participant's exercise experience and training goals. Also, the choice of exercises should promote muscle balance across joints and between opposing muscle groups (e.g., quadriceps and hamstrings). Selected weight-machine and free-weight exercises and the primary muscle groups strengthened are listed in table 13.3.

Exercises generally can be classified as single joint (i.e., body-part specific) or multijoint (i.e., structural). Dumbbell biceps curls and leg extensions are examples of single-joint exercises that isolate a specific body part (biceps and quadriceps, respectively), whereas squats and deadlifts are multijoint exercises that involve two or more primary joints. Exercises also can be classified as

Summary of the ACSM's Resistance Training Guidelines for Healthy Adults

- Perform 8 to 10 multijoint or compound exercises that involve more than one muscle group.
- Train each muscle group for 2 to 4 sets.
- Choose a resistance that allows 8 to 12 repetitions to be performed each set.
- Perform each repetition in a deliberate, controlled manner through the full ROM.
- Perform each exercise with proper technique and include both concentric and eccentric phases of the repetition.
- Maintain a regular breathing pattern that typically involves exhaling during the lifting phase and inhaling during the lowering phase.
- Train each major muscle group 2 or 3 nonconsecutive days · wk^{-1}.
- Periodically assess muscular strength so that a proper resistance is selected for each set.
- Progressively overload the muscles to create a greater training stimulus if continued gains in muscular fitness and mass are desired.

Adapted from American College of Sports Medicine 2010.

TABLE 13.3   Selected Weight-Machine and Free-Weight Exercises and the Primary Muscle Groups Strengthened

Weight-machine exercise	Free-weight exercise	Primary muscle groups strengthened
Leg press	Barbell squat	Quadriceps, gluteus maximus
Leg extension	Dumbbell lunge	Quadriceps
Leg curl	Barbell standing hip extension	Hamstrings
Chest press	Barbell bench press	Pectoralis major
Pec deck	Dumbbell fly	Pectoralis major
Front pull-down	Dumbbell pullover	Latissimus dorsi
Seated rows	Dumbbell one-arm row	Latissimus dorsi
Overhead press	Dumbbell press	Deltoids
Biceps curl	Barbell curl	Biceps
Triceps extension	Lying triceps extension	Triceps

A description of the proper exercise technique for each exercise is available elsewhere (7, 92).

closed kinetic chain or open kinetic chain. Closed-chain exercises are those in which the distal joint segment is stationary (e.g., squats), whereas open-chain exercises are those in which the terminal joint is free to move (e.g., leg extensions). Closed-chain exercises more closely mimic everyday activities and include more functional movement patterns (24).

Single-joint exercises and many machine exercises are often used by people who have limited experience resistance training or who simply enjoy this mode of training. This mode is also beneficial in activating specific muscles (e.g., during injury rehabilitation). With most machines, the path of movement is fixed and therefore the movement is stabilized. Conversely, exercises with free weights require additional muscles to stabilize the movement and are therefore more challenging. Also, dual-limb exercises with free weights (e.g., dumbbell lateral raises) may be particularly beneficial for people who need to strengthen a weaker limb. It is important to eventually incorporate multijoint exercises into a resistance training program to promote the coordinated use of multijoint movements.

Recently, the performance of single- and multijoint exercises on unstable surfaces (e.g., stability balls and wobble boards) has become popular. This type of training has been found to increase the activity of the lower-body musculature and the stabilizer muscles, but the magnitude of agonistic force production is reduced so lighter loads must be used (13). Although there are a multitude of exercises that can be performed under a variety of conditions, when participants learn a new exercise they should start with a light weight so that they can master the technique before adding weight to the bar. Regardless of the exercise type, the concentric and eccentric phases of each lift should be performed in a controlled manner with proper technique.

Another issue concerning choice of exercise is including exercises for abdominal and low-back musculature. It is not uncommon for beginners to focus on strengthening the chest and biceps and not spend enough time strengthening their abdominal muscles and low back. Strengthening the midsection not only may improve force output and enhance body control during free-weight exercises such as the squat, it also may decrease the incidence of low-back pain (44). Thus, prehabilitation exercises for the low-back and abdominal muscles should be included in all resistance training programs. In other words, as a preventive health measure, exercises that may be prescribed for the rehabilitation of an injury should be performed before injury occurs. Exercises such as abdominal curl-ups and back extensions are useful, but they only train the muscles that control trunk flexion and extension. Multidirectional exercises that involve rotational movements and diagonal patterns performed with body weight or a medicine ball on a stable or unstable surface can strengthen the abdominal muscles and lower back. Depending on the needs and goals of the person, other prehabilitation exercises (e.g., internal and external rotation for the rotator cuff) can be incorporated into the exercise session.

Order of Exercise

The order of resistance exercises within a training session may influence the quality of the exercise performance (84). Traditionally, exercises for large muscle groups are performed before exercises for smaller muscle groups, and multijoint exercises are performed before single-joint exercises. Following this order will allow participants to use heavier weights on the multijoint exercises because fatigue will be less of a factor. It is also helpful to perform more challenging exercises earlier in the workout when the neuromuscular system is less fatigued. However, in some cases (e.g., injury prevention or rehabilitation), it may be appropriate to reverse this order so that the smaller muscle groups are trained first. In general, it seems reasonable to follow the priority system of training in which exercises that will most enhance health and fitness are performed

Weekly Resistance Training Log

Name	10/23			10/25			10/27			Comments
	Wt (lb)	Rep	Set	Wt (lb)	Rep	Set	Wt (lb)	Rep	Set	
Leg press	150	10	2	150	11	2	150	12	2	
Leg curl	55	10	2	55	11	2	55	12	2	
Chest press	80	10	2	80	11	2	80	12	2	
Lat pull-down	80	10	2	80	11	2	80	12	2	
Biceps curl	30	10	2		11	2	30	11	2	
Triceps extension	40	10	2		11	2	40	12	2	Slight soreness in triceps
Kneeling trunk extension	No wt	10	2	No wt	11	2	No wt	12	2	
Abdominal curl	No wt	10	2	No wt	11	2	No wt	11	2	

early in the training session. Also, participants should perform power exercises such as plyometrics before strength exercises so that they can train for maximal power without undue fatigue. A sample resistance training program is illustrated in the Weekly Resistance Training Log.

Resistance Used

One of the most important variables in designing a resistance training program is the amount of weight used for an exercise (5, 35, 63). Gains in muscular strength and performance are influenced by the amount of weight lifted, which is highly dependent upon program variables such as exercise order, training volume, repetition velocity, and rest-interval length (51, 52). By definition, the amount of weight that can be lifted with proper technique for only 1 repetition is the 1-repetition maximum (1RM). Similarly, the amount of weight that can be lifted with proper technique for 10 but not 11 repetitions is the 10-repetition maximum (10RM). To maximize gains in muscle strength and performance, it is recommended that training sets be performed to volitional fatigue (i.e., unable to complete a repetition because of temporary fatigue) using the appropriate resistance.

The use of RM loads is a relatively simple method to prescribe resistance training intensity. Research studies suggest that RM loads of 6 or fewer have the greatest effect on developing muscle strength, whereas RM loads of 15 to 25 or more have the greatest effect on developing muscular endurance (19, 35). Although untrained people can make significant gains in muscle strength with lighter loads, it is believed that people with resistance training experience

RESEARCH INSIGHT

It is known that specific types of resistance training result in specific adaptations, but there is little information concerning specific intramuscular adaptations to various set and repetition combinations. Holm and colleagues (46) compared the effects of two 12 wk resistance training protocols in which the same subject trained one leg at 70% 1RM (heavy load) and the other leg at 15.5% 1RM (light load). MRI, 1RM performance measures, and muscle biopsies were measured pre- and posttraining. Heavy load training resulted in greater gains in quadriceps cross-sectional area and 1RM strength. Also, myosin heavy-chain IIx protein expression was decreased following heavy-load training but not light-load training. Although light-load resistance training was sufficient to induce muscle-mass accretion, the responses were inferior to heavy-load resistance training. These data demonstrate that adaptations to resistance training are linked to the intensity of the training program.

need to train with a heavier resistance to optimize training adaptations (5, 76). ACSM recommends a repetition range between 8 and 12 to enhance muscle strength and performance (see figure 13.7) (6). Using weights that exceed a person's 6RM capacity minimally affects muscular endurance, whereas training with very light weights (e.g., above 20RM) results in only small gains in maximal muscle strength. Since each repetition zone (e.g., 3-6, 8-12, 15-25) has advantages, the best approach is to systematically vary the resistance used in order to avoid training plateaus and to optimize training adaptations (17, 34).

A percentage of a person's 1RM also can be used to determine the resistance training intensity. If the 1RM on the chest press is 100 lb (45 kg), a training intensity of 70% would be 70 lb (32 kg). It is reasonable for beginners to use a training resistance of approximately 60% to 70% 1RM because they are mostly improving motor performance at this stage (5). As participants get stronger and gain training experience, heavier resistances (~80% 1RM) will be needed to optimize gains in muscular strength and performance (5, 76). Obviously, this method of prescribing resistance exercise requires testing the 1RM on all exercises in the training program. In many cases this is not realistic because of the time required to correctly perform 1RM testing on 8 to 10 exercises. Furthermore, maximal resistance testing for small-muscle-group exercises (e.g.,

biceps curls and lying triceps extensions) typically is not performed.

Fitness professionals should also be knowledgeable about the relationship between the percentage of 1RM and the number of repetitions that can be performed. In general, most people can perform about 10 reps using 75% of their 1RM. However, the number of repetitions that can be performed at a given percentage of the 1RM varies with the amount of muscle mass required to perform the exercise. For example, studies have shown that at a given percentage of the 1RM (e.g., 60%), adults can perform more repetitions of an exercise for large muscle groups such as the squat or leg press compared with an exercise for smaller muscle groups such as the arm curl or leg curl (45, 81). Therefore, prescribing a resistance training intensity of 70% of 1RM on all exercises warrants additional consideration because at 70% of the 1RM, a person may be able to perform 20 or more reps on a large-muscle-group exercise, which may not be ideal for enhancing muscle strength. If a percentage of the 1RM is used for prescribing resistance training, the prescribed percentage of the 1RM for each exercise may need to vary to maintain a desired training range (e.g., 8RM-10RM). Further, since self-selected intensities tend to be lower than what is recommended (39, 74), fitness professionals need to carefully prescribe the amount of weight used for each exercise to maximize training adaptations.

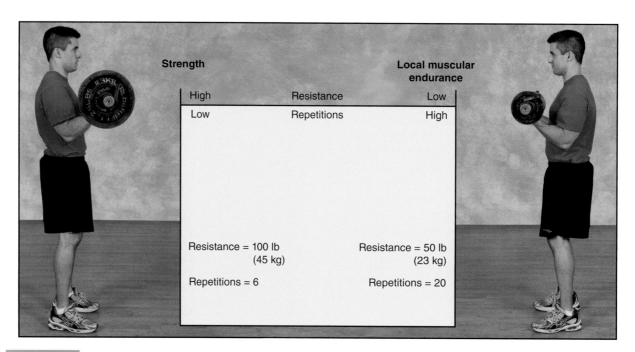

FIGURE 13.7 The strength–endurance continuum. The use of heavy weights and low repetitions has the greatest effect on strength and power, whereas the use of light weights and high repetitions has the greatest effect on local muscular endurance.

Training Volume

The number of exercises performed per session, the repetitions performed per set, and the number of sets performed per exercise all influence the training volume (5). For example, if a participant performs 3 sets of 10 reps with 100 lb (45 kg) on the bench press, the training volume for this exercise is 3,000 lb ($3 \cdot 10 \cdot 100 = 3,000$), or 1,361 kg. Altering the training volume can influence neural, hypertrophic, metabolic, and hormonal responses and adaptations to resistance training (5, 69). Although there has been much debate regarding training volume, it is important to remember that every training session does not need to be characterized by the same number of sets, repetitions, and exercises.

ACSM recommends that apparently healthy adults train each major muscle group with 2 to 4 sets to achieve muscular fitness goals (6). These sets may be for the same exercise or for different exercises affecting the same muscle group. Although training protocols using 1, 2, or 3 sets seem to be equally effective for untrained people during the first 2 to 3 mo of training if the programs are not periodized or varied over time (57, 61), the results of meta-analytical studies have found that multiple-set resistance training protocols are superior to single-set protocols for strength enhancement in untrained and trained populations (53, 76, 77, 96). Additional research is needed to explore the effects of various training volumes on muscular strength and performance; however, no comparative study has found single-set training to be superior to multiple-set training in trained or untrained people.

When fitness professionals design a resistance training program, they need to consider the person's training status and goals because of the numerous possibilities for program design. It seems reasonable for beginners and very deconditioned people to start with a single-set program of 10 to 15 reps of moderate intensity and gradually increase the number of sets depending on personal goals and time available for training. A single-set protocol reduces training time and may therefore increase the likelihood for exercise compliance in people who do not train regularly. However, it is also possible that a multiple-set protocol can be a time-efficient method of training. For example, instead of performing 1 set for each of 12 exercises during every workout, participants can perform 2 sets for each of 6 exercises or 3 sets for each of 4 exercises. With a careful selection of multijoint exercises, all muscle groups can be trained each exercise session regardless of the number of sets or exercises performed.

Nonetheless, it is important to point out that a dramatic increase in training intensity may increase the risk of overtraining. By gradually varying the sets, repetitions, and number of exercises (i.e., training volume), the training stimulus will remain effective and therefore the adaptations to the training program will be maximized. Periods of low-volume or single-set training can provide a needed variation for people who have been participating in a high-volume or multiple-set conditioning program for a prolonged time.

RESEARCH INSIGHT

A quantifiable relationship between program variables and strength improvements has been somewhat controversial. Rhea and colleagues (76) used meta-analytical techniques to combine and evaluate the treatment effects from 140 studies that included strength measures before and after a resistance training intervention. They reported that a training intensity of 60% 1RM elicits maximal strength gains in untrained people, whereas 80% 1RM is most effective in trained people. In addition, they found that 4 sets per muscle group elicited maximal gains in trained and untrained people. Although the importance of gradually increasing the demands placed on the body must not be overlooked, fitness professionals can use this information to make an informed decision regarding the time and effort needed to achieve training goals.

Rests Between Sets and Exercises

The rest interval between sets and exercises is an important but often overlooked training variable. In general, the length of the rest influences energy recovery and the training adaptations that take place. For example, if the primary goal of the program is to maximize gains in muscular strength, heavier weights and longer rests (e.g., 2-3 min) are needed, whereas if the goal is local muscular endurance, lighter weights and shorter rests (e.g., <1 min) are required. Obviously, training intensity, training goals, and fitness level will influence the length of the rest interval. For example, it has been shown that the number of repetitions performed is compromised with short rest intervals (<1 min), whereas performance can be maintained during a multiset protocol when 3 and 5 min rest intervals are used (75). As previously noted for the other program variables, the same rest interval does not need to be used for all exercises. In addition, fatigue resulting from a previous exercise should be considered when prescribing the rest interval. In general, resting 2 to 3 min between sets is recommended for exercises with heavier loads, although for assistance exercises a shorter rest interval of 1 to 2 min may suffice (5). Short rests (<30 sec between sets and exercises) are not recommended for beginners because of the discomfort and high blood lactate concentrations (10-14 mmol $\cdot$ L^{-1}) associated with this type of training (50). However, the rests can be shortened gradually over time to provide ample opportunity for the body to tolerate increased muscle and blood acid levels. For example, circuit training is a type of conditioning that is characterized by relatively short rest intervals between exercise stations.

Repetition Velocity

The velocity or cadence at which a resistance exercise is performed can affect the neural, hypertrophic, and metabolic adaptations to a training program (5). According to the principle of training specificity, gains in muscle strength and performance are specific to the training velocity (35). For example, fast-velocity plyometric training is more likely to enhance speed and power than are slow-velocity exercises on weight machines. However, there are two types of slow-velocity training (50). *Unintentional* slow velocities are used when a heavy resistance is lifted and the velocity is slow despite the attempt to exert maximal force. On the other hand, *intentional* slow velocities are used when a person trains with a submaximal load and purposefully performs the exercise at a slow velocity. Given that concentric force production is lower for an intentionally slower velocity compared with a moderate velocity, it appears that lighter loads performed at a slower velocity may not be optimal for maximizing strength development (48).

Since beginners need to learn how to perform each exercise correctly with a light resistance, it is generally recommended that untrained people perform exercises at a slow to moderate velocity (5). As they gain experience, they may use unintentional slow velocities with a heavier resistance to optimize strength gains. Of interest, it has been found that the intent to maximally accelerate the weight during training is essential for maximizing strength gains in trained people (14). Therefore, depending on training goals and experience, participants can perform a continuum of velocities, from unintentionally slow to fast, in order to maximize performance adaptations (5). It is likely that performing a variety of velocities within a training program provides the most effective stimulus.

Training Frequency

Training frequency typically refers to the number of training sessions per week. In general, a training frequency of 2 to 3 sessions · wk⁻¹ on nonconsecutive days is recommended (5). This training frequency allows for adequate recovery between sessions (48-72 hr between sessions) and has proven to be effective for enhancing muscle strength and performance (35). However, trained people who perform more advanced programs may need more time between sessions (76). Factors such as training volume, training intensity, exercise selection, and nutritional intake may influence the ability to recover from and adapt to the training program. For example, trained people who perform a split routine may resistance train 4 times · wk⁻¹, but they only train each muscle group twice per week; they might train muscles of the lower body on Monday and Thursday and muscles of the upper body on Tuesday and Friday. Although an increase in training experience does not necessitate an increase in training frequency, a higher frequency does allow for greater specialization characterized by more exercises and a higher weekly training volume.

Periodization

Periodization refers to systematic variation in a resistance training program. Since it is impossible to continually improve at the same rate over long-term training, properly varying the training variables can limit training plateaus, maximize performance gains, and reduce the likelihood of overtraining. Periodization is a process whereby fitness professionals regularly change the training stimulus in order to keep it effective. Though the concept of periodization has been part of program design for many years, our understanding of the benefits of periodized programs compared with nonperiodized programs for long-term progression has only recently been explored in the literature (5, 17, 34).

The concept of periodization, or program variation, is not just for athletes but for people with all levels of training experience who want to enhance their health and fitness. By periodically varying program variables such as choice of exercise, training weight (resistance), number of sets, rest intervals between sets, or any combination of these, long-term performance gains will be optimized and the risk of overuse injuries may be reduced (5). Moreover, it is reasonable to suggest that people who participate in well-designed periodized programs and continue to improve their health and fitness may be more likely to adhere to an exercise program over the long term.

For example, if a person's lower-body routine typically consists of leg presses, leg extensions, and leg curls, performing dumbbell lunges, hip abductions, and hip adductions on alternate workout days will likely add to the effectiveness and enjoyment of the resistance training program. Further, varying the volume and intensity of training can help to prevent training plateaus, which are common after the first 2 mo of training. Many times participants can avoid a strength plateau by varying the training intensity and volume to allow for ample recovery. In the long term, program variation with adequate recovery will result in even greater gains because the body will be challenged to adapt to even greater demands. The underlying concept of periodization is based on the theory that after a certain time, adaptations to a stimulus will no longer take place unless the stimulus is altered. Periodized resistance training has been shown to be superior to nonperiodized resistance training for promoting long-term training adaptations in strength and power (77).

Although there are many models of periodization, the general concept is to prioritize training goals and then develop a long-term plan that varies throughout the year. In general, the overall training plan is divided into time periods called **macrocycles** (about 1 yr), **mesocycles** (3-4 mo), and **microcycles** (1-4 wk), with each cycle having a specific goal (e.g., hypertrophy, strength, or power). The classic periodization model is referred to as a *linear model* because the volume and intensity of training gradually change over time (87). For example, at the start of a macrocycle, the training volume may be high and the training intensity may be low. As the year progresses, the volume decreases as the intensity increases.

Although the linear training model was originally designed for weightlifters and track and field athletes who wanted to peak for a specific competition, it can be modified by fitness professionals in order to enhance health and fitness. For example, people who routinely perform the same combination of sets and repetitions may benefit from gradually increasing the weight and decreasing the number of repetitions as strength improves. The classic periodized model is outlined in table 13.4. After the four-phase program is complete, people should be encouraged to participate in recreational activities or low-intensity resistance training to reduce the likelihood of overtraining. This period of restoration is called *active rest* and typically lasts for 1 to 3 wk. After active rest, participants can then return to the first phase of their training program with more energy and vigor.

A second model of periodization is referred to as an *undulating (nonlinear) model* because of the daily fluctuations in training volume and intensity. For example, a person may perform 2 sets of 10 repetitions with a moderate load on Monday, 3 sets of 6 repetitions with a heavy load on Wednesday, and 1 set of 15 repetitions with a light load on Friday. The heavy training days will maximally activate the trained musculature, and selected muscle fibers will not be maximally taxed on light and moderate training days. By alternating training intensities, the participant can minimize the risk of overtraining and maximize the potential for maintaining training-induced strength gains (41). A sample nonlinear periodized workout plan for a trained adult is presented in table 13.5. In addition, fitness professionals should consider a participant's vacation schedule or travel plans when incorporating active rest into the year-long training schedule. Periods of restoration lasting from 1 to 3 wk will allow for physical and psychological recovery from the resistance training. A detailed review of periodization and specific examples of periodized programs are available elsewhere (5, 17).

KEY POINT

Designing a safe and effective resistance training program involves an understanding of exercise science along with an appreciation of the art of prescribing exercise. The specific exercise, the order of exercise, the resistance used, the number of sets, the rest intervals between sets and exercises, the training velocity, and the training frequency are variables that contribute to the design of a resistance training program. Periodization is the systematic variation of program variables to optimize long-term training adaptations.

TABLE 13.4   Sample Linear Periodized Workout for Maximizing Strength Gains in Healthy Adults

	Phase 1 General preparation	Phase 2 Hypertrophy	Phase 3 Strength	Phase 4 Peaking
Intensity	12RM-15RM	8RM-12RM	6RM-8RM	4RM-6RM
Sets	1-2	2	2-3	3
Rest between sets	60-120 sec	60 sec	60-120 sec	120-180 sec

The workout is for major-muscle-group exercises performed each phase; each phase lasts about 6-8 wk. RM = repetition maximum.

TABLE 13.5   Sample Nonlinear Periodized Workout for a Trained Adult

	Monday	Wednesday	Friday
Intensity	8 RM -10RM	4 RM -6RM	13 RM -15RM
Sets	2	3	3
Rest between sets and exercises	2 min	3 min	1 min

This plan is for the major-muscle-group exercises performed each day.

Resistance Training Models for Healthy Adults

A crucial factor to consider when designing resistance training programs is a participant's training status or training age. Although any reasonable resistance training program will enhance the strength of untrained people, trained people improve at a slower rate and require more advanced programs in order to enhance muscular strength (5, 76). Thus resistance training programs designed for beginners may not be effective for trained participants who have at least 3 mo of experience with resistance training. Clearly, there is no single model of resistance exercise that will optimize training-induced adaptations in both untrained and trained people.

Therefore, it is reasonable for beginners to start with a general resistance training program and gradually progress to more advanced programs as performance and self-confidence in their ability to perform resistance exercise improve. However, as more advanced training programs are designed, fitness professionals must consider the additional time and effort that are required to make additional gains. For example, people with several years of training experience may need to devote a large amount of time to training in order to make relatively small gains. Although athletes may be willing to make this type of commitment for small changes in performance, others may be less willing to devote a large amount of time to resistance training.

RESEARCH INSIGHT

Although it has been reported that people must resistance train at an intensity of at least 60% 1RM to induce strength gains, data regarding self-selected training intensities are scarce. Ratamess and colleagues (74) examined the influence of resistance training with a personal trainer versus unsupervised resistance training on the self-selected intensities used by women during resistance training. Following self-selection trials on four exercises, each subject's 1RM was determined. The results showed that the average self-selected training intensity was 51% 1RM in the personal trainer group and 42% 1RM in the other group; additionally, 1RM values were also higher in the personal trainer group. Although resistance training under the supervision of a personal trainer leads to greater initial 1RM values and a self-selection of greater workout intensities, fitness professionals may need to prescribe an appropriate intensity in order to maximize performance adaptations.

Since long-term progression in resistance exercise requires a systematic manipulation of the program variables, fitness professionals need to make critical decisions regarding the exercise prescription. These decisions require a solid understanding of training-induced adaptations that take place in both beginners and nonbeginners. Beginners need limited variation, but as the program progresses, more variation and more complex training regimens are needed. General recommendations for enhancing muscular strength in beginners were summarized previously in this chapter. More advanced training programs are available elsewhere (17, 67, 88).

Overreaching and Overtraining

Fitness professionals need to balance the demands of training with adequate recovery between workouts in order to optimize training adaptations. A resistance training program characterized by an excessive frequency, volume, or intensity of training, combined with inadequate rest and recovery, eventually results in overtraining syndrome. In essence, overtraining syndrome may occur when the training stimulus exceeds the rate of adaptation. Overtraining syndrome typically includes a plateau or decrease in performance. Other observable manifestations of overtraining include decreased body weight, decreased appetite, sleep disturbances, decreased desire to train, muscle tenderness, and increased risk of infection (83, 86).

Overtraining on a short-term basis has become known as *overreaching* (37). Unlike overtraining syndrome, which can last for months, recovery from overreaching can occur within a few days. In fact, overreaching is sometimes a planned part of conditioning programs as participants train at higher volumes and intensities. Nevertheless, overreaching should be considered the first stage of overtraining and therefore warrants attention because not all people recover quickly from overreaching. Participants may need to decrease the intensity and volume of their training program to recover from overreaching.

A downfall of many fitness programs is not allowing adequate recovery between workouts. For example, if a person resistance trains on Monday, Wednesday, and Friday and jogs on Tuesday and Thursday, the chronic forces placed on the lower body can injure muscles and connective tissue and decrease performance in the weight room and on the track. Overtraining can result from poor programming characterized by frequent training sessions without adequate rest and recovery between workouts. From a practical perspective, it is important to consider a person's training age as well as all fitness activities regularly performed. Periodization can help to avoid overtraining and promote long-term gains in muscular fitness (17).

In addition, lifestyle factors such as sensible nutrition, proper hydration, and adequate sleep can influence how people adapt to fitness training.

KEY POINT

Resistance training programs should be characterized by an appropriate overload and progression combined with planned periods of rest and recovery. Although beginners can make relatively large gains in performance from a general training program, people with resistance training experience need more advanced programs in order to progress over the long term. Overreaching is often the first stage of the overtraining syndrome, which is characterized by a decrease in performance and other physical and psychological effects. Adequate rest and recovery between workouts can help to avoid overtraining syndrome.

Resistance Training Systems

Many resistance training systems can be used to enhance muscular fitness. Some systems have been scientifically proven to be effective, whereas others are based on anecdotal evidence. The wide variety of systems illustrates the types of programs that can be developed by manipulating program variables. Five of the most common resistance training systems are the single-set system, multiple-set system, circuit training system, preexhaustion system, and assisted training system.

Single-Set System

This system of resistance training is one of the oldest and consists of performing a single set of a predetermined number of repetitions (e.g., 8-12) until volitional fatigue. More recently, the single-set approach has become known as the high-intensity training (HIT) system. This time-efficient method of resistance training can be an effective method for people who have no resistance training experience or who have not trained for several years (85). Since the acute adaptations to resistance training (i.e., 6-12 wk) are primarily due to neuromuscular adaptations (79), a single-set system can be an appropriate method of training for beginners or very deconditioned people, especially since this approach may promote participation and improve compliance versus more time-consuming training systems.

Multiple-Set System

The multiple-set system is an effective training method for enhancing strength and power. This system of training became popular in the 1940s and originally consisted of 3 sets of 10 repetitions with increasing weights. For example, the classic multiple-set protocol used by Delorme in his pioneering rehabilitation work involved performing the first set of 10 repetitions at 50% of 10RM, the second set of 10 repetitions at 75% of 10RM, and the third set of 10 repetitions at 100% of 10RM (26). Over the years, many multiple-set programs using various combinations of sets and repetitions have been shown to be effective. For example, the pyramid system is a multiple-set system in which the weight increases progressively over several sets so that fewer and fewer repetitions can be performed (see table 13.6). For continued progression in a resistance training program, multiple sets should be used. However, in order to reduce the risk of overtraining, the total number of sets performed per training session should gradually increase. In addition, not all exercises need to be performed for the same number of sets.

Circuit Training System

This system of training involves performing a series of resistance exercises in a circuit with minimal rest (about 30 sec) between exercises (see figure 13.8). Generally, moderate weights are used (about 60% of 1RM), and 10 to 15 repetitions are performed at each exercise station. In addition to increasing muscular strength and local muscular endurance, circuit training also can improve CRF. However, gains in maximal oxygen consumption resulting from aerobic training are far greater than those resulting from circuit training. Starting with a 1 min rest between exercises and gradually reducing the rest to the desired range as the body adapts is recommended when a person is beginning circuit training. A sample circuit training program is illustrated in figure 13.8

Preexhaustion System

This training method consists of performing successive sets of two exercises for the same target muscle or muscle group. For example, after performing one set to volitional fatigue on the bench press, the participant immediately performs a set of dumbbell flys to facilitate chest development. This type of training forces the target muscle group (e.g., pectoralis major) to work longer and harder and is often used to increase muscle hypertrophy.

TABLE 13.6 Sample Light-to-Heavy Pyramid Training System

Set number	Repetitions	Intensity (%1RM)
1	10	75
2	8	80
3	6	85

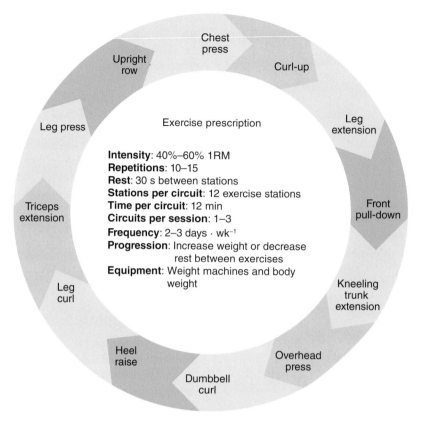

Exercise prescription

Intensity: 40%–60% 1RM
Repetitions: 10–15
Rest: 30 s between stations
Stations per circuit: 12 exercise stations
Time per circuit: 12 min
Circuits per session: 1–3
Frequency: 2–3 days · wk^{-1}
Progression: Increase weight or decrease rest between exercises
Equipment: Weight machines and body weight

FIGURE 13.8 Sample program for circuit resistance training.

Adapted, by permission, from V.H. Heyward, 2010, *Advanced fitness assessment and exercise prescription*, 6th ed. (Champaign, IL: Human Kinetics), 163

Assisted Training System

As the name implies, this method of training requires the assistance of another person who, after several repetitions of an exercise are performed to volitional fatigue, can provide just enough assistance to allow the lifter to complete 3 to 5 additional repetitions. Because muscles are stronger eccentrically than concentrically, assistance may not be needed during the eccentric phase of the forced repetitions. Although this advanced training system will enhance muscular fitness, it is not recommended for beginners because it typically results in muscle soreness attributable to the reliance on heavy eccentric muscle actions. Other training systems also may result in some muscle soreness, but assisted training increases the likelihood that soreness will result.

KEY POINT

A variety of resistance training systems can be used to enhance strength, power, and local muscular endurance. Although all training systems can be effective, the key is to match the system with the needs, goals, and abilities of each participant for long-term success. The resistance training system will influence the training-induced adaptations that take place.

Resistance Training for Special Populations

Resistance training can be a safe, effective, and beneficial method of conditioning for men and women of all ages and physical abilities. Although research on resistance training has focused predominantly on healthy adults, a growing body of evidence indicates that children, seniors, pregnant women, and people with certain chronic but stable conditions (e.g., high BP, diabetes, CHD) can participate safely in resistance training provided that appropriate training guidelines are followed.

Children

Despite previous concerns that children under 13 yr old would not benefit from resistance training because of inadequate levels of circulating androgens, studies conducted over the past decade clearly demonstrate that boys and girls can benefit from resistance training (15, 29, 56). ACSM (6), the Canadian Society for Exercise Physiology (12), and the National Strength and Conditioning Association (NSCA) (30) support children's participation in resistance training provided that the program is appropriately designed and supervised. In addition to increasing muscular strength and muscular endurance, regular participation in a resistance training program may favorably influence several measurable indexes of health, including body composition and BMD (11, 30). Further, because many aspiring young athletes who enter sport programs may not be prepared for the demands of training and competition, participation in a preseason conditioning program that includes resistance training may decrease the risk of sport-related injuries (43, 83).

A traditional concern associated with youth resistance training is that it may harm the developing musculoskeletal system. This myth seems to have come from an earlier report that suggested that children who performed heavy labor damaged their epiphyseal plates, which resulted in significant decreases in stature (47). However, this study did not control for other etiological factors, such as poor nutrition, that could be responsible for the reported growth arrest. Current observations indicate no evidence of a decrease in stature in young people who participate in resistance training in controlled environments (29, 56). In fact, the belief that resistance training is harmful to the immature skeleton of young weight trainers is inconsistent with current findings suggesting that childhood may be the time during which the bone-modeling process responds best to the mechanical loading of physical activities such as resistance training (11). Children and adolescents are now encouraged to participate regularly in 60 min or more of physical activity that includes aerobic activities as well as age-appropriate muscle-strengthening and bone-strengthening activities (92).

Another corollary of youth resistance training is its influence on body composition. As the number of overweight young people in the United States and other countries continues to increase (68), the effect of resistance training on body composition has received increased attention (32). Although aerobic exercise is typically prescribed for decreasing body fatness, researchers have reported that resistance training may be beneficial for treating children who are overweight (59, 80). Of interest is the finding that progressive resistance training has been found to significantly increase insulin sensitivity in overweight youth (80, 93). It appears that young people who are overweight enjoy resistance training because it is not aerobically taxing and it gives all participants a chance to experience success and feel good about their performance. Further study is warranted, but the first step in encouraging these youth to exercise may be to increase their confidence in their ability to be physically active, which in turn may lead to an increase in physical activity and a decrease in body fat.

RESEARCH INSIGHT

Safe and effective exercise programs are needed to treat children who are overweight. Shaibi and colleagues (80) examined the effects of 16 wk of progressive resistance training on overweight adolescents and reported a significant decrease in body fat and a significant increase in insulin sensitivity along with an impressive 96% exercise adherence rate. Because the increase in insulin sensitivity remained significant after adjustment for changes in total fat mass and total lean mass, the researchers speculated that resistance training may have resulted in qualitative changes in skeletal muscle that contributed to enhanced insulin action. These findings demonstrate that resistance training may be a valuable component of a multidisciplinary weight management program for children who are overweight.

Although there is no minimum age requirement for participating in a youth resistance training program, all children who participate should have the emotional maturity to accept and follow directions and understand the benefits and risks associated with this type of training. In general, if children are ready for organized sport, then they are ready for some type of resistance training. As a point of reference, many 7- and 8-yr-old boys and girls have participated in closely supervised resistance training programs (31). Although some observers may be concerned about the stress that resistance training places on the developing musculoskeletal system, the sport-specific forces placed on the joints of children may be greater in both duration and magnitude than those resulting from moderate-intensity resistance training. Further, injury to the epiphyseal plate or growth cartilage has not been reported in any prospective study on youth resistance training (29). Nevertheless, fitness professionals should follow age-specific training guidelines to decrease the likelihood of an accident or injury when young people perform resistance exercises.

Children should begin resistance training at a level that is commensurate with their physical abilities. No matter how big or strong a child is, adult training programs and philosophies (e.g., "No pain, no gain") should not be imposed on children. The focus of youth resistance training should be on learning proper technique for a variety of exercises. During each session, fitness professionals should listen to each child's concerns and closely monitor each child's ability to handle the prescribed training weight. Various combinations of sets and repetitions and a variety of training modes from child-sized weight machines to body-weight exercises have proven to be effective (21, 31). According to ACSM, children should perform 8 to 15 repetitions of a variety of exercises that use all the major muscle groups (5).

When working with children, remember that the goal of the program should not be limited to increasing muscle strength. Teaching children about their bodies and promoting a lifelong interest in physical activity are equally important. The following considerations for program design should be followed when developing resistance training programs for children:

- Parents or legal guardians should complete an HSQ for each child.

- Children with diseases or disabilities should have their exercise program tailored to their condition, symptoms, and functional capacity.

- Qualified instructors should supervise youth fitness activities.

- The exercise area should be free of clutter and adequately ventilated.

- Children should use a light weight or wooden dowel when learning a new exercise.

- Resistance should be increased only when the child can perform the desired number of repetitions with good form.

- Two or three nonconsecutive training sessions per week are recommended.

- The resistance training program should increase motor skill and fitness level.

Seniors

The number of men and women over the age of 64 in the United States is increasing, and research studies and clinical observations indicate that seniors can benefit from resistance training (4, 8, 55, 82, 95). Even people over the age of 90 can enhance their muscular fitness through resistance training (33). Regular participation in a resistance training program can help offset the age-related declines in bone, muscle mass, and strength that often make ADLs—such as climbing stairs—more difficult. Bones become more fragile with age because of a decrease in bone mineral content that results in an increase in bone porosity (66). Advancing age also is associated with a loss of muscle mass, or sarcopenia, which includes a proportional loss of both type I (slow-twitch) and type II (fast-twitch) fibers, with the type II fibers having the greatest loss in cross-sectional area (4). Evidence indicates that seniors who resistance train can improve muscle strength, muscle power, gait speed, and balance, which in turn can enhance overall function and reduce the potential for injuries caused by falls (33, 55, 82, 95). Moreover, there is emerging evidence for significant psychological and cognitive benefits from regular exercise participation by older adults (4). Fitness professionals should educate seniors on the benefits of resistance train-

ing because a majority of adults aged 65 and older do not participate regularly in strength-building activities (54).

Seniors can adapt readily to resistance training exercises. If the training intensity is adequate, they can make relative gains in strength that are equal to or greater than those of younger people. Of interest is the observation that resistance training trials comparing training intensities show strong resistance training effects in a dose–response manner, with high-intensity training being more effective than moderate- and low-intensity training in seniors (82). Research studies using CT and muscle-biopsy analysis have also reported evidence of muscle hypertrophy in seniors who resistance train, and others have reported that resistance training can increase the resting metabolic rate and BMD of older adults who resistance train (4, 33). Although both aerobic and resistance exercise are important for seniors, only resistance training can increase muscle strength and muscle mass. These potential benefits may be particularly important for seniors who are at increased risk for osteoporotic fractures. However, adults will retain the beneficial effects of resistance training only as long as they continue their exercise program. During prolonged inactivity, adaptive changes in skeletal muscle strength and bone will return to preexercise levels (28). This is sometimes referred to as the **principle of reversibility**.

Before starting a resistance training program, seniors should undergo preparticipation health screening since many have a variety of known, coexisting medical conditions. In addition, at least during the initial phase of training, fitness professionals should provide instruction and offer assistance as needed. Older adults should begin resistance training with minimal resistance during the first few weeks to allow time for musculoskeletal adaptation and to practice proper exercise technique (94). People who are very frail may need to perform muscle-strengthening activities before aerobic training because of their physical limitations. Although there are no specific recommendations for neuromuscular training, exercises that combine balance, agility, and proprioceptive training can be effective in reducing and preventing falls in older adults (6). Over time, exercises that gradually reduce the base of support (e.g., tandem stand and one-legged stand), stress postural muscle groups (e.g., heel stands and toe stands), and reduce sensory input (standing with eyes closed) can be sensibly incorporated into senior training programs provided that qualified supervision and instruction are available (6). ACSM recommends the following program design considerations for seniors who want to resistance train (6):

- Perform 10 to 15 repetitions for each of 8 to 10 exercises.

- Use a rating between moderate (5-6) and vigorous (7-8) on a scale of 0 to 10 for level of physical exertion.

- Maintain proper breathing patterns while exercising.

- Perform all exercises within a pain-free ROM.

- Individualize progression of all resistance training activities

- Gradually incorporate balance, agility, and proprioceptive training into the exercise program.

- Resistance train at least 2 days · wk^{-1}.

- Use behavioral strategies such as social support to enhance adherence.

Pregnant Women

Growing evidence suggests that regular exercise during a low-risk pregnancy poses little risk to either the mother or the fetus and improves overall maternal fitness and well-being (2, 23, 25, 62, 64). Indeed, regular exercise may reduce the risk of developing conditions associated with pregnancy, including pregnancy-induced hypertension and gestational diabetes mellitus (27, 70). Participation in a wide range of physical activities appears safe during and after pregnancy, but resistance training may be particularly beneficial because it enhances muscle strength, which allows expectant mothers to perform ADLs with greater ease and possibly minimizes low-back pain, which is common during pregnancy (2, 38). Along with moderate-intensity aerobic exercise, resistance training at an appropriate intensity, duration, and frequency may offer significant health value to women with an uncomplicated pregnancy.

Exercise is not advised for all women who are pregnant, especially those who have medical complications. Thus, pregnant women should undergo a medical evaluation with their personal physician or qualified medical care provider and ask about activities that may or may not be appropriate during pregnancy. The American College of Obstetricians and Gynecologists (ACOG) established the following absolute contraindications for exercise during pregnancy: hemodynamically significant heart disease, restrictive lung disease, incompetent cervix or cervical cerclage, multiple gestation at risk for premature labor, persistent second- to third-trimester bleeding, placenta previa after 26 wk of gestation, premature labor during the current pregnancy, ruptured membranes, and preeclampsia or pregnancy-induced hypertension (2).

Limited data are available regarding resistance training for pregnant women (10). General guidelines for resistance training are outlined in this chapter and recommendations for exercising while pregnant are discussed in chapter 17. General exercise recommendations include maintaining adequate hydration, wearing appropriate clothing, and exercising at a comfortable intensity. Also, since pregnancy requires an additional 300 kcal · day^{-1}, pregnant women who exercise should be particularly careful to maintain adequate calories and a well-balanced diet (2, 64).

The following ACSM program design considerations are appropriate for pregnant women who perform resistance training (6):

- Perform multiple repetitions (i.e., 12-15) to the point of moderate fatigue.

- Gradually increase the weight as strength improves.

- Practice proper breathing patterns while resistance training.

- Avoid isometric muscle actions and the Valsalva maneuver.

- Avoid exercise in the supine position after the first trimester.

- Avoid sports and activities that may cause a loss of balance or trauma to the mother or fetus.

- Exercise in a thermoneutral environment and stay hydrated.

- Stop exercise in the event of any discomfort or complications such as vaginal bleeding, dyspnea before exertion, dizziness, headache, chest pain, muscle weakness, calf pain or swelling, preterm labor, decreased fetal movement, or amniotic fluid leakage.

- Exercise in the postpartum period may begin about 4 to 6 wk after delivery.

Adults With Heart Disease

Cardiac rehabilitation programs traditionally have emphasized aerobic exercise to maintain and improve CRF. However, muscular strength and local muscular endurance are also important to prepare the patient for return to work and leisure activities (9, 94). Many ADLs, as well as most occupational tasks, place demands on the cardiovascular system that closely resemble resistance exercise. Because many cardiac patients are deconditioned and lack the strength and confidence to perform common activities involving muscular effort, adding resistance training to an overall physical activity program provides patients with an opportunity to restore or gain optimal physiologic, vocational, and psychosocial status. The AHA (94), ACSM (6), and AACVPR (1) recommend resistance training as part of a comprehensive cardiac rehabilitation program.

Research indicates that medically stable cardiac patients can safely engage in resistance training provided that the program is appropriately designed and carried out within the prescribed guidelines (1, 6, 9, 94). Regular participation in a resistance training program may favorably affect muscular strength, muscular endurance, cardiorespiratory endurance, cardiac risk factors, and psychosocial well-being. Training-induced gains in muscular strength also can decrease the rate–pressure product (and associated myocardial demands) during daily activities such as carrying groceries and gardening (9, 94). In general, improving physical fitness can improve a patient's quality of life and help older patients live independently.

Before patients begin a resistance training program, a qualified health care provider should review their health and medical history to identify any condition that may exclude participation. Although most low- to moderate-risk patients can safely participate in resistance training, the safety and appropriateness of training for patients with low fitness levels or severe left ventricular dysfunction may be more appropriate to take place in medically supervised environment. According to ACSM (6), contraindications for inpatient and outpatient cardiac rehabilitations include the following: unstable angina, resting SBP >200 mmHg or resting DBP >110 mmHg, orthostatic BP drop of 20 mmHg with symptoms, critical aortic stenosis, acute systemic illness or fever, uncontrolled dysrhythmias, uncontrolled

sinus tachycardia (>120 beats · min^{-1}), uncompensated CHF, third-degree AV block (without pacemaker), active pericarditis or myocarditis, recent embolism, thrombophlebitis, resting ST segment displacement (>2 mm), uncontrolled diabetes, severe orthopedic conditions, and other metabolic conditions such as thyroiditis or hypokalemia.

Recent recommendations indicate that most cardiac patients can begin resistance training 5 wk after MI or cardiac surgery provided that they participated in 4 wk of supervised endurance training in a cardiac rehabilitation program (66). Although patients can use elastic bands and light weights (1-5 lb, or 0.5-2 kg) in a progressive fashion immediately upon entry into an outpatient program, consistent participation in a cardiac rehabilitation program should precede a traditional resistance training program in which patients lift weights corresponding to 30% to 60% of their 1RM for 12 to 15 repetitions (6). Low-risk patients may gradually progress to 60% to 80% of their 1 RM for 8 to 12 repetitions (6). ACSM recommends that patients perform 8 to 10 exercises and train each major muscle group with 2 to 4 sets (6). Further, patients should maintain a regular breathing pattern and avoid sustained, tight gripping, which may evoke an excessive BP response. The decision to begin a resistance training program should be based on current health status as determined by a qualified health care provider. The guidelines for designing a resistance training program for cardiac patients are the same as those for older adults, namely, patients should start with a light weight and gradually progress as they adapt to the training program. For patients returning to work, exercise training should be specific to the muscle groups and energy systems used for occupational tasks in order to increase physical work capacity, improve safety, and enhance self-efficacy (6).

KEY POINT

Resistance training can be a safe and beneficial component of a comprehensive fitness program for people of all ages and those with medical conditions provided that appropriate guidelines are followed and qualified instruction is available. Despite previous concerns, children, seniors, pregnant women, and patients with heart disease can benefit from participation in a well-designed resistance training program. Participants should first be screened to identify those who may be contraindicated for resistance training, as determined by a qualified health care provider.

Program Design for People With Heart Disease

- A physician or other qualified health care provider should review the health and medical history.
- Begin with a light weight and focus on controlled movements for 12 to 15 repetitions.
- Following initial adaptations, progress to 8 to 12 repetitions with a heavier weights.
- Train each major muscle group for 2 to 4 sets.
- Include multijoint exercises that involve more than one muscle group.
- Progress slowly as the individual adapts to the training program.
- Train 2 to 3 times each week on nonconsecutive days.
- Maintain regular breathing and avoid straining.
- Stop exercise in the event of any warning signs or symptoms such as dizziness, dysrhythmias, unusual shortness of breath, or anginal discomfort.

STUDY QUESTIONS

1. What four principles determine the effectiveness of resistance training programs?

2. Provide three examples of free-weight exercises in which a spotter is required.

3. What physiological adaptations result from resistance training in healthy adults?

4. List four types of resistance training and provide an example of each method.

5. What are the advantages and disadvantages of resistance training with weight machines, free weights, and body-weight exercises?

6. Define *periodization* and provide an example of a linear and nonlinear resistance training program.

7. What program variables should be outlined when designing a resistance training program for children, adults, or seniors?

8. What are three resistance exercises that pregnant women should avoid after the first trimester?

9. When can low-risk cardiac patients begin resistance training, and what precautions should be followed to reduce the risk of an adverse event?

10. What resistance training system would be most appropriate for a deconditioned client, a healthy adult who wants to enhance general fitness, and a trained person who wants to increase muscle hypertrophy?

CASE STUDIES

You can check your answers by referring to appendix A.

1. A 25-yr-old member of your fitness center has been resistance training for 4 mo and claims to have made significant gains in strength. He performs 1 set of 12 to 15 repetitions on 8 weight machines twice per week. However, over the past 6 wk he noticed that he isn't making the strength gains that he used to. Since his goal is to get stronger and increase his muscle mass, how would you modify his training program to optimize his desired gains in muscular fitness over the long term?

2. A 48-yr-old female currently swims for 45 to 60 min, 3 to 4 days · wk^{-1}, at the local recreation center. Although she has been a swimmer for years, she was recently advised by her doctor to participate in weight-bearing physical activities to increase her musculoskeletal strength. However, she is somewhat concerned about lifting weights and states that she doesn't want to develop bulky muscles. Address her preconceived concerns regarding resistance training and modify her current exercise program to optimize gains in musculoskeletal strength.

3. The director of a local assisted-living center for seniors wants to offer a new activity class at the facility, and she asks you for guidance and recommendations. In addition to a walking program that is already established, she wants you to develop a proposal for a senior resistance training program that not only enhances muscular fitness, but is safe and enjoyable for men and women over 65 yr old who have no resistance training experience. The facility does not have weight machines, but it does have several pairs of lightweight (1-5 lb, or 0.5-2 kg) dumbbells and a variety of elastic bands. Comment on program design considerations for seniors that will enhance muscular fitness and reduce the risk of falling.

REFERENCES

1. American Association of Cardiovascular and Pulmonary Rehabilitation (AACVPR). 2006. *AACVPR cardiac rehabilitation resource manual.* Champaign, IL: Human Kinetics.

2. American College of Obstetricians and Gynecologists (ACOG). 2002. Exercise during pregnancy and the postpartum period. *International Journal of Gynecology and Obstetrics* 77:79-81.

3. American College of Sports Medicine (ACSM). 2007. *ACSM's health/fitness facility standards and guidelines.* 3rd ed. Champaign, IL: Human Kinetics.

4. American College of Sports Medicine (ACSM). 2009. Exercise and physical activity for older adults. *Medicine and Science in Sports and Exercise* 41:1510-1530.

5. American College of Sports Medicine (ACSM). 2009. Progression models in resistance training for healthy adults. *Medicine and Science in Sports and Exercise* 41:687-708.

6. American College of Sports Medicine (ACSM). 2010. *ACSM's guidelines for exercise testing and prescription.* 8th ed. Philadelphia: Lippincott Williams & Wilkins.

7. Baechle, T., and R. Earle. 2008. *Essentials of strength training and conditioning.* 3rd ed. Champaign, IL: Human Kinetics.

8. Baechle, T., and W. Westcott. 2010. *Fitness professional's guide to strength training for older adults.* Champaign, IL: Human Kinetics

9. Balady, G., M. Williams, P. Ades, V. Bittner, P. Comoss, J. Foody, B. Franklin, B. Sanderson, and D. Southard. 2007. Core components of cardiac rehabilitation/secondary prevention programs: 2007 update. *Journal of Cardiopulmonary Rehabilitation and Prevention* 27:121-129.

10. Barakat, R., A. Lucia, and J. Ruiz. 2009. Resistance exercise training during pregnancy and newborn's birth size: A randomized controlled trial. *International Journal of Obesity* 33:1048-1057.

11. Bass, S. 2000. The prepubertal years: A uniquely opportune stage of growth when the skeletal is most responsive to exercise? *Sports Medicine* 30(2): 73-78.

12. Behm, D., A. Faigenbaum, B. Falk, and P. Klentrou. 2008. Canadian Society for Exercise Physiology position paper: Resistance training for children and adolescents. *Applied Physiology Nutrition and Metabolism* 33:547-561.

13. Behm, D., and Anderson, K. 2006. The role of instability with resistance training. *Journal of Strength and Conditioning Research* 20:716-722.

14. Behm, D., and Sale, D. 1993. Intended rather than actual movement velocity determines the velocity specific training response. *Journal of Applied Physiology* 74:359-368.

15. Behringer, M., A. vom Heede, Z. Yue, and J. Mester. 2010. Effects of resistance training in children and adolescents: A meta-analysis. *Pediatrics* 126:e1199-e1210.

16. Bishop, D. 2003. Warm-up II: Performance changes following active warm-up and how to structure the warm-up. *Sports Medicine* 33:483-498.

17. Bompa, T., and G. Haff. 2009. *Periodization.* 5th ed. Champaign, IL: Human Kinetics.

18. Brown, L. 2000. *Isokinetics in human performance.* Champaign, IL: Human Kinetics.

19. Campos, G., T. Luecke, H. Wendeln, K. Toma, F. Hagerman, T. Murray, K. Ragg, N. Ratamess, W. Kraemer, and R. Staron. 2002. Muscular adaptations in response to three different resistance training regimens: Specificity of repetition maximum training zones. *European Journal of Applied Physiology* 88:50-60.

20. Chu, D. 1998. *Jumping into plyometrics.* 2nd ed. Champaign, IL: Human Kinetics.

21. Chu, D., A. Faigenbaum, and J. Falkel. 2006. *Progressive plyometrics for kids.* Monterey, CA: Healthy Learning.

22. Clarkson, P. 2006. Case report of exertional rhabdomyolysis in a 12-year-old boy. *Medicine and Science in Sports and Exercise* 38:197-200.

23. DeMaio, M., and E. Magann. 2009. Exercise and pregnancy. *Journal of the American Academy of Orthopedic Surgery* 17:504-514.

24. Davies, G. 1995. The need for critical thinking in rehabilitation. *Journal of Sport Rehabilitation* 4:1-22.

25. Davies, G., L. Wolfe, M. Mottola, and C. MacKinnon. 2003. Joint SOGC/CSEP clinical practice guideline: Exercise in pregnancy and the postpartum period. *Canadian Journal of Applied Physiology* 28:329-341.

26. DeLorme, T., and A. Watkins. 1948. Techniques of progressive resistance exercise. *Archives of Physical Medicine and Rehabilitation* 29:263-273.

27. Dempsey, J., C. Butler, and M. Williams. 2005. No need for a pregnant pause: Physical activity may reduce the occurrence of gestational diabetes mellitus and preclampsia. *Exercise and Sport Science Reviews* 33:141-149.

28. Drinkwater, B. 1995. Weight-bearing exercise and bone mass. *Physical Medicine and Rehabilitation Clinics of North America* 6:567-578.

29. Faigenbaum, A., and G. Myer. 2010. Resistance training among young athletes: Safety, efficacy and injury prevention effects. *British Journal of Sports Medicine* 44:56-63.

30. Faigenbaum, A., W. Kraemer, C. Blimkie, I. Jeffreys, L. Micheli, M. Nitka, and T. Rowland. 2009. Youth resistance training: Updated position statement paper from the National Strength and Conditioning Association. *Journal of Strength and Conditioning Research 23(Supplement 5): S60-S79.*

31. Faigenbaum, A., and W. Westcott. 2009. *Youth strength training.* Champaign, IL: Human Kinetics.

32. Faigenbaum, A., and W. Westcott. 2007. Resistance training for obese children and adolescents. *President's Council on Physical Fitness and Sports Research Digest* 8:1-8.

33. Fiatarone, M.A., E.C. Marks, N.D. Ryan, C.N. Meredith, L.A. Lipsitz, and W. Evans. 1990. High-intensity strength training in nonagenarians: Effects on skeletal muscle. *Journal of the American Medical Association* 263:3029-3034.

34. Fleck, S. 1999. Periodized strength training: A critical review. *Journal of Strength and Conditioning Research* 13:82-89.

35. Fleck, S., and W. Kraemer. 2004. *Designing resistance training programs.* 3rd ed. Champaign, IL: Human Kinetics.

36. Fletcher, I., and M. Monte-Colombo. 2010. An investigation into the possible physiological mechanisms associated with changes in performance related to acute response to different preactivity stretch modalities. *Applied Physiology Nutrition and Metabolism* 35:27-34.

37. Fry, A., and W. Kraemer. 1997. Resistance exercise overtraining and overreaching. *Sports Medicine* 23(2): 106-129.

38. Garshasbi, A., and S. Zadeh. 2005. The effect of exercise on the intensity of low back pain in pregnant women. *International Journal of Gynecology and Obstetrics* 88:271-275.

39. Glass, S., and D. Stanton. 2004. Self-selected resistance training intensity in novice weightlifters. *Journal of Strength and Conditioning Research* 18:324-327.

40. Goldberg, L., and P. Twist. 2007. *Strength ball training.* Champaign, IL: Human Kinetics

41. Hass, C., L. Garzarella, D. De Hoyos, and M. Pollock. 2000. Single versus multiple sets in long-term recreational

weightlifters. *Medicine and Science in Sports and Exercise* 32:235-242.

42. Hettinger, R., and E. Muller. 1953. Muskelleistung und muskeltraining (Muscle achievement and muscle training). *ArbeitsPhysiologie* 15:111-126.

43. Hewett, T., G. Myer, and K. Ford. 2005. Reducing knee and anterior cruciate ligament injuries among female athletes. *Journal of Knee Surgery* 18:82-88.

44. Hibbs, A., K. Thompson, D. French, A. Wrigley, and I. Spears. 2008. Optimizing performance by improving core stability and core strength. *Sports Medicine* 38:995-1008.

45. Hoeger, W., S. Barette, D. Hale, and D. Hopkins. 1987. Relationship between repetitions and selected percentages on the one repetition maximum. *Journal of Applied Sport Science Research* 1:11-13.

46. Holm, L., S. Reitelseder, T. Pedersen, S. Doessing, S. Petersen, A. Flyvbjerg, J. Andersen, P. Aagaard, and M. Kjaer. 2008. Changes in muscle size and MHC composition in response to resistance exercise with heavy and light loading intensity. *Journal of Applied Physiology* 105:1454-1461.

47. Kato, S., and T. Ishiko. 1964. Obstructed growth of children's bones due to excessive labor in remote corners. In *Proceedings of the International Congress of Sports Sciences,* ed. S. Kato, 476. Tokyo: Japanese Union of Sports Sciences.

48. Keeler, L., L. Finkelstein, W. Miller, and B. Fernhall. 2001. Early phase adaptations to traditional speed vs. super slow resistance training on strength and aerobic capacity in sedentary individuals. *Journal of Strength and Conditioning Research* 15:309-314.

49. Kerr, Z., C. Collins, and R. Comstock. Epidemiology of weight training related injuries presenting to United States emergency room departments, 1990-2007. *American Journal of Sports Medicine* 38:765-771.

50. Kraemer, W., B. Noble, B. Culver, and M. Clark. 1987. Physiologic responses to heavy resistance exercise with very short rest periods. *International Journal of Sports Medicine* 8:247-252.

51. Kraemer, W., and N. Ratamess. 2005. Hormonal responses and adaptations to resistance exercise and training. *Sports Medicine* 35:339-361.

52. Kraemer, W., and N. Ratamess. 2004. Fundamentals of resistance training: Progression and exercise prescription. *Medicine and Science in Sports and Exercise* 36:674-688.

53. Krieger, J. 2009. Single versus multiple sets of resistance exercise: A meta-regression. *Journal of Strength and Conditioning Research* 23:1890-1901.

54. Kruger, J., S. Carlson, and H. Kohl, 2006. Trends in strength training—United States, 1998-2004. *Morbidity and Mortality Weekly Report* 55:769-772.

55. Liu, C., and N. Latham. 2009 Progressive resistance training for improving physical function in older adults. Cochrane Database Systems Reviews, Issue 3. Art. No.: CD002759. doi: 10.1002/14651858.CD002759.pub2.

56. Malina, R. 2006. Weight training in youth—growth, maturation and safety: An evidenced-based review. *Clinical Journal of Sports Medicine* 16:478-487.

57. Marx, J., N. Ratamess, B. Nindl, L. Gotshalk, J. Volek, K. Dohi, J. Bush, A. Gomez, S. Mazzetti, S. Fleck, K. Hakkinen, R. Newton, and W. Kraemer. 2001. Low volume circuit versus high volume periodized resistance training in women. *Medicine and Science in Sports and Exercise* 33:635-643.

58. Mazzetti, S., W. Kraemer, J. Volek, N. Duncan, N. Ratamess, A. Gomez, R. Newton, K. Hakkinen, and S. Fleck. 2000. The influence of direct supervision of resistance training on strength performance. *Medicine and Science in Sports and Exercise* 32:1175-1184.

59. McGuigan, M.R., Tatasciore, M., Newton, R.U., et al. 2009. Eight weeks of resistance training can significantly alter body composition in children who are overweight or obese. *Journal of Strength and Conditioning Research* 23:80-85.

60. Mediate, P., and A. Faigenbaum. 2007. *Medicine ball training for all kids.* Monterey Bay, CA: Healthy Learning.

61. McGee, D., T. Jessee, H. Stone, and D. Blessing. 1992. Leg and hip endurance adaptations to three weight training programs. *Journal of Applied Sport Science Research* 6:92-95.

62. Melzer, K., Y. Schutz, M. Boulvain, and B. Kayser. 2010. Physical activity and pregnancy: Cardiovascular adaptations, recommendations and pregnancy outcomes. *Sports Medicine* 40:493-507.

63. Mikesky, A., C. Gidding, W. Mathews, and W. Gonyea. 1991. Changes in muscle fiber size and composition in response to heavy-resistance exercise. *Medicine and Science in Sports and Exercise* 23:1042-1049.

64. Morris, S., and N. Johnson. 2005. Exercise during pregnancy: A critical appraisal of the literature. *Journal of Reproductive Medicine* 50:181-188.

65. Myer, G., C. Quatman, J. Khoury, E. Wall, and T. Hewett. 2009. Youth vs. adult "weightlifting" injuries presented to United States emergency rooms: Accidental vs. non-accidental injury mechanisms. *Journal of Strength and Conditioning Research* 23:2054-2060.

66. Nelson, M., M. Fiatarone, C. Morganti, I. Trice, R. Greenberg, and W. Evans. 1994. Effects of high intensity strength training on multiple risk factors for osteoporotic fractures. *Journal of the American Medical Association* 272:1909-1914.

67. Newton, H. 2006. *Explosive lifting for sports.* Champaign, IL: Human Kinetics.

68. Ogden, C., M. Carroll, L. Curtin, M. Lamb, and K. Flegal. 2010. Prevalence of high body mass index in US children and adolescents, 2007-2008. *Journal of the American Medical Association* 303(3): 242-249

69. Peterson, M., M. Rhea, and B. Alvar. 2005. Applications of the dose response for muscular strength development: A review of meta-analytic efficacy and reliability for designing training prescription. *Journal of Strength and Conditioning Research* 19:950-958.

70. Pivarnik, J., H. Chambliss, J. Clapp, S. Dugan, M. Hatch, C. Lovelady, M. Mottola, and M. Williams. 2006. Impact of physical activity during pregnancy and postpartum on chronic disease risk. *Medicine and Science in Sports and Exercise* 38:989-1006.

71. Potach, D., and D. Chu. 2008. Plyometric training. In *Essentials of strength training and conditioning.* 3rd ed. Ed. T. Baechle and R. Earle, 413-456. Champaign, IL: Human Kinetics.

72. Quatman, C., G. Myer, J. Khoury, E. Wall, and T. Hewett. Sex differences in "weightlifting" injuries presenting to United States emergency rooms. *Journal of Strength and Conditioning Research* 23:2061-2067.

73. Radcliff, J. 2005. *High-powered plyometrics.* Champaign, IL: Human Kinetics.

74. Ratamess, N., A. Faigenbaum, J. Hoffman, and J. Kang. 2008. Self-selected resistance training intensity in healthy women: The influence of a personal trainer. *Journal of Strength and Conditioning Research* 22:103-111.

75. Ratamess, N., M. Falvo, G. Mangine, J. Hoffman, A. Faigenbaum, and J. Kang. 2007. The effect of rest interval length on metabolic responses to the bench press exercise. *European Journal of Applied Physiology* 100:1-17.

76. Rhea, M., B. Alvar, L. Brukett, and S. Ball. 2003. A meta-analysis to determine the dose response for strength development. *Medicine and Science in Sports and Exercise* 35:456-464.

77. Rhea, M., and B. Alderman. 2004. A meta-analysis of periodized versus nonperiodized strength and power training programs. *Research Quarterly for Exercise and Sport* 75:413-422.

78. Robbins, D. 2005. Postactivation potentiation and its practical application. *Journal of Strength and Conditioning Research* 19:453-458.

79. Rutherford, O.M., and D.D. Jones. 1986. The role of learning and coordination in strength training. *European Journal of Applied Physiology* 55:100-105.

80. Shaibi, G., M. Cruz, G. Ball, M. Weigensberg, G. Salem, N. Crespo, and M. Goran. 2006. Effects of resistance training on insulin sensitivity in overweight Latino adolescent males. *Medicine and Science in Sports and Exercise* 38:1208-1215.

81. Shimano, T., W. Kraemer, B. Sppiering, J. Volek, D. Hatfield, R. Silvestre, J. Vingren, M. Fragala, C. Maresh, S. Fleck, R. Newton, L. Spreuwenberg, and K. Hakkinen. 2008. Relationship between the number of repetitions and selected percentages of one repetition maximum in free weight exercises in trained and untrained men. *Journal of Strength and Conditioning Research* 20:819-823.

82. Steib, S., D. Schoene, and K. Pfeifer. 2009. Dose–relationship of resistance training in older adults: A meta-analysis. *Medicine and Science in Sports and Exercise* 42:902-914.

83. Stein, C., and L. Micheli. 2010. Overuse injuries in youth sports. *Physician and Sports Medicine* 38:102-108.

84. Spreuwenberg, L., W. Kraemer, B. Spiering, J. Volek, D. Hatfield, R. Silvestre, J. Vingren, M. Fragala, K. Hakkinen, R. Newtown, C. Maresh, and S. Fleck. 2006. Influence of exercise order in a resistance training exercise session. *Journal of Strength and Conditioning Research* 20:141-144.

85. Starkey, D.B., M.L. Pollock, T. Ishida, Y. Ishida, M. Welsch, W. Bechve, J. Graves, and M. Feigenbaum. 1996. Effect of resistance training volume on strength and muscle thickness. *Medicine and Science in Sports and Exercise* 28:1311-1320.

86. Stone, M., R. Keith, J. Kearney, S. Fleck, G. Wilson, and N. Triplett. 1991. Overtraining: A review of signs and symptoms. *Journal of Applied Strength and Conditioning Research* 5:35-50.

87. Stone, M.H., H. O'Bryant, and J. Garhammer. 1981. A hypothetical model for strength training. *Journal of Sports Medicine* 21:342-351.

88. Stone, M., M. Stone, and W. Sands. 2007. *Principles and practice of resistance training.* Champaign, IL: Human Kinetics.

89. Thompsen, A., T. Kackley, M. Palumbo, and A. Faigenbaum. 2007. Acute effects of different warm-up protocols with and without a weighted vest on jumping performance in athletic women. *Journal of Strength and Conditioning Research* 21:52-56.

90. Thompson, W. 2010. *ACSM's resources for the personal trainer.* 3rd ed. Philadelphia: Lippincott, Williams and Wilkins.

91. Thompson, W. 2010. Worldwide survey of fitness trends for 2011. *ACSM's Health and Fitness Journal* 14:8-17.

92. United States Department of Health and Human Services (HHS). *2008 Physical Activity Guidelines for Americans.* www.health.gov/paguidelines.

93. Van der Heijden, G., Z. Wang, Z. Chu, G. Toffolo, E. Manesso, P. Sauer, and A. Sunehag. 2010. Strength exercise improves muscle mass and hepatic insulin sensitivity in obese youth. *Medicine and Science in Sports and Exercise* 42:1973-1980.

94. Williams, M., W. Haskell, P. Ades, E. Amsterdam, V. Bittner, B. Franklin, M. Gulanick, S. Laing, and K. Stewart. 2007. Resistance exercise in individuals with and without cardiovascular disease: 2007 update. *Circulation* 116:572-584.

95. Williams, M., and K. Stewart. 2009. Impact of strength and resistance training on cardiovascular disease risk factors and outcomes in older adults. *Clinics in Geriatric Medicine* 25:703-714.

96. Wolfe, B., L. Lemura, and P. Cole. 2003. Quantitative analysis of single- vs. multiple-set programs in resistance training. *Journal of Strength and Conditioning Research* 18:35-47.

97. Yamaguchi, T., and K. Ishii. 2005. Effects of static stretching for 30 sec and dynamic stretching on leg power. *Journal of Strength and Conditioning Research* 19:677-683.

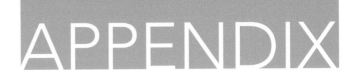

Selected Resistance Training Exercises for the Major Muscle Groups

Leg Press

Prime muscle movers: Quadriceps, gluteus maximus

Exercise technique: The exerciser starts in a sitting position with the knees bent at 90° and the feet placed about shoulder-width apart on the foot pad. The torso should be erect and the back should be pressed against the back of the seat. The participant extends the legs almost completely (without locking the knees) and then slowly returns to the starting position.

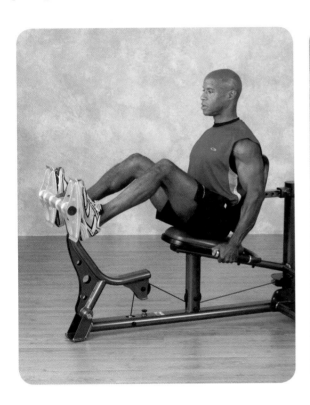
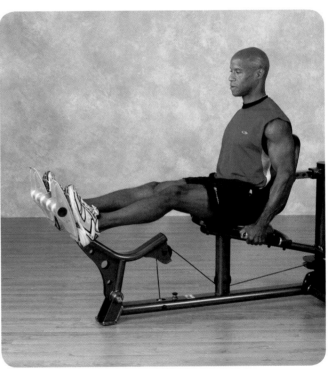

Leg Curl

Prime muscle movers: Hamstrings

Exercise technique: The participant faces the machine with one ankle in front of the pad. After grasping the handles and stabilizing the body, the participant bends the knee to lift the weight. Slowly return to the starting position and repeat the movement. Do not use momentum to complete the lift. After the desired number of repetitions, switch legs.

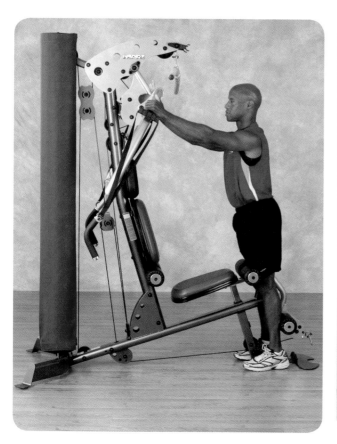 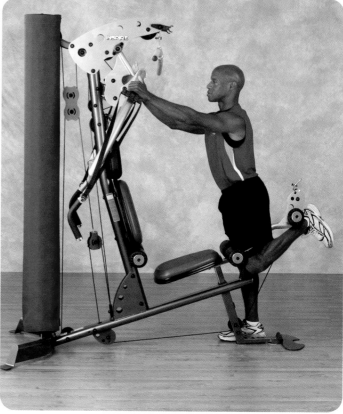

Dumbbell Heel Raise

Prime muscle movers: Gastrocnemius, soleus

Exercise technique: The participant stands, holding a dumbbell in the right hand and placing the left hand on a wall for support. The left foot is lifted off the floor. The participant raises the heel of the right foot as high as possible and then slowly lowers it to the starting position. This exercise should be performed on both sides of the body. The participant should concentrate on keeping the torso and knees straight to avoid upper-leg involvement. To increase the ROM, a 1 to 2 in. (2.5-5.0 cm) board or weight plate can be placed under the ball of the exercising foot. If this is too difficult, the exercise can be performed with both feet on the floor or board.

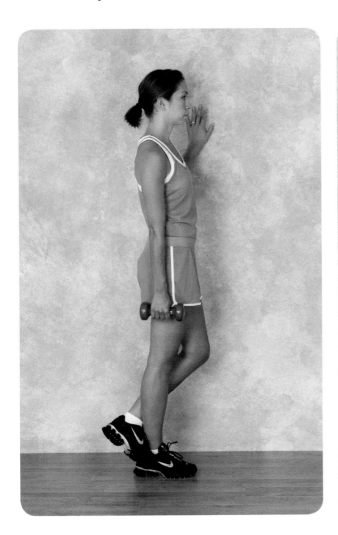
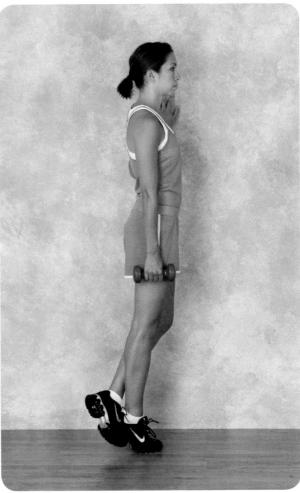

Bench Press

Prime muscle movers: Pectoralis major, anterior deltoid, triceps

Exercise technique: The participant lies flat on the bench and holds the barbell with a wider-than-shoulder-width grip directly above the chest, with arms straight and feet flat on the floor. The participant slowly lowers the barbell to the chest and then presses the barbell back up to the starting position. The barbell should not be bounced on the chest, and a spotter should stand by in case of a failed repetition.

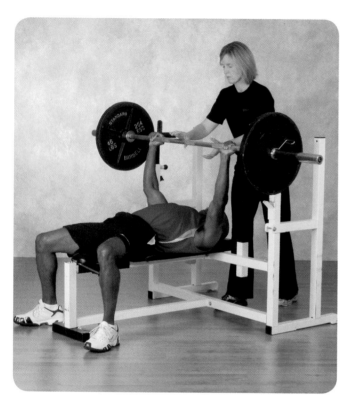 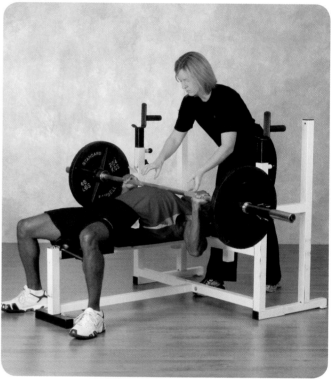

Front Pull-Down

Prime muscle movers: Latissimus dorsi, biceps

Exercise technique: The participant sits on the seat with the arms fully extended, places both knees under the exercise pad, and grips the bar underhand (palms toward the face) using a shoulder-width grip. The participant should lean slightly backward from the waist and maintain this position throughout the duration of the exercise to avoid getting hit by the bar. The bar is pulled down just under the chin and then returned slowly until the arms are fully extended.

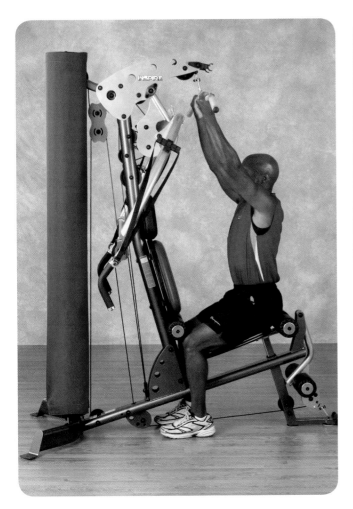
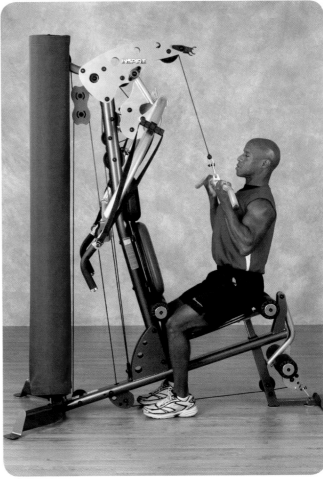

Dumbbell Overhead Press

Prime muscle movers: Deltoids, triceps

Exercise technique: In the standing position, the participant holds a dumbbell in each hand at shoulder level with palms facing forward. The participant presses the weights overhead to a straight-arm position and then slowly returns to the starting position. The participant should not bend or sway the back to complete a repetition.

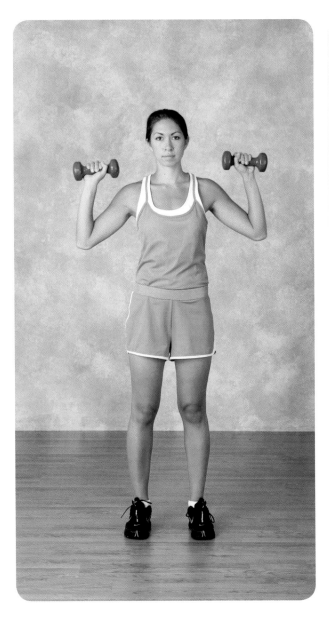
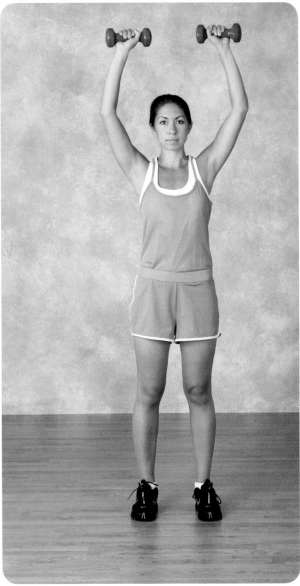

Dumbbell Curl

Prime muscle movers: Biceps

Exercise technique: The participant stands with a dumbbell in each hand (palms facing forward) and the arms at the sides of the body. The participant bends the elbows to bring the weights toward the shoulders and then slowly returns to the starting position. The back should not be bent or swayed to complete a repetition.

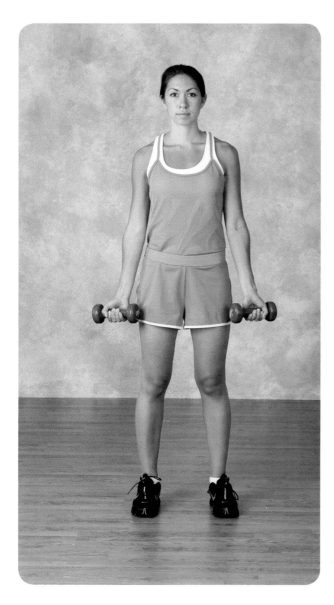 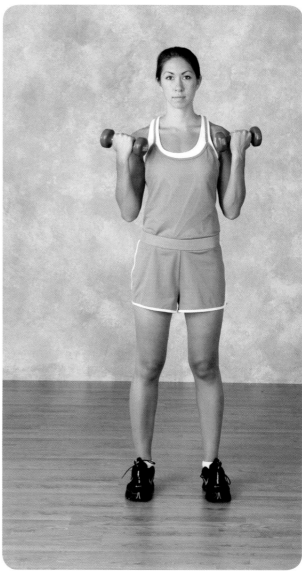

Lying Triceps Extension

Prime muscle movers: Triceps

Exercise technique: The participant lies flat on the back on an exercise bench and holds a dumbbell in each hand with arms straight over shoulders and palms facing each other. The participant lowers both dumbbells to the side of the head by bending only at the elbows and then slowly returns to the starting position. The upper arm should not be swayed to complete a repetition.

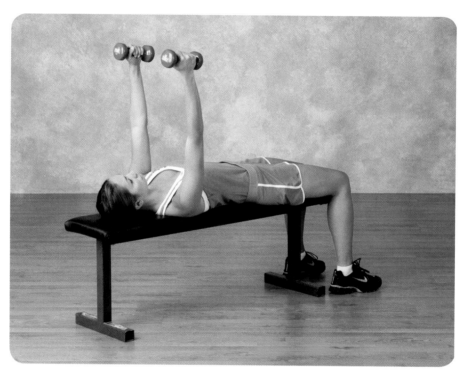

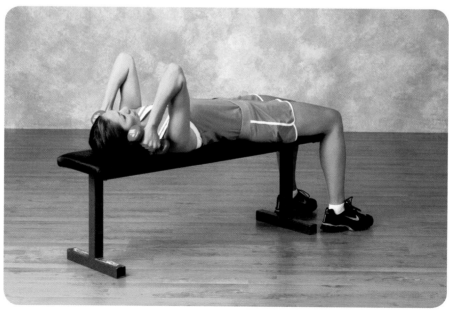

Kneeling Trunk Extension

Prime muscle mover: Erector spinae

Exercise technique: The participant kneels on the floor and supports the body on both hands and knees. The participant extends the right leg backward until it is parallel to the floor, pauses briefly, returns to the starting position, and then extends the left leg backward. To make this exercise more challenging, the participant can raise the left arm parallel to the floor while extending the right leg (and vice versa).

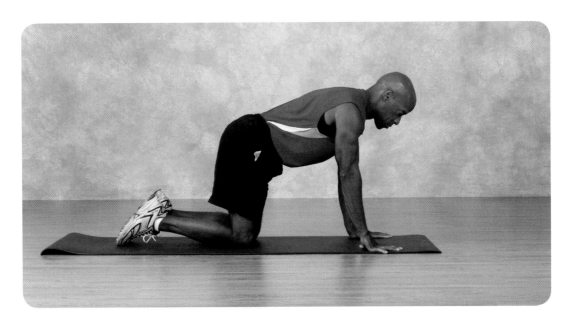

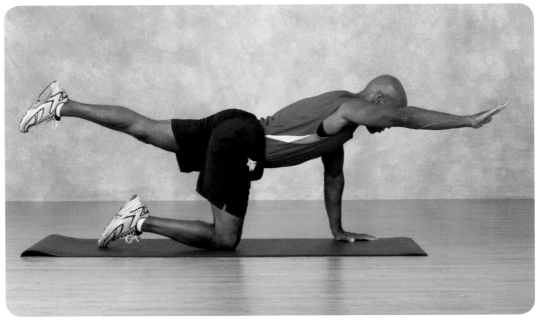

Abdominal Curl

Prime muscle mover: Rectus abdominis

Exercise technique: The participant lies flat on the back with the knees bent, feet about 12 to 15 in. (30.5-38.0 cm) from the buttocks, and hands placed on the thighs (or across the chest). Leading with the chin, the participant lifts the shoulders and upper back off the mat (about 30°-45°) while moving the hands toward the knees, pauses briefly, and then returns to starting position. If the hands are placed behind the head, the participant must not pull the head forward with the hands.

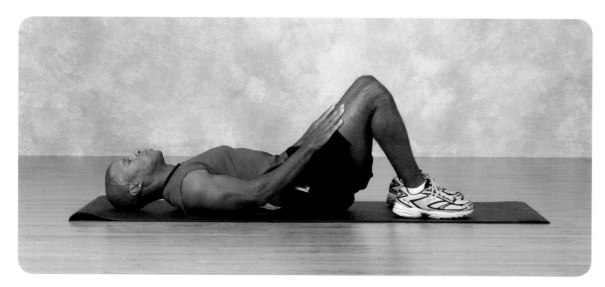

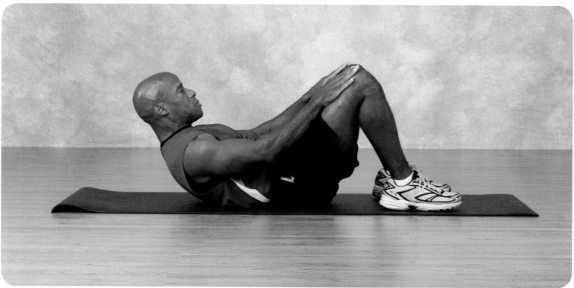

Exercise Prescription for Flexibility and Low-Back Function

Wendell Liemohn

OBJECTIVES

The reader will be able to do the following:

1. Describe motion segments and the shock absorbers of the spine, and explain the role of the facet joints.

2. Differentiate between functional and structural spinal curves and describe limitations that each may impose on exercise programs.

3. Explain why it is important that the muscles of the trunk be able to control pelvic positioning.

4. Differentiate between the low-back problems typically seen in adults and those seen in youth.

5. Describe how the anatomical limitations of ROM should be a factor when prescribing ROM exercises.

6. Identify the components of core stability (CS).

7. Explain how the muscles of the trunk work together as a dynamic corset.

8. Describe exercises that will increase the strength and endurance of muscles that are fundamental to the development of CS.

9. Explain why CS requirements can differ for an office worker and a competitive athlete.

10. Explain why flexibility is important to having a healthy spine.

Low-back pain is one of the most common complaints among adults in the United States; it accounts for more hours lost from work than any other type of occupational injury and is the most frequent cause of activity limitation in people under the age of 45. This chapter begins with a review of select anatomical and biomechanical aspects of the trunk and spine. The types of low-back problems seen in adults versus those seen in young people are then explored. A discussion follows on potential stresses to the spine and how they can produce symptoms related to low-back pain. This is followed by a discussion on core stability (CS). The last section describes exercises that can improve low-back function.

Anatomy of the Spine

The lumbar spine and sacrum are depicted in figure 14.1; their anatomy is important to understanding the spine and low-back pain. When low-back pain is discussed, the fundamental unit of the lumbar spine is the **motion segment**, which consists of two vertebrae and their intervening **disc** (figure 14.2). The bodies of the vertebrae and their intervening disc are sometimes referred to as the *anterior aspect* of the motion segment. The posterior aspect of the motion segment is attached to the anterior aspect by the pedicles; the latter provide the lateral boundary of the foramen (vertical passageway) for the spinal cord and its nerves. In addition to the transverse and spinous processes, the posterior elements of the vertebrae include the superior and inferior articular processes, and each of their junctions is referred to as a *zygapophyseal joint,* or **facet joint**. In addition to assisting in supporting loads on the spine, the

facet joints control the amount and direction of vertebral movement.

A series of ligaments additionally reinforces the vertebrae of the spine. The anterior and posterior longitudinal ligaments provide stability for the anterior portion of the motion segments; they run the length of the spine on the anterior and posterior surfaces of the bodies of the vertebrae as well as the intervertebral discs. The ligaments that support the posterior aspect of the motion segment include the

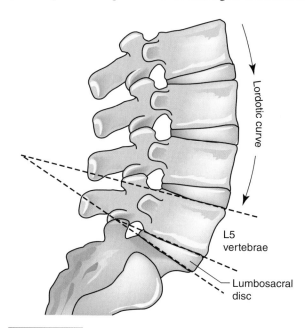

FIGURE 14.1 The lordotic curve is a result of the wedge shapes of the lumbosacral disc and the L5 vertebra.

Adapted, by permissions, from W. Liemohn, 2001, *Exercise prescription and the back* (New York, NY: McGraw-Hill), 6. ©The McGraw-Hill Companies.

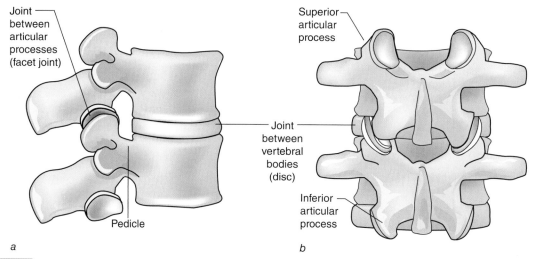

FIGURE 14.2 Lumbar vertebral motion segment. Note how the facet joints (i.e., the junction of the superior and inferior articular processes) are positioned to provide stability and control the amount and direction of movement. Nerves of the lumbar plexus and the sacral plexus exit the spinal cord between the pedicles.

Adapted, by permissions, from W. Liemohn, 2001, *Exercise prescription and the back* (New York, NY: McGraw-Hill), 8. ©The McGraw-Hill Companies.

ligamentum flavum, which is located immediately behind the spinal cord and serves as its posterior boundary. Also reinforcing the posterior aspect of the motion segments are the facet-joint capsular ligaments that span the synovial joints formed by the superior and inferior articular processes between each vertebral pair. The posterior aspects of each motion segment are reinforced further by the interspinous and supraspinous ligaments, which are attached to the spinous processes. All of these ligaments have pain receptors; therefore, a sprain to any of them can signal a potential back problem.

The discs enable each vertebra to be more mobile (figure 14.3). Each intervertebral disc consists of a centrally placed nucleus (nucleus pulposus) surrounded by a sheath of connective-tissue fibers (annulus fibrosis peripherally and

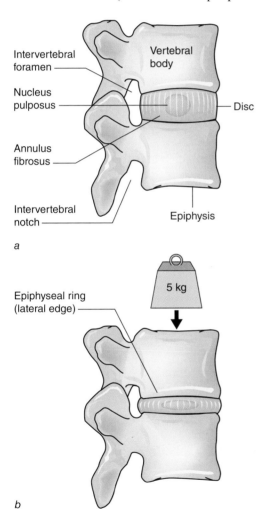

Intervertebral foramen

Vertebral body

Nucleus pulposus

Disc

Annulus fibrosus

Intervertebral notch

Epiphysis

a

Epiphyseal ring (lateral edge)

5 kg

b

FIGURE 14.3 Discs allow flexibility and act as shock absorbers. *(a)* In adults, most low-back problems start in the disc. *(b)* When weight is added (in this case perpendicular to the disc), the force is absorbed in all directions; however, if the external force is applied obliquely, the pressure within the disc is away from the direction of the applied force.

Adapted from Liemohn 2001.

vertebral end plates superiorly and inferiorly), somewhat analogous to a jelly donut (i.e., the central nucleus is the jelly and the peripheral annulus fibrosis and vertebral end plates are the surrounding donut). Intervertebral discs act as spacers and shock absorbers, and when compressive forces are placed on the spine (e.g., when a person carries a load), the nucleus of the disc exerts pressure in all directions to help absorb the force. Force absorption can also be transferred from the nucleus pulposus through the vertebral end plates into the trabeculae of adjacent vertebrae.

The disc most vulnerable to injury in the low back is the one between the fifth lumbar vertebra and the sacrum (the L5-S1 disc). Its load is greater than that of any other disc. The disc that is the second most often injured in the low back is the one between L4 and L5. Except for their periphery, the discs do not have pain receptors; however, if the nucleus of a disc breaks through its normal boundaries (e.g., distends or ruptures its annulus), the peripheral pain receptors of the disc will respond. (The pain receptors in the ligaments of the spine can also quickly tell the body when something is wrong in a ligament or in an adjacent damaged disc that exceeds its normal confines.) If a disc is diseased or injured, its ability to withstand stress is adversely affected and the motion segment to which it belongs may become unstable. (Note that disc pathology also occurs in the cervical spine. Although there can be traumatic causes, poor sitting posture such as forward bending of the neck can contribute to this condition.)

The disc is avascular (i.e., without a blood supply), and its nutrition is enhanced by motion in the spine (motion enables the disc to absorb nutrients through the vertebral end plates). Long-term bed rest and smoking both decrease nutrition to the disc (3). However, when we sleep, discs imbibe fluid and actually become tighter than they were at the end of the day. For this reason back injuries often occur in the morning, when these fuller discs permit less movement. Thus, slow warm-ups before strenuous exercise or work are especially important in the morning or following sleep.

The curvatures of the spine as viewed from the side are described as **lordotic** when they are concave and **kyphotic** when they are convex; cervical and lumbar curves are normally lordotic and the thoracic curve is kyphotic. Exaggerations of these curves are not desirable. For example, an increased anterior (or forward) pelvic tilt increases the lordotic curve in the lumbar area, which increases the stresses on ligaments, discs, vertebrae, and the musculature of the spine. A small lumbar lordotic curve is natural and, along with the cervical lordosis and thoracic kyphosis, assists the discs in cushioning compressive forces occurring in the spine during ADLs. The neutral spine concept is based on a balance of these curves. Although some believe that an excessive lordosis is a risk factor for low-back pain, not all research supports this contention. Factors such as being overweight, wearing high heels, and lacking appropriate muscle length or strength can affect the degree of lordosis. Tightness in the hip flexors (i.e., the psoas) can increase the lordotic curve by causing an anterior pelvic tilt; conversely, tightness in the hamstrings can reduce the lordosis (see figure 10.6).

KEY POINT

The fundamental unit of the spine is the motion segment, which consists of two vertebrae and their intervening disc. The spinal discs absorb shock to the vertebral column by exerting pressure in all directions. Most back problems begin in the disc, and the disc most often injured is the one between L5 and S1. Natural curvatures of the spine assist the discs in cushioning compressive forces. Although the facet joints aid in supporting loads, one of their primary responsibilities is controlling the amount and direction of spinal movement, such as that seen in rotation.

Spinal Movement

Chapter 10 provides a general review of constraints on spinal movement. This section discusses flexion, spinal curvature, extension, and lateral movement. First, a few general points should be raised. McGill (21) contends that there is little quantitative data supporting the contention that trunk flexibility is important to back health. Further-

more, he contends that exercises such as bringing the knees to the chest (from supine) to toe touches (from standing) are silly stretches and can be detrimental to spine health. Moreover, Biering-Sorensen (4) pointed out that greater spine mobility is associated with some spine problems. Nevertheless, there is general agreement that most successful programs emphasize stabilization exercises with a neutral spine, and to facilitate the latter, one must have good mobility at both the hip and knee joints.

Flexion

The flexion movements seen in curl-up exercises are discussed in chapter 3. In these exercises, each lumbar vertebra rotates from its backward tilted position to a neutral or **end-ROM** position (i.e., the lumbar spine straightens). After the lumbar spine is straightened, no further spinal flexion can take place (see figure 10.4). If a curl-up movement is continued until a full sit-up position is reached, the movement must occur at the hip joint; then the muscles crossing this joint (i.e., psoas and iliacus) are the prime movers as the abdominal muscles contract statically. The drawbacks to this type of movement are discussed later in this chapter.

Functional and Structural Spinal Curves

Spinal curves are **functional** if the curve can be removed by assuming a posture that takes away the force responsible for the curve. Figure 14.4 shows how leg posture affects the

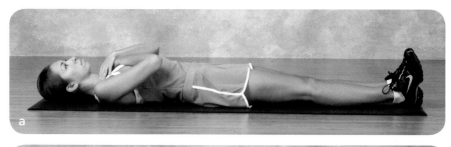

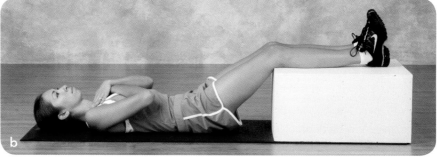

FIGURE 14.4 (a) When the supine posture is assumed, the pull of the psoas muscle can produce an exaggerated lordotic curve. (b) When the legs are supported, the psoas relaxes and the lordotic curve flattens if it is a functional curve. However, if the lordosis is a structural curve, a curve similar to that seen in (a) would be seen in (b) despite the absence of muscle tension.

pull of the psoas musculature on the lumbar spine (figure 14.4a); when the paired psoas are relaxed (figure 14.4b), the lordotic curve is reduced. Habitually tight hip flexors, however, can cause an anterior tilt of the pelvis and thus reduce ROM at the hip joint. If this happens, a functional curve may eventually become **structural**; such curves can result from assuming an unhealthy posture over several years. A structural curve is not easy to straighten. For example, if the individual in figure 14.4b had a structural lumbar lordosis, the lordotic curve would be retained even if the legs were supported.

A person with a structural lumbar lordosis would have extreme difficulty performing crunches due to lack of mobility in the **lumbosacral area**. Although this person might be able to do sit-ups by using the hip flexors while the feet are held down, this motion could exacerbate the problem. It would be far better for the fitness professional to provide a substitute abdominal exercise such as iso-metric holds.

Extension

As discussed in chapter 10, spinal extension movements and postures are not used as often as spinal flexion ones in most ADLs; therefore, it should not be any surprise that, with aging, there is often a greater loss in extension ROM than in flexion ROM. For example, an individual sitting for many hours each day at a desk often assumes a slumping posture for much of this time, and an increase in thoracic kyphosis and rounded shoulders and a decrease in the lumbar curve might result from continuing poor postures (see figure 10.1a). If this person does not extend the spine or retract the shoulders periodically, the capability of doing these movements may decrease and the poor posture may become structural. Moreover, sitting postures can be more stressful on the spine than standing postures because the lordotic curve is often diminished. For example, people may hang on their ligaments (i.e., the posterior ligaments of the lumbar and thoracic spine) or use the back musculature to hold this posture (figure 10.1a) or sit with a balanced posture (10.1b). Most individuals spend much more time sitting, whether at a desk, at a work station, or in a vehicle, than they do standing. The end result is that greater com-pressive forces can be placed on intervertebral discs if the lumbar curve is not maintained. Keeping the spine in a neutral position (e.g., midway between maximum flexion and extension) is much more desirable; many CS training activities emanate from this position.

Lateral Flexion and Rotation

Because some of the most forceful stresses placed on the discs occur during movements that combine bending and rotation, exercises involving these movements should always be done under muscle control. In other words, exercises involving intervertebral movement should *not*

be ballistic (e.g., movements in which momentum plays a major role). If the movement results from momentum rather than muscle control, normal end-ROM may be exceeded and connective-tissue structures such as spinal ligaments or discs may be damaged. As mentioned, one can be particularly vulnerable at the beginning of the day since the discs imbibe tissue fluid while recumbent in sleeping postures, resulting in tighter discs that are more vulnerable to sprain or other injury.

Lateral Curvatures

When the spine is viewed from the back, ideally a straight vertical line is seen; however, minor lateral deviations are prevalent and may relate to something so nominal as hand dominance. (Figure 10.4 presents a screening test that may help determine if a scoliosis is present). Therapeutic exer-cise alone is not very effective in correcting major lateral curves (e.g., scoliosis); moreover, inappropriate exercise prescription can worsen a scoliotic condition. Therefore, it is imperative that fitness professionals obtain advice from a physical therapist, a physiatrist, an orthopedic surgeon, or other appropriate medical personnel before prescrib-ing exercises in an attempt to correct a scoliotic curve. In young people with a scoliosis, bracing is the mainstay of nonoperative therapy. However, because bracing is not always effective for young people and rarely is effective for adults, internal fixation devices may be implanted surgically (6). The exercise program for patients who have a scoliosis and either external bracing or internal fixation would have to incorporate the limitations that either device places on ROM and general mobility. It is imperative that the fitness professional get advice from an appropriate medical source before prescribing exercises for someone who has scoliosis.

KEY POINT

Functional curves can be removed by assuming a posture that reduces the force that caused the curve. Structural curves usually develop over several years and are not easily removed.

Mechanics of the Spine and the Hip Joint

For this discussion, refer to figures 10.4 and 10.5. As shown in figure 10.5, the muscles crossing the hip joint can be viewed as guy-wires bracing the pelvis. If any of these guy-wires are too tight, the abdominal musculature has difficulty controlling pelvic positioning. The person in figure 10.5 is displaying a good neutral spine posture, in which the convex curves in the thoracic and sacral areas are balanced by the concave curves in the cervical and lumbar areas. Energy expenditure is minimal because body segments are in balance. If the convex and concave curves were not in balance, the individual in the figure would have to contract the muscles more and hang on the ligaments (e.g., if head were tilted forward).

Because the sacrum (in the pelvis) is the foundation for the 24 vertebrae stacked on it, pelvic positioning is important to the integrity of the spine. Tightness in the hamstrings can severely affect the ability of the pelvis to tilt anteriorly and thus can diminish pelvic ROM. If the body subsequently is subjected to an unplanned stress (e.g., stepping in a hole or slipping on ice), body parts are obligated to give with the resulting force. If the hamstrings cannot give, connective-tissue structures of the spine may have to absorb the stress. Tightness of the hip flexors, although not apt to occur concurrently with tightness of the hamstrings, can also be detrimental to low-back function. If there is tearing or other damage to spinal ligaments, discs, or both, a step toward an acute low-back problem has been made. A shortened IT band or a tightened piriformis also might create a problem; however, it has been contended that piriformis syndrome is usually caused by other pathology (31). More in-depth discussions of biomechanical stresses to the spine appear elsewhere (2, 5, 14, 20, 25, 26, 29-31).

KEY POINT

The pelvis serves as the foundation for the spine, so the ability of the trunk muscles to control pelvic positioning is essential for maintaining a neutral spine and a healthy back. If either the hip flexors or hip extensors are too tight, posture may be compromised.

Low-Back Pain: A Repetitive Motion Injury

Even though some people might remember a specific movement that they believe caused their low-back problem, this is not generally the case. Rather, the analogy of the straw that breaks the camel's back usually describes the occurrence of a **low-back problem**.

Low-Back Problems in Adults

It has been contended that most cases of acute low-back pain in adults are caused by damage to the intervertebral discs (8). However, one incorrect movement seldom causes injury to a disc. Low-back pain such as a disc injury typically is caused by a succession of inappropriate movements occurring over time; because of this, low-back pain often is called a *repetitive microtrauma condition* or a *repetitive motion injury*.

If you take a paper clip and bend it once, it is still quite strong; however, its molecular makeup has changed and it will never be the same again. The paper clip can be further bent and remain strong, but with each successive bend it becomes weaker, and with continual bending it eventually breaks. Similarly, if you use poor biomechanics to lift an object, the one poor maneuver is not apt to cause a back problem. If these poor biomechanics are repeated hundreds of times, however, connective-tissue structures of the spine can weaken and eventually yield to even a nominal stress (e.g., bending to the floor to pick up a paper clip). It might not be until this time that acute symptoms are noted.

Cumulative repetitive microtrauma affects the homeostasis of the disc, and eventually it adversely alters the disc's pivotal responsibility as a shock absorber of the spinal unit. For example, minor tears in the periphery of the disc can be painful and can forewarn of more serious problems. Bogduk (5) suggests that injuries such as these are comparable to spraining an ankle. However, if the jelly-like nucleus leaks out of its normal confines through the annulus fibrosis (or the vertebral end plates), an unstable motion segment could result. This process is analogous to a radial tire losing air pressure and thus negatively affecting cornering ability. When a disc is affected, specific movements may be exceedingly painful and exceed normal ROM, and the condition is apt to worsen without appropriate intervention. Thus, what started as a minor problem can evolve into a major one. The key is to never let the problem get started. Maintaining good physical fitness and strengthening the trunk musculature with appropriate exercises can help maintain a neutral spine posture and decrease the chances of having low-back pain.

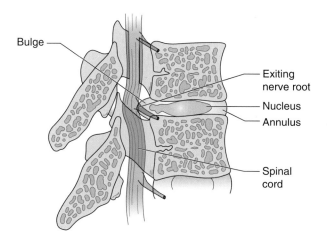

FIGURE 14.5 A herniated disc is shown between two lumbar vertebra. As depicted, this herniation can affect the nerve exiting at this level as well as compress other nerves passing to lower levels.

Reprinted, by permission, from S.J. Shultz, P.H. Houglum, and D.H. Perrin, 2010, *Examination of musculoskeletal injuries,* 3rd ed. (Champaign, IL: Human Kinetics), 198.

Low-Back Problems in Youth

In young people, low-back problems are not typically seen in the disc but rather in the part of the vertebrae posterior to the spinal cord, including the superior and inferior articular processes (refer to figure 14.2). The part of a vertebra between the superior and inferior articular processes is called the **pars interarticularis**. Stress to this area can lead to complications such as **spondylolysis** and **spondylolisthesis** (figure 14.6). The former condition is essentially a stress fracture in the pars interarticularis on one side; sometimes it evolves into a frank (complete) fracture on both sides of a spinous process, either because the bone does not unite properly or because it fails to withstand the stress to which it is subjected. Then the condition is called *spondylolisthesis,* and the body of the vertebra above may displace anteriorly over the vertebra below. This injury usually occurs at the lumbosacral junction (i.e., L5 slips over S1).

Although the causes of spondylolisthesis might be genetic, stresses resulting from activities such as weightlifting or gymnastics could also be the cause. Appropriate coaching and guidance in youth athletic activities are important for avoiding unhealthy stresses on growing bones. Not all cases of spondylolysis and spondylolisthesis necessarily begin before skeletal maturity. Although the exact age of onset might be unknown, spondylolisthesis is seen in professional football players (28) and has also been cited as the most likely cause of low-back pain in patients under 26 yr of age; however, it is rarely the sole cause of low-back pain in people over 40 (6).

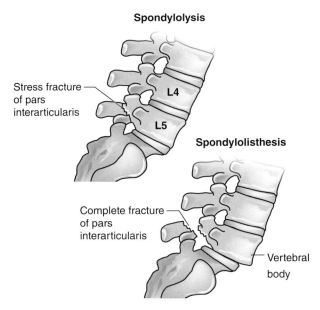

Spondylolysis

Stress fracture of pars interarticularis

L4

L5

Spondylolisthesis

Complete fracture of pars interarticularis

Vertebral body

FIGURE 14.6 In spondylolysis, there is a stress fracture of the pars interarticularis on only one side. In spondylolisthesis, there is a bilateral fracture of the pars accompanied by an anterior displacement of the vertebral body.

Repetitive hyperextension can also damage the facet joints. These are synovial joints and their articular cartilage can be subject to injury in this type of movement. Although this type of stress to tissue may happen in young people, damage to articular cartilage could eventually lead to arthritic problems.

KEY POINT

Low-back pain is often referred to as a *repetitive microtrauma* or *repetitive motion injury* because its development occurs over time as opposed to resulting from one traumatic incident. Low-back problems in adults usually originate in the disc; if low-back problems occur in young people, they usually originate in the posterior elements of the vertebrae.

Exercise Considerations: Preventive and Therapeutic

Although CS training is often used to train athletes to better perform in their particular sports, CS is also emphasized in low-back pain prevention and in therapeutic programs. For example, stepped-up versions of therapeutic exercises often can be used as prophylactic (preventive) exercises. Ideally ROM, strength, or both should be improved before their deficiencies cause a problem.

Range of Motion and Low-Back Function

As discussed in chapter 10, ROM deficiencies at the hip joint may be viewed as a prognostic indicator of low-back pain. Although lack of ROM in the spine is less apt to causally relate to low-back pain, a negative correlation has been seen between excessive flexibility of the spine and subsequent back injuries (22).

As displayed in figure 3.9, a limited degree of spinal mobility in the sagittal plane (e.g., flexion, extension) and the coronal plane (e.g., lateral flexion) is present in the cervical and lumbar segments. Although rotation is restricted in the lumbar and thoracic regions, a considerable amount is present in the cervical region, particularly between C1 and C2.

Spinal extension is often ignored or misinterpreted in exercise programs. Although it is acknowledged that ballistic extension (and ballistic rotation) are totally inappropriate, as discussed in chapter 10, slow and controlled extension movements are appropriate and should be included in exercise programs. People who avoid exercise and have an occupation that requires little in the way of movement are destined to lose ROM at a much faster rate than comparable individuals who exercise or who are in an occupation that demands mobility. People who do not participate in strength training, ROM training, or other physical activity on a regular basis are going to experience deficits in both parameters commensurate with the lifestyle chosen.

Core Stability

The trunk is sometimes referred to as the *core* of the body, and the musculature of the spine and the abdominal wall is positioned to contribute to CS, also called *spinal stabilization*. CS has received much attention in recent years; in addition to core strength, it includes core coordination and endurance. CS results when the passive structures of the spinal column (i.e., the vertebrae, discs, rib cage, pelvis, and all associated connective tissue) are stabilized by the active component (i.e., the musculature). The efficacy of functionally progressive CS exercises was compared with manually applied physical therapy in 160 patients with chronic low-back disorder (11). Data were collected after the 6 mo training programs and also 2 yr after intervention. The CS subjects had a significantly greater reduction in both pain and dysfunction symptoms than those subjects receiving manually applied physical therapy; the latter group did, however, perform better than the 40 controls who received an educational booklet.

Good CS can enhance performance in athletic as well as work-related activities. The CS requirements for an athlete (e.g., football player) obviously far exceed the CS requirements for a person in a sedentary job. The former needs much more strength; however, both the athlete and the office worker require coordination and endurance commensurate with the requirements of the activities in which they participate.

The large muscles of the spine that contribute to CS include the erector spinae, multifidus, and quadratus lumborum (see figure 14.7). The other trunk muscles that contribute to CS include the rectus abdominis, internal and external obliques, transversus abdominis, and quadratus lumborum. The importance of the transversus abdominis and the quadratus lumborum in CS has been emphasized in the past few years (5, 9, 12, 13, 21). Again we can use the concept of guy-wires. In this case the larger muscles located more peripherally are in a position to react to greater turning moments to which the body is subjected as in contact sports or work-related activity; collectively, these muscles strive to keep the spine in a relatively neutral position.

There are some extremely small muscles that are close to the spinal column; these include the intertransversarii mediales, interspinales, and rotatores. Even though anatomy books present specific actions for each, their small physiologic cross-sectional area doubtfully enables any significant contribution to movement. However, Nitz and Peck (24) state that these muscles have a much richer density of muscle spindles (4.5-7.3 times more) than the multifidus. Bogduk (5) and McGill (23) contend that these muscles can act as vertebral position sensors and play a vital role in maintaining core stability by providing

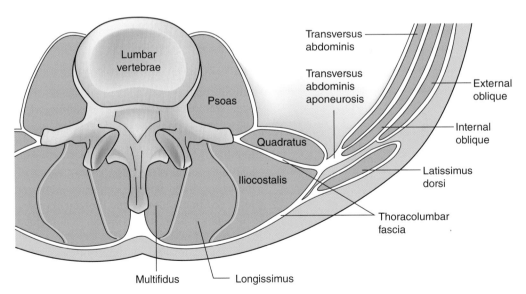

FIGURE 14.7 Cross section of the major muscles of the trunk that contribute to CS. Note how the transversus abdominis (TA) attaches to the connective-tissue sheath that houses the erector spinae (iliocostalis and longissimus) and multifidus; with the obliques, the TA envelops the rectus abdominis anteriorly as its sides meet at the linea alba. Although the internal oblique also attaches to this sheath, its attachment is narrow and hence it cannot exert as much of a lateral stabilizing force (hoop tension) as the TA exerts.

feedback on the amount of contraction needed by other muscles. The contention that coordination is important to CS has also been supported by other research (1, 7, 12).

Although much literature indicts weakened abdominal musculature as a prime cause of low-back pain, the musculature of the spine is proportionately weaker than the abdominal musculature in low-back patients, particularly in terms of endurance (4, 20). This notwithstanding, the strength of the abdominal muscles is also vital to a healthy spine; therefore, the exercises that are discussed later include strengthening exercises for all the major trunk muscles believed to be important for CS.

Exercises Involving Core Muscles

One CS exercise that has gained popularity in recent years both as a therapeutic exercise in the clinic as well as an exercise that can be used in conditioning programs is the quadruped (see figure 14.8). Although it is not considered a challenging strength-building exercise for the back musculature, it can improve the endurance of these important muscles; moreover, the compression force that it places on the discs is only about 30% of MVC (22). When the contralateral limbs are raised, the quadruped exercise becomes more difficult and requires additional bracing; this raises

the MVC of the extensors about 10%, but the contraction is unilateral. However, the lateral abdominal muscles are also active if the exercise is performed correctly (i.e., the trunk is virtually motionless and the hips and shoulders are kept level—good technique cannot be overemphasized). This exercise, as well as many other CS exercises, can be made more challenging by performing it on a stability ball (10, 17, 18, 22). For example, performing the crunch on a stability ball involves the lateral abdominal muscles much more than if the same exercise were done on a mat.

A muscle of the spine that once received little emphasis but now is deemed important to spine function and core stability is the quadratus lumborum (see figure 14.9). Because its origin is on the posterior part of the iliac crest and the iliolumbar ligament and its insertion is on the last rib and the transverse processes of the upper four lumbar vertebrae, it is well positioned to stabilize (i.e., control forces to which the body is subjected) the core in the frontal plane. McGill (22) contends that contraction of the quadratus lumborum is virtually isometric. An exercise that develops not only the quadratus lumborum but also the lateral abdominal muscles is the horizontal isometric bridge (see appendix at the end of this chapter). Because this exercise involves only nominal contraction of the psoas, it does not place much compressive pressure on the intervertebral discs of the lumbar vertebrae (figure 14.9); moreover, it emphasizes both strength and endurance.

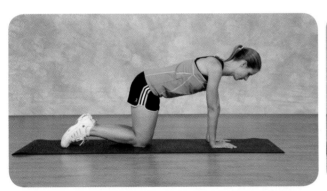
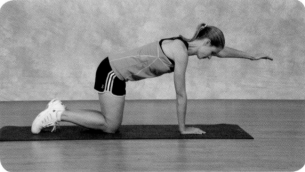
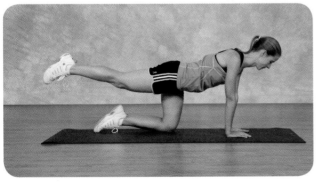
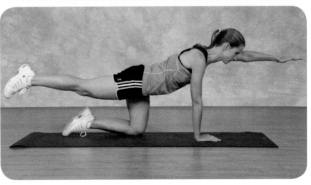

FIGURE 14.8 The quadruped exercise strengthens abdominal, buttocks, and back muscles. The progression begins by first raising the arms (unilaterally). When the exerciser can perform this while keeping other body parts motionless, the legs can be raised alternately. The most difficult exercise of this sequence is raising the contralateral limbs while keeping other body parts motionless.

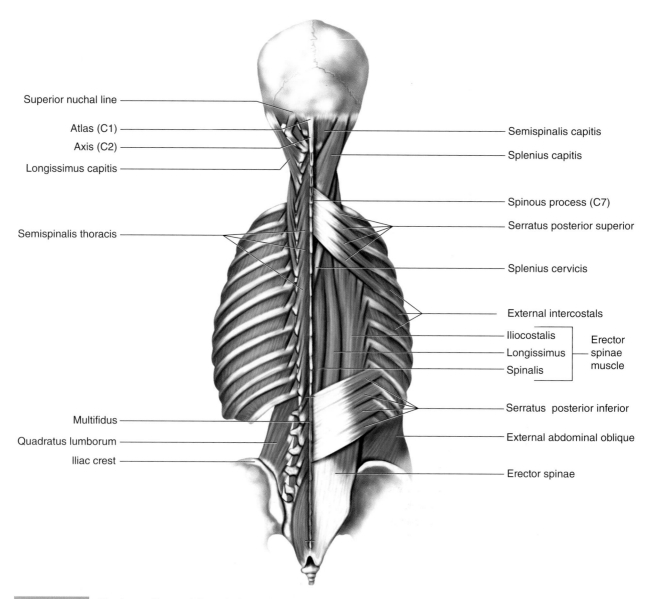

FIGURE 14.9 The inner fibers of the quadratus lumborum are positioned to control movement of the lumbar vertebrae in the frontal plane; this control is important to having a healthy back. (The fibers of the psoas, not pictured, run laterally to the lumber vertebrae on each side; and by their insertion on the lessor trochanters of each femur, are aligned to exert strong compression forces on the lumbar intervertebral discs in select abdominal strengthening exercises. Some of these exercises can be detrimental to the discs and to low-back functioning.)

Reprinted from R. Behnke, 2006, *Kinetic anatomy,* 2nd ed. (Champaign, IL: Human Kinetics).

Another common exercise for developing spinal musculature is back extension on the Roman chair. In a review of research on exercise intervention for chronic low-back pain in which randomized, controlled trial designs were followed, only three studies were found, and each emphasized development of extensor muscles of the spine with the use of this equipment (16). This is a difficult exercise because it can place a compressive force on the intervertebral discs that exceeds 53% of MVC (21); however, in the studies we reviewed, each patient's exercise period was closely monitored by a physical therapist (16). A modification of this equipment, called the *variable-angle Roman chair,* is appropriate for people who are too weak to use a regular Roman chair, have an acute low-back pain condition, or are recovering from surgery. When undertaking trunk extension exercises to develop back extensor muscle strength, exercisers should never exceed their normal lordosis when doing the trunk raise (i.e., the exerciser should not hyperextend the spine). However, depending on the specific diagnosis of the spine malady, extension-biased exercises might be appropriate for one diagnosis and contraindicated for another.

RESEARCH INSIGHT

CS is dependent upon coordination as well as strength. This makes it a difficult construct to measure because with the coordination element, scores could be expected to improve with practice before becoming consistent. In our first research (15) in this area, we used four balance activities that could be performed on an old stability platform designed to measure standing balance. For two of the four tests, stability reliability was high (>0.90). After seeing our research, Lafayette Instrument Company provided us with a prototype stability platform that was computer driven and large enough to permit any subject to assume the quadruped position (see figure 14.10). In research using this platform (19), we administered the quadruped test with alternate arm raises that the San Francisco Spine Institute used in their Dynamic Lumbar Stabilization Program (27). Although stability reliability coefficients were again high (0.85), we found that 3 days of testing were required since there was nominal improvement in balance scores from testing days 2 and 3. In 2008, Hibbs (12) stated that there is no gold standard for measuring CS; our test would appear to warrant consideration.

KEY POINT

CS training is now emphasized in most low-back training as well as in rehabilitation programs; many CS exercises also emphasize coordination. Lack of strength and endurance in the back musculature is often seen in people with low-back pain, and the back musculature often is proportionately weaker than the abdominal musculature. In part, this might be attributable to neglecting extensor muscle strength in exercise programs. When performing dynamic extension exercises, the participant should not exceed the normal lumbar lordosis. Some of the exercises designed to improve the strength and endurance of the spinal muscles are also good exercises for the lateral abdominal muscles.

Exercises Involving the Abdominal Wall

Even though the back musculature may be disproportionately weaker in people with low-back pain, it is still imperative that the abdominal muscles not be neglected. For example, the rectus abdominis is in a position to directly control the tilt of the pelvis (figure 10.5), an important consideration in maintaining a healthy spine. The rectus abdominis is emphasized in crunch-type activities. When performing these activities, it is only necessary to lift the shoulders off the exercise surface. It is critical to minimize the role of the hip flexors (e.g., the paired psoas) in any trunk flexion exercise, particularly for people who are less fit. Many people believe that bending the knees reduces the role of the psoas muscles, but this is not so, particularly if the feet are supported (e.g., held by another person). Moreover, the psoas muscles place extreme compressive forces on the discs of the lumbar-motion segments of the vertebral column in activities such as sit-ups or bilateral leg lifts (2, 14).

Posterior rotation of the pelvis is often incorporated into abdominal strengthening exercises, but for someone with disc disease, it is not always appropriate. Posterior rotation of the pelvis typically removes the lumbar lordosis, and such movement can prompt the nucleus of the intervertebral disc to migrate posteriorly. If the disc is damaged, pressure can be placed on the damaged tissue and its pain receptors or even on spinal nerves. McGill (22) suggests that to rectify this potential problem, the exerciser should keep one leg extended while bending the contralateral knee and should place the palm of one hand on the exercise surface under the lumbar lordotic curve (i.e., the small of the back).

In standard crunch-type activities, the rectus abdominis does most of the work. The lateral abdominal muscles (i.e.,

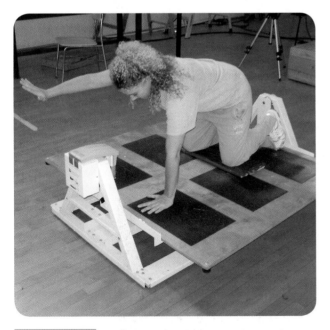

FIGURE 14.10 In our CS test, only the arms were alternately raised rhythmically as the subject attempted to maintain balance. Although this is not an easy task on a stability platform, it is the easiest of the quadruped exercise series when performed on a mat or the floor.

transversus abdominis, internal and external obliques) also should be developed because they can enhance the anterior and posterior muscle groups due to their attachments. Because strong lateral abdominal muscles can brace and corset the trunk, they can help prevent undesirable rotary motion in addition to protecting the back as heavy objects are lifted. From a biomechanical perspective, the lateral abdominal muscles are vital to attain and maintain a healthy low back.

Exercises that enhance the lateral musculature also include diagonal crunches and isometrics. Besides doing the diagonal curl dynamically, the participant can perform it isometrically by using challenging isometric holds (e.g., holds lasting 5-30 sec). Although isometric exercises may be considered passé for limb movements because they lack specificity of training, in reality isometrics are most specific to the stabilization of the spine (23). The horizontal isometric side bridge is also an excellent exercise. Strong lateral abdominal muscles make it much easier to stabilize and brace the spine, and people with a strong core will be much less susceptible to the repetitive microtrauma that can lead to serious cases of low-back pain.

Two excellent studies discussed trunk flexion exercises from a cost–benefit perspective (2, 14). In essence, these studies determined the %MVC of select muscles used in common abdominal strengthening activities. Concurrently they determined either indirectly or directly the amount of compressive force each exercise placed on intervertebral discs, which indicates psoas activity. Ideally, there should be a high %MVC of the abdominal muscles, which would be a benefit. However, a high level of psoas activity would be a cost because the paired psoas can put an extreme amount of compressive force on the spine and damage the discs. The strengthening exercises for trunk flexion presented in the appendix of this chapter were selected because the MVC of the psoas was found to be relatively low and the MVC of one or more of the abdominal muscles was high (14). However, another consideration should be factored

into exercise selection: the client's physical fitness level. Some exercises may benefit athletes in excellent condition but harm nonathletes; thus, sometimes the quality of the movement should be considered along with the physical condition of the exerciser.

Prophylactic Exercises for Enhancing Low-Back Function

Even though many injuries and diseases of the low back can be treated conservatively with therapeutic exercise, the diversity and complexity of low-back problems are such that they preclude making a simple diagnosis and presenting an exercise regimen for that diagnosis. Moreover, arming a person with a set of therapeutic exercises when the person does not concurrently understand the nuances of various low-back conditions could be dangerous. Because it is beyond the scope of this chapter to discuss these countless nuances, the emphasis in this discussion is on sound exercises that enhance low-back function. Nevertheless, the exercises in the appendix are often used by physical therapists in treating low-back patients. For in-depth information on this subject, many other sources are available (2, 8, 10, 14, 16-18, 21, 22, 25, 29, 31).

Exercises to Enhance Flexibility

The appendix of this chapter describes exercises recommended for low-back flexibility. The guy-wire concept discussed in chapter 10 (see figure 10.5) is helpful to consider when exploring exercises for low-back flexibility. Although the trunk musculature (e.g., the abdominal muscles and the erector spinae) is crucial to controlling pelvic positioning, the ability to control the pelvis may be reduced or negated if either the hip flexors or the hip extensors are too tight. The bottom line is that good hip mobility is fundamental to having a healthy spine; ideally any disparities between the left and right hip joints with respect to ROM (and strength) are nominal. Several exercises that can be used to improve ROM in joints and structures relevant to the low back are presented in the appendix.

Exercises to Develop Trunk Musculature

Although by no means all inclusive, the appendix of this chapter also describes exercises recommended for developing the musculature of the trunk. A key point to remember with spinal extension movements is that exercisers should not exceed their normal lumbar lordosis when moving into extension.

Posterior pelvic tilts and crunches are common exercises for developing the abdominal musculature. As previously mentioned, when individuals do these exercises, the rectus abdominis often does most of the work and the lateral abdominal muscles are minimally involved.

KEY POINT

In people with low-back problems, the back musculature often is proportionately weaker and has less endurance than the abdominal musculature has; in part, this might be attributable to neglect of the extensor muscles in exercise programs. When trained, the trunk musculature works together as a dynamic corset as the lateral abdominal muscles tie together the flexors and extensors of the spine to facilitate a strong core. Although the erector spinae, multifidus, and rectus abdominis are important trunk muscles, the lateral abdominal muscles and the quadratus lumborum warrant special attention to develop a strong core.

KEY POINT

Maintenance of hip ROM is essential for a healthy spine. An exerciser should not exceed the normal lordotic curve when doing active back extension exercises. The ROM capabilities of the trunk are nominal, which should be kept in mind when setting up exercise programs for clients. Isometric holds can nicely supplement regular crunches and diagonal crunches.

KEY POINT

The reader should realize that disc pathology also occurs in the cervical spine. Poor sitting posture can contribute to this condition; however, in cervical dysfunction, a motion segment of the neck corresponding to the brachial plexus is the site of the problem rather than the lumbar-sacral plexus.

STUDY QUESTIONS

1. What constitutes a motion segment? What part of the motion segment provides a cushioning element? Which joints of a motion segment are synovial joints?

2. Describe the difference between a structural and a functional spinal curve.

3. Which muscles are important in controlling pelvic position?

4. The low-back problems seen in youth and in adults usually differ. Discuss the major differences.

5. Explain why strength is important to CS.

6. Explain how ROM could affect CS.

7. Teamwork between muscles is important to CS. Give two examples of this teamwork.

8. Although muscles seldom are solely responsible for a movement (i.e., they tend to act as part of a team), describe a good exercise for developing each of the following muscles: quadratus lumborum, rectus abdominis, transversus abdominis, and erector spinae.

9. Explain why CS requirements can differ for an office worker and a competitive athlete.

10. Why is having good flexibility and ROM important to spinal health?

CASE STUDIES

You can check your answers by referring to appendix A.

1. An exercise leader is using a double-leg-lowering task with a group of relatively fit adults, ostensibly to improve the strength of the abdominal muscles. When questioned about the use of this exercise, he advises you that physical therapists have often used a similar activity to test the abdominal strength of their patients, even those who have low-back pain. Discuss the appropriateness or inappropriateness of such an exercise. For whom would it be least appropriate and possibly even contraindicated?

2. An exercise leader is using the sit-and-reach (or standing toe-touch) exercise, presumably to improve hip flexibility. Because she is aware that ballistic stretches are usually contraindicated, she strongly warns her group to perform the exercise with slow and easy stretches. Discuss the appropriateness or inappropriateness of these directions.

3. An exercise leader prescribes oblique (diagonal) curls that require the exerciser to maintain a 15 sec isometric contraction after at least one shoulder blade is raised from the exercise surface. Discuss the appropriateness or inappropriateness of this activity.

REFERENCES

1. Akuthota, V. 2008. Core stability exercise principles. *Current Sports Medicine Reports* 7:39-44.

2. Axler, C.T., and S.M. McGill. 1997. Low back loads over a variety of abdominal exercises: Searching for the safest abdominal challenge. *Medicine and Science in Sports and Exercise* 29(6): 804-811.

3. Battie, M.C., T. Videman, K. Gill, G.B. Moneta, R. Nyman, J. Kaprio, and M. Koskenvut. 1991. Smoking and lumbar

intervertebral disc degeneration: An MRI study of identical twins. *Spine* 16(9): 1015-1021.

4. Biering-Sorensen, F. 1984. Physical measurements as risk indicators for low-back trouble over a one-year period. *Spine* 9(2): 106-119.

5. Bogduk, N. 1998. *Clinical anatomy of the lumbar spine and sacrum.* London: Churchill Livingstone.

6. Borenstein, D.G., and S.W. Wiesel. 1989. *Low back pain—Medical diagnosis and comprehensive management.* Philadelphia: Saunders.

7. Borghuis, J., L. Hof, & K. Lemmink. 2008. The importance of sensory-motor control in providing core stability: Implications for measurement and training. *Sports Medicine* 38:893-916.

8. Cailliet, R. 1988. *Low back pain syndrome.* Philadelphia: Davis.

9. Crisco, J.J., and M.M. Panjabi. 1991. The intersegmental and multisegmental muscles of the spine: A biomechanical model comparing lateral stabilising potential. *Spine* 16(7): 793-799.

10. Fritz, J.M., and G.E. Hicks. 2001. Exercise protocols for low back pain. In *Exercise prescription and the back,* ed. W. Liemohn, 167-181. New York: McGraw-Hill Medical.

11. Goldby, L.J., A.P. Moore, J. Doust, and M.E. Trew. 2006. A randomized controlled trial investigating the efficiency of musculoskeletal physiotherapy on chronic low back disorder. *Spine* 31(10): 1083-1093.

12. Hibbs, A.E. 2008. Optimizing performance by improving core stability and core strength. *Sports Medicine* 38:996-1008.

13. Hodges, P.W. 2003. Core stability exercise in chronic low back pain. *Orthopedic Clinics of North America* 34:245-254.

14. Juker, D., S. McGill, P. Kropf, and T. Steffen. 1998. Quantitative intramuscular myoelectric activity of lumbar portions of psoas and the abdominal wall during a wide variety of tasks. *Medicine and Science in Sports and Exercise* 30(2): 301-310.

15. Liemohn, W.P., T.A. Baumgartner, and L.H. Gagnon. 2005. Measuring core stability. *Journal of Strength Conditioning Research* 19(3): 583-586.

16. Liemohn, W., and L.H. Gagnon. 2001. Efficacy of therapeutic exercise in low back rehabilitation. In *Exercise prescription and the back,* ed. W. Liemohn, 229-240. New York: McGraw-Hill Medical.

17. Liemohn, W., and M. Miller. 2001. Low back pain incidence in sports. In *Exercise prescription and the back,* ed. W. Liemohn, 99-134. New York: McGraw-Hill Medical.

18. Liemohn, W., and G. Pariser. 2002. Core strength: Implications for fitness and low back pain. *ACSM's Health and Fitness Journal* 6(5): 10-16.

19. Liemohn, W.P., T.A. Baumgartner, S.R. Fordham, and A. Srivatsan. 2010. Quantifying core stability: A technical report. *Journal of Strength Conditioning Research* 24(2): 575-579.

20. Luoto, S., M. Heliovaara, H. Hurri, and H. Alaranta. 1995. Static back endurance and the risk of low back pain. *Clinical Biomechanics* 10:323-324.

21. McGill, S. 2002. *Low back disorders: Evidence-based prevention and rehabilitation.* Champaign, IL: Human Kinetics.

22. McGill, S. 2004. *Ultimate back fitness and performance.* Waterloo, ON: Wabuno.

23. McGill, S. 2004. Mechanics and pathomechanics of muscles acting on the lumbar spine. In *Kinesiology: The mechanics and pathomechanics of human movement,* ed. C.A. Oatis, 563-575. Philadelphia: Lippincott Williams & Wilkins.

24. Nitz, A.J., and D. Peck. 1986. Comparison of muscle spindle concentrations in large and small human epaxial muscles acting in parallel combinations. *American Journal of Surgery* 52:273-277.

25. O'Sullivan, P.B., L. Twomey, and G.T. Allison. 1997. Dynamic stabilization of the lumbar spine. *Critical Reviews in Physical and Rehabilitation Medicine* 9(3-4): 315-330.

26. Porterfield, J.A., and C. DeRosa. 1998. *Mechanical low back pain—Perspective in functional anatomy.* Philadelphia: Saunders.

27. San Francisco Spine Institute. 1989. *Dynamic lumbar stabilization program.* San Francisco: San Francisco Spine Institute.

28. Sinaki, M., M.P. Lutness, D.M. Ilstrup, C.P. Chu, and R.R. Gramse. 1989. Lumbar spondylolisthesis: Retrospective comparison and three-year follow-up of two conservative treatment programs. *Archives in Physical Medicine and Rehabilitation* 70(8): 594-598.

29. Waddell, G. 1998. *The back pain revolution.* Edinburgh, UK: Churchill Livingstone.

30. White, A.A., and M.M. Panjabbi. 1990. *Clinical biomechanics of the spine.* Philadelphia: Lippincott Williams & Wilkins.

31. Zuhosky, J.P., and J.L. Young. 2001. Functional physical assessment for low back injuries in the athlete. In *Exercise prescription and the back,* ed. W. Liemohn, 67-88. New York: McGraw-Hill Medical.

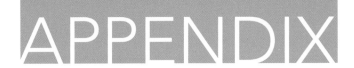

Flexibility, Strength, and Endurance Exercises to Improve Low-Back Function

Stretching Exercises to Maintain and Improve Range of Motion

Although proper stretching should include both upper and lower extremities in addition to the trunk, the exercises presented in the appendix have a direct relationship to low-back function. Following this section is a somewhat more cursory section on additional stretching exercises.

Here are a few guiding principles:

1. The need for proper stretching appears to have a strong relationship to age; however, genotypes do differ.

2. Proper stretching before *and* after activity may help improve ROM, enhance performance, and decrease injuries and postexercise muscle soreness.

3. If a gentle warm-up (e.g., walking, easy jogging) does not precede stretching, it is important to begin the stretching regimen slowly.

4. Stretching to symmetry is particularly important when working with the lower extremities. If you think of the body as a kinetic chain, would not any link out of sync with its left or right counterpart potentially have an impact on a superior link? If the forepart of one foot has a valgus deviation, could not that potentially affect the ankle, knee, hip, and spine? (This is not only relevant to ROM but also to strength.) Upper-extremity deviations tend to be much more forgiving.

5. Do not bounce when stretching or let momentum carry the body part beyond its normal ROM.

6. The muscles that particularly need to be warmed up and stretched are the hamstrings, quadriceps, calves (gastrocnemius and soleus), hip flexors, and shoulder muscles. Of course, for some activities and conditions, other muscle groups would need stretching, too.

7. Hold each stretch for 10 to 30 sec and repeat 3 to 4 times in the exercise session. For problematic areas, repeated sessions may be desired.

Hip Flexor Stretch (Standing)

The participant grasps the contralateral ankle and raises the leg while keeping the trunk straight as the foot is pulled toward the buttocks (the free hand may be placed against the wall or other support if desired) *(a)*. Note incorrect technique of individual on the right *(b)*; tilting the pelvis precludes stretching the hip flexors.

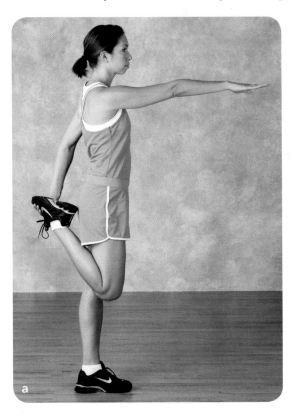
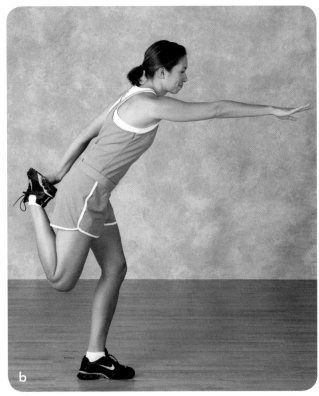

Hip Flexor Stretch (Supine)

The participant assumes the Thomas test position and pulls the contralateral leg back as far as possible. This posterior rotation of the pelvis can place added tension on the contralateral hip flexors.

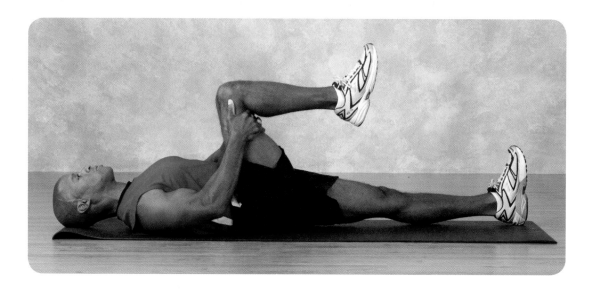

Iliotibial Band Stretch

With hips stacked, the exerciser places the ankle of the lower leg on the lateral distal thigh. By outwardly rotating the thigh of the lower leg, the IT band of the upper leg is stretched. If the IT band is tight, gravity alone may be an effective stretch from this position, and the lower leg is not needed.

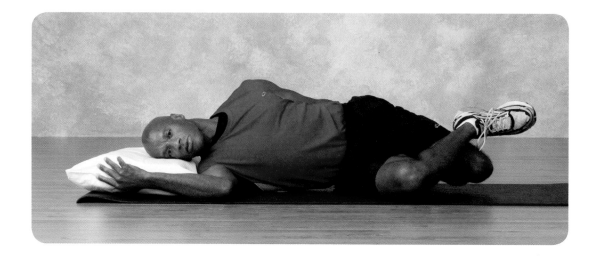

Piriformis Stretch

The piriformis of the right leg is stretched in this maneuver. This posturing is markedly similar to that achieved while sitting at a chair and placing the lateral malleolus (ankle) of one leg on the distal femur of the contralateral leg.

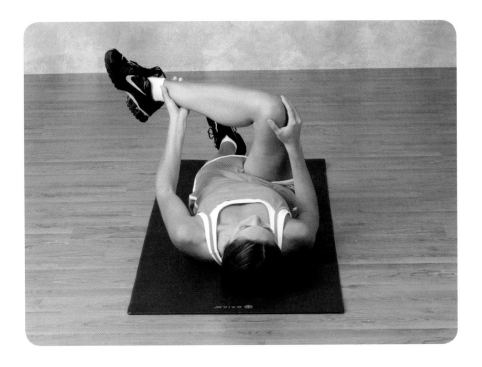

Cailliet Stretch

The exerciser should lean forward (with neutral spine) until tension is felt in the hamstrings and then hold this position. The sequence is repeated for each leg 3 to 4 times. If the hamstrings are tight (e.g., sacral angle less than 80°), stress could be placed on structures of the spine. To avoid this, the back should be kept straight and the movement emphasis should be at the hip joint.

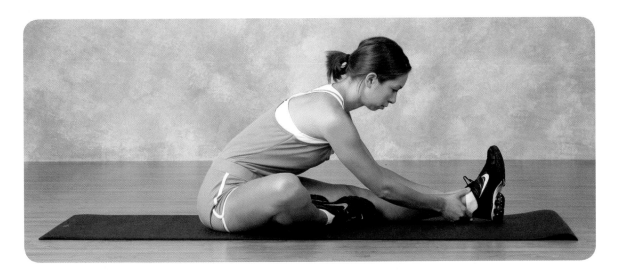

Step or Chair Stretch

The hamstrings can be isolated in the stretch if the movement is made only at the hip joint *(a)*. Although the hamstrings can also be stretched in *(b)*, the soft-tissue structures of the lower back are also stretched. This stretch is more effective if the trunk is splinted (i.e., neutral spine or normal standing posture) so that movement only occurs at the hip joint. An appropriate stretch for the low back is the mad cat stretch, introduced in the next section.

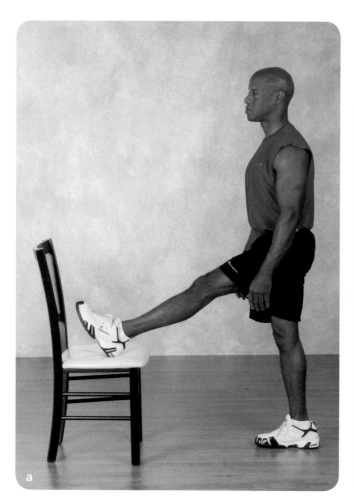
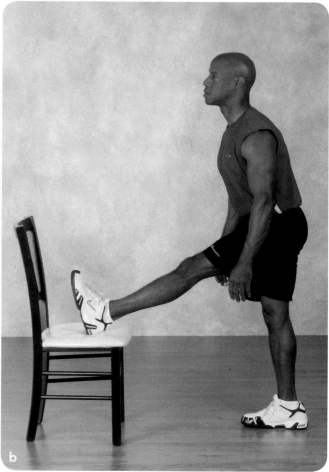

Stretching Exercises to Maintain Range of Motion

This section includes a few examples of stretching exercises relevant to spinal function. Without adequate warm-up of this area of the body, an individual can be most vulnerable to injury. It is particularly important to execute all movements slowly and under total control; ballistic exercises are contraindicated.

Mad Cat Stretch

This exercise involves slowly cycling through full spinal flexion to full extension. It is not used for increasing ROM but rather for maintaining mobility of the spine. Because the spinal loading is minimal, it would be a particularly appropriate morning exercise when the discs tend to be distended and tight.

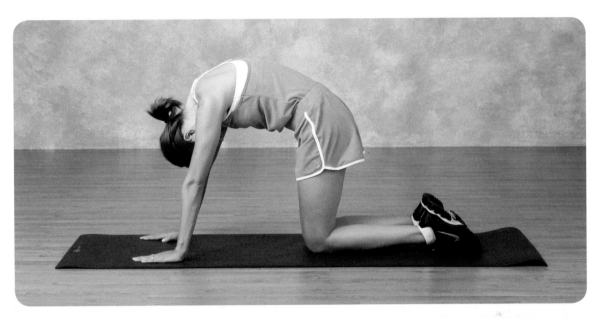

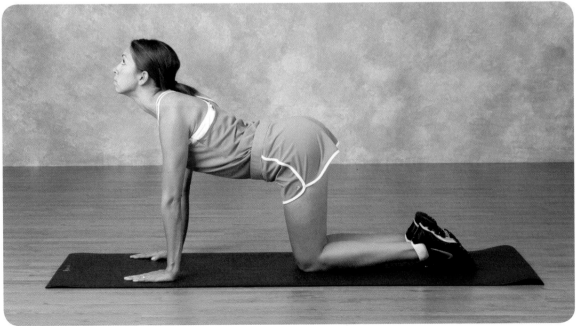

Trunk Flexion

The participant pulls one *(a)* and eventually both *(b)* knees toward the shoulders. This exercise is not for people with disc symptoms because in some flexion movements, the nucleus of the disc could be pushed posteriorly.

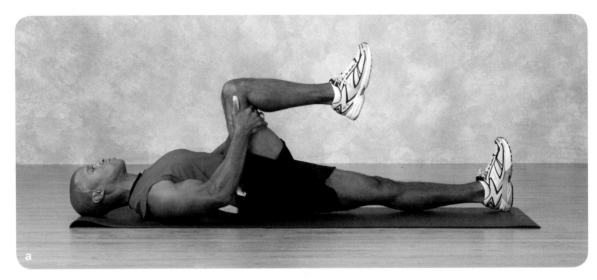

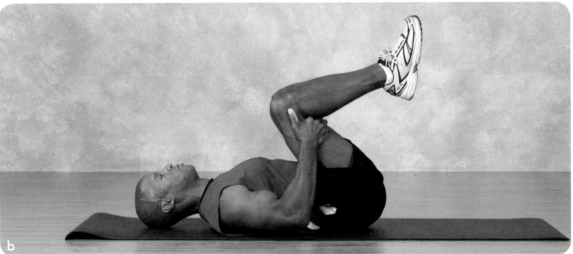

Trunk Extension

The exerciser places the hands under the shoulders and slowly extends the arms while keeping the pelvis in contact with the floor (back muscles are kept relaxed).

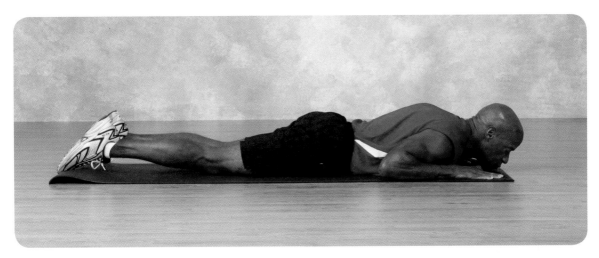

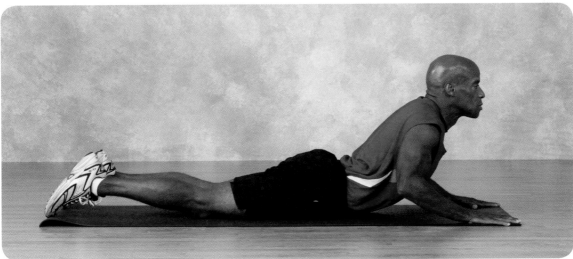

Trunk Strength and Endurance Exercises

In these exercises, as in any other resistance training exercises, overload must be achieved. Strength can be developed by doing, for example, 10 to 15 repetitions of each exercise (or until overload is reached); however, workouts can also be varied by doing most of the exercises with 30 to 60 sec isometric holds and fewer repetitions. The latter can be advantageous for developing trunk muscle endurance, which is critical for attaining good CS.

Quadruped

Initially this exercise is done one limb at a time (e.g., alternately raise each arm, then alternately raise each leg), and then after these tasks are mastered, the activity is advanced and the exerciser concurrently raises contralateral limbs. It can be done dynamically or isometrically. Throughout the execution of this exercise there should be no movement in the axial skeleton (i.e., no extraneous movement of the hips or shoulders). Abdominal bracing and CS requirements are increased when contralateral limbs are raised. When back patients perform this exercise, it is important that they do so in pain-free ROM and that the shoulders and hips remain level (i.e., no bobbing or other trunk movement during this exercise). (See also figures 14.8 and 14.10)

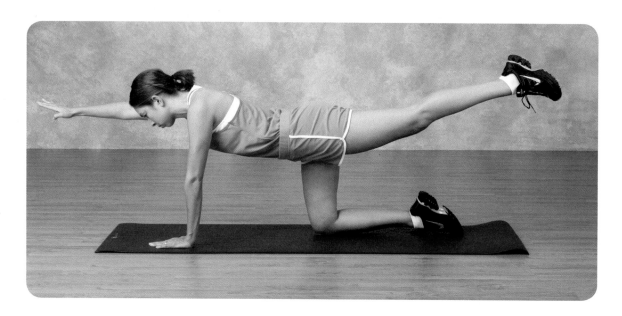

Roman Chair

This is an effective exercise for the lumbar erector spinae and the multifidus. For people with less strength, the activity depicted in (b) is more appropriate. The compressive forces on the discs are lower in (b) than in (a); nevertheless, even the exercise depicted in (b) might be too difficult for some individuals.

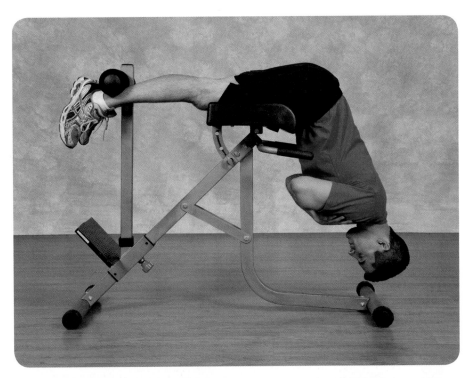

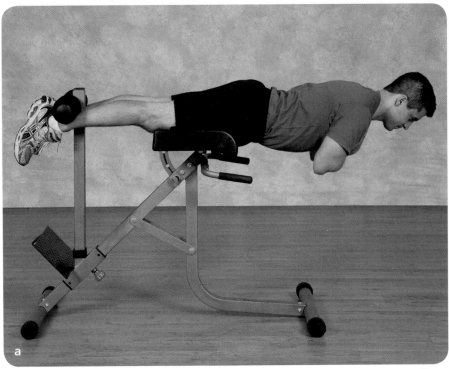

a

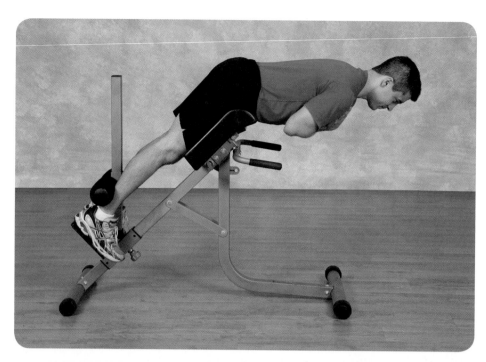

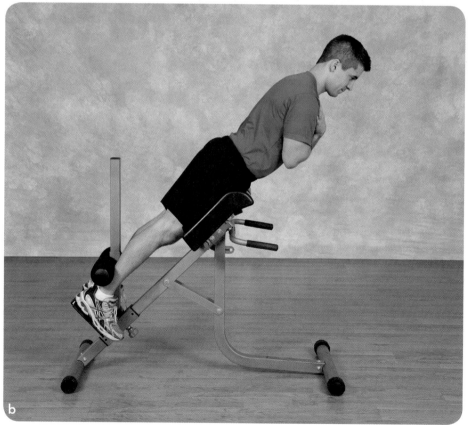

Posterior Pelvic Tilt

This exercise can be done by itself or as the first phase of a crunch. The participant posteriorly rotates the pelvis from starting position *(a)* until the low back is snug against the floor *(b)*. (This exercise may not be appropriate for individuals with disc pathology.)

For the following abdominal wall exercises, research is cited that indicates the degree of MVC seen for the musculature involved. As discussed previously, it is desirable to minimize psoas activity as much as possible while concurrently maximizing abdominal wall activity. The only exercises included here are those that best meet these criteria. Other exercises may be appropriate for a specific population.

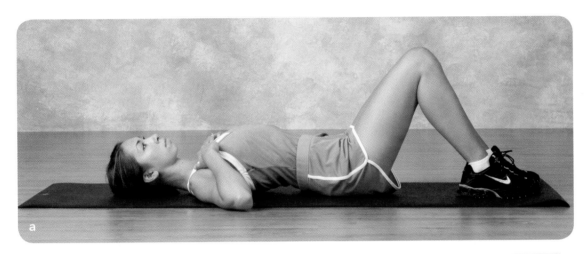

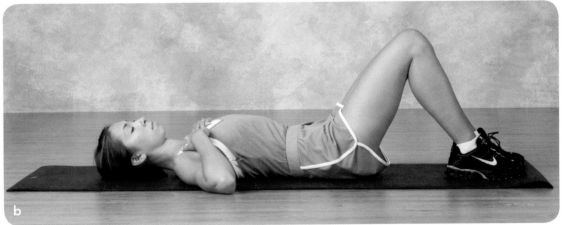

Crunch or Partial Curl-Up

Once the shoulders are raised from the floor, the normal lordosis has been straightened and movement should cease *(a)*. If the movement continues, it will occur at the iliofemoral joint and the movers will be the hip flexors, because the abdominal muscles contract isometrically to stabilize the trunk. The crunch also can be performed with the thighs vertical *(b)*. A minimum of 10 to 15 repetitions should be the goal. Two or 3 sets may be repeated, and isometric holds of 5 sec or more can be incorporated with the up position. MVC: psoas—7% to 10%, rectus abdominis—62%, external oblique—68%, internal oblique—36%, transversus abdominis—12% (14).

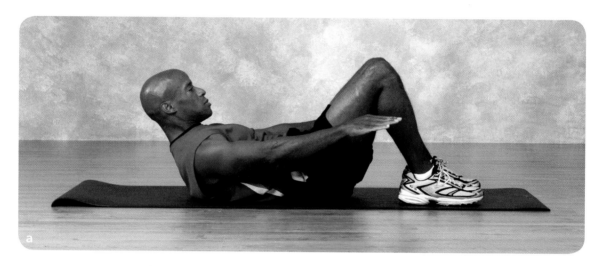

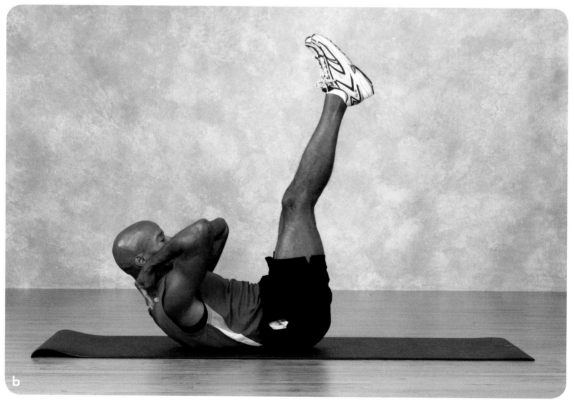

Cross Curl-Up

This exercise ensures greater involvement of the internal and external oblique musculature. A minimum of 10 to 15 repetitions should be the goal. Two or 3 sets may be repeated, and isometric holds of 5 sec or more can be incorporated with the up position. MVC: psoas—4% to 5%, rectus abdominis—62%, external oblique—68%, internal oblique—36%, transversus abdominis—12% (14).

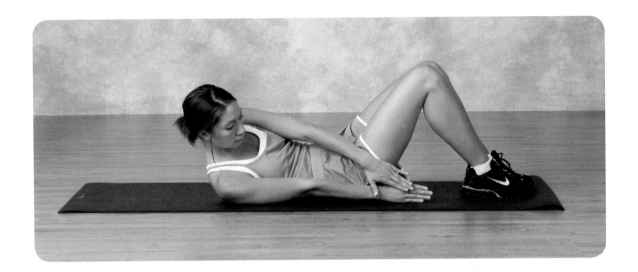

Flexor Endurance Exercise

This exercise can be used as a somewhat novel test, as proposed by McGill (22). The subject assumes a sit-up posture (knees and hips at 90°) resting against a 60° support; by starting from this angle, the psoas is not a factor. The subject holds this position as the support is moved back 10 cm (4 in.); the score is the number of seconds held until the back touches the support.

Horizontal Isometric Side Bridge

This exercise can be done with either the knees or the feet on the floor. The latter is more difficult and increases the spine load over the figures cited. MVC: psoas—12% to 21%, rectus abdominis—21%, external oblique—43%, internal oblique—36%, transversus abdominis—39% (14).

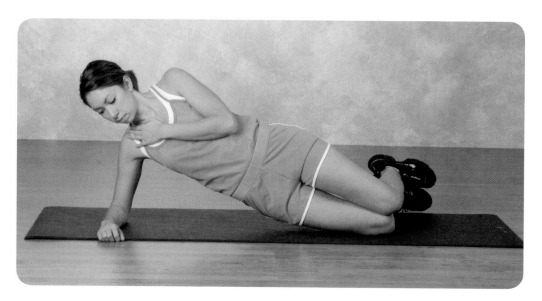

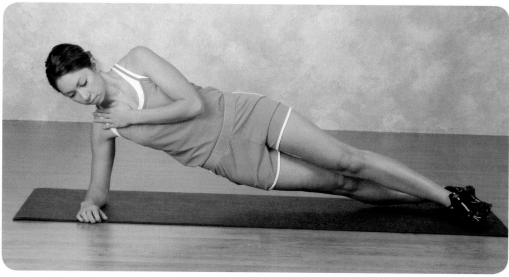

Dynamic Side Bridge

This exercise is the horizontal isometric side bridge without the isometric hold. It can be done with the knees or the feet on the floor. The latter is more difficult and also increases the spine load over the figures cited. In the dynamic version of this bridge exercise, the hips are raised and lowered rhythmically. MVC (dynamic version): psoas—13% to 26%, rectus abdominis—41%, external oblique—44%, internal oblique—42%, transversus abdominis—44% (14).

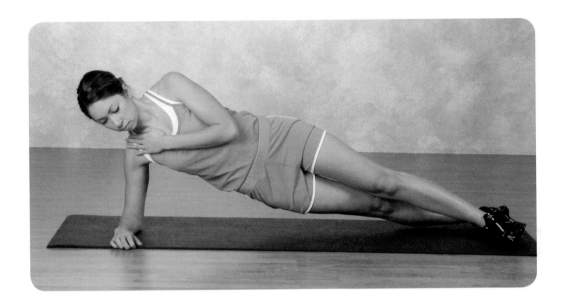

Special Considerations

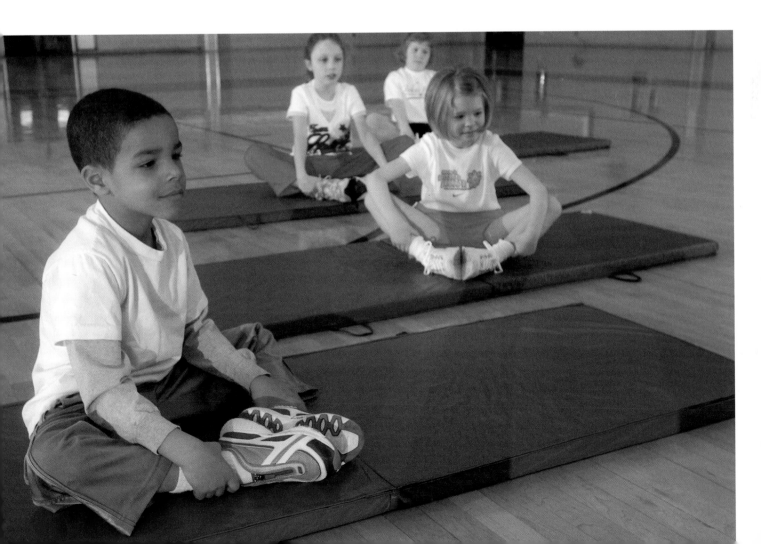

PART V

This section is based on several inter-related factors:

- Physical activity benefits people of both sexes, all ages, and a variety of medical conditions.
- Recommendations for physical activity need to address unique factors that can have a bearing on the exercises selected for the individual (age, medical condition, and so on).
- Fitness professionals are increasingly expected to work with individuals with a variety of clinical conditions.

In chapters 15, 16, and 17 we explain special characteristics and health challenges for children, older adults, and women. In chapters 18, 19, 20, and 21, we provide recommendations to promote safe and effective physical activity for people experiencing some of the major health problems of today, including

- heart disease (chapter 18);
- obesity, the new public health epidemic (chapter 19);
- diabetes (chapter 20); and
- pulmonary disease (chapter 21).

Any one of these topics could make a complete book in and of itself. Our purpose is to help fitness professionals appreciate the importance of these populations, understand the role of physical activity in the quality of life for all people, and provide practical guidelines for special screening, testing, supervision, and activity modifications for each population.

Exercise and Children and Youth

The reader will be able to do the following:

1. Compare the responses of children and youth with those of adults for both acute and chronic exercise.

2. Describe health-related physical fitness testing for children and youth.

3. List the health-related benefits realized by children and adolescents who participate in physical activity.

4. Describe special precautions for exercise participation and testing of children and youth.

5. Describe the public health physical activity guidelines for children and youth.

6. Contrast the public health physical activity guidelines for children and youth with those for children and youth with disabilities.

7. Describe the physical activity guidelines for children from birth to 5 yr of age.

8. Describe the characteristics of structured exercise programs consistent with achieving CRF, strength, body composition, and bone health goals in children and youth.

9. Identify the types of social and psychological benefits derived from participation in physical activity.

Evidence shows that physical activity is essential for attaining the highest quality of life throughout the life span; however, most of the experimental research on how exercise affects fitness has been conducted on young adults, and most of the epidemiological research on how physical activity improves health outcomes has emphasized older adults. One of the common conclusions drawn from the research is that regular physical activity needs to be integrated with one's lifestyle, and it is recommended that this active lifestyle begin early in life. Although the correlations for tracking physical activity across various ages are not very high, Malina (16) concludes, "Allowing for the different methods for estimating habitual physical activity, change associated with normal growth and maturation, and lack of control for important covariates in studies of tracking, physical activity tracks reasonably well from childhood into young adulthood" (p. 7). There is increasing evidence that physical activity enhances the health and fitness of children and youth; that evidence served as the basis for the U.S. Physical Activity Guidelines (40).

In the United States, there is increasing emphasis on motivating people of all ages to begin and continue regular physical activity (39). In addition, physical fitness testing for children and youth is part of many physical education programs.

This chapter deals with physical activity programs for children and youth, the role of fitness testing, and activity guidelines for health and fitness. We focus on school-aged children and youth. Although only briefly covered in this chapter, physical development is vital in preschoolers (11, 19, 21). The emphases of activity during the first years of life are primarily on motor development and healthy growth and are very individualized.

KEY POINT

Regular physical activity is essential for attaining the highest quality of life throughout the life span. Children and youth need physical activity as an integral part of their lifestyle.

Response to Exercise

This section reviews the immediate (acute) and long-term (chronic) effects of physical activity on children and youth. It also compares the exercise responses of children and youth with those of adults (see chapter 4).

Acute Effects

There are a variety of similarities and differences between children and adults in how they respond to acute and chronic (e.g., endurance training) exercise (2, 14, 29, 45).

Children are similar to adults in

- $\dot{V}O_2$max in ml · kg^{-1} · min^{-1} (endurance tasks can be performed well),
- phosphocreatine and ATP (children can deal well with very brief, intense exercise), and
- ventilatory threshold.

Children are higher than adults in

- maximal HR,
- ventilation at a given absolute $\dot{V}O_2$, and

Children are lower than adults in their

- capacity to generate ATP via glycolysis (children have a lower capacity to do intense activity lasting 10-90 sec),
- absolute energy production (kcal · min^{-1}; this is due to differences in body size).
- ability to dissipate heat via evaporation and acclimatize to heat (children have an increased potential for heat-related illness),
- ability to deal with cold (due to a higher ratio of surface area to mass and less subcutaneous fat),
- economy of walking and running (children require more oxygen to walk or run at the same speed; standard equations listed in chapter 6 for estimating energy expenditure of walking and running cannot be used for children),
- BP response to exercise,
- RPE (for most children, their RPE is lower at the same HR or %HRmax), and
- oxygen deficit (children achieve the steady state faster than adults).

KEY POINT

Children are well suited for intermittent activities but should use caution in extreme environmental conditions.

Chronic Effects

Children and youth experience many of the same health and fitness benefits from regular physical activity and structured exercise programs that adults experience.

- Gains in $\dot{V}O_2$max due to endurance training are slightly lower (5%-15%) in children compared with adults.
- Strength gains are independent of age in children and youth.

- In prepubertal children, most of the gain is due to neural adaptations.
- In older adolescents and adults, strength gains are due to both hypertrophy and neural adaptations (see chapter 13 for more on this).

An active lifestyle seems to be natural for children, and activity is a normal and essential part of the growth and development that take place during these years (11, 20). This chapter emphasizes the fitness and health aspects of activity for children and youth, but achieving fundamental motor skills (e.g., moving, throwing, catching) is also an important aspect of the active lifestyle for this age group (45).

KEY POINT

Regularly active youth not only prepare for maintaining active lifestyles as adults but also derive health and fitness benefits during their childhood and adolescence.

Special Considerations

Children and youth with various medical problems need special attention (5). Young children need to be protected from overemphasizing a specific sport or activity and the intense training that often accompanies it, which can lead to physical or emotional problems. Children and youth should be encouraged to choose a variety of activities in an enjoyable and fun atmosphere. Young children do not adapt well to extreme environmental conditions; thus, more precautions need to be taken when exercising in very hot or cold conditions (1, 2, 3, 45).

Although exercise-related deaths are rare in children, when they do occur, they are most often linked to congenital heart defects (i.e., abnormalities of the heart resulting in imperfect oxygenation of the blood as manifested by cyanosis and breathlessness) or acquired myocarditis (i.e., inflammation of the myocardium). Children with these conditions should avoid intense activities. Children (as well as adolescents and adults) with other medical conditions (see chapters 18-21) need to modify their activities, but in almost all cases activity can still be healthful. These children and their parents should work with health care professionals to reasonably modify activities (e.g., longer warm-up and cool-down, lower intensity).

KEY POINT

Children and young people should be screened for cardiovascular problems that might cause exercise-related deaths. Other medical problems can be addressed by modifying activities. The fitness professional should encourage children to enjoy a variety of activities with less emphasis on intense training for competition in one specific sport.

Testing

Concern for the fitness of children and youth goes back over a century. Park's (22) historical review of the topic of fitness and fitness testing indicates that leaders of physical education from the latter part of the 19th century were

Benefits of Regular Physical Activity: Children and Youth

Strong Evidence

1. Improved cardiorespiratory and muscular fitness for boys and girls
2. Improved bone health
3. Improved cardiovascular and metabolic biomarkers (impact is greater in those at higher risk)
   - Insulin sensitivity (increased)
   - HDL-C (increased)
   - Type 2 diabetes (lower risk)
4. Favorable body composition

Moderate Evidence

Reduced symptoms of anxiety and depression

Reprinted from U.S. Department of Health and Human Services, 2008, *Physical activity guidelines advisory report.*

convinced of the connections among exercise, fitness, and health. Not surprisingly, fitness testing was part of physical education. Initially, testing in the United States was concerned more with anthropometry and strength, and it sometimes included a medical exam. Tests of motor ability also were developed, but it was a long time before a national battery of fitness tests for young people became a reality.

The driving force for promoting fitness in the United States in the first half of the 20th century was war or the threat of war, attributable to the concern raised when a large number of young men could not pass a fitness exam for induction into the armed forces. In the early 1950s, a new alarm was sounded when a study showed that a large percentage of American children could not pass basic flexibility and power tests. In response to this concern, President Eisenhower established the President's Council on Youth Fitness. Soon after that, the American Association for Health, Physical Education and Recreation (AAHPER) published its Youth Fitness Test, with fitness items such as the pull-up, sit-up, shuttle run, standing broad jump, 50 yd (45.7 m) dash, softball throw for distance, and 600 yd (548.6 m) run-walk. This test battery focused on skill-related fitness with an emphasis on muscular power (22).

In the early 1980s, the publications of *Healthy People* and of *Promoting Health/Preventing Disease: Objectives for the Nation* shifted the focus to health-related fitness. In support of this focus, the American Alliance of Health, Physical Education, Recreation and Dance (AAHPERD) published the *Health-Related Physical Fitness Test Manual*

for testing fitness components related to health, including the 1 mi (1.6 km) run for CRF, skinfold measurements to evaluate body composition, and the sit-and-reach and the sit-up test to evaluate low-back function. Following this publication, the introduction of criterion-referenced standards was advocated to focus on health-related goals rather than normative standards that compare one child with another (22). For more on this, see the sidebar Cardiorespiratory Fitness Standards for Children.

Physical Fitness

There are two major physical fitness tests for children and youth (see table 15.1), namely, the Fitnessgram (10) and the test by the President's Council on Physical Fitness and Sports (PCPFS) (24). Both assess CRF, muscular strength and endurance, and flexibility. The Fitnessgram and the health-related part of the PCPFS test also check body composition. In addition, the PCPFS test includes a test of agility.

The Fitnessgram and the health-related portion of the PCPFS test use health criteria as standards for the tests, whereas the physical fitness portion of the PCPFS test uses percentiles (by age and sex) for its standards.

Clinical Testing

Although fitness professionals are rarely involved in the diagnostic testing of children, a brief overview is appropriate given that fitness professionals may be directly involved in the delivery of the exercise program (see Exercise is

Cardiorespiratory Fitness Standards for Children

Determining the best way to evaluate fitness in children has been a concern for educators and scientists for the past century (22). One of the most important questions related to fitness tests is the type of standards to use in making judgments about a child's level of fitness. Normative standards such as percentile scores have traditionally been used to describe where children stand relative to their peers (e.g., 75th percentile—see chapter 11). The current thinking, especially for health-related fitness tests (e.g., 1 mi [1.6 km] walk or run test, skinfold test) is that criterion-referenced standards might be more appropriate. Criterion-referenced standards attempt to describe the minimum level of fitness consistent with good health, regardless of what percentile that might be in a normative data set.

For example, Blair et al. (7) showed that in adults, $\dot{V}O_2max$ values associated with a low risk of disease were not that high (i.e., 35 ml $\cdot$ kg^{-1} $\cdot$ min^{-1} for men and 30 ml $\cdot$ kg^{-1} $\cdot$ min^{-1} for women 20 to 39 yr of age). This information was used in setting the criterion-referenced standards for the Fitnessgram, the fitness evaluation program developed by the Cooper Institute. $\dot{V}O_2max$ standards were set at 42 ml $\cdot$ kg^{-1} $\cdot$ min^{-1} for boys aged 5 to 17 yr. For girls, the values were set at 40 ml kg^{-1} min^{-1} for ages 5 to 9 yr, with a decrease of 1 ml $\cdot$ kg^{-1} $\cdot$ min^{-1} per year until age 14, where the 35 ml $\cdot$ kg^{-1} $\cdot$ min^{-1} value held until age 17. Once these standards were set, the investigators had to translate those ml $\cdot$ kg^{-1} $\cdot$ min^{-1} values into equivalent 1 mi (1.6 km) run times, the actual test the children would take. The investigators had to consider the percent of maximal aerobic power the children would perform at during the run and the fact that economy of running improves with age. The result is that we now have standards that are used nationwide to classify children as to whether they have a sufficient level of CRF consistent with a low risk of disease (12).

TABLE 15.1 Physical Fitness Tests

Fitness component	Fitnessgram[a]	PCPFS[b] fitness	PCPFS health-related
Cardiorespiratory	1 mi (1.6 km) run[c]	1 mi (1.6 km) run[d]	1 mi (1.6 km) run[d]
Muscular strength and endurance	Curl-up; push-up	Curl-up; push-up[e]	Curl-up; push-up
Flexibility	Sit-and-reach[e]; trunk lift	Sit-and-reach[f]	Sit-and-reach
Body composition	Skinfolds or BMI	—	BMI
Agility	—	Agility run	—

PCPFS = President's Council on Physical Fitness and Sports; BMI = body mass index.

[a]Cooper Institute for Aerobic Research (10)

[b]President's Council on Physical Fitness and Sports President's Challenge (24)

[c]Or PACER (10)

[d]Shorter distances for younger children (24)

[e]Uses one leg at a time (10)

[f]Or V-sit (24)

Medicine, www.exerciseismedicine.org/fitpros.htm). In addition to the contraindications to exercise testing listed for adults in chapter 7, Zwiren (45) provided the following reasons not to test children:

- Dyspnea at rest (or forced expiratory volume <60% of predicted value)
- Acute renal disease or hepatitis
- Insulin-dependent diabetes (in subjects who do not take insulin as prescribed) or ketoacidosis
- Acute rheumatic fever with carditis
- Severe pulmonary vascular disease
- Poorly compensated heart failure
- Severe aortic or mitral stenosis
- Hypertrophic cardiomyopathy with syncope

Cardiorespiratory Fitness

Measuring $\dot{V}O_2$max in children using the cycle ergometer or the treadmill has a sound historical foundation (4, 26). The GXT format is used for children, and the test (initial grade and speed on the treadmill, increments per stage) must match the child in the same way as tests are matched to adults (see chapter 7). Treadmill testing may be easier because the child's shorter attention span can interfere with a cycle protocol. In addition, local muscle fatigue may shorten a cycle ergometer test before the child reaches maximum aerobic power. If a cycle is used for young children, the handlebars, seat height, crank length, and resistance scale must be adjusted (45). Many laboratories use the Bruce protocol, with 2 min stages, or a Balke protocol in which a speed of 3 to 3.5 mi · hr^{-1} (4.8-5.6 km · hr^{-1}) for walking or 5 mi · hr^{-1} (8.1 km · hr^{-1}) for running is constant and the grade is increased 2% per stage (1).

A variety of cycle ergometer protocols exist to test children, with the initial work rate and the work rate increment per stage based on characteristics of the child (1, 42). To set the values,

- the James protocol uses body surface area,
- the Strong protocol uses weight, and
- the McMaster protocol uses height.

In all cases, shorter, lighter children begin at a lower work rate with smaller increments per stage compared with taller, heavier children. This is similar to the YMCA cycle ergometer protocol for adults described in chapter 7 in that a smaller person would have a higher HR response to the first fixed work rate and would progress through the test with smaller increments per stage. Karila et al. (15) recommended an individual approach based on the child's predicted $\dot{V}O_2$max, from which a maximal power output can be calculated. Then these procedures are followed:

- The child maintains a cadence of 60 rpm, and the test typically lasts 11 min.
  - It begins with a 3 min warm-up at 20% of the calculated maximal power output.
  - The remaining 80% of the calculated power output is divided by 8 to obtain 1 min increments.
- A 2 min recovery follows the test at the warm-up intensity, plus 3 min of passive recovery.

These investigators also have a treadmill protocol that follows a similar pattern once the initial speed is selected.

What is important to remember is that there is no one best test for everyone in all circumstances. Depending on the clinical issue that the child brings to the table (e.g.,

U.S. Physical Activity Guidelines for Children and Adolescents

1. Children and adolescents (6-17 yr old) should do 60 min (1 hr) or more of physical activity daily:

    o *Aerobic:* Most of the 60 min · day^{-1} should be either moderate- or vigorous-intensity aerobic physical activity, and it should include vigorous-intensity physical activity at least 3 days · wk^{-1}.

    o *Muscle strengthening:* As part of their 60 min of daily physical activity, children and adolescents should include muscle-strengthening physical activity on at least 3 days · wk^{-1}.

    o *Bone strengthening:* As part of their 60 min of daily physical activity, children and adolescents should include bone-strengthening physical activity on at least 3 days · wk^{-1}.

    It is important to encourage young people to participate in physical activities that are appropriate for their age, that are enjoyable, and that offer variety.

2. Children and adolescents with disabilities

    o are more likely to be inactive than those without disabilities,

    o should work with their health care provider to understand the appropriate types and amounts of physical activity,

    o should meet the guidelines (see number 1, above) when possible, and

    o should be as active as possible and avoid being inactive when the guidelines cannot be met.

Reprinted from U.S. Department of Health and Human Services, 2008, *Physical activity guidelines advisory report.*

KEY POINT

Fitness testing of children and adolescents is part of many school and youth agency programs. The emphasis has usually been on field tests of health-related components of physical fitness. Children and youth with various diseases can be tested with a GXT, with the protocol selected based on their clinical condition.

asthma, cystic fibrosis, obesity, congenital heart disease), one test format will be preferred over another (25).

Recommendations for Physical Activity

Children and youth enhance their health and well-being through regular physical activity. At a time when many adult diseases are increasingly diagnosed in young people, we must be concerned with health throughout the life span. Risk factors for heart disease are increasingly appearing in young people, including obesity, hypertension, and type 2 diabetes (39). The recent increase in childhood obesity is considered a public health epidemic (34, 37). Both healthy and unhealthy behaviors often begin early in life and are

more difficult to acquire or change as age progresses. Thus, encouraging children and youth to incorporate physical activity into their daily life may provide the basis for a lifetime of this healthy habit (16). It is now well established that regular physical activity can reduce the risk of developing a wide variety of health problems at all ages (38-40).

Currently, the trend is to emphasize the physical activity behavior more than the fitness test scores. The major question is, what kinds of physical activities should children do?

Most motor skills (e.g., throwing, jumping, running, riding bikes, swimming) develop during childhood. Children are inherently active, and one of the most important elements adults must provide for them is an opportunity to play (11, 20). The need for children to develop motor skills must be kept in mind when attending to fitness goals (45).

Both the Fitnessgram and the President's Council (10, 24) recognize the behavior of physical activity (through the Activitygram and the Presidential Active Lifestyle Award). This allows teachers and youth leaders to reward both the behavior of regular physical activity and the physical fitness outcomes. The Activitygram (10) provides a profile of the type, amount, and intensity of activity. It recommends at least 45 min (in three segments) for children and 30 min (in two segments) for adolescents. The Presidential Active Lifestyle Award (24) provides an award for participating in at least 60 min of activity 5 days · wk^{-1} for 6 out of 8 wk. As an alternative, children can count their daily activity steps using a pedometer (girls' goal: 11,000; boys' goal: 13,000). Both are based on the child's self-report of activity. The Activitygram provides more information about the type of activity, although the Presidential Active Lifestyle Award is easier to use.

There are three major reasons for emphasizing an active lifestyle for children and youth:

- Enhancing health and fitness
- Beginning an active lifestyle that can be continued throughout life
- Reducing risks for health problems throughout life

Exercise Prescription for Children and Adolescents

In the past, physical activity recommendations were separated for children and adolescents (9, 23), but in the *2008 U.S. Physical Activity Guidelines*, they were combined (see U.S. Physical Activity Guidelines for Children and Adolescents; 40). What follows is a brief description of each guideline related to fitness goals.

Cardiorespiratory Fitness

In general, the same exercise prescription for CRF for adults (see chapter 11) can be used for children. For example, in the *Physical Activity Guidelines Advisory Committee Report* (41), the review of the literature used to write the *2008 U.S. Physical Activity Guidelines*, gains in $\dot{V}O_2$max were achieved in structured exercise programs in which the intensity was ≥80% HRmax, done 3 to 4 days · wk^{-1}, for 30 to 60 min · day^{-1}, over the course of 1 to 3 mo (41). However, the actual gains in $\dot{V}O_2$max are typically less than those seen in adults. This suggests that the focus should be on health-related benefits of aerobic exercise rather than simply $\dot{V}O_2$max. When the focus is on health-related benefits, using a variety of continuous physical activities (e.g., cycling, running, in-line skating), team sports (e.g., basketball, soccer), individual and dual sports (e.g., tennis, racquetball), and recreational activities (e.g., hiking) can contribute to energy expenditure and its associated benefits. Parents, schools, and communities must provide opportunities for children to have safe places to walk, run, and cycle; provide organized programs for children to learn and play sports; and focus on personal achievement rather than winning at all costs.

KEY POINT

Children should focus on health-related physical activity with a variety of endurance activities appropriate for their age. Long durations of inactivity should be avoided.

Strength

Both boys and girls can improve muscular strength and endurance by participating in formal resistance training programs. In the *Physical Activity Guidelines Advisory Committee Report* (41), the typical program associated with strength gains included the following characteristics: intensity of 75% 1RM, 2 to 3 days · wk^{-1} with a day of rest between sessions, done over 8 to 12 wk. Safety precautions must be taken, however, because children are anatomically, physiologically, and psychologically immature (6, 28, 45). Chapter 13 discusses resistance training programs, including those for children. Here we highlight some of the more important considerations for children:

- Have the parent or legal guardian complete a health history for each child.
- Children with diseases or disabilities should have their exercise program tailored to their condition, symptoms, and functional capacity.
- Ensure that trained personnel supervise each session.
- Adapt equipment to children.
- Teach proper lifting techniques.
- Have children perform 1 or 2 sets of 8 to 10 exercises (8-15 repetitions per set) and include major muscle groups.
- Increase resistance only when the child can perform the desired number of repetitions in good form.
- Individualize progression of all resistance activities.
- Do 2 or 3 nonconsecutive sessions each week.
- Encourage other activities.

KEY POINT

Children can benefit from resistance training. Such training should emphasize safety, supervision for proper form, and muscular endurance (i.e., less resistance and more repetitions).

Body Composition

In the *Physical Activity Guidelines Advisory Committee Report* (41), physical activity programs that included 30 to 60 min of moderate- to vigorous-intensity activity done 3 to 5 days · wk^{-1} were effective in reducing adiposity and visceral obesity in those who were overweight or obese. Keep in mind that when working with overweight or obese children who are sedentary, it is necessary to use a progression model when introducing the physical activity, just as you would do for a sedentary adult (40).

Bone Health

In the *Physical Activity Guidelines Advisory Committee Report* (41), studies that demonstrated gains in BMD in children included the following types of activities: jumping, weight-bearing activities (e.g., running), games, and resistance exercises. These were better than weight-supported activities such as swimming and cycling (41). The evidence suggests that one of the best times to influence bone health is during puberty and the premenarchal years. The effect of such exercises on bone health is realized over many months of training, in contrast to the gains in CRF and strength that can be realized in shorter amounts of time.

All of the fitness component can be positively affected by following the physical activity recommendations of the U.S. Physical Activity Guidelines (40). Doing more vigorous activity would have a greater effect on these fitness outcomes, and in addition, those children and adolescents who do at least 360 min $\cdot$ wk^{-1} of physical activity have good health risk profiles.

All of the previously described guidelines are for children and adolescents aged 6 to 17 yr. What about the younger crowd? See Physical Activity Guidelines for Children: Birth to Age 5.

Transition From Childhood to Adolescence

Rowland (27) pointed out that the motivation for activity shifts from a biological one in children to a more psychosocial one in adolescence. Many of the adolescent psychosocial factors negatively influence physical activity, resulting in the well-known decline in physical activity, especially among females. Although the recommendations for physical activity are essentially the same as those for adults (33), the strategy for enhancing motivation must target these adolescent psychosocial factors (30). Youth sport can fill the need for appropriate motivation (35). In 2007 and 2008, over 3 million girls and over 4 million boys participated in high school sport (44). Physical activity

KEY POINT

Young people gain physical, social, and psychological benefits through participation in physical activity, especially when it includes mastery of motor and sport-specific skills. Adults play a major role in providing opportunities for children to be physically active.

Physical Activity Guidelines for Children: Birth to Age 5

An overriding recommendation is that adults responsible for the well-being of infants and young children should be aware of the importance of physical activity and facilitate the development of the child's movement skills. Infants (birth-12 mo) should

- interact with parents and caregivers in daily physical activities dedicated to exploring their environment and promoting the development of movement skills, and
- be active in a safe environment.

Toddlers (12-36 mo) should

- accumulate at least 30 min of structured physical activity per day,
- engage in at least 60 min and up to several hr of unstructured physical activity per day,
- not be sedentary for more than 60 min at a time,
- develop movement skills, and
- be active in safe indoor and outdoor areas.

Preschoolers (3-5 yr) should

- accumulate at least 60 min of structured physical activity per day,
- engage in at least 60 min and up to several hr per day of unstructured physical activity,
- not be sedentary for more than 60 min at a time,
- develop competence in fundamental movement skills, and
- be active in safe indoor and outdoor areas.

Adapted from NASPE 2009.

Developmental Assets Attained Through Sport-Specific Activity Programs

Psychological Assets

- Self-determined motivation toward physical activity
- Positive values toward physical activity
- Feelings of self-determination, autonomy, and choice
- Positive identity, body image, and self-esteem
- Perceived physical competence and self-efficacy
- Positive affect and stress relief
- Moral identity, empathy, and social perspective-taking
- Cognitive functioning and intellectual health
- Hope and optimism about the future

Social Assets

- Support from significant adults and peers
- Feelings of social acceptance
- Close friendship and friendship quality
- Leadership, teamwork, and cooperation
- Respect, responsibility, courtesy, and integrity
- Sense of civic engagement and contribution to community
- Resistance to peer pressure to engage in risky behavior

programs that promote mastery of motor and sport-specific skills contribute to a wide variety of psychological and social assets (8, 43) (see sidebar Developmental Assets Attained Through Sport-Specific Activity Programs).

The best way to attain these outcomes is through the involvement of physical activity leaders (e.g., coaches, fitness professionals), family members, health care providers, fellow participants and friends, and community leaders (43). Children are dependent on adults for a physically active lifestyle, be it though safe parks and playgrounds, bike trails, sidewalks, or, of course, physical education programs.

Increasing the percentage of children involved in school-based physical education is a major goal of *Healthy People 2020* (39). As Morrow and Jackson (18) have indicated, physical education helps promote physical activity for children and adolescents. A number of programs, such as Coordinated School Health (17), SPARK (31), and PATH (13), have shown that physical education programs can have a positive effect on both children (31) and youth (13). In addition, the increased time spent on physical education does not diminish achievement in other subject areas (32). Finally, a principal recommendation from the evidenced-based review of physical activity and youth was to restore daily physical education programs and after-school intramural programs to address the lack of physical activity in adolescents (36). In the United States, we must invest in our children when we can influence their physical activity—when they are at school. If we don't invest the money now, we will pay a penalty in the form of higher disease-related costs in the years ahead.

STUDY QUESTIONS

1. How do children compare with adults in terms of $\dot{V}O_2max$ (per kg body weight), maximal HR, ability to produce ATP through glycolysis, and absolute energy production during exercise?

2. Describe some of the health-related benefits derived when children and adolescents participate in physical activity.

3. What common field test is used to assess CRF in children and youth?

4. What are criterion-referenced fitness standards?

5. Describe the 2008 U.S. Physical Activity Guidelines for children and adolescents aged 6 to 17 yr. How do they compare with the adult standards?

6. What are the physical activity guidelines for children and adolescents with disabilities?

7. How much physical activity is recommended for infants and toddlers?

8. List some of the social and psychological benefits children and adolescents experience as a result of participation in physical activity.

CASE STUDIES

You can check your answers by referring to appendix A.

1. A parent has read that for major strength gains, weightlifters should use a resistance that can be lifted for only 3 to 6 repetitions. He knows that strength is important for some of the sports his 9-yr-old son wants to play, so he asks for your advice. What do you tell him?

2. A parent's group is recommending that additional reading and math be included in the schools by reducing time for physical education and recess. The school board has asked you to respond to this recommendation. How do you respond?

3. A friend is considering not allowing her daughter to participate in sports in school because of the risk of injury. Although that risk is real, what information could you provide to indicate the benefits of participation in school sports?

REFERENCES

1. American College of Sports Medicine (ACSM). 2006. *ACSM's guidelines for exercise testing and prescription.* 7th ed. Philadelphia: Lippincott Williams & Wilkins.

2. American College of Sports Medicine (ACSM). 2006. Prevention of cold injuries during exercise. *Medicine and Science in Sports and Exercise* 38:2012-2029.

3. American College of Sports Medicine (ACSM). 2007. Exertional heat illness during training and competition. *Medicine and Science in Sports and Exercise* 39:556-572.

4. Åstrand, P.-O. 1952. *Experimental studies of physical working capacity in relation to sex and age.* Copenhagen: Ejnar Munksgaard.

5. Bar-Or, O. 1995. Health benefits of physical activity during childhood and adolescence. *PCPFS Research Digest* 2(4).

6. Bar-Or, O., and R.M. Malina. 1995. Activity, fitness, and health of children and adolescents. In *Child health, nutrition, and physical activity,* ed. L.W.Y. Cheung and J.B. Richmond, 79-123. Champaign, IL: Human Kinetics.

7. Blair, S.N., H.W. Kohl III, R.S. Paffenbarger Jr., D.G. Clark, K.H. Cooper, and L.W. Gibbons. 1989. Physical fitness and all-cause mortality. *Journal of the American Medical Association* 262:2395-2401.

8. Bunker, L.K. 1998. Psycho-physiological contributions of physical activity and sports for girls. *PCPFS Research Digest* 3(1).

9. Centers for Disease Control and Prevention (CDC). 1997. Guidelines for school and community programs to promote lifelong physical activity among young people. *Morbidity and Mortality Weekly Report* 44(RR-6): 1-36.

10. Cooper Institute for Aerobic Research. 2005. *Fitnessgram: Test administration manual.* 3rd ed. Champaign, IL: Human Kinetics.

11. Corbin, C.B., R.P. Pangrazi, and G.C. LaMasurier. 2004. Physical activity for children: Current patterns and guidelines. *PCPFS Research Digest* 5(2).

12. Cureton, K.J., and G.L. Warren. 1990. Criterion-referenced standards for youth health-related fitness tests: A tutorial. *Research Quarterly for Exercise and Sports* 61:7-19.

13. Fardy, P., and A. Azzollini. 1998. The PATH program. In *Active youth: Ideas for implementing CDC physical activity promotion guidelines,* 81-85. Champaign, IL: Human Kinetics.

14. Hebestreit, H.U., and O. Bar-Or. 2005. Differences between children and adults for exercise testing and exercise prescription. In *Exercise testing and exercise prescription for special cases.* 3rd ed. Ed. J.S. Skinner, 68-84. Baltimore: Lippincott Williams & Wilkins

15. Karila, C., J. de Blic, S. Waernessyckle, M.-R. Benoist, and P. Scheinmann. 2001. Cardiopulmonary testing in children: An individualized protocol for workload increase. *Chest* 120:81-87.

16. Malina, R.M. 2001. Tracking of physical activity across the life-span. *PCPFS Research Digest* 3(14).

17. McKenzie, F.D., and J.B. Richmond. 1998. Linking health and learning: An overview of coordinated school health programs. In *Health is academic: A guide to coordinated school health programs,* ed. E. Marx, S. Frelick Wooley, and D. Northrop, 1-14. New York: Teachers College Press.

18. Morrow Jr., J.R., and A.W. Jackson. 1999. Physical activity promotion and school physical education. *PCPFS Research Digest* 3(7).

19. National Association for Sport and Physical Education (NASPE). *Active start: A statement of physical activity guidelines for children birth to age five.* 2009. Reston, VA: Author.

20. National Association for Sport and Physical Education (NASPE). 2004. *Physical activity for children: A statement of guidelines for children ages 5-12.* 2nd ed. Reston, VA: Author.

21. National Center for Education in Maternal and Child Health. 2001. *Bright futures in practice: Physical activity.* Arlington, VA: Author.

22. Park, R.S. 1989. *Measurement of physical fitness: A historical perspective.* Washington, DC: ODPHP National Health Information Center.

23. Pate, R. 1998. Physical activity for young people. *PCPFS Research Digest* 3(3).

24. President's Council on Physical Fitness and Sports. 2005. *President's Challenge Physical Activity and Fitness Award Program.* Washington, DC: Author.

25. Regamey, N., and A. Moeller. 2010. Paediatric exercise testing. *European Respiratory Monograph* 47:291-309.

26. Robinson, S. 1938. Experimental studies of physical fitness in relation to age. *Arbeitsphysiologie* 10:251-323.

27. Rowland, T.W. 1999. Adolescence: A "risk factor" for physical inactivity. *PCPFS Research Digest* 2(4).

28. Rowland, T.W. 1990. *Exercise and children's health.* Champaign, IL: Human Kinetics.

29. Rowland, T.W. 2005. *Children's exercise physiology.* Champaign, IL: Human Kinetics.

30. Sallis, J.F. 1994. Influences on physical activity of children, adolescents, and adults or determinants of active living. *PCPFS Research Digest* 1(7).

31. Sallis, J.F., T.L. McKenzie, J.E. Alcaraz, B. Kolody, N. Faucette, and M. Hovell. 1997. The effects of a 2-year physical education program (SPARK) on physical activity and fitness on elementary school students. *American Journal of Public Health* 87:45-50.

32. Sallis, J.F., T.L. McKenzie, B. Kolody, M. Lewis, S. Marshall, and P. Rosegard. 1999. Effects of health-related physical education on academic achievement: Project SPARK. *Research Quarterly for Exercise and Sport* 70:127-134.

33. Sallis, J.F., K. Patrick, and B.L. Long. 1994. An overview of international consensus conference on physical activity guidelines for adolescents. *Pediatric Exercise Science* 6:299-301.

34. Satcher, D. 1998. Opening remarks. *Childhood obesity: Causes and prevention* (CNPP-6). Washington, DC: USDA Center for Nutrition Policy and Promotion.

35. Seefeldt, V.D., and M.E. Ewing. 1997. Youth sports in America: An overview. *PCPFS Research Digest* 2(11).

36. Strong, W.B., R.M. Malina, C.J.R. Blimkie, S.R. Daniles, R.K. Dishman, B. Gutin, A.C. Hergenroeder, A. Must, P.A. Nixon, J.M. Pivarnik, T. Rowland, S. Trost, and F. Trudeau. 2005. Evidenced-based physical activity for school-age youth. *Journal of Pediatrics* 146:732-737.

37. U.S. Department of Agriculture (USDA). 1999. *Childhood obesity: Causes and prevention. Symposium proceedings* (CNPP-6). Washington, DC: USDA Center for Nutrition Policy and Promotion.

38. U.S. Department of Health and Human Services (HHS). 1996. *Physical activity and health: Report of the Surgeon General.* Atlanta: HHS, CDC, National Center for Chronic Disease Prevention and Health Promotion.

39. U.S. Department of Health and Human Services (HHS). 2010. *Healthy people 2020.* Washington, DC: Author.

40. U.S. Department of Health and Human Services (HHS). 2008. *2008 Physical Activity Guidelines for Americans.* www.health.gov/paguidelines/guidelines/default.aspx.

41. U.S. Department of Health and Human Services (HHS). 2008. Physical Activity Guidelines Advisory Committee Report 2008. www.health.gov/paguidelines/committeereport.aspx.

42. Washington, R.L., J.T. Bricker, B.S. Alpert, S.R. Daniels, R.J. Deckelbaum, E.A. Fisher, S.S. Gidding, J. Isabel-Jones, R.-E.W. Kavey, G.R. Marx, W.B. Strong, D.W. Teske, J.H. Wilmore, and M. Winston. 1994. Guidelines for exercise testing in the pediatric age group. *Circulation* 90:2166-2179.

43. Weiss, M.R., and D.M. Wiese-Bjornstal. 2009. Promoting positive youth development through physical activity. *Research Digest* 10:3.

44. Women's Sport Foundation. 2008. Gender equality in athletics: 2007-2008 high school and college statistics. www.womenssportsfoundation.org/Content/Articles/Issues/General/123/2007_2008-Gender-Equity-in-Athletics.aspx.

45. Zwiren, L.D. 2001. Exercise testing and prescription considerations throughout childhood. In *ACSM's resource manual for guidelines for exercise testing and prescription.* 4th ed. Ed. J.L. Roitman, 520-528. Philadelphia: Lippincott Williams & Wilkins.

Exercise and Older Adults

OBJECTIVES

The reader will be able to do the following:

1. Describe the changes in the number of people older than 65 yr that will take place during the first three decades of the 21st century, and provide a brief profile of older adults, indicating factors that affect the delivery of fitness-related programs.

2. Describe the typical changes in $\dot{V}O_2max$, strength, body composition, and flexibility that occur with age and the effect of exercise training on each.

3. Describe modifications to exercise tests to accommodate typical limitations seen in older adults.

4. Describe functional tests used to evaluate the components of fitness.

5. Explain why it is necessary to address individual differences in older adults regarding exercise prescription.

6. Provide current physical activity guidelines for CRF, muscular fitness, and flexibility for older adults.

A constant theme throughout this text is the importance of physical activity and exercise in leading a healthy life. This message is especially important for older people, the fastest growing segment of the U.S. population. The baby boom generation (those born between 1946 and 1960) was a spike in the birth rate in the United States after World War II, and these individuals are now coming to full maturity. Figure 16.1 shows the changes in the number of people over age 65, projected to the year 2030 (30). The number actually doubles between 2000 and 2030 because of the baby boomers. In addition, because of advances in hygiene and medicine over the past century, life expectancy has increased in general and with it the numbers of people living to advanced ages. Shephard (23) described the following age classifications and characteristics of those aged 40 and older:

- Middle age—40 to 65 yr; 10% to 30% loss of biological functions
- Old age—also called *young old age*; 65 to 75 yr; further loss of function
- Very old age—75 to 85 yr; substantial impairment in function but can still lead an independent life
- Oldest old age—over 85 yr; institutional or nursing care typically needed

Currently, there are 17 times more people in the 75-to-84 age group and 47 times more people in the 85+ age group than there were in 1900 (30). These latter age groups already have had a major effect on health delivery systems, financing of health care, family issues in caring for parents and grandparents, and general concerns about quality of life for those contemplating retirement. These changes also affect the role of the fitness professional in providing appropriate physical activity and exercise programs to increase and maintain health and fitness in older adults. Are fitness clubs ready to welcome older participants when the focus has been on younger, healthier age groups? Are personnel trained to serve the special needs of older adults? This chapter summarizes important health and fitness information related to this age group. We recommend consulting the following references to gain a more complete understanding: *Physical Dimensions of Aging* (25), ACSM's "Exercise and Physical Activity for Older Adults" (1), and Holloszy and Kohrt's review on aging and exercise in the *Handbook of Physiology* (14).

Overview

A variety of demographic and physiological characteristics of the older population (>65 yr of age) affect the planning of fitness facilities, the programming options available, and the kinds of emergencies to anticipate. The following information, from *A Profile of Older Americans: 2009* (30), provides some insights into the population as a whole:

- There are four times as many widows (8.8 million) as widowers (2.2 million) in this age group.
- The majority live in a family setting; however, as the population ages, the number living alone or in an institution increases.
- In 2008, 41.8% of older white Americans rated their health as excellent or very good, versus 25.1% of African Americans and 28.0% of Hispanics.

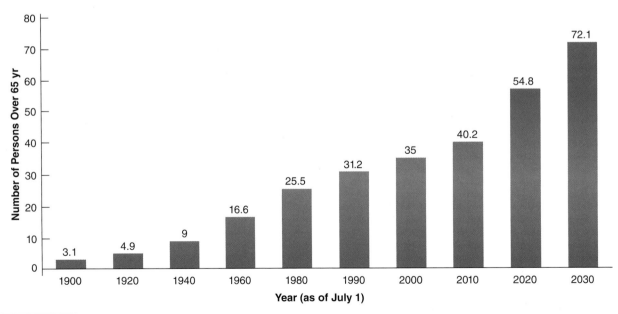

FIGURE 16.1 Number of persons aged 65 yr and older from 1900 to 2030. Increments in years are uneven.

From U.S. Department of Health and Human Services 2009.

- Physical activity limitations increase with age, with 37% reporting a severe disability. There is a strong link between disability and reported health status, with 64% percent of those with a major disability having fair or poor health status. The disabilities interfered with their capacity to carry out ADLs and instrumental activities of daily living (IADLs), that is, preparing meals, shopping, doing housework, and so on.

- Most older adults have at least one chronic condition and many have several. These include hypertension (41%), arthritis (49%), heart disease (31%), cancer (22%), and diabetes (18%).

This brief demographic profile indicates that fitness programs must address health-screening issues, the need for socialization, joint-protective activities, prevention and treatment of chronic diseases, and pragmatic goals to maintain independent living (23). However, these characteristics (i.e., type and severity of disease, physical limitations, fitness) are not uniformly distributed across the older population, and fitness professionals must attend to individual differences. We address this issue in the sections dealing with exercise prescription.

KEY POINT

The number of older adults in the United States is increasing as the baby boom generation comes to full maturity. Older participants present special challenges to fitness professionals because of chronic disease conditions and physical activity limitations. Programs must focus on preventing and reducing the progression of chronic diseases as well as increasing or maintaining fitness to allow for independent living.

Effects of Aging on Fitness

There is no question that physiological function decreases with age; however, some functions age faster than others. Further compounding the problem, each person displays a unique rate of aging that is influenced by genetic and environmental (e.g., education, health care, economic status, nutrition, exercise) factors (25). Consequently, it is not uncommon to find a person who is intellectually young but physically old or a 70-yr-old who has the physiological capacity of a 50-yr-old.

In general, the common chronic diseases that contribute to morbidity in older adults respond to exercise interventions in a manner similar to that of younger adults. Endurance training

- improves blood lipids (linked more to a reduction in body fatness than an increase in exercise),

- lowers BP to the same degree as shown for younger individuals with hypertension, and

- improves glucose tolerance and insulin sensitivity (1).

As described earlier in the text, the primary fitness components (CRF, muscular fitness, body composition, and flexibility) affect our ability to perform work and engage in recreational pursuits at any age. Although natural changes in these fitness components occur with age, the evidence is overwhelming that regular physical activity and exercise maintains fitness at considerably better levels than does a sedentary lifestyle. The following sections address each fitness component.

Cardiorespiratory Fitness

Figure 16.2 shows that maximal aerobic power ($\dot{V}O_2$max) decreases at the rate of about 1% per year in healthy men and women after the age of 20 (14). This decrease is due to both inactivity and weight gain as well as to aging (1). Some studies show that this rate of decline is reduced by half in men who maintain a vigorous exercise program, but not without exception (2, 14). Women show a 10% decline per decade independent of activity status (7); however, trained women, as expected, have a higher $\dot{V}O_2$max at any age compared with their sedentary counterparts (9). It should be no surprise that the decrease in $\dot{V}O_2$max affects endurance performance. Average running speed in distance races decreases about 1% per year, suggesting a link between the decrease in $\dot{V}O_2$max and performance in distance running. However, a variety of other factors (e.g., running economy, lactate threshold, joint trauma) also might affect running performance (14).

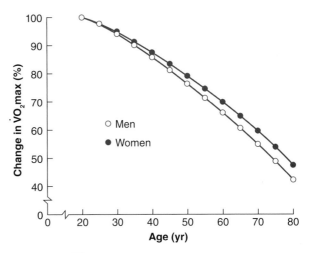

FIGURE 16.2 Percent change in $\dot{V}O_2$max with age in men and women.

Adapted from J.O. Holloszy and W.M. Kohrt, 1995, Exercise. In *Handbook of physiology, Section II: Aging,* edited by E.J. Mason (Bethesda, MD: American Physiological Society), 633-666. Used with permission.

The fact that all people experience a decline in V̇O₂max with age means that by the time of retirement, the ability to engage in routine physical activities has been compromised. This reduced capacity for work can further reduce physical activity, setting up a vicious cycle leading to lower and lower levels of CRF. This may result in the inability to perform ADLs, which affects quality of life and the ability to live independently (25).

Maximal oxygen uptake (see chapter 4) equals the product of maximal cardiac output (maximal HR · maximal SV) and maximal oxygen extraction (systemic arteriovenous oxygen difference). There is no question that maximal HR decreases with age (e.g., 220 − age) and is the major contributor to the age-related decrease in maximal cardiac output. The Frank–Starling mechanism (greater stretch of the ventricle due to higher venous return) appears to compensate for the lower maximal HR in middle age and so reduces the magnitude of change in maximal cardiac output, but this mechanism is less effective in old age (1, 14). Maximal oxygen extraction is also lower in the elderly compared with younger sedentary adults, but this decrease is probably attributable more to their level of inactivity than to a true aging effect.

The good news is that endurance training increases V̇O₂max about 10% to 30% in previously sedentary older adults, an increase similar to that of younger adults (1, 14). The increase in V̇O₂max is due to an increase in both maximal cardiac output and oxygen extraction in older men but is due almost entirely to an increase in oxygen extraction in older women. This may be related to the observation that older women show little or no increase in left ventricle mass, end diastolic volume, or maximal SV after endurance training. The increase in oxygen extraction is due to increases in capillary number and mitochondrial enzymes, the same as in younger adults (14).

KEY POINT

V̇O₂max decreases about 1% per year in sedentary men and women because of a decrease in both maximal cardiac output and maximal oxygen extraction. Endurance training increases V̇O₂max in older adults just as it does in younger adults. The greater V̇O₂max results from gains in both maximal cardiac output and oxygen extraction in men but is due solely to an increase in oxygen extraction in women.

Muscular Strength and Endurance

Muscular strength begins to decline at about age 30, but the majority of the decrease occurs after age 50, when it falls at the rate of 15% per decade, with a more rapid decline of 30% per decade after age 70 (16, 22). The loss of strength relates directly to a loss of muscle mass (sar-

copenia), with the latter attributable primarily to a loss of muscle fibers (motor units) and secondarily to an atrophy of those muscle fibers (primarily type II) that remain (see figure 16.3). However, the distribution of fiber types is maintained across age, as is strength per cross-sectional area of muscle (1, 14, 16, 22).

Maintaining muscle mass is important not only for preserving the ability to carry out daily activities but also for its link to RMR (see chapter 12) and the risks of type 2 diabetes and hypertension (2, 22). Considerable evidence shows that an intense (80% 1RM) resistance training program increases both muscle mass and strength in 60- to 96-yr-old individuals (8, 12). These training programs resulted in modest increases in muscle fiber area (10%-30%) but very large increases (>100%) in 1RM strength. The disproportionate increase in strength is similar to what is observed when young adults participate in intense resis-

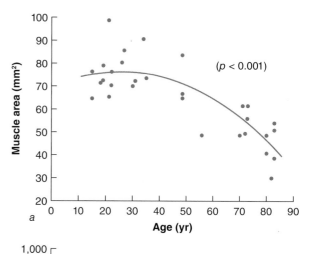

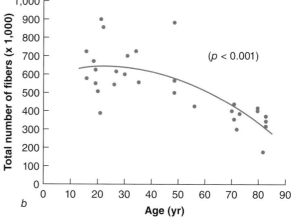

FIGURE 16.3 *(a)* Relationship between age and muscle area of whole vastus lateralis muscle cross sections. *(b)* Relationship between total number of fibers and age in whole vastus lateralis muscle.

Adapted, by permission, from M.A. Rigers and W.J. Evans, 1993, "Changes in skeletal muscle with aging: Effects of exercise training," *Exercise and Sport Sciences Reviews* 21: 65-102.

tance training programs (see chapter 13) and is ascribed to neural adaptations. There is also evidence that resistance training can increase $\dot{V}O_2$max in this population (11). For the frail elderly, it is even recommended that resistance training should precede aerobic conditioning because they must be able to rise from a chair and maintain balance and posture in order to walk (1).

> ## KEY POINT
>
> Muscular strength decreases with age because of a loss of motor units (muscle mass) as well as a reduction in the size of the remaining muscle fibers. Intense resistance training (80% 1RM) causes large (>100%) increases in strength; this is attributable primarily to neural factors, because fiber size increases only 10% to 30%.

Body Composition

Chapters 8 and 12 provided details about health risks, measurement issues, and fitness programs for body composition. In general, body fatness increases from about 16% (males) and 25% (females) in 25-yr-olds to 28% (males) and 41% (females) in 75-yr-olds. This amounts to a gain of about 10 kg of fat for both groups during that time. Fat-free mass is stable until about age 40 but decreases 3% (males) and 4% (females) per decade between age 40 and 60 and 6% (males) and 10% (females) per decade from age 60 to 80 (14). As mentioned, exercise can play an important role in battling sarcopenia.

Evidence indicates that the increase in body fat relates to a sedentary lifestyle rather than to an increase in food intake or an aging effect. Cross-sectional and longitudinal studies on older male and female athletes suggest that regular vigorous exercise is associated with maintaining a stable weight during aging (14). However, observations of highly trained athletes indicate that body fatness still increases about 2% per decade. Consequently, vigorous exercise attenuates, but does not prevent, the increase in body fatness that accompanies age. Importantly, when body composition in older adults changes due to exercise, most of the body fat is lost from central stores, which reduces the risk of metabolic and cardiovascular diseases (14). Exercise is also important in dealing with the loss of BMD with age, but there is more to that story (see the sidebar Bone).

> ## KEY POINT
>
> An increase in body fat with age is attributed more to a decrease in physical activity than to an increase in caloric intake. Vigorous exercise is associated with maintaining a stable body weight with increasing age, and exercise intervention results in the loss of body fat from central stores, which is associated with reduced risk of cardiovascular and metabolic diseases.

Flexibility

The ability to move a joint through its normal ROM is an important factor related to the ability to carry out daily

Bone

BMD (bone mineral density), a measure of bone mass, decreases with age at about the same rate as the fat-free mass; however, in women bone loss accelerates after menopause (14). Accelerated bone loss is a major concern because the risk of fractures increases as BMD decreases. A general recommendation is to maximize BMD through adequate calcium intake and physical activity before age 30 and then reduce the rate of loss from that point in time (3, 5). Hormone levels (estrogen and testosterone), calcium intake, and physical activity affect the rate of loss of BMD. The higher rate of loss of BMD after menopause can be prevented by hormone-replacement therapy, but some women may choose not to use this therapy because of an increased risk of CHD and cancer (19). In addition, there are certain drugs (e.g., bisphosphonates) that can prevent bone loss. Vigorous exercise, calcium intake, and vitamin D are important in maintaining BMD. Older adults need additional calcium (see chapter 5) to help maintain BMD and possibly to realize the full benefits of increased physical activity. The most effective exercise programs for bone health in older women include activities that

- involve a wide variety of muscle groups and movement directions,
- are weight bearing (e.g., walking, jogging),
- strengthen most muscle groups, and
- generally exceed 75% of maximal capacity for both strength and endurance.

However, in older adults with severe osteoporosis, impact-producing exercises and those that involve forward spinal flexion should be avoided (1, 5). Please see chapter 17 for more on women's health.

activities and to the risk of low-back problems (see chapter 10). Joint motion is influenced by the condition of the muscle, connective tissues, and cartilage associated with the joint. In general, the increase in collagen cross-linkages in tendons and ligaments and a degradation of articular cartilage contribute to decreased joint ROM with age (1). However, in evaluating the health of a joint, it is difficult to separate aging effects from those associated with chronic inactivity.

Because of the variability in the number of subjects, the types of research design, and the methods of assessment in studies investigating the effect of training on flexibility, it is difficult to provide a general profile of the training effect as was done for $\dot{V}O_2$max and strength (1, 20, 25). However, general programs of physical activity as well as special ROM exercise programs have been shown to improve flexibility in people who are very old (1, 23). Clearly, additional research is needed in this area.

KEY POINT

Possessing adequate flexibility throughout old age contributes to the ability to perform ADLs and maintain independence. Flexibility can be improved through general programs of physical activity and special ROM exercises.

Special Considerations Regarding Exercise Testing

Age is a risk factor because the likelihood of developing serious conditions increases with age. The passage of time allows the consequences of poor health behaviors (e.g., smoking, high-fat diet, inactivity) to add up and manifest themselves as major medical problems (e.g., lung cancer, atherosclerosis, glucose intolerance). Consequently, fitness professionals must follow the ACSM guidelines for risk stratification (3) closely when working with the elderly (1).

Risk stratification provides guidance for test selection and personnel requirements. Clearly, with the higher incidence of CVD in the older age groups, diagnostic exercise testing may be used as part of a medical exam. However, standard submaximal CRF tests (see chapter 7) may be used as part of a fitness assessment. Independent of the reason for testing, modifications may be necessary to address certain limitations (3, 7, 24):

Instrumentation

- A cycle ergometer may be a better choice for those with arthritis of the knee or hip or those with balance problems.

- Tracking cadence may be a problem unless an electronic cycle ergometer is available.

- If a treadmill is used, additional practice may be needed, with emphasis on slow walking speeds.

Intensity and progression

As mentioned in chapter 7, for deconditioned people with low $\dot{V}O_2$max values, the initial intensity of a GXT should be low, increments per stage should be small, and perhaps the time (3 versus 2 min) per stage should be longer so the person can achieve a steady state.

Exercise Prescription

The U.S. Surgeon General's report on physical activity and health (27) documented that many adults do not participate in any leisure-time physical activity. Clearly, the general recommendation that adults should participate in moderate-intensity physical activity for at least 150 min · wk^{-1} is an essential message for all ages, but especially for older people who are positioned to benefit substantially from an increase in physical activity (1, 18). However, only 39% of those over 65 yr meet the public health recommendations for physical activity (13). When working with this age group, the fitness professional needs to keep in mind that an activity that is moderate work for a younger, fitter adult may be classified as very heavy for an older adult (see figure 11.9) (15).

Older adults are not all the same, and fitness professionals must treat them as unique individuals. The only thing two 65-yr-old men in the same fitness class may have in common is their age! They may differ substantially in their health risk (chronic diseases), CRF ($\dot{V}O_2$max), and experience with exercise. Scientists and clinicians (10, 21, 25) have developed a variety of classification schemes to deal with this reality; Rimmer's (21) classification scheme is representative of these:

- Level I *Healthy:* No major medical problems; in relatively good condition for age; has exercised the past 5 yr.

- Level II *Ambulatory, nonactive:* No major medical problems; has never participated in a structured exercise program.

- Level III *Ambulatory, disease failure:* Diagnosed as having severe CAD, arthritis, diabetes, or COPD.

- Level IV *Frail elderly:* Relies on partial assistance from professional staff for ADLs; can stand or walk short distances, usually less than 100 ft (30.5 m) with an assistive device; spends most of the day sitting.

- Level V *Wheelchair dependent:* Relies on total assistance from professional staff for ADLs; cannot stand or walk.

These classifications of abilities and problems should be viewed as a continuum rather than as discrete categories.

As a person moves across the continuum, the following occurs:

Risk of disease increases

- Need for supervision by medical personnel is greater.
- Use of medication increases.
- Testing moves from fitness to diagnostic to functional (see the sidebar Functional Testing).

Fitness level decreases

- Range of suitable fitness activities decreases.
- Fitness professionals must be creative and adapt conventional activities to the limitations of the participant.
- Fitness professionals must incorporate socialization as part of the activity.

Personnel needs change

- Personnel need more education in gerontology, pathophysiology, and pharmacology.
- Staff mix may include fitness, nursing, physical therapy, and therapeutic recreation personnel.

Given the variation that exists among people in this age group, it should be no surprise that physical activity recommendations are equally diverse. These recommendations are discussed in the next sections of the chapter.

Aerobic Activity for Health and Cardiorespiratory Fitness

Physical activity recommendations for older adults were addressed in both the *2008 U.S. Physical Activity Guidelines* (28) and in the 2009 update of the ACSM position stand, "Exercise and Physical Activity for Older Adults" (1). What follows is a summary of those recommendations for health and fitness outcomes from the U.S. Physical Activity Guidelines (28).

- The following physical activity guidelines are the same for adults and older adults:
  - All older adults should avoid inactivity, some activity is better than none, and older adults who participate in any amount of physical activity gain some health benefits.
  - For substantial health benefits, older adults should do at least 150 min · wk^{-1} of moderate-intensity physical activity, 75 min · wk^{-1} of vigorous-intensity aerobic activity, or an appropriate combination of both. The physical activity

Functional Testing

A common method to evaluate the capabilities of older adults involves a series of performance tests that are linked to underlying fitness components. The Senior Fitness Test, developed by Rikli and Jones (20), uses the following tests to evaluate the various fitness components:

Chair stand—Number of times within 30 sec a person can stand from a seated position with arms folded across the chest (assesses lower-body strength).

Arm curl—Number of curls that can be completed in 30 sec with a 5 lb (2.3 kg; women) or 8 lb (3.6 kg; men) dumbbell while the participant is seated (assesses upper-body strength).

6 min walk—Number of yards the participant can walk in 6 min around a 50 yd (46 m) course (assesses aerobic endurance).

2 min step—Number of full steps the participant can complete in 2 min, raising knee to midway between knee and hip while standing in place. This is an alternative to the 6 min walk.

Chair sit-and-reach—Number of inches between extended fingertips and tips of toes when the participant is sitting in a chair with legs extended and hands reaching toward toes (assesses lower-body flexibility).

Back scratch—Number of inches between the extended middle fingers when the participant reaches with one hand over the shoulder and the other hand up the back (assesses upper-body flexibility).

8 ft up and go—Number of seconds required to get up from a seated position, walk 8 ft (2.4 m), turn, and return to the seated position (assesses agility and dynamic balance).

Height and weight—Used to calculate BMI.

These tests have been shown to be valid and reliable, and normative data are provided for men and women aged 60 to 94 yr (20). These practical and easy tests can be used to track progress over the course of a training program or to document loss of function that might necessitate additional medical attention.

should be done in bouts of at least 10 min, and the total amount should be spread throughout the week.

- On a scale of 0 to 10 for level of physical exertion, use 5 to 6 for moderate-intensity activity and 7 to 8 for vigorous-intensity activity.

- For additional and more extensive health benefits, older adults should increase their aerobic physical activity to 300 min · wk^{-1} of moderate-intensity activity or 150 min · wk^{-1} of vigorous-intensity activity. Additional health benefits can be gained by going beyond this amount.

- The following guidelines are just for older adults:

  - If older adults cannot do 150 min of moderate-intensity activity because of chronic conditions, they should be as active as their abilities and conditions allow.

  - Older adults should determine their level of effort for physical activity relative to their level of fitness.

  - Older adults with chronic conditions should understand how their conditions affect their ability to do regular physical activity safely.

Consistent with the breadth of these guidelines and the diversity of the older adult population, special attention must be given to progression. The physical activity must be suited to each individual, with an emphasis on a conservative approach for the most deconditioned older adults. Although a formal program of activities aimed at improving CRF should be built on a base of regular moderate-intensity activities, some older individuals may need to begin with light-intensity activities (1). As with any workout, it should begin with a formal warm-up and end with a cool-down, during which flexibility exercises can be done.

It is crucial to adapt the activities to the abilities of the group. Those at the high end of the fitness continuum can participate in a wide variety of activities similar to those used for younger adults. Those who have the $\dot{V}O_2$max of cardiac patients (5-7 METs) can follow an exercise routine that would not be too different from those used in a cardiac rehabilitation program (see chapter 18). However, prescribing activities for those at the low end of the functional continuum, in whom $\dot{V}O_2$max may be only 2 to 4 METs, demands special creativity and attention to safety. Exercises can be done standing with support, seated on a chair, or in the water (4, 20). Because of the prevalence of joint-related problems, exercise modes should be chosen that do not aggravate the problem. The need for additional assistance with balance and attention to safety regarding the risk of a fall should be incorporated into the routine (see the sidebar Balance and Falls).

The general exercise prescription for older adults is similar to what was described in chapter 11 for the typically sedentary person (2, 3):

- **Intensity:** THR can be used to set the exercise intensity, but measured maximal HR is preferred to predicted maximal HR. Intensity guidelines are similar to those for younger adults, but the low end of the THR zone should be emphasized at the beginning of the program, and RPE or an equivalent relative intensity scale should be used to determine whether the intensity is suitable.

- **Duration:** If the client is extremely deconditioned, the exercise sessions should be divided into segments (5-10 min) that can be done throughout the day (or within the context of a single class). Some participants may not be able to exercise continuously for 30 min.

Balance and Falls

Loss of balance can lead to a fall, with dire consequences. The lower bone density in elderly people predisposes them to fractures, and about half are unable to return to regular walking after a fracture (25). The ability to maintain balance is influenced by a variety of factors, such as strength, vision, proprioception, medications, illnesses, flexibility, and environmental hazards (25). Considerable information shows that exercise programs improve balance and reduce falls, but not without exception (1, 23). In older adults at greater risk for falling, the research shows that regular physical activity is safe and reduces the risk of falls. However, due to inadequate research there is no firm recommendation regarding intensity, frequency, and type of balance exercises (1). That said, successful programs include balance training, moderate-intensity strength training for 90 min · wk^{-1}, and moderate-intensity walking for about 1 hr · wk^{-1}. Exercises may include backward walking, sideways walking, heel walking, toe walking, and standing from a seated position. A progression can begin with handrails for support until the exercises can be done without support. Tai chi exercises may be useful in this regard (28, 29). However, medications, environmental hazards, and vision also must be addressed to reduce the risk of falls (25).

- **Frequency:** Even though the recommendation is given in minutes per week, there is no question that the total volume of activity should be spread over the course of the week, and as mentioned previously, over the course of a day if the person cannot do a single 30 min bout of moderate-intensity physical activity. Formal vigorous-intensity exercise sessions should be done 3 to 4 times each week, with a rest day between exercise days.

The National Institute on Aging provides information and examples of exercises that address all of the fitness components for this population (www.nia.nih.gov/Health-Information/Publications/ExerciseGuide/default.htm).

Muscular Strength and Endurance

The exercise prescription for increasing strength is described in chapter 13. It is highlighted here (1, 3, 28):

- Instruct participants on safety, proper lifting technique, and breathing.
- Begin with minimal resistance for the first 8 wk to allow for gradual adaptations.
- Participants should perform 8 to 10 exercises that use the major muscle groups.
- Participants should stay within the pain-free ROM.
- Participants should not exercise if an arthritic joint is painful or inflamed (see the sidebar Osteoarthritis).
- Each set should involve 8 to 12 repetitions that elicit an RPE of about 12 to 13 (e.g., somewhat hard) or a 5 to 6 on the 10-point scale.
- Participants should perform the workout at least twice a week on nonconsecutive days.

Flexibility

A flexibility program should involve all joints with the goal to maintain their normal ROM. However, there are few studies that compare or contrast various ROM exercises and their flexibility outcomes, and as a result there is little consensus on the frequency, duration, or type of exercise (static versus dynamic) to use (1). That said, the results do suggest that flexibility can be increased in major joints by doing ROM exercises specific to the joint (see chapter 14 for more information). Tai chi and yoga programs can be used to achieve and maintain flexibility goals. However, for most people, flexibility goals can be achieved within the context of a regular exercise class. Elements of a flexibility program include the following (3):

- Movements should be performed as a regular part of the warm-up and cool-down, the same as for younger participants.
- Doing stretching exercises after a workout when the muscles are warm is more effective.
- Static stretches are preferred, although others can be done (1).
- For static stretches, use slow movements through pain-free ROM, with stretches held for 15 to 60 sec; do ≥4 repetitions per muscle group.
- Stretching should be performed ≥ 2 days $\cdot$ wk^{-1}.

Psychological Health and Well-Being

This chapter has focused on the fact that regular participation in physical activity is associated with better health (lower risk of chronic diseases) and fitness (cardiovascular function, strength, body composition, and flexibility) during aging. However, regular participation in physical activity also has been shown to improve psychological health and well-being (1, 6, 26, 31). Short-term benefits due to a single exercise session include enhanced relaxation and mood state, enhanced social and cultural integration, and empowerment to be more independent (31). The most recent review of the long-term benefits shows that physical activity (1)

- improves overall psychological well-being (mediated through effects on self-concept and self-esteem),
- decreases risk of clinical depression and anxiety,
- decreases risk of cognitive decline and dementia,
- improves cognitive performance in previously sedentary adults, and
- has a positive impact on quality of life.

This is a good example of how regular physical activity affects the whole person, leading to a more active and fulfilling life.

KEY POINT

The exercise prescription for older adults is similar to that for younger adults, with additional attention to risk stratification, level of CRF, and limitations related to chronic or degenerative (e.g., osteoarthritis) diseases. Exercises should be selected to minimize joint trauma, provide an additional measure of safety against falling, and accomplish fitness goals in a socially supportive environment.

Osteoarthritis

Osteoarthritis, a common problem in many older adults, is a degenerative joint disease associated with damage to the articular cartilage that lines joint structures. The swelling and pain associated with osteoarthritis affect joint ROM and may prevent some individuals from participating in physical activity. A variety of over-the-counter and prescription medications can reduce pain and inflammation and allow participation in physical activity. Activity programs should not excessively load the involved joint (e.g., participants with a knee or hip problem should perform stationary cycling or pool work instead of jogging or stair-climbing). Select the modes that provide the least discomfort; poor choices may cause pain and lead to noncompliance. Gradual warm-up and flexibility exercises should be included, and the intensity and duration of the endurance exercise program should be at the low end of the spectrum. Resistance training should begin with only 2 to 3 reps and gradually progress to 10 to 12 reps, using pain threshold as a guide (3, 17).

STUDY QUESTIONS

1. By the year 2030, how many people in the United States will be over the age of 65 yr compared with the year 2000?

2. Briefly describe the kinds of chronic conditions that exist in older adults that are less common in younger adults.

3. What happens to $\dot{V}O_2$max, muscular strength, and body fatness with age?

4. How might you have to modify a fitness test for CRF to accommodate the problems present in older adults?

5. What are some functional tests to evaluate flexibility, muscular endurance, and CRF?

6. Would you implement the same exercise program for all 65-yr-old adults? Why or why not?

7. Present the newest physical activity guidelines for older adults that address health and CRF, muscular strength, and flexibility.

8. If older adults cannot meet the activity guidelines you just stated, they should do nothing. Do you agree? Why or why not?

9. Discuss the role that progression plays in implementing physical activity programs for older adults, with specific emphasis on how to deal with duration and intensity in deconditioned individuals.

10. What are some psychological benefits that older adults experience as a result of regular participation in physical activity?

CASE STUDIES

You can check your answers by referring to appendix A.

1. A 67-yr-old male who has been actively involved in jogging and tennis most of his life has developed arthritis in his left knee. The problem has caused him to reduce his jogging, and his lack of fitness, as he calls it, is affecting his tennis game, which he is determined to continue. He comes to your health club for testing and advice about what he can do to increase and maintain his fitness. How do you address his concerns?

2. A 55-yr-old woman does 3 workouts every week, with an emphasis on vigorous aerobic exercise in a competitive masters swim class. Her doctor is concerned that her bone density is decreasing in spite of the exercise, and she comes to you for help. What do you recommend to address this concern?

3. A 70-yr-old woman has been referred to you for advice. She indicates that she has not been able to comfortably do her ordinary activities, and she would like your help. What tests do you perform, and what physical activities do you recommend to improve her CRF and muscle endurance to help her regain her confidence in doing routine activities?

REFERENCES

1. American College of Sports Medicine (ACSM). 2009. Exercise and physical activity for older adults. *Medicine and Science in Sports and Exercise* 41:1510-1530.

2. American College of Sports Medicine (ACSM). 1998. The recommended quantity and quality of exercise for developing and maintaining cardiorespiratory and muscular fitness, and flexibility in healthy adults. *Medicine and Science in Sports and Exercise* 30:975-991.

3. American College of Sports Medicine (ACSM). 2010. *ACSM's guidelines for exercise testing and prescription.* 8th ed. Baltimore: Lippincott Williams & Wilkins.

4. American Council on Exercise. 1998. *Exercise for the older adult.* Champaign, IL: Human Kinetics.

5. Bloomfield, S.A., and S.S. Smith. 2003. Osteoporosis. In *ACSM's exercise management for persons with chronic diseases and disabilities.* 2nd ed. Eds. J. L. Durstine and G. E. Moore, 222-229. Champaign, IL: Human Kinetics.

6. Chodzko-Zajko, W.J. 1998. Physical activity and aging: Implications for health and quality of life in older persons. *PCPFS Research Digest* 3(4).

7. Criswell, D.S. 2001. Human development and aging. In *ACSM's health and fitness certification review,* eds. J.L. Roitman and K.W. Bibi, 31-47. Baltimore: Lippincott Williams & Wilkins.

8. Fiatarone, M.A., E.C. Marks, N.D. Ryan, C.N. Meredith, L.A. Lipsitz, and W.J. Evans. 1990. High-intensity strength training in nonagenarians. *Journal of the American Medical Association* 263:3029-3034.

9. Fitzgerald, M.D., H. Tanaka, Z.V. Tran, and D.R. Seals. 1997. Age-related declines in maximal aerobic capacity in regularly exercising vs. sedentary women: A meta-analysis. *Journal of Applied Physiology* 83:160-165.

10. Fitzgerald, P.L. 1985. Exercise for the elderly. *Medical Clinics of North America* 69:189-196.

11. Frontera, W.R., C.N. Meredith, K.P. O'Reilly, and W.J. Evans. 1990. Strength training and determinants of $\dot{V}O_2$max in older men. *Journal of Applied Physiology* 68:329-333.

12. Frontera, W.R., C.N. Meredith, K.P. O'Reilly, H.G. Knuttgen, and W.J. Evans. 1988. Strength conditioning in older men: Skeletal muscle hypertrophy and improved function. *Journal of Applied Physiology* 64:1038-1044.

13. Haskell, W.L., I.M. Lee, R.R. Pate, K.E. Powell, S.N. Blair, B.A. Franklin, C.A. Macera, G.W. Heath, P.D. Thompson, and A. Bauman. 2007. Physical activity and public health: Updated recommendations for adults from the American College of Sports Medicine and the American Heart Association. *Medicine and Science in Sports and Exercise* 39:1423-1434.

14. Holloszy, J.O., and W.M. Kohrt. 1995. Exercise. In *Handbook of physiology, section 11: Aging,* ed. E.J. Masoro, *pp.* 633-666. New York: Oxford Press.

15. Howley, E.T. 2001. Type of activity: Resistance, aerobic and leisure versus occupational physical activity. *Medicine and Science in Sports and Exercise* 33:S364-S369.

16. Kraemer, W.J., S.J. Fleck, and W.J. Evans. 1996. Strength and power training: Physiological mechanisms of adaptations. *Exercise and Sport Sciences Reviews* 24:363-397.

17. Minor, M.A., and D.R. Kay. 2003. Arthritis. In *ACSM's exercise management for persons with chronic diseases and disabilities,* eds. J.L. Durstine and G.E. Moore, 210-216. Champaign, IL: Human Kinetics.

18. Pate, R.R., M. Pratt, S.N. Blair, W.L. Haskell, C.A. Marcera, and C. Bouchard. 1995. Physical activity and public health: A recommendation from the Centers for Disease Control and Prevention and the American College of Sports Medicine. *Journal of the American Medical Association* 273:402-407.

19. Petit, M.A., J.M. Hughes, and J.M. Warpeha. 2007. Exercise prescription for people with osteoporosis. In *ACSM's resource manual for guidelines for exercise testing and prescription,* 6th ed. Ed. J.K. Ehrman, 635-650. Baltimore: Lippincott Williams & Wilkins.

20. Rikli, R.E., and C.J. Jones. 2001. *Senior fitness test manual.* Champaign, IL: Human Kinetics.

21. Rimmer, J.H. 1994. *Fitness and rehabilitation programs for special populations.* Dubuque, IA: Brown & Benchmark.

22. Rogers, M.A., and W.J. Evans. 1993. Changes in skeletal muscle with aging: Effects of exercise training. *Exercise and Sport Sciences Reviews* 21:65-102.

23. Shephard, R.J. 1997. *Aging, physical activity, and health.* Champaign, IL: Human Kinetics.

24. Skinner, J.S. 2005. Aging for exercise testing and exercise prescription. In *Exercise testing and exercise prescription for special cases.* 3rd ed. Ed. J.S. Skinner, 85-99. Baltimore: Lippincott Williams & Wilkins.

25. Spirduso, W.W., K.L. Francis, and P.G. MacRae. 2005. *Physical dimensions of aging.* 2nd ed. Champaign, IL: Human Kinetics.

26. Spirduso, W.W., and D.L. Cronin. 2001. Exercise dose-response effects on quality of life and independent living in older adults. *Medicine and Science in Sports and Exercise* 33:S598-S608.

27. U.S. Department of Health and Human Services (HHS). 1996. *Physical activity and health: A report of the Surgeon General.* Washington, DC: Author.

28. U.S. Department of Health and Human Services (HHS). 2008. *2008 Physical Activity Guidelines for Americans.* www.health.gov/paguidelines/guidelines/default.aspx.

29. U.S. Department of Health and Human Services (HHS). 2008. Physical Activity Guidelines Advisory Committee Report 2008. www.health.gov/paguidelines/committeereport.aspx.

30. U.S. Department of Health and Human Services (HHS). 2009. *A profile of older Americans: 2009.* Washington, DC: Author.

31. World Health Organization (WHO). 1997. *A summary of the physiological benefits of physical activity for older persons.* Geneva: Author.

Exercise and Women's Health

The reader will be able to do the following:

1. Describe the risks and benefits of exercise during pregnancy, and suggest ways to alter exercise to make it more comfortable and safe for pregnant women.

2. Describe osteoporosis and its risk factors, and prescribe exercise to promote bone health.

3. Define the female athlete triad, and describe how a fitness professional might assist someone exhibiting signs of the triad.

Women and

men share many of the same obstacles to good health (e.g., CVD, type 2 diabetes, obesity). Likewise, the benefits of exercise that combat these diseases are similar for men and women, as are exercise guidelines. However, some conditions are faced exclusively or primarily by women. In this chapter, we examine three of these: pregnancy, osteoporosis, and the female athlete triad.

Pregnancy and Exercise

Pregnancy places enormous demands on a woman's body. Concern about the safety of the fetus and the mother leads to questions about whether exercise is wise during pregnancy. Fortunately, there is substantial evidence that for healthy pregnant women, exercise is safe and beneficial during this critical time (4). Although difficult to document, proposed benefits of exercise during pregnancy include greater psychological well-being, less fatigue, and shorter and easier delivery (6, 25). Exercise during pregnancy can be helpful in avoiding excessive gestational weight gain (21), and leading an active life before and during early pregnancy is associated with a lower risk of developing gestational diabetes mellitus (22).

However, some conditions require that exercise be approached cautiously. Pregnant women with cardiovascular, pulmonary, or metabolic disease, as well as those with severe obesity or who are considerably underweight, should seek physician guidance concerning exercise (11). The contraindications for exercise during pregnancy as determined by ACOG (5) are shown in Contraindications for Exercise During Pregnancy. In addition, the Canadian Society for Exercise Physiology (CSEP) has created the Physical Activity Readiness Medical Examination (PAR-med-X) for Pregnancy. This tool screens for potential medical problems and assists with exercise prescription and can be found on the CSEP website (www.csep.ca/forms.asp).

Potential Problems of Exercising During Pregnancy

Concerns about exercise during pregnancy target four crucial areas: heat dissipation, oxygen delivery, nutrition supply, and premature delivery. During the first trimester, the fetus is particularly vulnerable to developmental defects caused by excessive heat. Although the body's core temperature can increase with exercise, there are no known links between a greater prevalence of birth defects and exercise. An increase in the woman's blood volume provides adequate blood for heat dissipation, exercise, and nourishment of the fetus. Increases in skin blood flow also help protect against excessive changes in body temperature (25). Additionally, the temperature at which sweating begins decreases as pregnancy progresses, providing another protective mechanism against higher core temperatures (11).

Concern that vigorous exercise could compromise uterine blood flow is also unsubstantiated. The increase in maternal blood volume coupled with a decrease in systemic vascular resistance results in an increase in cardiac output, providing adequate blood flow, and therefore oxygen, to the fetus (6, 25). The fact that fetal HR is only modestly, if at all, affected by exercise provides evidence that this type of physical activity does not significantly distress the fetus (6, 25). Because of the nutritional demands of pregnancy, greater caloric consumption is needed. The nutritional demands of exercise and fetal development must be adequately met by the exercising woman. For most women, the energy demands of pregnancy are approximately 300 kcal · day^{-1} (4). Evidence that exercise does not compromise the nutritional needs of the developing fetus comes from studies showing little difference between the weights of newborns from exercising and nonexercising mothers (6, 25).

Another major concern is that exercise may cause premature delivery. For normal pregnancies, there is no evidence that the length of the pregnancy is affected by exercise (6, 25). Care should be taken, however, to avoid activities (e.g., contact sports) in which injury could lead to fetal injury or premature delivery (5).

Exercise Testing and Prescription During Pregnancy

Maximal exercise testing should be avoided unless it is medically necessary and under the direction of a physician (4). Submaximal exercise testing, with termination <75% HRR, can be used if specific information is required for exercise prescription (4). Moderate and even vigorous exercise can be performed safely by previously active pregnant women. The type, intensity, frequency, and duration of activity should conform to the woman's health and comfort. The U.S. Physical Activity Guidelines (24) and ACSM (4) suggest that healthy pregnant women should accumulate at least 150 min · wk^{-1} of moderate-intensity activity. Encourage regular (at least 3 days · wk^{-1}) rather than periodic exercise (4). Intensity can be gauged with RPE, with a recommended range of 12 to 14 (4). Suggested HR ranges for moderate-intensity exercise based on age can also be used in exercise prescription (see table 17.1).

Although the physiological response patterns described in chapter 4 generally hold true for pregnant women, the variables themselves (e.g., HR, oxygen consumption) are changed due to the increased metabolic demands (8, 15). For example, HR, SV, and minute ventilation at rest and during exercise are higher than they were before pregnancy. These variables change throughout the pregnancy to meet the needs of the mother and the growing fetus (15).

Because of the demands of pregnancy, the mode of exercise should be based on comfort and convenience. Some women find that non-weight-bearing exercises such as swimming and stationary cycling are more comfortable,

Contraindications for Exercise During Pregnancy

Absolute Contraindications

Hemodynamically significant heart disease

Restrictive lung disease

Incompetent cervix or cerclage

Multiple gestation at risk for premature labor

Persistent second- or third-trimester bleeding

Placenta previa after 26 wk of gestation

Premature labor during current pregnancy

Ruptured membranes

Preeclampsia or pregnancy-induced hypertension

Relative Contraindications

Severe anemia

Unevaluated maternal cardiac arrhythmia

Chronic bronchitis

Poorly controlled type 1 diabetes

Extreme morbid obesity

Extreme underweight (BMI <12 kg · m^{-2})

History of extremely sedentary lifestyle

Intrauterine growth restriction

Poorly controlled hypertension

Orthopedic limitations

Poorly controlled seizure disorder

Poorly controlled hyperthyroidism

Heavy smoker

Adapted, by permission, from OCOG Committee on Obstetric Practice, 2002, "Committee opinion #267: Exercise during pregnancy and the postpartum period," *Obstetrics and Gynecology* 1: 171. Obstetrics and gynecology by AMERICAN COLLEGE OF OBSTETRICIANS AND GYNECOLOGIST Reproduced with permission of LIPPINCOTT WILLIAMS & WILKINS in the format Journal via Copyright Clearance Center.

especially as pregnancy advances. During the postpartum stage, the return to activity should be gradual and based on individual response. A pregnant client should take the following precautions when exercising (4, 5, 24).

- Avoid exercise in a supine position after the first trimester. The enlarged uterus can apply pressure to the surrounding blood vessels and limit venous return.

- Take steps to avoid heat injury. To prevent hyperthermia, avoid exercising in hot and humid environments, ensure adequate hydration (before, during, and after exercise), and dress appropriately for the heat.

- Limit exposure to falling and impact injury. Although completely eliminating the risk is impos-

sible, do not participate in competitive contact sports (e.g., soccer, boxing) and activities where trauma risk is great (e.g., skydiving, waterskiing). As pregnancy advances, center of gravity and balance change; therefore, exercise that requires rapid changes in direction may be more problematic than it was before pregnancy.

- Be aware that joint laxity increases during pregnancy. The release of relaxin allows the pelvis to undergo the changes needed during pregnancy and delivery. However, this hormone also leads to greater laxity in other joints. Follow the precautions in the previous point to help prevent joint injury.

- Resistance training can be used during pregnancy, but observe the following precautions: (a) Avoid the Valsalva maneuver during lifting, (b) keep the program at low to moderate intensity (resistance should be low enough that at least 12 repetitions can be completed without fatigue), and (c) use slow and steady rather than ballistic movement patterns. For more information on resistance training during pregnancy, see chapter 13.

- Avoid exercise in which extremes in air pressure occur. Scuba diving should be avoided because it puts the fetus at risk for decompression sickness. Exercise at altitudes over 6,000 ft (1,829 m) could be potentially dangerous and should be performed with caution.

- Be aware of the body's warning signs (5). Each woman should closely monitor her body for signs or symptoms that something may be wrong. If any of the following occur, stop exercise and consult a physician:

    Vaginal bleeding

    Dyspnea before exertion

    Dizziness

    Headache

    Chest pain

    Muscle weakness

    Calf pain or swelling

    Preterm labor

    Decreased fetal movement

    Amniotic fluid leakage

KEY POINT

Exercising during pregnancy is safe and beneficial for most women. Protecting against traumatic impact, heat injury, musculoskeletal injury, and overexertion is the key to planning safe exercise programs for pregnant women.

TABLE 17.1 Heart Rates Corresponding to Moderate-Intensity Exercise in Pregnant Women

Age (yr)	HR range (beats · min^{-1})
Under 20	140-155
20-29	135-150
30-39	130-145
40 or older	125-140

Adapted from Davis, Wolfe, Mottola, and MacKinnon 2003.

Osteoporosis

Osteoporosis is a disease characterized by fragile bones. Approximately 10 million Americans over age 50 have osteoporosis, and another 34 million have low bone mass, or **osteopenia**, and are at risk for developing osteoporosis (23). Osteoporotic fractures account for nearly $20 billion in medical expenses each year (19). The most common sites for osteoporotic fractures are the hip, vertebrae, and wrist. Bone strength is determined by **bone mineral density (BMD)** and the structural integrity of the bone. BMD is measured by dual-energy X-ray absorptiometry (DXA; see chapter 8) and reflects the amount of bone mineral per unit area (g · cm^{-2}). BMD accounts for about 70% of bone strength and is highly correlated with resistance to fractures (17). Structural integrity is determined by the microarchitecture of the bone and is much more difficult to assess, requiring invasive testing of bone (1). Because of the low risk, the ease, and the availability of DXA, it has become the preferred method for diagnosing osteoporosis.

According to World Health Organization (WHO) guidelines, *osteoporosis* is defined as a BMD that is 2.5 standard deviations below the mean for young white women. When BMD is in the osteoporotic range, fracture risk is high. Common pharmaceutical treatments for osteoporosis are selective estrogen receptor modulators, hormone-replacement therapy (for women), and bisphosphonates. These drug interventions slow bone loss, and some even increase BMD. More information about osteoporosis and its treatment can be found at the website of the National Institute of Arthritis and Musculoskeletal and Skin Diseases (www.niams.nih.gov).

Risk Factors for Osteoporosis

Osteoporosis can affect both males and females across all ages and ethnicities. However, older women, particularly of Caucasian and Asian descent, are especially at risk. Half of all women 50 yr or older will experience an osteoporotic fracture in their lifetime (19). Bone accumulates during childhood and generally peaks in early adult life (14). Although BMD declines somewhat during the middle adult years, the most rapid loss in women occurs in the years surrounding menopause (14). The decline in estrogen levels around the time of menopause is the reason for the rapid bone loss, which can be as great as 3% to 5% of bone mass each year. In men, bone loss is typically slow but steady from the time of peak accumulation until death. In general, men are less likely than women to experience osteoporotic fractures because their peak BMD is higher than women's. However, men are not completely protected from osteoporosis. Some estimate that 1 in 4 men over age 50 will experience an osteoporotic fracture (18). In addition to sex, race is a factor in determining peak bone mass. Peak BMD is generally higher in individuals of African descent compared with those of European and Asian ancestry (17).

Risk Factors for Osteoporosis

Female

Older age

Estrogen deficiency

Caucasian or Asian race

Low weight or BMI

Diet low in calcium

Alcohol abuse

Inactivity

Muscle weakness

Family history of osteoporosis

Smoking

History of fracture

Sometimes osteoporosis results from other medical conditions or is related to use of prescription medications; examples include endocrine disorders, gastrointestinal diseases, nutritional deficiencies, and the long-term use of glucocorticoid medications. Because of the many factors that lead to low bone density, people of all ages, including children, can develop osteoporosis. Low intake of calcium and vitamin D can limit the accumulation of bone during childhood, and it is estimated that only 25% of boys and 10% of girls achieve the recommended levels for calcium intake (17). Attaining a peak bone density that is lower than expected increases the risk of osteoporosis in later life. The International Osteoporosis Foundation (IOF) has developed a screening tool to assess risk for osteoporosis. This simple, online test, designed to help identify people at particularly high risk for osteoporosis, is found in the sidebar IOF One-Minute Osteoporosis Risk Test. When BMD is known, an estimate of one's 10 yr fracture risk can be calculated using FRAX®, an assessment measure published by the WHO. In addition to BMD, the FRAX® algorithm includes biological factors (e.g., age, sex), family history, and lifestyle factors (e.g., alcohol use). Information on the screening tool and FRAX® can be found at the IOF website (www.iofbonehealth.org).

Exercise in Prevention and Treatment of Osteoporosis

One of the primary means for preventing osteoporosis is maximizing bone accumulation during childhood and adolescence. In addition to adequate calcium and vitamin D intake, physical activity is important for developing strong bones. Studies demonstrate that children who exercise regularly have higher bone mineral levels than their sedentary peers, and this increase in bone carries over into adulthood (3). The primary goal for children is to participate in activities that maximize bone accrual.

The research examining exercise as a tool to increase bone density among adults has produced mixed results. Although some studies have demonstrated gains in bone density with exercise, others have shown that exercise has little effect. The wide variety among research protocols is one reason for the mixed results. Some common elements among studies that yielded the most profound effect on adult bone health are moderate to vigorous activity, adequate calcium intake (1,000-1,500 mg · day^{-1}) in conjunction with exercise, and movements that involve either impact loading or resistance training. For older adults, exercise alone may not be adequate to prevent age-related bone loss; however, exercise is essential in slowing this potentially devastating condition. Older adults with osteoporosis should be encouraged to engage in exercises designed to lower the risk of falling (e.g., balance and resistance training) in order to help protect against osteoporotic fractures.

Exercise Prescription for Bone Health

Exercise for children and adolescents helps maximize bone density. Regular participation in high-intensity loading activities should be encouraged. ACSM recommends the following (3):

- Mode: activities and sports that involve weight bearing and jumping (e.g., volleyball, gymnastics) and moderate resistance training

- Intensity: high-loading forces in jumping; moderate (<60% 1RM) resistance training

- Frequency: at least 3 days · wk^{-1}

- Duration: 10 to 20 min (multiple bouts per day if possible)

IOF One-Minute Osteoporosis Risk Test

Your Family History

- Has either of your parents been diagnosed with osteoporosis or broken a bone after a minor fall (a fall from standing height or less)? Yes No
- Did either of your parents have a "dowager's hump"? Yes No

Your Personal Clinical Factors

- Are you 40 years old or older? Yes No
- Have you ever broken a bone after a minor fall, as an adult? Yes No
- Do you fall frequently (more than once in the last year) or do you have a fear of falling because you are frail? Yes No
- After the age of 40, have you lost more than 3 cm in height (just over an inch)? Yes No
- Are you underweight, (is your Body Mass Index less than 19 kg/m²)? Yes No
- Have you ever taken corticosteroid tablets (cortisone, prednisone, etc.) for more than 3 consecutive months (corticosteroids are often prescribed for conditions like asthma, rheumatoid arthritis, and some inflammatory diseases)? Yes No
- Have you ever been diagnosed with rheumatoid arthritis? Yes No
- Have you been diagnosed with an over-reactive thyroid or over-reactive parathyroid glands? Yes No

For Women

- For women over 45, did your menopause occur before the age of 45? Yes No
- Have your periods ever stopped for 12 consecutive months or more (other than because of pregnancy, menopause, or hysterectomy)? Yes No
- Were your ovaries removed before age 50, without you taking hormonal replacement therapy? Yes No

For Men

- Have you ever suffered from impotence, lack of libido or other symptoms related to low testosterone levels? Yes No

Your Lifestyle Factors

- Do you regularly drink alcohol in excess of safe drinking limits (more than 2 units per day)? Yes No
- Do you currently, or have you ever, smoked cigarettes? Yes No
- Is your level of physical activity less than 30 minutes per day (housework, gardening, walking, running, etc.)? Yes No
- Do you avoid, or are you allergic to milk or dairy products, without taking any calcium supplements? Yes No
- Do you spend less than 10 minutes per day outdoors (with part of your body exposed to sunlight), without taking vitamin D supplements? Yes No

If you answered *yes* to one or more of these questions, it is possible that you are at increased risk for osteoporosis, and consultation with your physician is recommended.

Reprinted with permission from the International Osteoporosis Foundation, *Millennium one-minute osteoporosis risk test.* (Nyon, Switzerland) Available: www.iofbonehealth.org.

For nonosteoporotic adults, loading exercises and muscle-building activities promote bone health. An excellent example of this type of program is described by Metcalfe and colleagues (16). Using the evidence available, ACSM recommends the following approach to preserve bone during adulthood (3):

- Mode: weight-bearing aerobic exercise, jumping activities (e.g., basketball), and resistance exercise
- Intensity: moderate to high loading forces
- Frequency: weight-bearing endurance exercise 3 or 4 times · wk⁻¹; resistance exercise 2 or 3 times · wk⁻¹

- Duration: 30 to 60 min, combining weight-bearing and resistance exercise

Exercise Testing and Prescription for Individuals With Osteoporosis

For individuals with osteoporosis, precautions should be taken with both exercise testing and prescription. The benefits versus the risks of exercise testing must be weighed, and physician presence during maximal exercise testing is recommended (18). For individuals with severe kyphosis that limits forward vision or balance, stationary cycling may be a better choice than treadmill walking (4). Those with compression fractures may find cycle ergometry less painful than walking. Testing muscular strength can be important in designing programs for osteoporotic clients; however, maximal exertion and exercises that involve significant spinal flexion should be avoided because of the risk of compression fractures. Tests of balance and functionality can be useful in designing programs to reduce the risk of falling. Improving functional muscle strength and balance is important in reducing the risk of falls.

Exercise prescription for the osteoporotic client must be individualized and based on the severity of disease and the presence of other conditions. In general, exercise prescription should include aerobic activity, exercises that strengthen muscle, and activities that improve balance. This combination incorporates three major components: cardiovascular health, bone health, and reduced risk of falling. It is common for individuals with osteoporosis to be deconditioned, so initial exercise prescription may involve low-intensity activity and slow progression. Ultimately, one should attempt to reach the following exercise levels (4):

- Mode: weight-bearing aerobic exercise (walking, stair-climbing) and resistance exercise

- Intensity: moderate-intensity aerobic exercise (40% to 59% HRR); moderate loading force for resistance exercise (60%-80% 1RM)

- Frequency: weight-bearing endurance exercise 3 to 5 days · wk^{-1}; resistance exercise 2 or 3 days · wk^{-1}

- Duration: 30 to 60 min, combining weight-bearing and resistance exercise

Explosive, high-impact activities generally should be avoided by people with osteoporosis. Clients should be counseled to note any new pain, and this information should be carefully considered in modifying exercise. Exercises that improve balance should also be incorporated into the overall exercise program. Tai chi is an example of activity that can be used to improve balance and functional ability. See chapter 24 for more information on this and other types of mind–body exercises. For more details on exercise testing and prescription for osteoporotic clients, see Smith, Wang, and Bloomfield (19).

KEY POINT

Osteoporosis, a disease characterized by fragile bones, affects millions of Americans. Although males and females of all ages can develop osteoporosis, it is most commonly seen in postmenopausal women. Healthy eating practices and an active lifestyle are keys to promoting bone health. Exercises that involve impact loading or resistance training appear most beneficial for promoting bone development. Special care should be taken when testing and prescribing exercise for osteoporotic clients. Building strength, endurance, and balance should be special considerations when planning exercise for those with osteoporosis.

Female Athlete Triad

The female athlete triad includes three interrelated components: energy availability, bone health, and menstrual status (2). As shown in figure 17.1, athletes at the healthy end of the continuum eat healthy diets with an adequate number of calories to meet energy needs; have normal menstrual cycles; and have healthy, strong bones. Unfortunately, athletes who continually underconsume calories may have irregular or absent menses (amenorrhea) and compromised BMD (osteoporosis). If left untreated, this condition can produce significant health consequences, including glycogen depletion, anemia, and electrolyte imbalances (2).

The precipitating factor in the female athlete triad is low energy availability (with or without disordered eating). Anorexia nervosa and bulimia nervosa are two eating disorders commonly associated with the female athlete triad. However, among athletes who develop the triad, the

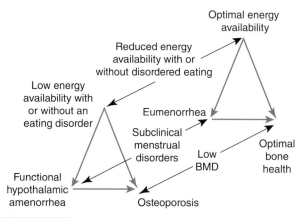

FIGURE 17.1 Female athlete triad.

Adapted, by permission, from American College of Sports Medicine, 2007, "Position stand on the female athlete triad," *Medicine and Science in Sports and Exercise* 39:1867-1882.

range of unhealthy eating practices varies. Some athletes clearly present with eating disorders, whereas others limit calories without meeting the strict clinical definitions of an eating disorder (2, 12). The unhealthy eating pattern with insufficient calories and nutritional density leads to amenorrhea. The estrogen deficiency seen in amenorrhea leads to osteopenia and potentially even osteoporosis. This loss of bone puts the athlete at great risk for stress fractures and for osteoporotic compression fractures.

In the general adult population, anorexia nervosa occurs at a rate of 0.5% to 1% and bulimia nervosa occurs at a rate of 2% to 4% (13). Although it is difficult to determine the percentage of athletes struggling with unhealthy eating practices, the prevalence of these eating disorders among athletes seems to be at least as high as that for the general population and is often found to be higher, particularly in sports with an emphasis on thinness (2). A meta-analysis found that some athletes are at particular risk for eating disorders (elite athletes, dancers, athletes in sports that emphasize thinness), whereas others (nonelite status, athletes in sports that do not emphasize thinness) may actually have some protection from unhealthy eating (20). Several studies have reported that one-third to one-half of elite female athletes report habits indicative of disordered eating (2). When left untreated, eating disorders can lead to seriously deteriorating health and potentially even death (see chapter 12).

Amenorrhea, or lack of menses, is clinically divided into two categories. **Primary amenorrhea** is characterized by the absence of menarche (i.e., first menses) in girls aged 16 or older. When there is a lack of menses for 3 or more consecutive months in females after menarche, it is classified as **secondary amenorrhea**. The cause of amenorrhea can be difficult to establish and involves a complex interaction among the hypothalamus, pituitary gland, and ovaries. Because of inadequate stimulation, the ovaries do not function normally, resulting in lower-than-normal estrogen and progesterone levels. The high prevalence of irregular menstruation has been observed in athletic women for a number of years, but the consequences on bone largely were ignored until Drinkwater and colleagues' landmark study (10) in which the bones of young amenorrheic athletes were found to be comparable in density to those of postmenopausal women. To help protect against bone loss, physicians sometimes treat amenorrheic athletes by replacing the missing endogenous estrogen with oral contraceptives, but the results of this treatment is minimal at best (2). Restoring a healthy eating pattern and achieving a normal weight are keys to assisting bone health (2).

Recognizing the signs of disordered eating (see chapter 12) is necessary before successful intervention. Often coaches and athletes are ill informed about the female athlete triad. Therefore, education is an important first step in battling this condition. Successful intervention for the female athlete triad requires a multidisciplinary approach that includes input from medical, nutritional, and psychological professionals (2, 12). Screening and diagnosis of the female athlete triad falls under the scope of practice for physicians and mental health professionals (2). The preparticipation physical or annual exam is an opportune time to screen for the triad.

Prevention of the female athlete triad takes effort on the part of many individuals: coaches, parents, nutritionists, health care providers, and officials providing oversight for sport governing bodies. Creating an environment that values optimal health as well as athletic performance is key. To create a healthy environment for female athletes, the National Athletic Trainers' Association (NATA) makes several recommendations including that ideal weight and body fat percentage be deemphasized and that public discussion of results from body composition testing be avoided (7). For more information on eating disorders, refer to chapter 12.

KEY POINT

The female athlete triad is characterized by low energy availability, amenorrhea, and osteoporosis. Anorexia nervosa and bulimia nervosa are eating disorders frequently seen in the female athlete triad and can lead to significant health impairment and even death if left untreated. Intervention for the female athlete triad should be multidisciplinary and should include psychological counseling.

STUDY QUESTIONS

1. What are the benefits of exercising during pregnancy?
2. What special precautions should a pregnant woman take when exercising?
3. What are the relative and absolute contraindications to exercise for pregnant women?
4. What is the standard exercise recommendation for pregnant women?
5. What is osteoporosis?
6. What are risk factors for osteoporosis?

7. What exercise recommendations for children will help promote good bone development?

8. What precautions should be taken when testing clients with osteoporosis?

9. What is the standard exercise prescription for a person with osteoporosis?

10. Describe the female athlete triad.

11. What steps might help prevent the female athlete triad?

CASE STUDIES

You can check your answers by referring to appendix A.

1. A sedentary 52-yr-old woman with a family history of osteoporosis comes to your facility for information on exercise to promote bone health. Her doctor says she is in generally good health and does not have osteoporosis, but there are signs that her bones are weaker than when she was younger (i.e., osteopenia). What type of exercise do you recommend?

2. Janice is an active, healthy, 32-yr-old woman who is pregnant for the first time. She is in her first trimester. Although she has been a runner for years, she has been told by her mother-in-law that she should give up running while pregnant. Her doctor told her she is perfectly healthy to continue running. What is your advice?

3. Samantha is a 17-yr-old runner who has dreams of someday competing in an Olympic marathon. You have been helping to plan her workouts for the past year, and you notice some disturbing signs: Her weight has decreased dramatically, she is constantly battling stress fractures, her mood is negative and characterized by self-criticism, and her performance times are worse than a few months earlier. What do you do?

REFERENCES

1. American College of Sports Medicine (ACSM). 1995. Position stand: Osteoporosis and exercise. *Medicine and Science in Sports and Exercise* 27:i-vii.

2. American College of Sports Medicine (ACSM). 2007. Position stand: The female athlete triad. *Medicine and Science in Sports and Exercise* 39:1867-1882.

3. American College of Sports Medicine (ACSM). 2004. Physical activity and bone health. *Medicine and Science in Sports and Exercise* 36:1985-1996.

4. American College of Sports Medicine (ACSM). 2010. *ACSM's guidelines for exercise testing and prescription.* 8th ed. Baltimore: Lippincott Williams & Wilkins.

5. American College of Obstetricians and Gynecologists (ACOG). 2003. Exercise during pregnancy and the postpartum period. *Clinical Obstetrics and Gynecology* 46:496-499.

6. Artal, R., C. Sherman, and N.A. DiNubile. 1999. Exercise during pregnancy. *Physician and Sportsmedicine* 27:51-60+.

7. Bonci, C.M., L.J. Bonci, L.R. Granger, C.L. Johnson, R.M. Malina, L.W. Milne, R.R. Ryan, and E.W. Vanderbunt. 2008. National Athletic Trainers' Association position statement: Preventing, detecting, and managing disordered eating in athletes. *Journal of Athletic Training* 43:80-108.

8. Coe, D.P., and M.A. Fiatarone-Singh. 2010. Exercise prescription in special populations: women, pregnancy, children and the elderly. In *ACSM's resource manual for guidelines for exercise testing and prescription.* 6th ed. Ed. J.K. Ehrman, 665-695. Baltimore: Lippincott Williams & Wilkins.

9. Davies, G.A., L.A. Wolfe, M.F. Mottola, and C. MacKinnon. 2003. Joint SOGC/CSEP clinical practice guideline: Exercise in pregnancy and the postpartum period. *Canadian Journal of Applied Physiology* 28:330-341.

10. Drinkwater, B.L., K. Nilson, C.H. Chesnut, W.J. Bremner, S. Schainholtz, and M.B. Southworth. 1984. Bone mineral content of amenorrheic and eumenorrheic athletes. *New England Journal of Medicine* 311:277-281.

11. Heffernan, A.E. 2000. Exercise and pregnancy in primary care. *Nurse Practitioner* 25:42, 49, 53-56, 59-60.

12. Hobart, J.A., and D.R. Smucker. 2000. The female athlete triad. *American Family Physician* 61:3357-3364, 3367.

13. Johnson, M.D. 1994. Disordered eating. In *Medical and orthopedic issues of active and athletic women*, ed. R. Agostini, 141-151. Philadelphia: Hanley & Belfus.

14. Khan, K., H. McKay, P. Kannus, D. Bailey, J. Wark, and K. Bennell. 2001. *Physical activity and bone health.* Champaign, IL: Human Kinetics.

15. Melzer, K., Y. Schutz, M. Boulvain, and B. Kayser. 2010. Physical activity and pregnancy: cardiovascular adaptations, recommendations and pregnancy outcomes. *Sports Medicine* 40:493-507.

16. Metcalfe, L., T. Lohman, S. Going, L. Houtkooper, D. Ferriera, H. Flint-Wagner, T. Guido, J. Martin, J. Wright, and E. Cussler. 2001. Postmenopausal women and exercise for prevention of osteoporosis: The Bone, Estrogen, Strength Training (BEST) study. *ACSM's Health and Fitness Journal* 5:6-14.

17. National Institutes of Health (NIH). 2000. Osteoporosis prevention, diagnosis, and therapy. NIH Consensus Development Conference. Bethesda, MD: Author.

18. Petit, M.A., J.M. Hughes, and J.M. Warpeha. 2010. Exercise prescription for people with osteoporosis. In *ACSM's resource manual for guidelines for exercise testing and prescription*. 6th ed. Ed. J.K. Ehrman, 635-650. Baltimore: Lippincott Williams & Wilkins.

19. Smith, S.S., C.H.E. Wang, and S.A. Bloomfield. 2009. Osteoporosis. In *ACSM's exercise management for persons with chronic diseases and disabilities*, 3rd ed., ed. J.L. Durstine, G.E. Moore, P.L. Painter, and S.O. Roberts, 270-279. Champaign, IL: Human Kinetics.

20. Smolak, L., S.K. Murnen, and A.E. Ruble. 2000. Female athletes and eating problems: A meta-analysis. *International Journal of Eating Disorders* 27:371-380.

21. Streuling, I., A. Beyerlein, E. Rosenfeld, H. Hofmann, T. Schulz, and R. von Kries. 2011. Physical activity and gestational weight gain: A meta-analysis of intervention trials. *British Journal of Obstetrics and Gynaecology* 118:278-284.

22. Tobias, D.K., C. Zhang, R.M. van Dam, K. Bowers, and F.B. Hu. 2011. Physical activity before and during pregnancy and risk of gestational diabetes mellitus. *Diabetes Care* 34:223-229.

23. U.S. Department of Health and Human Services (HHS). 2004. *Bone health and osteoporosis: A report of the Surgeon General*. Rockville, MD: HHS, Office of the Surgeon General.

24. U.S. Department of Health and Human Services (HHS). 2008. *2008 Physical Activity Guidelines for Americans*. www.health.gov/paguidelines/guidelines/default.aspx.

25. Wang, T.W., and B.S. Apgar. 1998. Exercise during pregnancy. *American Family Physician* 57:1846-1852, 1857.

Exercise and Heart Disease

David R. Bassett, Jr.

The reader will be able to do the following:

1. Describe the atherosclerotic process and the resulting outcome if blood flow becomes obstructed in the arteries of the heart, brain, or periphery.

2. Quantify the magnitude of CVD as a health problem in the United States and list the various subcategories of CVD.

3. Identify the various patient populations found in cardiac rehabilitation programs.

4. Describe the physiological and mental health benefits of exercise for individuals with CVD.

5. Explain what is meant by secondary prevention of CHD.

6. Describe tests that can help diagnose the presence or absence of CHD, including those that use exercise and nonexercise challenges to stress the heart.

7. Describe how to prescribe aerobic exercise (frequency, intensity, and duration) in cardiac rehabilitation programs.

8. Discuss special considerations in prescribing exercise intensity for individuals who are taking beta-blocker medications.

Coronary heart disease (CHD) is a major problem in the United States and other industrialized nations. This chapter provides the fitness professional with a basic understanding of the development of CHD, the types of patients found in cardiac rehabilitation programs, the benefits of exercise for a cardiac population, and the special considerations for exercise prescription in this group. It is not a comprehensive guide to exercise in cardiac rehabilitation; a number of excellent texts provide more complete information on the topic (3, 5, 14).

Atherosclerosis

Atherosclerosis refers to an accumulation of lipid deposits in the large and medium-sized arteries (figure 18.1), a process that provokes fibrosis and calcification. The atherosclerotic process begins early in life, as evidenced by studies of soldiers killed in the Korean War. Approximately three-fourths of the 300 soldiers examined (mean age 22.1 yr) had some degree of blockage in their coronary arteries (8). It is believed that the atherosclerotic process begins when the **endothelial cells** lining the artery become damaged because of smoking, toxic agents, or high BP (see Hypertension sidebar). When lipoproteins are deposited at the damaged site, plaque formation (or atherosclerosis) occurs. Eventually, these deposits impede blood flow in the affected arteries, sometimes to the point of complete occlusion (21).

Consequences of Atherosclerosis

Atherosclerosis can occur in various arteries throughout the body and have various results. Blockages in the coronary arteries lead to **myocardial ischemia** (reduced blood flow to the heart) and in severe cases to **myocardial infarction**

(MI). If the blood vessels in the brain become occluded, a **stroke** will result. Blockages in the peripheral leg vessels can result in **claudication**, or intermittent muscle pain that occurs with exertion.

Cardiovascular Disease

In the United States, CVD is the leading cause of death, with 831,272 people dying from CVD (including congenital cardiovascular defects) in 2006. CHD accounts for 51% of these deaths, with stroke (17%), hypertensive disease (7%), and CHF (7%) making up most of the other leading causes (4). (CVD refers to any disease of the heart and the blood vessels or circulation, while CHD is a more specific condition resulting from reduced blood flow in the coronary arteries.) The death rate attributable to coronary artery disease (CAD) has declined in recent decades, but it remains a problem of huge proportions. According to the AHA, approximately 1,255,000 Americans will have a coronary attack this year. About 785,000 of these will be first heart attacks, and the rest will be recurrent attacks. Of those experiencing a heart attack, 80% will survive, and some of the survivors will be referred to cardiac rehabilitation programs (4). Although CVD is often thought of as a man's disease, it is the leading cause of death in women as well as men.

> **KEY POINT**
>
> Atherosclerosis is a disease that starts early in life and leads to blockages in the arteries of the heart, brain, or peripheral muscles. If a blockage occurs in a coronary artery, myocardial ischemia or infarction results. There is a high prevalence of such health problems in the United States.

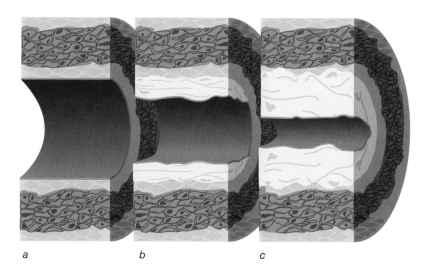

a   b   c

FIGURE 18.1 Stages of atherosclerosis: *(a)* normal artery, *(b)* partially blocked artery, and *(c)* significantly blocked artery.

Hypertension

Hypertension, or high BP, greatly increases the risk of developing CVD. It is estimated that 75 million people in the United States have hypertension (4), defined as a BP of 140/90 or higher. **Stage 1 hypertension** is defined as an SBP of 140 to 159 mmHg or a DBP of 90 to 99 mmHg. For those who have this type of hypertension, a variety of nonpharmacological approaches to reducing BP are often recommended at first; however, if their BP is not normalized with lifestyle changes, medications may be prescribed. Dietary change includes reducing sodium intake, which has been shown to independently lower SBP and DBP by 5 and 3 mmHg, respectively (13,15). Obesity is linked to hypertension, and research shows that a loss of 1 kg of body weight decreases SBP and DBP by 1.6 and 1.3 mmHg, respectively (13, 15). Also, participating in an endurance exercise program has been shown to decrease SBP and DBP by 7 and 6 mmHg, respectively, in hypertensive individuals (1).

Stage 2 hypertension (SBP of 160-179 mmHg or DBP of 100-109 mmHg) is more serious, and it is typically controlled through medication (see chapter 25). **Stage 3 hypertension** refers to a persistent elevation in BP (SBP >180 mmHg or DBP >110 mmHg) with target-organ damage. This may include damage to the heart (such as enlargement of the left ventricle), damage to the kidneys leading to renal insufficiency, and damage to the eyes caused by small hemorrhages in the blood vessels.

The standard ACSM exercise prescription for improving $\dot{V}O_2$max (see chapter 11) also reduces BP in previously hypertensive individuals (1, 13). In addition, endurance exercise at moderate intensities (40%-60% $\dot{V}O_2$max) has been shown to reduce BP. Moderate-intensity exercise should be done frequently and for durations long enough to expend a large number of calories. Furthermore, for people with higher BPs who are taking medication, this type of exercise program along with changes in diet, smoking, and body weight can lower BP. In these cases, BP should be checked frequently so medications can be reduced as needed. Gradually establishing appropriate diet and exercise habits improves the chance that a person will maintain an appropriate BP once it has been normalized.

Populations in Cardiac Rehabilitation Programs

Cardiac rehabilitation programs include people who have experienced angina pectoris, MI, **coronary artery bypass graft (CABG)**, and angioplasty (10,11). **Angina pectoris** refers to the chest pain attributable to ischemia of the ventricle resulting from an occlusion of one or more of the coronary arteries. The pain appears when the oxygen requirement of the heart (estimated by the double product SBP · HR) exceeds a value that coronary blood flow can meet. The ischemia can be transient and may subside once the oxygen demand of the heart returns to normal.

MI patients have heart damage (death of ventricular muscle fibers) caused by the occlusion of one or more of the coronary arteries. The degree to which ventricular function is affected depends on the mass of the ventricle permanently damaged. Individuals who have experienced an MI usually take medications (beta-blockers) to reduce the work of the heart and control the irritability of the heart tissue so that dangerous arrhythmias (irregular heartbeats) do not occur. Generally, these individuals experience a training effect similar to that of people who have not had an MI.

CABG patients have had surgery to bypass one or more blocked coronary arteries. In this procedure, a blood vessel is sewn into existing coronary arteries above and below the blockage in order to reroute the blood flow (see figure 18.2). People with chronic angina pectoris before CABG find a relief of symptoms, with 50% to 70% experiencing no more pain. Generally, with an increased blood flow to the ventricle, left ventricular function and the capacity for work improve (22). These patients benefit from systematic exercise training because most are deconditioned before surgery as a result of activity restrictions related to chest pain.

Some CHD patients undergo a special procedure, **percutaneous transluminal coronary angioplasty (PTCA)**, to open occluded arteries. In this procedure, the chest is not opened; instead, a balloon-tipped catheter (a long, slender tube) is inserted into the coronary artery, where the balloon is inflated to push the plaque back toward the arterial wall (see figure 18.3). These patients tend not to have as severe CHD as those who undergo CABG. For these patients, PTCA has some advantages, including being less invasive, requiring a shorter hospital stay (1-2 days instead of 6-9 days), and costing less (11). However, with PTCA the coronary artery becomes reoccluded in approximately one-third to one-half of patients within 6 mo of the procedure (12).

To help prevent reocclusion, **intracoronary stents** are often used to help keep the lumen of the coronary artery open. A stent is composed of a metal mesh that is inserted into the artery on a balloon catheter and positioned in the area of obstruction. Some stents slowly release a drug that helps to prevent restenosis; these are known as drug-eluting

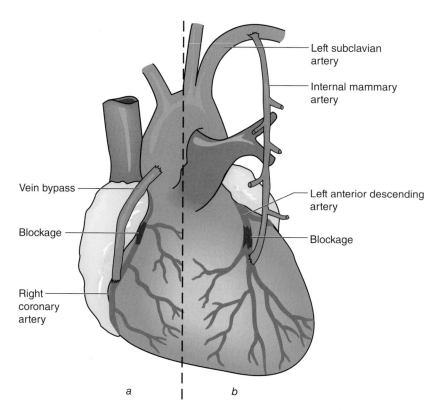

FIGURE 18.2 Coronary artery bypass surgery. *(a)* CABG using saphenous vein and *(b)* CABG using mammary artery. Blood flow is rerouted around the site of obstruction by taking a blood vessel from another part of the body and sewing it to the affected coronary artery, distal to the site of the obstruction. Blood vessels typically used in the procedure are the saphenous (leg) vein and the mammary artery.

Reprinted from *Pathophysiology: Clinical concepts of disease processes*, 4th ed, S.A. Price and L.M. Wilson, p. 439. Copyright 1992. By permission of Lorraine Wilson.

stents. The balloon is first inflated to increase the lumen size, and then it is deflated and pulled back while the stent remains embedded in the artery. The main disadvantage of metal stents is that they increase the risk of blood clots; hence, anticoagulation therapy is needed to reduce this risk (6).

> **KEY POINT**
>
> CHD is treated by CABG, angioplasty, or intracoronary stent. Patients who have undergone these procedures are candidates for a hospital-based cardiac rehabilitation program.

Evidence for Exercise Training

Fifty years ago, the most common advice given to patients who had experienced an MI was to take several weeks of complete bed rest (3). Today, however, exercise training is an ordinary part of treatment for people with CHD. Cardiac rehabilitation programs use a multidisciplinary approach of education and exercise to help clients with heart disease return to normal function within the limits of their disease (14).

There is no question that patients with CHD have improved cardiovascular function as a result of exercising. This is evidenced by higher $\dot{V}O_2$max values, higher work rates achieved without ischemia (as shown by angina pectoris or ST segment changes), and an increased capacity for prolonged submaximal work (7, 19, 21). Moderate reductions in body fat, BP, total cholesterol, serum triglycerides, and LDL-C have been shown to occur with regular exercise, along with increases in HDL-C. The improved lipid profile is a function of more than the exercise alone, given that weight loss and the saturated-fat content of the diet can modify these variables.

A major focus of cardiac rehabilitation programs is to reduce the occurrence of subsequent MIs (3). This is referred to as **secondary prevention** of CHD. The Framingham Heart Study has shown that people who have experienced one heart attack are at increased risk of a second heart attack. Further, the likelihood of recurrence clearly is associated with many of the same risk factors that caused atherosclerosis in the first place. Thus, cardiac rehabilitation personnel must monitor BP, blood cholesterol levels, and smoking in their patients. In general, research has shown that a cardiac rehabilitation program involving exercise results in a 20% to 25% reduction in all-cause and cardiovascular mortality after an MI. This is good news,

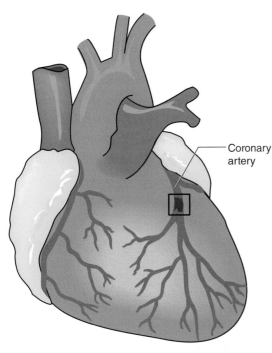

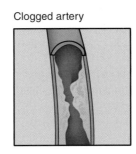

Clogged artery

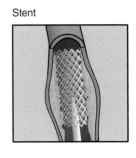

Stent

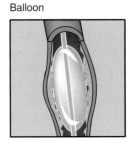

Balloon

Coronary artery

FIGURE 18.3 Percutaneous transluminal coronary angioplasty (PTCA). The cardiologist locates a clogged section of a coronary artery by injecting a contrast dye into the artery, allowing it to be seen on an X-ray machine. A guide wire is inserted into a femoral artery and is pushed up to the heart, where it is used to position the balloon catheter at the site of obstruction inside the coronary artery. The balloon is temporarily inflated, increasing the lumen size and capacity for blood flow. The balloon catheter is then deflated and removed. In some cases, a metal stent is placed inside the coronary artery to help keep it open. The stent is expanded by inflation pressure, and it remains inside the patient.

because it indicates that such patients derive a substantial benefit from participating in cardiac rehabilitation. In addition, patients gain an improved sense of well-being (14).

One of the most exciting developments in cardiac rehabilitation in recent years is the demonstration that lifestyle modification can reverse CAD. Ornish and colleagues (18) conducted a series of studies in which they showed that a program consisting of a strict vegetarian diet, yoga, meditation, smoking cessation, and physical activity reversed the atherosclerotic process. Patients in this study showed actual reversal of blockages in their coronary arteries, lending credibility to the idea that this condition can, in some cases, be treated with nonsurgical interventions. The lifestyle intervention group had more regression of CHD after 5 yr than after 1 yr, while the control group (which made more modest changes in lifestyle) showed continued

KEY POINT

Cardiac rehabilitation programs help people with heart disease regain their fitness and return to normal, everyday activities. The benefits of such programs include increased work capacity and reduced cardiovascular risk factors. Cardiac rehabilitation programs generally lower the risk of a second heart attack.

progression of atherosclerosis and more than twice as many cardiac events.

Special Diagnostic Tests to Detect Coronary Heart Disease

Testing a patient with CHD is much more involved than testing the apparently healthy person. There are some classes of patients with CHD for whom exercise or exercise testing is inappropriate and dangerous (2). (See chapter 7 for absolute and relative contraindications to exercise.) In others, however, the benefits of a **graded exercise test (GXT)** outweigh the risks. Diagnostic exercise testing is nearly always performed in a hospital environment with a physician present. A 12-lead ECG is monitored at discrete intervals during the GXT, and three leads are displayed continuously on an oscilloscope. BP, RPE, and various signs and symptoms also are noted. Emergency equipment includes a defibrillator, supplemental oxygen, and emergency medications. Personnel trained and certified in advanced cardiac life support (ACLS) are on hand to provide assistance if needed.

Treadmill tests commonly used in diagnostic exercise testing are the Naughton, Balke, Bruce, and Ellestad protocols, named after their developers (2). These protocols are all GXTs that increase speed or grade at regular intervals to increase the exercise intensity. For those who are unable to perform treadmill exercise, a cycle test or arm ergometer test may be used. The criteria for terminating the GXT focus on various pathological signs (e.g., ST segment depression on the ECG) or symptoms (e.g., angina pectoris) rather than on achieving some percentage of age-adjusted maximal HR (2). A subjective angina scale may be used to assess the severity of the symptoms (see table 18.1).

Other tests of heart function include radionuclide procedures, typically administered in conjunction with either exercise or pharmacological (nonexercise) stress tests (5, 6, 16). In the latter case, the pharmacologic agents provoke myocardial ischemia through either increased myocardial oxygen demand or coronary vasodilation. For instance, thallium-201 (a radioactive substance) can be injected intravenously to assess myocardial perfusion. Thallium is taken up by well-perfused myocardium similarly to the way potassium is taken up. Ischemic myocardium tends not to take up the thallium, thus identifying areas of the heart with poor blood flow. Another technique involves a radioisotope that binds to the red blood cells (technetium-99m), which is useful for cardiac blood pool imaging. This allows the end-systolic volume (ESV) and end-diastolic volume (EDV) to be measured, and the ejection fraction then can be computed as follows: Ejection fraction = (EDV − ESV) ÷ EDV. A normal ejection fraction is 55% to 70%, but a person with a severely damaged myocardium may have an ejection fraction of only 30%. Ventricular wall motion abnormalities also can be identified (6).

The most definitive tests for CHD are **coronary angiography** and **positron emission tomography (PET)** scans. In angiography, a cardiac catheter is inserted into the femoral artery and pushed all the way up the aorta until it reaches the entrance to a coronary artery, where the curved tip of the catheter guide allows it to be inserted into the artery. A contrast dye is injected through the catheter into the coronary artery. By viewing an image of the coronary arteries on a screen, the cardiologist can measure the degree of occlusion (narrowing) that exists (see figure 18.4). PET scans use [18F]deoxyglucose or [13N]ammonia. These substances allow the level of myocardial cell metabolism to be assessed. Metabolically active areas, indicative of good perfusion, can be distinguished from underperfused areas by color.

KEY POINT

Special types of diagnostic tests can determine whether a patient has CHD. Using GXTs on the treadmill (with close monitoring of the ECG and BP) is a common method of detecting signs and symptoms of heart disease. Radionuclide tests can more definitively confirm the presence or absence of heart disease.

Typical Exercise Prescription

Fitness professionals who work in health clubs and YMCAs often encounter clients who have gone through a cardiac rehabilitation program. Thus, it is important to have an understanding and appreciation of what these clients have experienced during their recovery process. In addition, many individuals with a master's degree in exercise physiology can, with the proper training, find jobs in cardiac rehabilitation. As part of a team of medical

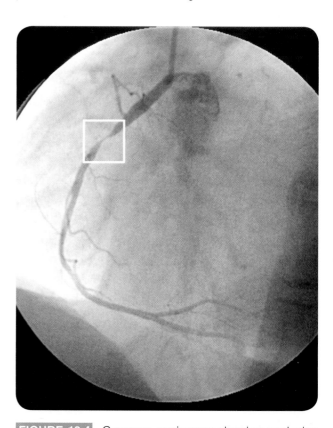

FIGURE 18.4 Coronary angiogram showing occlusion (narrowing) of a coronary artery. A catheter has been inserted into a coronary artery and radiographic contrast dye injected to allow the artery to be seen.

Courtesy of David R. Bassett Jr.

TABLE 18.1 Angina Rating Scale

1	Mild, barely noticeable
2	Moderate, bothersome
3	Moderately severe, very uncomfortable
4	Most severe or most intense pain ever experienced

This scale is used in rating the subjective pain associated with myocardial insufficiency.

Adapted from American College of Sports Medicine 2006.

professionals that includes physicians, nurses, dieticians, physical therapists, and clinical psychologists, the fitness professional can play an important role in helping patients to resume a healthy life after a heart event (20). A fitness professional working in cardiac rehabilitation must be vigilant about monitoring the signs and symptoms of heart disease. This involves knowing how to read an ECG, take BP readings, and administer the angina rating scale (refer back to table 18.1). Fitness professionals should be trained in emergency procedures and preferably should achieve certification in ACLS.

The details of how to design and implement cardiac rehabilitation programs, from the first steps taken after patients are confined to bed to the time that they return to work and beyond, are provided in the AACVPR guidelines (3). This section briefly introduces these programs.

Cardiac rehabilitation programs are organized in progressive phases of programming to meet the needs of clients and their families. Phase I (the acute phase) begins when a patient arrives in the hospital step-down unit after leaving the intensive or coronary care unit (14). Within 1 to 3 days of the MI or revascularization procedure, the patient has already been taught the risk factors for atherosclerotic disease and begun the rehabilitation process. Patients are exposed to orthostatic or gravitation stress by intermittently sitting and standing. Later, bedside activities and slow ambulation (i.e., walking) in the hallways are recommended (3).

Phases II and III refer to outpatient exercise programs conducted in a hospital environment. Rhythmic activities using large muscle groups are recommended for physical conditioning; these activities include treadmill exercise, cycle ergometry, combined arm and leg exercise, rowing, and stair-climbing. Light to moderate resistance training is accomplished with free weights (dumbbells) and elastic tubing. Special care must be taken when prescribing upper-body exercises to clients who have undergone CABG procedures because of limitations related to the chest incision. See chapter 13 for more details on resistance training in cardiac populations.

Recommendations for aerobic exercise programming in outpatient cardiac rehabilitation (phases II and III) are as follows, with patients progressing on an individual basis (9-11):

- Frequency: 3 to 4 days $\cdot$ wk^{-1}
- Intensity: 40% to 75% of $\dot{V}O_2$max or HRR
- Duration: 20 to 40 min $\cdot$ day^{-1}
- 5 to 10 min of warm-up and cool-down exercises

Fitness professionals who work in cardiac rehabilitation must have knowledge of cardiovascular medications (for a description of these, see chapter 25). Patients who are on beta-blockers require special consideration, because the Karvonen formula for computing THR range is invalid if the client was not on beta-blockers at the time of testing. For these patients, a THR is sometimes computed by adding 20 to 30 beats $\cdot$ min^{-1} to the client's standing, resting HR. However, in view of the wide differences in physiological responses to beta-blockade, another approach is to use RPE ratings around *somewhat hard*, which correspond to 11 to 14 on the original Borg RPE scale (3).

In phase II, clients are monitored carefully for vital signs (HR, BP, ventilation), and the ECG is monitored at a central observation station via telemetry (radio signals). A single-channel recording of 6 to 10 patients can be monitored simultaneously on a computer screen, and in the event of arrhythmias or ST segment changes, a rhythm strip is printed out. The rate–pressure product (SBP $\cdot$ HR) is sometimes used as an indicator of myocardial oxygen demand. After training, the rate–pressure product at a fixed work rate is reduced, allowing the cardiac patient to exercise at higher work rates before the onset of angina (20). In addition to exercise classes, patient education classes are offered, and they cover topics such as healthy eating, stress management, cardiovascular medications, and principles of behavior modification. Phase II programs typically last about 12 wk and are covered by health insurance.

Phase III programs are hospital-based programs in which outpatients are encouraged to continue their exercise regimens and are provided access to continuing health care and patient education. In these cases, the client's ECG usually is not monitored by telemetry, but clients continue to follow an individualized exercise prescription and attend patient education classes. Eventually, clients may enter the maintenance phase and move to a phase IV program in a nonhospital setting (e.g., sports medicine clinic).

For heart patients who are unable to attend a traditional cardiac rehabilitation outpatient program due to geography or finances, there are other options. Many hospitals offer rehabilitation programs following a distance-education model and can even monitor a client's ECG over the Internet. In addition, a group called Mended Hearts (http://mendedhearts.org/) offers support-group meetings and online resources to help clients with heart disease and their families deal with the physical and emotional effects of heart disease.

KEY POINT

Cardiac rehabilitation programs are divided into four phases. Phase I is the acute phase, performed while the patient is still in the hospital. Phases II and III are conducted on an outpatient basis, and phase IV is the maintenance phase. Cardiac patients can benefit from aerobic and resistance training, but working with this population requires special knowledge of their medical conditions.

STUDY QUESTIONS

1. Define *atherosclerosis*, and list three alterable cardiovascular risk factors that promote the atherosclerotic process.

2. Describe what will happen if an atherosclerotic plaque leads to a blockage in blood flow to a carotid artery, coronary artery, or femoral artery.

3. Where does CVD rank among causes of death in the United States today? What are four subcategories of CVD?

4. Describe the effects of aerobic exercise on people with hypertension. What are some other recommended treatments for hypertension?

5. List four specific patient populations who are commonly referred to cardiac rehabilitation programs.

6. What evidence is there that exercise training can be beneficial for individuals with CHD?

7. One of the goals of any cardiac rehabilitation program is secondary prevention of CHD. Explain what this means.

8. Identify diagnostic tests that can be used to detect the presence of CHD.

9. Outline the recommendations for aerobic exercise programming in phase II and phase III cardiac rehabilitation in terms of frequency, intensity, duration, and mode. Is weight training recommended?

10. Why is the Karvonen formula often not very useful in establishing a THR for a cardiac patient?

CASE STUDIES

You can check your answers by referring to appendix A.

1. John is a 46-yr-old male. He is an insurance executive who is married with two children. John is active in his church and plays golf on the weekends. He went to see his cardiologist because he experienced recent fatigue with chest pain on exertion. He has never smoked but he consumes 1 to 2 alcoholic drinks a day. His medical history reveals a blood cholesterol level of 263 mg $\cdot$ dl^{-1}, a triglyceride level of 195 mg $\cdot$ dl^{-1}, and an HDL-C value of 45 mg $\cdot$ dl^{-1}. Considering his sex, age, symptoms, and risk factors, what do you think is the likelihood he has CHD? What would be a reasonable next step to diagnose the presence or absence of CHD?

2. Jane is a 61-yr-old retired female. She recently underwent a left heart catheterization, which revealed significant occlusion in the left anterior descending artery and the circumflex artery. Therefore, a balloon angioplasty procedure was performed. Approximately 2 wk later, she performed a GXT with the following results:

Protocol: Balke (3.3 mi $\cdot$ hr^{-1}, or 5.3 km $\cdot$ hr^{-1})

Resting: HR = 72 beats $\cdot$ min^{-1}, BP = 130/72 mmHg

End point: stage 3 for 1 min (approximately 7 METs)

HR = 126 beats $\cdot$ min^{-1}, BP = 160/90 mmHg

Reason for termination: Fatigue

No ST segment depression, no reported symptoms

Jane was taking atenolol (a beta-blocker) at the time of her test, and her physician instructed her to continue taking this medication. She was referred to the cardiac rehabilitation center for supervised exercise and risk-factor modification. List some types of exercise that would be appropriate for her. In addition to the mode, be sure to recommend an appropriate frequency, intensity, and duration of exercise.

3. Ralph is a 65-yr-old male who had CABGs on two coronary arteries (left anterior descending and circumflex). Both arteries were 75% occluded at the time of his surgery, which involved a sternectomy. His sternum was cut and separated, and the saphenous vein in his leg was harvested to obtain the grafting material; the sternum was then closed and fastened with stainless steel wires that are still in his chest. Ralph has completed phase I cardiac rehabilitation and has now been referred to an outpatient cardiac rehabilitation program 3 wk postoperative. He has inquired about a weight training program as part of his 12 wk phase II cardiac rehabilitation. What type of resistance training program would you design for this cardiac patient?

REFERENCES

1. American College of Sports Medicine (ACSM). 2004. Position stand: Exercise and hypertension. *Medicine and Science in Sports and Exercise* 36(3): 533-553.

2. American College of Sports Medicine (ACSM). 2010. *ACSM's guidelines for exercise testing and prescription.* 8th ed. Baltimore: Lippincott Williams & Wilkins.

3. American Association for Cardiovascular and Pulmonary Rehabilitation (AACVPR). 2004. *Guidelines for cardiac rehabilitation and secondary prevention programs.* 4th ed. Champaign, IL: Human Kinetics.

4. American Heart Association (AHA). 2010. *Heart and stroke statistics—2010 update.* Dallas: Author.

5. Brubaker, P.H., L.A. Kaminsky, and M.H. Whaley. 2002. *Coronary artery disease: Essentials of prevention and rehabilitation programs.* Champaign, IL: Human Kinetics.

6. Brubaker, P.H. 2008. Contemporary approaches to cardiovascular disease diagnosis. In *Pollock's textbook of cardiovascular disease and rehabilitation*, 83-94. Champaign, IL: Human Kinetics.

7. Clausen, J.P. 1977. Circulatory adjustments to dynamic exercise and physical training in normal subjects and in patients with coronary artery disease. In *Exercise and the heart,* ed. E.H. Sonnenblick and M. Lesch, 39-75. New York: Grune & Stratton.

8. Enos, W., R. Holmes, and J. Beyer. 1953. Coronary disease among United States soldiers killed in action in Korea. *Journal of the American Medical Association* 152:1090-1093.

9. Franklin, B.A., J.E. Trivax, and T.E. Vanhecke. 2008. Coronary artery disease, myocardial infarction, and angina pectoris. In *Pollock's textbook of cardiovascular disease and rehabilitation*, 271-284. Champaign, IL: Human Kinetics.

10. Franklin, B.A. 2009. Myocardial infarction. In *ACSM's exercise management for persons with chronic diseases and disabilities. 3rd ed.* Ed. J.L. Durstine and G.E. Moore, 49-57. Champaign, IL: Human Kinetics.

11. Franklin, B.A. 2009. Revascularization: CABGS and PTCA or PCI. In *ACSM's exercise management for persons with chronic diseases and disabilities. 3rd ed. E*d. J.L. Durstine, G.E. Moore, P.L. Painter, and S.O. Roberts, 58-65. Champaign, IL: Human Kinetics.

12. Grines, C.L. 1996. Aggressive intervention for myocardial infarction: Angioplasty, stents, and intra-aortic balloon pumping. *American Journal of Cardiology* 78:29-34.

13. Hagberg, J.M. 1990. Exercise, fitness, and hypertension. In *Physical activity, fitness, and health,* ed. C. Bouchard, R.J. Shephard, and T. Stephens, 993-1005. Champaign, IL: Human Kinetics.

14. Hillegass E.A., and W.C. Temes. 2001. Therapeutic interventions in cardiac rehabilitation and prevention. In *Essentials of cardiopulmonary physical therapy.* 2nd ed. Ed. E.A. Hillegass and H.S. Sadowsky, 676-726. Philadelphia: Saunders.

15. Kaplan, N.M. 1994. *Clinical hypertension.* 6th ed. Baltimore: Williams & Wilkins.

16. McCullough, P.A. 2010. Diagnostic procedures for cardiovascular disease. In *ACSM's resource manual for guidelines for exercise testing and prescription.* 6th ed. Ed. J.K. Ehrman, 360-374. Baltimore: Lippincott Williams & Wilkins.

17. Nagelkirk, P. 2010. Pathophysiology and treatment of cardiovascular disease. In *ACSM's resource manual for guidelines for exercise testing and prescription.* 6th ed. Ed. J.K. Ehrman, 109-118. Baltimore: Lippincott Williams & Wilkins.

18. Ornish, D., L.W. Scherwitz, and J.H. Billings. 1998. Intensive lifestyle changes for reversal of coronary heart disease. *Journal of the American Medical Association* 280:2001-2007.

19. Pollock, M.L., and J.H. Wilmore. 1990. *Exercise in health and disease.* 2nd ed. Philadelphia: Saunders.

20. Schairer, J.R., R.A. Jarvis, amd S.J. Keteyian. 2010. Exercise prescription in patients with cardiovascular disease. In *ACSM's resource manual for guidelines for exercise testing and prescription.* 6th ed. Ed. J.K. Ehrman, 559-574. Baltimore: Lippincott Williams & Wilkins.

21. Thompson, P.D. 1988. The benefits and risks of exercise training in patients with chronic coronary artery disease. *Journal of the American Medical Association* 259:1537-1540.

22. Wenger, N.K., and J.W. Hurst. 1984. Coronary bypass surgery as a rehabilitative procedure. In *Rehabilitation of the coronary patient,* Ed. N.K. Wenger and H.K. Hellerstein, 115-132. New York: Wiley.

Exercise and Obesity

OBJECTIVES

The reader will be able to do the following:

1. Define *obesity* and describe its health risks.

2. Describe the role that exercise plays in preventing and treating obesity.

3. Explain the modifications to standard testing procedures necessary for clients who are obese.

4. Write an exercise prescription for someone who is obese.

Obesity is characterized by excessive adiposity. It can be documented by examining the relationship between height and weight (e.g., BMI) or by evaluating percent body fat (%BF). Because BMI requires simple measurements and, for the majority of adults, closely relates to body fatness, it has become the clinically preferred method of assessing obesity (see chapter 8). Generally accepted guidelines classify a BMI of 30 kg · m⁻² or higher as obese (9). The following are subclasses of obesity:

- Class I obesity—30.0 to 34.9 kg · m⁻²
- Class II obesity—35.0 to 39.9 kg · m⁻²
- Class III (extreme) obesity—40 kg · m⁻² or higher

Although there are no universally agreed-upon standards for classifying obesity from %BF, a %BF of >38% for females and >25% for males generally is considered to be obese (28). Another tool used to screen for obesity is WC (waist circumference; see chapter 8 for more details). Adiposity located in the abdominal region is strongly linked with chronic disease risk; therefore, a WC of ≥102 cm (40 in.) in men or ≥88 cm (35 in.) in women is used to classify individuals with abdominal obesity (9).

Potential Causes

Although consuming calories in excess of daily caloric need is an easily identified culprit in the etiology of obesity, this condition is much more complex than suggested by that simple explanation. Both biological (e.g., genetic predisposition attributable to lower-than-normal metabolic rate) and psychological (e.g., poor body image) factors can contribute to obesity and can pose significant obstacles when a person attempts to lose weight (9, 10). Some studies show that genetics contribute around 25% to 40% of the variation in body composition (7), but others argue that genetics are responsible for 50% to 70% of this variation (5). Many biological factors have been identified as possible mechanisms that predispose a person to obesity. These factors include leptin (a protein), activity of the sympathetic nervous system, several neuropeptides, and some hormones (5). Suggested pathways through which these factors work include lowering resting metabolic rate, influencing eating behaviors, and slowing the rate of fat oxidation. Because of the attention recently focused on the genetic roots of obesity, individuals who are obese can become discouraged from attempting to lose weight. Although biological factors clearly contribute to obesity, the imbalance between energy intake and expenditure ultimately leads to fat accumulation. Educating clients on the role of appropriate nutrition and exercise in maintaining a healthy weight is an important aspect of the fitness professional's responsibilities.

The prevalence of obesity in the United States and in many countries around the world increased dramatically during the last part of the 20th century (21). The U.S. prevalence of obesity rose from 13.4% in the early 1960s to 33.8% in 2007 (11, 12). Figure 19.1 shows the increase in BMI and WC in recent decades. Recent national surveys reveal that 68% of American adults now have a BMI of 25 kg · m⁻² or higher and thus are classified as overweight or obese (11). Certain minority groups appear particularly at risk for overweight and obesity, with non-Hispanic blacks and Mexican Americans having prevalence rates of 73.8% and 78.8%, respectively, for BMI ≥25 kg · m⁻² (11). According to criteria for waist circumference, 38.3% of men and 59.9% of women have abdominal obesity (27).

Another disturbing trend is the increasing rate of obesity among children. Recent national surveys (2007-2008) reveal that 31.7% of American children are overweight (at or above the 85th percentile for BMI), 16.9% are obese (at or above the 95th percentile for BMI), and 11.9% are extremely obese (at or above the 97th percentile for BMI) (26). Some researchers have linked the rising prevalence of childhood obesity to an increase in inactive leisure pursuits such as television viewing (16, 29). The rapid increase in obesity in the United States over the last four decades supports the contention that lifestyle choices (i.e., diet and physical activity), not genetics, are primarily responsible for the increasing prevalence of obesity.

The increasing prevalence of obesity is important because of the negative health complications that accompany it. Obesity is linked with increased mortality and

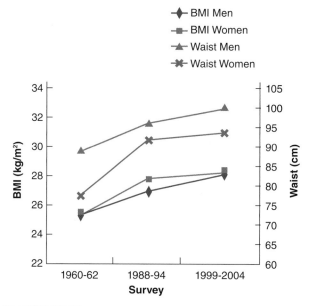

FIGURE 19.1 Changes in BMI and WC for men and women (6, 27).

morbidity rates. Diseases and conditions associated with obesity include CHD, CHF, stroke, type 2 diabetes, hypertension, dyslipidemia, gallbladder disease, osteoarthritis, some cancers (e.g., breast, colon), sleep apnea, and respiratory problems (24). Women who are obese are more likely to experience menstrual irregularities and complications with pregnancy (24). Estimates of annual U.S. deaths attributable to obesity range from 112,000 (13) to 300,000 (3). Deaths due to CVD, diabetes, and kidney disease are particularly related to obesity (14). Recent reviews of the costs related to obesity reveal the toll this condition places on the economy (33, 42). It is estimated that the medical costs of an obese person are 30% higher than those of a person of normal weight (42). In the United States, it is estimated that the cost of overweight and obesity is approximately $114 billion and accounts for 5% to 10% of health care spending (33).

Clearly, obesity results in major personal as well as financial strains. The serious effects of overweight and obesity are reflected by the issuance of *The Surgeon General's Call to Action to Prevent and Decrease Overweight and Obesity* (34) and *The Surgeon General's Vision for a Healthy and Fit Nation* (36). These reports outline the problem of overweight and obesity and call for both public and private commitments to address this health concern.

KEY POINT

Obesity is a complex condition with biological and lifestyle links. One-third of U.S. adults are classified as obese, and the prevalence has risen dramatically in recent decades. Comorbidities of obesity include type 2 diabetes, CHD, stroke, and some cancers. In the United States the economic cost of obesity is more than $100 billion per year.

Physical Activity in Prevention and Treatment of Obesity

The rapid increase in obesity prevalence appears linked to both low physical activity and excessive energy intake (32). This suggests that increasing physical activity and reducing caloric intake will lower rates of obesity. Although the evidence is indirect, an overview of cross-sectional and prospective studies suggests that active people are less likely to be obese, and those who maintain an active lifestyle are least likely to become obese over time (2, 8, 20). A recent international consensus meeting concluded that 45 to 60 min of daily moderate activity is needed to prevent obesity (30). However, estimating energy intake and expenditure on a population level is crude, the studies do not always agree, and much additional research is needed to clarify these issues. Despite the need for more research, there is general agreement in the medical (31) and public health (34) communities that both exercise and dietary modification should be used in treating patients who are obese.

A number of studies have used exercise as a means for treating obesity. Most of these trials were short term, and many had design flaws that limit the conclusions that can be drawn. In general, well-controlled, randomized control trials typically have found modest weight reduction when exercise is used to treat obesity (2, 14, 35). Slightly greater weight loss typically is seen when caloric restriction is combined with exercise. There is also evidence that a combination of dietary restriction and exercise is better at helping maintain weight loss than is either method alone (17, 39). The data from the National Weight Control Registry (NWCR) suggest that regular aerobic exercise is common among those who successfully maintain significant weight loss (40, 41). See the Research Insight for more information on the characteristics of people who are successful at maintaining weight loss. Exercise recommendations for individuals who are obese can be found later in this chapter.

RESEARCH INSIGHT

The NWCR was established in 1994 to provide insight into ways that people successfully lose weight and then maintain weight loss (40, 41). Approximately 5,000 people participate in the NWCR, with an average weight loss of 30 kg maintained for 5.5 yr. About half of these participants used commercial weight-loss programs, whereas the others lost weight without formal guidance. Several interesting facts have been gathered from these successful losers: (1) The vast majority (over 85%) report using exercise in their weight-loss programs, (2) the most common dietary approach involved choosing a diet low in total calories and low in fat (<25% of calories from fat), (3) most participants weighed themselves frequently to provide feedback on the success of their behaviors, (4) a typical exercise routine was 1 hr · day^{-1} of moderate physical activity, and (5) walking was the most frequently reported exercise (80% of participants), while about 29% used resistance training. An overwhelming majority (>90%) of NCWR participants report that their weight loss has been associated with higher energy levels, better mobility, improved mood, higher self-confidence, and overall better quality of life. For more information on the NWCR, visit its website (www.nwcr.ws).

Special Medical Screening

Several conditions frequently coexist with obesity (e.g., type 2 diabetes, hypertension) (9). The high prevalence of these comorbidities requires that fitness professionals carefully screen participants who are obese before performing exercise testing. Health histories and pretesting screenings should be designed to identify any comorbidities (see chapter 2). These conditions as well as the person's overall physical condition will determine the types of exercise testing needed before exercise programming. Once the initial health history screening is completed, the ACSM risk stratification (1) can be used to determine the need for medical clearance and physician supervision of exercise tests.

Medications

As with all clients, a person who is obese should provide documentation of medications. Because of the wide-ranging comorbidities that can exist with obesity, a variety of medications may be prescribed. It is common to find clients who are obese and who take several medications, including those for hypertension and glucose control. Before exercise testing and prescription, fitness professionals should consider the possible effect of these medications.

Prescription medications for weight loss or weight control are available for individuals under a physician's care (24). Four medications are approved by the FDA for weight loss: phentermine, diethylpropion, phendimetrazine, and orlistat. Orlistat can be obtained through a physician's prescription (Xenical) or over-the-counter (Alli). Orlistat interferes with the absorption of fat in the digestive system and commonly results in weight loss and improved blood lipid profile. There is a slight chance of liver injury from using orlistat, but more common side effects are oily discharge and fecal urgency. Phentermine, diethylpropion, and phendimetrazine are appetite suppressants and are approved for short-term use (up to 12 wk) with a prescription. Sleeplessness, nervousness, and increased BP are sometimes reported while using these medications.

Over-the-counter weight-loss aids and herbal supplements are also taken frequently by people desiring weight loss. In 2004, the FDA banned ephedrine alkaloids (ephedra) in over-the-counter products because of the reported occurrence of tachycardia, hypertension, strokes, and heart attacks. It is beyond the scope of this chapter to review all products used to promote weight loss. Fitness professionals should encourage clients to be wise consumers of such products by learning about the potential side effects and discussing these substances with their physicians.

Exercise Testing

Typically, standard testing modes and protocols can be used when testing people who are obese; however, the initial intensity as well as the incremental increases should reflect the individual's fitness and activity level (see chapter 7). This is particularly important because of the severe deconditioning that often exists with obesity. With severe obesity or when ambulation is problematic, it may be preferable to use cycle or arm ergometry for testing. However, when walking is the exercise of choice for programming, treadmill testing provides useful insight into the velocity that the client can maintain during walking. This can be helpful information when designing a workout with a targeted caloric expenditure.

Surgical Procedures for Weight Loss

For individuals with extreme obesity (BMI >40 kg · m^{-2}) who have been unsuccessful in previous weight-loss attempts and who have serious comorbid conditions, **bariatric surgery** may be an option (22, 23, 25, 31). There are a variety of surgical options (25), but all modify the gastrointestinal system so that food intake is restricted and nutrient uptake is diminished. These procedures often lead to significant weight loss, but they also have a number of serious side effects (23, 25). These surgeries require major modifications in eating patterns. Once patients recover from surgery, exercise programming is recommended. The dietary planning and exercise programming for these patients should be overseen by medical professionals.

The physiological response to exercise typically is similar in people who are obese and people who are normal weight, except that excessive weight often reduces cardiorespiratory function. However, comorbidities, especially hypertension and type 2 diabetes, can alter the exercise or postexercise response. For more information on testing clients who are obese, refer to the review by Wallace and Ray (37).

Exercise Prescription

Weight loss, greater fitness, and improved chronic disease risk factors are the focus of exercise programs for individuals who are obese. ACSM guidelines state that all adults, including those who are obese, should exercise on most, if not all, days of the week for a minimum of 150 min · wk^{-1} in order to protect against chronic disease (1). However, evidence indicates that an even greater caloric expenditure (i.e., 200-300 min · wk^{-1}) may be most beneficial for long-term weight control (1, 2). Some groups advocate 45 to 60 min of daily moderate activity to prevent weight gain and 60 to 90 min for individuals who were previously obese in order to prevent weight regain (15, 30). The Physical Activity Guidelines for Americans encourage people who are using exercise for weight loss or weight control to accumulate 300 min · wk^{-1} of moderate-intensity exercise, or 150 min · wk^{-1} of vigorous-intensity activity (35). When first beginning an exercise program, participants may be unable to exercise this long, so an initial focus of programming is to build enough endurance to sustain aerobic activity to reach these duration goals. Accumulating activity in shorter bouts throughout the day is also an option.

ACSM recommends the following approach to exercise for weight loss (1):

- Frequency: 5 to 7 days · wk^{-1}.
- Intensity: initially moderate (40%-60% HRR), with progression to higher intensity (50%-75% HRR).
- Duration: progress from short, easily tolerated bouts to 45 to 60 min · day^{-1}. Multiple daily bouts can be used with bout duration of 10 min or longer.
- Type: aerobic exercise targeting large muscle groups. Resistance exercise is recommended as a supplement to aerobic activity.

Designing exercise programs for individuals who are obese requires some special considerations. One of the primary aims of any exercise program should be safety. For participants who are obese, avoiding orthopedic injuries is a particular concern because of the additional loading to joints. Therefore, low-impact activities (water exercise, cycling, and walking) are preferable when individuals who are obese begin to exercise regularly. After some weight loss and conditioning occur, they may participate in higher impact sports and activities. Another safety concern is thermoregulation (37). Because of excessive body fatness and the increased energy demands of activity, keeping the body cool during exercise can be problematic for people with a lot of body fat. They should be encouraged to exercise at cool times of the day or in temperature-controlled environments. They should also maintain hydration by drinking adequate amounts of water.

Resistance training also may be an important component of the overall exercise program. Although resistance training typically does not burn off a large number of calories, it can serve important functions in weight loss (2). During weight loss, both lean and fat tissues typically diminish. However, lean tissue may be maintained, or at least muscle loss can be minimized, by using resistance training during caloric restriction. Maintaining muscle mass benefits both functional capacity and metabolic rate. Compared with fat, muscle is a metabolically active tissue, so maintaining lean mass helps minimize decreases in metabolic rate.

Individuals who are obese rarely begin exercise without also setting goals related to weight loss (although exercise provides benefits even in the absence of weight loss; see Exercise Without Weight Loss). Fitness professionals should assist the client in developing healthy weight-loss goals. An appropriate goal is 0.5 to 1 kg · wk^{-1}. For example, reducing caloric intake by 500 kcal · day^{-1} and expending an additional 300 kcal · day^{-1} creates a caloric deficit that approximates a 0.7 kg loss in 1 wk: 7(500 + 300) = 5,600 kcal · wk^{-1}. Typically, diets with fewer than 1,200 kcal · day^{-1} are not recommended without physician supervision. A well-planned, low-fat diet with a caloric deficit of 500 to 1,000 kcal · day^{-1} gradually reduces weight without sacrificing nutritional needs (2). An appropriate distribution of macronutrients along with the necessary amounts of vitamins and minerals should be included in the dietary planning (see chapter 5). Diets that are low in fat, particularly saturated fat, not only are effective for weight loss but also are associated with long-term weight maintenance. See chapter 12 for additional information on weight-loss and management strategies. Individuals who are overweight and obese should reduce body weight by at least 5% to gain health benefits such as lower BP and a more favorable blood lipid profile. For some individuals, an even greater reduction in body weight may optimize health improvement (2).

Long-term adherence to exercise is problematic for people who have been sedentary and are obese. Fitness professionals should help clients overcome perceived barriers to living an active lifestyle. Commonly reported barriers are feeling too fat to exercise, believing that their health is too poor for exercise, and believing that an injury or disability precludes participation in exercise

Exercise Without Weight Loss

Even without weight loss, exercise benefits people who are overweight. These benefits (e.g., an improved blood lipid profile, lower BP, better stress management) are much the same as those seen in people who are normal weight. Although both reducing weight and improving fitness optimize health benefits, participation in regular exercise significantly protects against disease even when the person remains overweight. Data from the Cooper Clinic in Dallas have demonstrated that fitness protects against early death in people who are overweight (38). Because of these findings, it is important to emphasize an active lifestyle, even if weight loss is not an outcome.

(4). Fitness professionals should provide education about the risks of leading an inactive life, the health benefits of regular exercise (which occur independent of body weight), and the variety of exercise options available. A dialogue between the fitness professional and client determines program needs, client likes and dislikes, and level of support needed to increase adherence. These discussions can lead to decisions about the specific nature of the exercise routine (e.g., structured versus lifestyle, intermittent versus continuous) (18, 19). Look for opportunities to increase energy expenditure through structured exercise (e.g., taking brisk 30 min walks) and lifestyle activity (e.g., substituting active for sedentary leisure pursuits). When it comes to long-term adherence, finding an approach that fits the needs of the client is critical.

KEY POINT

Prudent weight-loss goals for clients who are overweight and obese range from 0.5 to 1.0 $kg \cdot wk^{-1}$. Daily or near-daily moderate aerobic activity is suggested. Although 30 $min \cdot day^{-1}$ of moderate-intensity exercise is a minimum goal, better success is seen with 45 to 90 min. People who are obese can use both aerobic exercise and resistance training. For weight loss, exercise programs should be combined with a low-fat, reduced-calorie diet. When prescribing exercise, emphasize avoiding musculoskeletal injuries and heat injury as well as finding ways to improve adherence.

STUDY QUESTIONS

1. What are potential causes of obesity?
2. Describe how the prevalence of obesity has changed over the past 50 years.
3. Describe the costs associated with obesity, both in terms of dollars and excess deaths.
4. Compare the exercise recommendation for health benefits with the exercise recommendation for weight control.
5. What is the National Weight Control Registry (NWCR)? What useful information has been obtained from this resource?
6. What special considerations should be applied when screening obese patients prior to exercise testing?
7. What special considerations should be applied to administering exercise tests to obese clients?
8. What medications have FDA approval for use in weight loss?

CASE STUDIES

You can check your answers by referring to appendix A.

1. Marsha is a 51-yr-old female who comes to your fitness facility and expresses interest in purchasing a membership. She is responding to a series of advertisements that your facility is using to attract people interested in weight loss. Your screening reveals the following:

   o Her height is 5 ft 5 in. (165 cm) and her weight is 240 lb (109 kg).

   o Her blood pressure is 152/88 mmHg.

   o She has never exercised regularly, has a desk job, and has no active leisure pursuits.

   o It has been more than 3 yr since she had a medical examination.

○ There is a history of heart disease on her father's side of the family, and her mother developed type 2 diabetes after menopause.

    a. What, if any, medical screening do you recommend before this client enrolls in your facility's programs?

    b. What fitness testing do you suggest for her?

    c. Assuming that no medical conditions are revealed with the screening and initial testing, describe a diet and exercise program that Marsha could use to achieve her weight-loss and fitness goals.

2. You have a new client, Kevin. He is a healthy, somewhat active 38-yr-old man who is coming to you for advice on exercise and maintaining a healthy weight. Kevin's BMI is 25.5. He reports that over the past 2 yr he has lost more than 75 lb (34 kg) using a commercial weight-loss plan. He is beginning to feel diet burnout and his weight has crept up 5 lb (2.3 kg) over the past month. What exercise and other lifestyle advice would you provide?

3. Shala comes to you for help in becoming more active. She is a 32-yr-old woman who underwent bariatric surgery 6 mo earlier. Her doctor has cleared her for moderate-intensity activity and has encouraged her to become more active. Shala has never been active. Her BMI is still in the extreme obesity range, and you noticed that she was breathless from just walking in from her car. What are the initial steps to take in helping Shala?

REFERENCES

1. American College of Sports Medicine (ACSM). 2010. *ACSM's guidelines for exercise testing and prescription.* 8th ed. Baltimore: Lippincott Williams & Wilkins.

2. American College of Sports Medicine (ACSM). 2009. Appropriate physical activity intervention strategies for weight loss and prevention of weight regain for adults. *Medicine and Science in Sports and Exercise* 41(2): 459-471.

3. Allison, D.B., K.R. Fontaine, J.E. Manson, J. Stevens, and T.B. VanItallie. 1999. Annual deaths attributable to obesity in the United States. *Journal of the American Medical Association* 282:1530-1538.

4. Ball, K., D. Crawford, and N. Owen. 2000. Too fat to exercise? Obesity as a barrier to physical activity. *Australian and New Zealand Journal of Public Health* 24:331-333.

5. Beamer, B.A. 2003. Genetic influences on obesity. In *Obesity: Etiology, assessment, treatment and prevention,* ed. R.E. Anderson, 43-56. Champaign, IL: Human Kinetics.

6. Beydoun, M.A., and Y. Wang. 2009. Gender-ethnic disparity in BMI and waist circumference distribution shifts in U.S. adults. *Obesity* 17:169-176.

7. Bouchard, C., L. Perusse, C. Leblanc, A. Tremblay, and G. Theriault. 1988. Inheritance of the amount and distribution of human body fat. *International Journal of Obesity* 12:205-215.

8. DiPietro, L. 1999. Physical activity in the prevention of obesity: Current evidence and research issues. *Medicine and Science in Sports and Exercise* 31:S542-S546.

9. Expert Panel on the Identification, Evaluation and Treatment of Overweight and Obesity in Adults. 1998. Executive summary of the clinical guidelines on the identification, evaluation, and treatment of overweight and obesity in adults. *Archives of Internal Medicine* 158:1855-1867.

10. Faith, M.S., P.E. Matz, and D.B. Allison. 2003. Psychosocial correlates and consequences of obesity. In *Obesity: etiology, assessment, treatment, and prevention,* ed. R.E. Andersen, 17-31. Champaign, IL: Human Kinetics.

11. Flegal, K.M., M.D. Carroll, C.L. Ogden, and L.R. Curtin. 2010. Prevalence and trends in obesity among U.S. adults, 1999-2008. *Journal of the American Medical Association* 303(3): 235-241.

12. Flegal, K., M. Carroll, C. Ogden, and C. Johnson. 2002. Prevalence and trends in obesity among U.S. adults, 1999-2000. *Journal of the American Medical Association* 288:1723-1727.

13. Flegal, K.M., B.I. Graubard, D.F. Williamson, and M.H. Gail. 2005. Excess deaths associated with underweight, overweight, and obesity. *Journal of the American Medical Association* 293:1861-1867.

14. Flegal, K.M., B.I. Graubard, D.F. Williamson, and M.H. Gail. 2007. Cause-specific excess deaths associated with underweight, overweight, and obesity. *Journal of the American Medical Association* 298:2028-2037.

15. Food and Nutrition Board, Institute of Medicine. 2002. *Dietary reference intakes for energy, carbohydrate, fiber, fat, fatty acids, cholesterol, protein, and amino acids.* Washington, DC: National Academies Press.

16. Gortmaker, S., A. Must, A. Sobel, K. Peterson, G.A. Colditz, and W.H. Dietz. 1996. Television viewing as a cause of increasing obesity among children in the United States. *Archives of Pediatric Adolescent Medicine* 150:356-362.

17. Grundy, S.M., G. Blackburn, M. Higgins, R. Lauer, M.G. Perri, and D. Ryan. 1999. Physical activity in the prevention and treatment of obesity and its comorbidities: Roundtable consensus statement. *Medicine and Science in Sports and Exercise* 31:S502-S508.

18. Jakicic, J.M. 2003. Exercise in the treatment of obesity. *Endocrinology and Metabolism Clinics of North America* 32:967-980.

19. Jakicic, J.M. 2003. Exercise strategies for the obese patient. *Primary Care* 30:393-403.

20. Jebb, S.A., and M.S. Moore. 1999. Contribution of a sedentary lifestyle and inactivity to the etiology of overweight and obesity: Current evidence and research issues. *Medicine and Science in Sports and Exercise* 31:S534-S541.

21. Khan, L.K., and B.A. Bowman. 1999. Obesity: A major global public health problem. *Annual Review of Nutrition* 19:xiii-xvii.

22. Maggard, M.A., L.R. Shugarman, M. Suttorp, M. Maglione, H.J. Sugarman, E.H. Livingston, N.T. Nguyen, Z. Li, W. Mojica, L. Hilton, S. Rhodes, S.C. Morton, and P.G. Shekelle. 2005. Meta-analysis: Surgical treatment of obesity. *Annals of Internal Medicine* 142:547-559.

23. National Heart, Lung, and Blood Institute. 1998. *Clinical guidelines on the identification, evaluation, and treatment of overweight and obesity in adults.* NIH Publication No. 98-4083. Bethesda, MD: National Institutes of Health—National Heart, Lung, and Blood Institute.

24. National Institute of Diabetes and Digestive and Kidney Diseases. 2010. *Prescription medications for the treatment of obesity.* NIH Publication No. 07-4191. Original publication November 2004, updated December 2010.

25. National Institute of Diabetes and Digestive and Kidney Diseases. 2009. *Bariatric surgery for severe obesity.* NIH Publication No. 08-4006.

26. Ogden, C.L., M.D. Carroll, L.R. Curtin, M.M. Lamb, and K.M. Flegal. 2010. Prevalence of high body mass index in U.S. children and adolescents, 2007-2008. *Journal of the American Medical Association* 303:242-249.

27. Okosun, I.S., K.M.D. Chandra, A. Boev, J.M. Boltri, S.T. Choi, D.C. Parrish, and G.E.A. Dever. 2004. Abdominal adiposity in U.S. adults: Prevalence and trends, 1960-2000. *Preventive Medicine* 39:197-206.

28. Ratamess, N. Body composition status and assessment. 2010. In *ACSM's resource manual for guidelines for exercise testing and prescription.* 6th ed. Ed. J.K. Ehrman, 264-281. Baltimore: Lippincott Williams & Wilkins.

29. Robinson, T.N. 1998. Does television cause childhood obesity? *Journal of the American Medical Association* 279:959-960.

30. Saris, W.H.M., S.N. Blair, M.A. van Baak, S.B. Eaton, P.S.W. Davies, L. Di Pietro, M. Fogelholm, A. Rissanen, D. Schoeller, B. Swinburn, A. Tremblay, K.R. Westerterp, and H. Wyatt. 2003. How much physical activity is enough to prevent unhealthy weight gain? Outcome of the IASO 1st Stock Conference and consensus statement. *Obesity Reviews* 4:101-114.

31. Snow, V., P. Barry, N. Fitterman, A. Qaseem, and K. Weiss. 2005. Pharmacologic and surgical management of obesity in primary care: A clinical practice guideline for the American College of Physicians. *Annals of Internal Medicine* 142:525-531.

32. Stubbs, C.O., and A.J. Lee. 2004. The obesity epidemic: Both energy intake and physical activity contribute. *Medical Journal of Australia* 181:489-491.

33. Tsai, A.G., D.F. Williamson, and H.A. Glick. 2011. Direct cost of overweight and obesity in the USA: A quantitative systematic review. *Obesity Reviews* 12:50-61.

34. U.S. Department of Health and Human Services (HHS). 2001. *The Surgeon General's call to action to prevent and decrease overweight and obesity.* Rockville, MD: U.S. GPO.

35. U.S. Department of Health and Human Services (HHS). 2008. *2008 Physical Activity Guidelines for Americans.* www.health.gov/paguidelines/guidelines/default.aspx.

36. U.S. Department of Health and Human Services (HHS). 2010. *The Surgeon General's vision for a healthy and fit nation.* Rockville, MD: U.S. GPO.

37. Wallace, J.P., and S. Ray. 2009. Obesity. In *ACSM's exercise management for persons with chronic diseases and disabilities.* 3rd ed. Ed. J.L. Durstine, G.E. Moore, P.L. Painter, and S.O. Roberts, 192-200. Champaign, IL: Human Kinetics.

38. Welk, G.J., and Blair, S.N. 2000. Physical activity protects against the health risks of obesity. *PCPFS Research Digest* 3:1-7.

39. Wing, R.R. 1999. Physical activity in the treatment of adulthood overweight and obesity: Current evidence and research issues. *Medicine and Science in Sports and Exercise* 31:S547-S552.

40. Wing, R.R., and Hill, J.O. 2001. Successful weight loss maintenance. *Annual Review of Nutrition* 21:323-341.

41. Wing, R.R., and S. Phelan. 2005. Long-term weight loss maintenance. *American Journal of Clinical Nutrition* 82(suppl): 222S-225S.

42. Withrow, D., and D.A. Alter. 2010. The economic burden of obesity worldwide: a systematic review of the direct costs of obesity. *Obesity Reviews.* doi: 10.1111/j.1467-789X.2009.00712.x.

Exercise and Diabetes

OBJECTIVES

The reader will be able to do the following:

1. Define *diabetes mellitus* and describe the characteristics of type 1 and type 2 diabetes.

2. Describe the role that exercise plays in the prevention and treatment of type 2 diabetes.

3. Describe special considerations in exercise testing for clients with diabetes.

4. Describe special considerations in exercise prescription for clients with diabetes.

Diabetes mellitus refers to metabolic diseases characterized by **hyperglycemia** (i.e., elevated plasma glucose). The criteria used to diagnose diabetes are fasting blood glucose levels, the blood glucose response to ingesting carbohydrate, and/or the hemoglobin A1c (i.e., glycosylated hemoglobin) level (see table 20.1). Hemoglobin A1c is a form of hemoglobin that is typically found in low concentrations but exists in higher concentrations when blood glucose is constantly higher than normal. Thus, hemoglobin A1c reflects overall blood glucose control during the past 2 to 3 mo.

The cause of hyperglycemia varies depending on the form of diabetes present, with the most common forms being type 1 and type 2 diabetes. **Type 1 diabetes**, accounting for 5% to 10% of cases of diabetes, is characterized by a deficiency of insulin often attributable to an autoimmune destruction of the insulin-producing beta cells of the pancreas. In **type 2 diabetes**, the insulin receptors become insensitive or resistant to insulin and, because glucose cannot move readily into the cells, hyperglycemia results. Although there are other forms of diabetes mellitus (e.g., gestational diabetes), type 1 and type 2 account for the vast majority of cases. Regardless of the type, a number of complications may result from diabetes. These complications typically affect the blood vessels and nerves and include vision impairment, kidney disease, peripheral vascular disease, atherosclerosis, and hypertension (6). The economic burden (direct and indirect costs) of diabetes in the United States in 2007 was estimated at $174 billion (3).

Approximately 24 million Americans have diabetes, and of this number, more than 5.5 million people are unaware that they are diabetic (9). Between 90% and 95% of the cases are type 2 diabetes (9). This form of diabetes has both lifestyle and genetic roots. Many people with type 2 diabetes are relatively inactive and overweight or obese, particularly with excessive abdominal fat. Other risk factors include a family history of type 2 diabetes, older age, and belonging to an ethnic minority (prevalence is higher among Hispanics, Native Americans, and African Americans compared with Caucasians). Type 2 diabetes frequently coexists with other conditions such as hypertension and dyslipidemia. Although type 2 diabetes can appear at any age, the highest rates are seen among people aged 60 yr and older (9, 15). However, there is an increasing prevalence of type 2 diabetes among children, and this trend seems to be linked to increasing obesity rates (9, 15).

Comparison of Type 1 and Type 2 Diabetes

Type 1 diabetes results from a lack of insulin. The most common cause is autoimmune destruction of the insulin-producing beta cells of the pancreas, leading to lack of insulin. Without insulin, the cells are unable to take in glucose. Unlike type 2 diabetes, type 1 diabetes often appears early in life and is more closely linked to genetic than lifestyle factors. People with type 1 diabetes require insulin injections. There are many types of insulin, and

TABLE 20.1 Criteria for Diagnosis of Prediabetes, Diabetes, and Gestational Diabetes

Prediabetes	FPG: 100 mg · dl^{-1} (5.6 mmol · L^{-1}) to 125 mg · dl^{-1} (6.9 mmol · L^{-1})
	PG 2 hr after OGTT: 140 mg · dl^{-1} (7.8 mmol · L^{-1}) to 199 mg · dl^{-1} (11 mmol · L^{-1})
	A1c: 5.7-6.4%
Diabetes	FPG: ≥126 mg · dl^{-1} (7.0 mmol · L^{-1})
	PG 2 hr after OGTT: ≥200 mg · dl^{-1} (11.1 mmol · L^{-1})
	Random PG: ≥200 mg · dl^{-1} (11.1 mmol · L^{-1}) (in patient with diabetic symptoms)
	A1c: ≥6.5%
Gestational diabetes	FPG: ≥92 mg · dl^{-1} (5.1 mmol · L^{-1})
	PG 1 hr after OGTT: ≥180 mg · dl^{-1} (10.0 mmol · L^{-1})
	PG 2 hr after OGTT: ≥153 mg · dl^{-1} (8.5 mmol · L^{-1})

FPG = fasting plasma glucose (no caloric intake for at least 8 hr); PG = plasma glucose; OGTT = oral glucose tolerance test using 75 g glucose load; A1c = hemoglobin A1c.

Data from American Diabetes Association 2011.

they vary by how rapidly they begin working, their peak time of action, and how long they continue to work. Insulins used to treat diabetes are listed in table 20.2. Some people with type 2 diabetes also require insulin injections. More often, however, they take other types of prescription medications to lower blood glucose. Many types of medications are used for this purpose (see table 20.3). For more information on medications used to treat diabetes mellitus, see the websites of the American Diabetes Association (ADA) (www.diabetes.org) and the National Institute of Diabetes and Digestive and Kidney Diseases (NIDDK) (www.niddk.nih.gov).

Type 2 diabetes is characterized by **insulin resistance**, a condition in which the body's insulin receptors no longer respond normally to insulin. Thus glucose entry into cells is impaired and hyperglycemia results. Plasma insulin levels of people with type 2 diabetes may be normal, suppressed, or elevated depending on the individual. Regardless, type 2 diabetes is considered a disease of relative insulin deficiency because the insulin available is inadequate to maintain normal glucose concentrations. Although some people with type 2 diabetes can control their disease through exercise and weight loss, others require medications such as oral hypoglycemic agents and possibly even insulin injections (see table 20.3).

Type 2 diabetes usually develops over time, first appearing as **impaired fasting glucose** (100-125 mg · dl^{-1}) or **impaired glucose tolerance (IGT)**. Impaired glucose tolerance is a condition in which the increase in blood glucose after ingestion of carbohydrate is higher than normal and remains elevated longer than normal. A glucose level of 140 to 199 mg · dl^{-1} 2 hr after an oral glucose tolerance test indicates impaired glucose tolerance. Examples of normal and abnormal blood glucose responses are shown in figure 20.1. A person with either impaired fasting glucose or impaired glucose tolerance is classified as having **prediabetes**. Without intervention, prediabetes generally evolves into type 2 diabetes. It is estimated that at least 57 million Americans have prediabetes (9).

KEY POINT

Diabetes mellitus is characterized by hyperglycemia. Approximately 24 million Americans have diabetes mellitus, and the economic cost is approximately $174 billion each year. Type 1 diabetes results from a lack of insulin production. Type 2 diabetes, the most common form of diabetes, is characterized by the cells becoming insensitive to insulin. Risk factors for type 2 diabetes include older age, a family history of type 2 diabetes, excess weight, and inactivity.

TABLE 20.2 Forms of Insulin Used to Control Diabetes Mellitus

Type of insulin	Onset of action	Peak	Duration
Rapid acting	15 min	30-90 min	3-5 hr
Short acting	30-60 min	2-4 hr	5-8 hr
Intermediate acting	1-3 hr	8 hr	12-16 hr
Long acting	1 hr	Lowers evenly for 24 hr	20-26 hr
Premixed (intermediate + short acting)	30-60 min	Varies	10-16 hr
Premixed (intermediate + rapid acting)	5-15 min	Varies	10-16 hr

TABLE 20.3 Medications Used to Control Type 2 Diabetes

Class of medication	Example	Mode of action
Sulfonylureas	Glyburide/Diabeta	Stimulates insulin production and release
Biguanides	Metformin/Glucophage	Reduces glucose release from liver
Alpha-glucosidase inhibitors	Acarbose/Precose	Slows absorption of carbohydrate
Thiazolidinediones	Rosiglitazone/Avandia	Increases insulin sensitivity
Meglitinides	Repaglinide/Prandin	Stimulates insulin production and release
Dipeptidyl peptidase-4 inhibitor	Sitagliptin/Januvia	Increases insulin release and inhibits glucagon release (helpful in managing hemoglobin A1c levels)

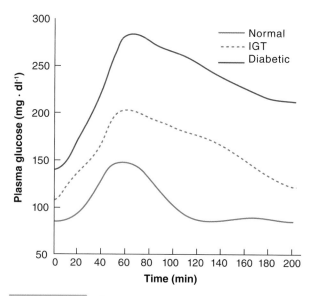

FIGURE 20.1 Comparison of glucose response with carbohydrate ingestion.

- Lower fasting blood glucose concentrations
- Better glucose tolerance (less of a spike in glucose after eating)
- Improved insulin sensitivity (more glucose uptake with a given amount of insulin)
- Weight control (increased lean mass and reduced fat mass)
- Improved lipid profiles
- Reduction in BP for those with hypertension
- Lower risk of CVD
- Stress management (stress can affect glucose control via increased levels of catecholamines)

KEY POINT

Exercise has been shown to be effective in preventing and treating type 2 diabetes. Regardless of the type of diabetes, exercise benefits people with diabetes in a number of ways.

Exercise for Clients With Diabetes

Exercise can provide many benefits to individuals with type 1 or type 2 diabetes. This is particularly true because of the strong link between diabetes and CVD and the role that exercise plays in reducing CVD risk. Unfortunately, people with diabetes are much less likely to exercise than their nondiabetic peers (17). Although exercise will not prevent or cure type 1 diabetes, exercise should be encouraged in this population for a number of reasons (4). Exercise improves insulin sensitivity and reduces disease risk for people with diabetes, much like in the population without diabetes. Because of the high rate of CVD among people with diabetes, exercise can promote overall well-being. Exercise protects against CAD, dyslipidemia, hypertension, and obesity. Increased physical activity and improved physical fitness also promote psychological health and quality of life.

Exercise helps prevent and treat type 2 diabetes. Inactivity and obesity are common characteristics of people with type 2 diabetes. Research has shown that individuals who are regularly active are 30% to 50% less likely to develop type 2 diabetes compared with their inactive counterparts (8). Additionally, people who have impaired glucose tolerance are less likely to develop type 2 diabetes if they begin to exercise regularly (2, 13). Evidence is mounting that people with type 2 diabetes experience better glucose tolerance and improved insulin sensitivity through regular exercise (2, 10). There are a number of reasons why exercise can benefit the treatment of type 2 diabetes (12, 16), including the following:

Screening and Testing Clients With Diabetes

Medical clearance should be required of all clients with diabetes mellitus to ensure that they can safely perform exercise (1). Individuals should discuss with their physicians how to modify their insulin dosage and/or other diabetes medications with exercise. Because exercise increases glucose uptake from peripheral tissues regardless of insulin levels, hypoglycemia may result if insulin intake is not adjusted (see the next section for tips on avoiding hypoglycemia). Diabetes is a primary risk factor for the development of CVD, so clients with diabetes should be screened carefully for signs and symptoms of disease (chapter 2). If the exercise prescription is to be more vigorous than brisk walking, it is recommended that participants, particularly sedentary and older people, undergo a GXT with ECG monitoring and a full medical screening with particular attention to diabetes-related complications (e.g., CAD, retinopathy, nephropathy) before beginning an exercise program (2).

People with type 2 diabetes frequently are overweight and hypertensive and have a poor blood lipid profile; therefore, they may be taking a number of medications that can influence the exercise response. For people who have had diabetes for a number of years, peripheral neuropathy may be a problem. Damage to the sensory nerves in the feet can lead to ulcerations, and if there is damage to blood vessels, healing can be slow. Because of these and other issues, conducting a thorough medical history is particularly important with these clients.

Guidelines for Higher-Risk Clients With Diabetes

Diabetic individuals who meet one of the following criteria should undergo diagnostic exercise tests (e.g., ECG stress testing) before beginning any exercise programming:

- Older than 40 yr
- Older than 30 yr with diabetes more than 10 yr
- Older than 30 yr and hypertensive
- Older than 30 yr and a smoker
- Older than 30 yr and dyslipidemic
- Older than 30 yr with retinopathy
- Older than 30 yr with nephropathy, including microalbuminuria
- Anyone with known or suspected CAD, cerebrovascular disease, peripheral artery disease, autonomic neuropathy, or advanced nephropathy with renal failure

Adapted, by permission, from American College of Sports Medicine and American Diabetes Association, 2010, "Joint position statement: Exercise and type 2 diabetes," *Medicine and Science in Sports and Exercise* 42:2282-2303.

KEY POINT

Because of the increased risks for exercise-related complications associated with diabetes mellitus, physician clearance should be obtained before exercise testing. The type of tests will depend on the client's needs.

The type of testing performed before exercise programming depends on the person (1, 2, 14). Diagnostic exercise stress testing under the supervision of a physician may be necessary for individuals with numerous risk factors. The protocol will depend on the client's age and functional ability. Submaximal exercise testing can be used to estimate aerobic power (see chapter 7). However, autonomic neuropathy can cause unusual HR and BP responses during exercise.

The decision of whether to perform exercise testing on clients with diabetes should be made in consultation with the client's physician. Generally, before the client begins a moderate or vigorous exercise program, exercise testing with CAD screening is recommended (14). It is also recommended that high-risk patients be tested before any program (see Guidelines for Higher-Risk Clients With Diabetes). Some low-risk participants will be able to begin low-intensity programs (<39% HRR) without stress testing. For additional information on testing clients who have diabetes, see *ACSM's Resource Manual for Guidelines for Exercise Testing and Prescription* (14) and *ACSM's Exercise Management for Persons With Chronic Diseases and Disabilities* (12).

Exercise Prescription

The goals of exercise programming for clients with diabetes (e.g., increasing aerobic power, reducing disease risk, increasing flexibility, increasing muscular strength and endurance) are similar to those for clients who do not have diabetes, with the exception of increased attention to improving glucose control. The basic elements of exercise prescription should be applied for clients with diabetes but with special considerations, as outlined in the following sections.

Type 1 Diabetes

A person with type 1 diabetes must carefully consider modifying insulin dosage and carbohydrate ingestion before beginning an exercise program. Increasing the intake of carbohydrate or reducing insulin dosage is often necessary to maintain glucose control and to avoid hypoglycemia that can result from exercise. The adjustment in carbohydrate intake and insulin dosage depends on the intensity and duration of activity. Glucose should be measured before initiating an exercise session. If glucose is <100 mg · dl^{-1}, carbohydrate (20-30 g) should be ingested before beginning exercise (1). If glucose is >300 mg · dl^{-1} but without ketosis, participants can undertake moderate-intensity exercise only if they are feeling well and are well hydrated; otherwise exercise should be delayed (1, 2).

For the client with type 1 diabetes who was previously inactive, progression should be slow, with careful monitoring of blood glucose and symptoms of cardiovascular and metabolic distress. Initially, supervised exercise is recommended. After the person is able to maintain glucose control with exercise, unsupervised exercise is acceptable. However, it is always preferable that clients with diabetes do not exercise alone because of the need to have someone nearby in case of a hypoglycemic event. Symptoms of hypoglycemia include dizziness, nausea, headache, confusion, and irritability (1). The following precautions should be observed for avoiding exercise-induced hypoglycemia:

- Measure blood glucose immediately before and 15 min after exercise (also during exercise if the exercise lasts longer than 30 min).
- Consume carbohydrate if glucose is <100 mg · dl^{-1}.
- Avoid exercising during times of peak insulin action.
- Reduce insulin dose (and inject into inactive areas) on days of planned exercise.
- Consume carbohydrate (5-30 g) after exercise, particularly after high-intensity, glycogen-depleting exercise. Hypoglycemia can appear several hours after exercise, so monitoring after exercise is crucial.
- Avoid exercise late at night, because hypoglycemia could occur while sleeping.
- Extend the warm-up and cool-down if needed.

Regular (3 or more times a week) aerobic exercise is recommended to maximize blood glucose control. The intensity of the exercise should match the characteristics of the client. Although moderate-intensity resistance exercise is safe for most people with diabetes, those with advanced complications (e.g., kidney disease, vision impairment) should avoid heavy lifting, where extreme BP elevation is possible. The ADA provides specific examples of recommended and discouraged exercises depending on the severity of the disease (4).

Dehydration due to polyuria can be problematic for diabetic clients. Dehydration can lead to a number of complications, including poor thermoregulatory control. Diabetic clients should be encouraged to maintain adequate hydration and watch for signs of heat or cold illness (see chapters 4, 7, and 26).

Because peripheral neuropathy can lead to ulcerations of the feet, good foot care is essential. Properly fitting and supportive shoes are particularly important for clients with diabetes who are engaging in weight-bearing exercise. For those with advanced peripheral neuropathy, low-impact and potentially non-weight-bearing exercises are more appropriate (4). Clients may find ACSM's exercise guide for people with diabetes helpful (7).

General recommendations for aerobic exercise with diabetic patients are as follows (1):

- Type: Rhythmic, large-muscle-group activities dependent on personal preferences and needs
- Intensity: 50% to 80% $\dot{V}O_2R$ or HRR; RPE 12 to 16
- Frequency: 3 to 7 days · wk^{-1}
- Time: 20-60 min in bouts of at least 10 min

In the absence of retinopathy, recent laser treatments, or other contraindications (1), resistance exercise is also recommended for diabetic patients. General guidelines are as follows (1):

- Type: Based on individual needs, with particular emphasis on avoiding major increases in blood pressure (avoid static contractions and sustained gripping; avoid Valsalva maneuver)
- Intensity: 2 to 3 sets of 8 to 12 repetitions (60%-80% of 1RM)
- Frequency: 2 to 3 days · wk^{-1}
- Time: 8-10 complex (multijoint) exercises with major muscle groups (upper and lower body) stressed

Type 2 Diabetes

The ADA and ACSM recommend that individuals with type 2 diabetes engage in both endurance and resistance training, unless significant complications or limitations exist (1, 2). Individuals should accumulate at least 150 min · wk^{-1} in moderate-intensity exercise (1, 2). When possible, additional minutes (e.g., 150-300 min · wk^{-1}) should be encouraged in order to achieve additional benefits. For those who are overweight or obese, aerobic activity should focus on caloric expenditure and weight control. Although at least 3 nonconsecutive days of exercise per week are recommended, individuals may choose to engage in daily physical activity to maximize glucose control and caloric expenditure (1).

Moderate-intensity exercise is generally recommended (1, 2), although the participant's characteristics should be considered when determining intensity. Activity at higher intensities is acceptable for those who are conditioned and choose more vigorous exercise. Because of the possibility of autonomic neuropathy, using HR to monitor exercise intensity may be problematic. Therefore, RPE may be a better choice for self-monitoring exercise intensity (see chapter 7). Exercise intensity and duration should be balanced to achieve goals for caloric expenditure. Typically, exercise sessions lasting at least 10 min are suggested, with physical activity accumulating to 30 to 60 min each day. The mode of aerobic exercise should fit the client's needs and abilities. Walking is the mode of choice for many, but for those with peripheral nerve damage, other modes (e.g., swimming, nonimpact exercise equipment) may be preferable.

General recommendations for aerobic exercise with type 2 diabetic patients are as follows (1):

- Type: Rhythmic, large-muscle-group activities dependent on personal preferences and needs
- Intensity: 50% to 80% $\dot{V}O_2R$ or HRR; RPE 12 to 16
- Frequency: 3 to 7 days · wk^{-1}
- Time: 20 to 60 min in bouts of at least 10 min

Resistance training also is suggested for many people with type 2 diabetes (1, 2). Resistance training maintains or even increases muscle mass and assists with glucose tolerance and insulin sensitivity. The program should focus on major muscle groups (8-10 exercises) and consist of 2 to 3 sets of 8 to 12 repetitions (see chapter 13). This routine should be performed at least 2 days $\cdot$ wk^{-1}. People without advanced complications can follow more aggressive programs. However, for those with eye or kidney damage resulting from diabetes, particular caution should be taken to avoid extreme BP elevations (4).

In the absence of retinopathy, recent laser treatments, or other contraindications (1), resistance exercise is recommended for diabetic patients. General guidelines are as follows (1):

- Type: Based on individual needs, with particular emphasis on avoiding major increases in blood pressure (avoid static contractions and sustained gripping; avoid Valsalva maneuver)
- Intensity: 2 to 3 sets of 8 to 12 repetitions (60%-80% of 1RM)
- Frequency: 2 to 3 days $\cdot$ wk^{-1}
- Time: 8 to 10 complex (multijoint) exercises with major muscle groups (upper and lower body) stressed

Because many clients with type 2 diabetes have a history of being relatively inactive and are often overweight, beginning and then maintaining an active lifestyle presents particular challenges. Creating a supportive environment is critical to the success of these clients. Early in the exercise program, it is particularly important to provide information on the benefits of a lifetime commitment to exercise. The program should progress slowly, be based on realistic goals, and incorporate the client's needs and desires. Additional information on increasing adherence to exercise can be found in chapter 23 and in the ACSM and ADA position statement on exercise and type 2 diabetes (2).

KEY POINT

Exercise prescription for the client with diabetes must take into account special needs caused by the disease. Careful monitoring of blood glucose levels is needed to help avoid hypoglycemic events. For individuals with type 2 diabetes, a minimum goal for aerobic activity should be 150 min $\cdot$ wk^{-1} of moderate-intensity exercise. Resistance training can be used with clients who have diabetes as long as the client avoids damage to already weakened blood vessels.

Metabolic Syndrome

Metabolic syndrome (also called *syndrome X)* is a condition in which a number of CAD risk factors exist together. People with metabolic syndrome have a much higher risk for atherosclerotic CVD. In order to be diagnosed with metabolic syndrome, a person must have at least three of the following (11):

- Abdominal obesity: WC ≥102 cm (men) or ≥88 cm (women)
- High triglycerides: ≥150 mg $\cdot$ dl^{-1}, or drug treatment
- Low HDL-C: <40 mg $\cdot$ dl^{-1} (men) or <50 mg $\cdot$ dl^{-1} (women), or drug treatment
- Elevated BP: ≥130/85 mmHg, or drug treatment
- Elevated fasting glucose: ≥100 mg $\cdot$ dl^{-1}, or drug treatment

It is estimated that more than a quarter of American adults have metabolic syndrome. Without intervention, chronic disease risk (e.g., CVD, diabetes) is much higher for these individuals. The approach to control metabolic syndrome depends on the symptoms that are present. Since abdominal obesity is common, weight loss is frequently suggested (7%-10% weight loss the first year and then continued reduction to reach a BMI of <25 kg $\cdot$ m^{-2}) (10). Physical activity is also commonly recommended because of the effect of regular exercise on all characteristics of metabolic syndrome.

Exercise testing for individuals with metabolic syndrome should follow the screening guidelines outlined in chapter 2. It is critical to screen for CVD risk factors and make decisions based on findings. See chapter 19 for more information about testing clients who are obese.

Exercise prescription for people with metabolic syndrome should include aerobic, resistance, and flexibility components as outlined in chapters 11, 13, and 14. Information on exercise prescription for obese clients is included in chapter 19. Achieving a healthy body weight and managing CVD risk factors are vital for clients with metabolic syndrome.

STUDY QUESTIONS

1. List the two major types of diabetes.
2. What are the similarities and differences between type 1 and type 2 diabetes?
3. What is prediabetes?
4. What are the diagnostic criteria for diabetes?
5. What characteristics in a diabetic client will lead you to recommend ECG stress testing prior to exercise prescription?
6. What are general aerobic exercise recommendations for diabetic clients?
7. What are general resistance training recommendations for diabetic clients?
8. What precautions should be taken to avoid hypoglycemia?
9. What is metabolic syndrome?

CASE STUDIES

You can check your answers by referring to appendix A.

1. Mr. Conner is a 40-yr-old man who, in response to doctor's orders, appears at your medical wellness facility for exercise programming. He recently sought the care of his physician after experiencing fatigue and headaches. Mr. Conner's physician ordered a series of tests, including a diagnostic exercise stress test. Here are Mr. Conner's test results:

   Weight = 265 lb (120 kg)

   Cholesterol = 270 mg · dl^{-1}

   Fasting glucose = 132 mg · dl^{-1}

   Height = 5 ft 9.5 in. (177 cm)

   LDL-C = 190 mg · dl^{-1}

   BP = 148/94 mmHg

   No smoking

   HDL-C = 32 mg · dl^{-1}

   $\dot{V}O_2$max = 22 ml · kg^{-1} · min^{-1}

   High stress

   Previously inactive

   No ischemia with GXT

2. Mr. Conner was diagnosed with type 2 diabetes, placed on medication to lower his cholesterol, and placed on a diuretic to lower his BP. He was told to begin to exercise and lose weight in an attempt to lower his blood glucose.

   a. Design a 3 mo supervised exercise program for Mr. Conner.

   b. What are reasonable weight-loss goals for Mr. Conner? What recommendations will you make to help him achieve these goals?

   c. What additional support systems will you recommend to help Mr. Conner achieve success with his exercise and weight-loss goals?

REFERENCES

1. American College of Sports Medicine (ACSM). 2010. *ACSM's guidelines for exercise testing and prescription.* 8th ed. Baltimore: Lippincott Williams & Wilkins.

2. American College of Sports Medicine (ACSM) and American Diabetes Association (ADA). 2010. Joint position statement: Exercise and type 2 diabetes. *Medicine and Science in Sports and Exercise* 42:2282-2303.

3. American Diabetes Association (ADA). 2008. Economic costs of diabetes in the U.S. in 2007. *Diabetes Care* 31:596-615.

4. American Diabetes Association (ADA). 2004. Physical activity/exercise and diabetes. *Diabetes Care* 27:S58-S62.

5. American Diabetes Association (ADA). 2011. Standards of medical care in diabetes—2011. *Diabetes Care* 34(suppl 1): S11-S62.

6. American Diabetes Association (ADA). 2011. Diagnosis and classification of diabetes mellitus. *Diabetes Care* 34(suppl 1): S62-S69.

7. Barnes, D.E. 2004. *Action plan for diabetes: Your guide to controlling blood sugar.* Champaign, IL: Human Kinetics.

8. Bassuk, S.S., and J.E. Manson. 2005. Epidemiological evidence for the role of physical activity in reducing risk of type 2 diabetes and cardiovascular disease. *Journal of Applied Physiology* 99:1193-1204.

9. Centers for Disease Control and Prevention (CDC). 2008. National diabetes fact sheet: General information and national estimates on diabetes in the United States, 2007. Atlanta: HHS.

10. Eriksson, J.G. 1999. Exercise and the treatment of type 2 diabetes mellitus: An update. *Sports Medicine* 27:381-391.

11. Grundy, S.M., J.L. Cleeman, S.R. Daniels, K.A. Donato, R.H. Eckel, B.A. Franklin, D.J. Gordon, R.M. Krauss, P.J. Savage, S.C. Smith, J.A. Spertus, and F. Costa. 2005. Diagnosis and management of the metabolic syndrome: An American Heart Association/National Heart, Lung, and Blood Institute scientific statement (executive summary). *Circulation* 112:285-290.

12. Hornsby, W.G., and A.L. Albright. 2009. Diabetes. In *ACSM's exercise management for persons with chronic diseases and disabilities.* 3rd ed. Ed. J.L. Durstine, G.E. Moore, P.L. Painter, and S.O. Roberts, 182-191. Champaign, IL: Human Kinetics.

13. Kriska, A. 2000. Physical activity and the prevention of type 2 diabetes mellitus: How much for how long? *Sports Medicine* 29:147-151.

14. Maynard, T. 2010. Diagnostic procedures in patients with metabolic disease. In *ACSM's resource manual for guidelines for exercise testing and prescription.* 6th ed. Ed. J.K. Ehrman, 391-403. Baltimore: Lippincott Williams & Wilkins.

15. U.S. Department of Health and Human Services (HHS). 2000. *Healthy People 2010: Understanding and improving health.* Washington, DC: U.S. GPO.

16. Verity, L. 2010. Exercise prescription in patients with diabetes. In *ACSM's resource manual for guidelines for exercise testing and prescription.* 6th ed. Ed. J.K. Ehrman, 600-616. Baltimore: Lippincott Williams & Wilkins.

17. Zhao, G., E.S. Ford, C. Li, and A.H. Mokdad. 2008. Compliance with physical activity recommendations in U.S. adults with diabetes. *Diabetic Medicine* 25:221-227.

Exercise
and Pulmonary Disease

David R. Bassett, Jr.

OBJECTIVES

The reader will be able to do the following:

1. Describe the differences between chronic obstructive lung diseases and restrictive lung diseases.

2. Define the underlying physiological problems associated with asthma, emphysema, bronchitis, and cystic fibrosis.

3. List physiological and mental health benefits of exercise for individuals with pulmonary disease.

4. Describe how pulmonary function testing can be used to diagnose chronic obstructive lung diseases versus restrictive lung diseases.

5. Describe how signs (e.g., dyspnea) and symptoms (e.g., hypoxemia) of pulmonary disease are monitored during a GXT.

6. Describe how to prescribe aerobic exercise (frequency, intensity, and duration) in pulmonary rehabilitation programs.

7. Identify the benefits of upper-body training in pulmonary rehabilitation.

8. Discuss the use of supplemental oxygen therapy and pursed-lip breathing for individuals with COPD.

9. List the common categories of medications used to treat pulmonary disease as well as examples of each category, and discuss the probable effect of these medications on exercise performance.

Pulmonary diseases can be subdivided into two major categories. In **chronic obstructive pulmonary diseases (COPDs)**, the airflow into and out of the lungs is impeded. In restrictive lung diseases, the expansion of the lungs is reduced because of conditions involving the chest cavity or parenchyma (lung tissue). Some pulmonary diseases are genetically inherited (e.g., cystic fibrosis), but in other cases a history of cigarette smoking, environmental pollutants, or occupational exposure to silica, coal dust, or asbestos is the primary contributing factor. All pulmonary diseases show a disruption in the exchange of gases between the ambient air and the pulmonary capillary blood. As a result, $\dot{V}O_2$max is reduced, the work of breathing is increased, and the ability to perform exercise is limited.

Chronic Obstructive Pulmonary Diseases

COPDs cause a reduction in airflow that can dramatically affect a person's ability to perform daily activities. Characteristics of COPDs include expiratory flow obstruction and shortness of breath on exertion. These diseases include chronic bronchitis, emphysema, and bronchial asthma. All of these diseases obstruct airflow, but the underlying reason for obstruction differs for each (5):

- Bronchial asthma is caused by bronchial smooth muscle contraction and increased airway reactivity.

- Chronic bronchitis results from persistent production of sputum attributable to a thickened bronchial wall with excess secretions.

- Emphysema is caused by loss of elastic recoil of alveoli and bronchioles and enlargement of those pulmonary structures.

- Cystic fibrosis is a genetic disorder that results in excessive mucous production in the airways, which hinders ventilation of the lungs.

In 2006, 12.1 million Americans were estimated to have COPD (15). Unfortunately, the mortality rates associated with COPDs have increased over the past two decades. Chronic bronchitis and emphysema are not reversible. The patient with COPD perceives an inability to perform normal activities without dyspnea, but, tragically, by the time this occurs the disease is well advanced (5). COPD is the fourth leading cause of death in the United States, accounting for 124,583 deaths in 2006 (15).

Asthma

An estimated 20.5 million people in the United States have asthma; 30% are children under the age of 18 (3). It is a con-dition that can reverse itself, and it varies from wheezing and slight breathlessness to severe attacks that may result in suffocation. Causes of asthma include allergic reactions to antigens such as dust, pollen, smoke, and air pollution. Nonspecific factors such as emotional stress and exercise as well as viral infections of the bronchi, sinuses, or tonsils can also result in asthma. People with exercise-induced asthma may have normal resting pulmonary function but experience bronchospasms during exercise. In some cases, no specific cause of the asthma can be identified. Treatment involves bronchodilators (often administered by inhalers) and other drugs that thin the mucous secretions and help eject them (expectorants) (8).

Exercise-induced asthma is a reactive airway disease affecting between 4% and 20% of the U.S. population (20). With this condition, exercise tends to cause the bronchioles to constrict. One method of diagnosing exercise-induced asthma is to have a patient run for 6 to 8 min on the treadmill at 85% to 90% of maximal HR (2). The forced expiratory volume in 1 sec (FEV_1) is measured before exercise and 3 to 9 min after exercise. A positive test occurs when the postexercise FEV_1 is 15% below the pretest value (2).

People with exercise-induced asthma can usually engage in exercise training (18). In fact, some notable Olympians like Jackie Joyner-Kersee (gold medalist in heptathlon, 1988 and 1992) and Amy Van Dyken (gold medalist in four swimming events, 1996) have had this condition. Oral inhalers, such as Ventolin and Flovent, are helpful for managing exercise-induced asthma. Other strategies to improve exercise tolerance include exercising in warm, moist environments rather than in cold, dry ones. Many people with asthma tolerate swimming better than running. In addition, a long warm-up can lessen the airway constriction that is more likely to occur with sudden, strenuous exercise (2, 20).

Chronic Bronchitis

According to data from the U.S. National Center for Health Statistics, 9.5 million Americans were diagnosed with chronic bronchitis in 2006 (3). Bronchitis is characterized by inflammation of the bronchi, anatomical structures that carry air from the trachea to the lungs. Symptoms of chronic bronchitis include a cough, often with the production of sputum (i.e., mucous that is coughed up from the respiratory tract). Airflow into the lungs is restricted due to inflammation of the airways and excess mucous production. Upon exertion, a patient with chronic bronchitis may experience wheezing and dyspnea (shortness of breath) (16).

The most common risk factor for chronic bronchitis is cigarette smoking. Chronic bronchitis can also be caused by air pollution, secondhand smoke, occupational exposure to airborne irritants, and genetic factors (15). Chronic bronchitis is much more serious than acute bronchitis.

About 90% of the time, acute bronchitis results from an acute virus such as the common cold or flu. Over time, acute bronchitis goes away and it normally does not pose a problem for long-term health.

The most important treatment for bronchitis is to stop smoking, if the patient is a smoker. This helps relieve symptoms and halt progression of the disease. Treatment for chronic bronchitis often involves the administration of a bronchodilator (e.g., albuterol), typically through the use of an inhaler. Short-term steroid therapy can reduce inflammation of the bronchial tubes. Good hydration is essential, since it will help to remove bronchial secretions, and over-the-counter medicines such as Mucinex and Robitussin may also help in that regard. If the patient suffers from hypoxemia, supplemental oxygen can help to increase arterial oxygenation and relieve symptoms of dyspnea (4).

Emphysema

An estimated 4.1 million Americans have reported being diagnosed with emphysema (3). Emphysema is characterized by destruction of the alveolar walls and enlargement of air spaces distal to the terminal bronchioles. As a result, the lung loses its elasticity and the airways tend to collapse on exhalation. Symptoms include coughing and severe shortness of breath upon exertion. The inability of the lungs to saturate the arterial blood with oxygen leads to hypoxemia (11).

Cigarette smoking is the most common cause of emphysema, just as with chronic bronchitis. Other causes of emphysema include environmental air pollutants and, in rare cases, a hereditary deficiency of alpha-1 antitrypsin. (Alpha-1 antitrypsin inhibits neutrophil elastase, a compound that breaks down the fibroelastic network of the lungs.) Patients with emphysema may have a barrel-shaped chest due to hyperinflation of the lungs. Breathing rate is often rapid and the tidal volume is smaller than normal (16).

Treatment for emphysema cannot cure or reverse the lung damage. Smoking cessation and prevention of respiratory infections with antibiotics are important in medical management of emphysema. Supplemental oxygen is often needed, and this can be administered for 18 to 24 hr $\cdot$ day^{-1}. Bronchodilators are sometimes given to relax and open the airways, and corticosteroids are used to reduce inflammation of the respiratory tract. Expectorants can help loosen the mucous secretions, enabling the patient to cough them up.

Cystic Fibrosis

Cystic fibrosis, another type of COPD, is a recessively inherited genetic disorder. Three decades ago, most cystic fibrosis patients died in childhood, but better treatments have prolonged life expectancy by 20 yr (14). In Caucasian children, 1 in 2,500 is born with the condition, although the disease is rare in Asians and African Americans (14).

Thick mucous secretions by the exocrine glands affect many systems in the body. In fact, clinical diagnosis is based on excessive chloride concentration in the sweat. In the lungs, the mucous secretions plug the airways, causing inflammation and chronic bacterial infections. Treatment for cystic fibrosis consists of having patients lie with the head facing downhill while percussion is used to enhance mucous drainage. In addition, aerobic exercise has been shown to help clear the lungs and prevent bacterial infections. The increased use of antibiotics is yet another reason that survival of cystic fibrosis patients has increased dramatically in recent years (16).

KEY POINT

COPDs reduce the capacity for airflow during respiration. Bronchitis and emphysema are irreversible. Bronchial asthma is an intermittent condition caused by restriction of airways; it can be relieved with bronchodilator medications. Cystic fibrosis is a fatal disease that results from a genetic defect.

Restrictive Lung Diseases

Restrictive lung diseases have many causes, including diseases of the rib cage and spine such as kyphoscoliosis and pectus excavatum (sunken chest). Other causes include pulmonary edema, pulmonary **embolism**, exposure to toxic substances (coal workers' pneumoconiosis, silicosis, asbestosis), chemotherapy, and radiation therapy. Often, these inflame the interstitium and fibrotic tissue develops. Various types of neuromuscular diseases (spinal cord injury, amyotrophic lateral sclerosis or Lou Gehrig's disease, Guillain-Barré syndrome, tetanus, and myasthenia gravis) can also cause restrictive lung disease. Obesity and pregnancy can restrict lung expansion because of the abdomen pushing up into the thoracic cavity. In general, people with restrictive lung diseases have reduced residual volume (RV), inspiratory reserve volume (IRV), expiratory reserve volume (ERV), forced vital capacity (FVC), and maximal tidal volume (TV) (see figure 21.1). Breathing is more difficult because the respiratory muscles must work harder to inflate the lungs (9).

KEY POINT

Restrictive lung diseases have numerous causes, but all are characterized by the reduced capacity to expand the lungs. Thus, smaller lung volumes, assessed through pulmonary function testing, typically are seen in people with these diseases.

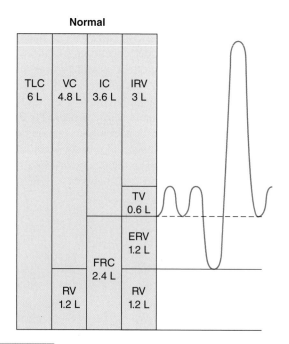

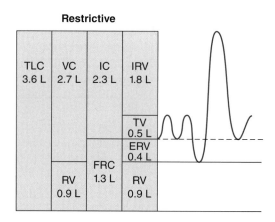

FIGURE 21.1 Lung volumes in a person with restrictive lung disease versus a person with normal pulmonary function. Lung volumes are total lung capacity (TLC), vital capacity (VC), inspiratory capacity (IC), inspiratory reserve volume (IRV), tidal volume (TV), functional residual capacity (FRC), expiratory reserve volume (ERV), and residual volume (RV).

Reprinted from *Essentials of cardiopulmonary physical therapy,* 2nd ed., edited by E.A. Hillegass and H.S. Sadowsky, p. 186, Copyright 2001, with permission from Elsevier.

Evidence for Exercise

Pulmonary rehabilitation programs are often found alongside cardiac rehabilitation programs in many hospitals. Most pulmonary rehabilitation programs focus on people with COPD, although people with other types of pulmonary disease may also benefit from exercise (4). Support for pulmonary rehabilitation programs is limited by the fact that patients typically show little or no improvement in $\dot{V}O_2$max, tests of lung function, and mortality rates. As a result, many insurance providers are reluctant to pay for pulmonary rehabilitation because they view it as medical management rather than a way to restore the patient to normal function (as much as possible).

However, most pulmonary rehabilitation patients do improve in functional outcomes, including symptom-limited GXT, symptoms of dyspnea, quality of life, and

KEY POINT

Patients with lung diseases can benefit from a pulmonary rehabilitation program. Although patients usually demonstrate little improvement in $\dot{V}O_2$max and pulmonary function tests, they do improve in their ability to carry out tasks and in other measures of quality of life.

frequency of hospitalization (4). Thus, pulmonary rehabilitation should be viewed as a desirable part of the patient's medical treatment (11, 12). The overall goals are to improve the patient's general health, to optimize oxygen saturation, to make ADLs more easily accomplished, and to improve self-efficacy (4).

Testing and Evaluation

In most instances, **pulmonary function testing** is carried out for diagnostic purposes and to assess the severity of the disease (17). Computerized spirometry systems measure lung volumes and flow parameters. In COPD, the principal measure is **forced expiratory volume (FEV₁)**, which reflects the maximum volume of air that can be moved in 1 sec (see figure 21.2). Sometimes forced expiratory volume is expressed as FEV₁/VC, where **VC (vital capacity)** is the volume of air that can be breathed out when going from maximal inhalation to maximal exhalation. Because of airway obstruction, individuals with COPD have a decreased ability to exhale quickly; if the FEV₁ is below 80% of the expected value, the test is considered abnormal (7). In addition, if the value of FEV₁/VC is below 0.70, it is considered indicative of COPD. In restrictive lung disease, the lung volumes (e.g., RV, IRV, ERV, FVC, and maximal TV) are smaller than normal because lung expansion is limited. People with restrictive lung disease compensate by

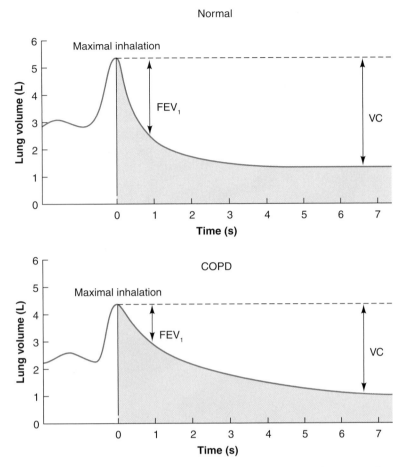

FIGURE 21.2 Pulmonary function test showing the volume versus time curves in a normal person and a person with obstructive lung disease. FEV_1 = forced expiratory volume in the first second of exhalation; VC = vital capacity.

taking faster, smaller breaths, which reduces the work that the respiratory muscles must perform to inflate the lung.

Exercise tests are often administered to assess the patient's ability to exercise. The test may be a standard GXT on a treadmill or cycle ergometer or a simple 6 or 12 min walk test on a flat surface. In a pulmonary patient, exercise capacity is limited more by the lungs than the cardiovascular system. As a result, these patients typically experience **hypoxemia** (low arterial oxygen content) and **dyspnea** (shortness of breath). Measurements of maximal ventilation rates ($\dot{V}_E$max), obtained during the final minute of an exercise test, are also clinically useful. $\dot{V}_E$max is typically 60% to 70% of the maximal voluntary ventilation (MVV), although in COPD patients it may approach 80% to 100%. MVV can be measured via a special spirometry test, or it can be predicted from the following formula: MVV = $FEV_1 \cdot 40$.

A **pulse oximeter** is used to assess the percent saturation of hemoglobin in the arterial blood (S_aO_2) of pulmonary patients (figure 21.3). This noninvasive device shines a light beam through the finger or earlobe. The absorption characteristics of oxygenated and deoxygenated hemoglobin in the red or infrared region are used to assess the arterial

oxygen saturation (www.oximetry.org/pulseox/principles.htm). Values for S_aO_2 below 90% indicate that the client needs supplemental oxygen to increase the driving force for diffusion of oxygen into the lungs. Frequently, a dyspnea rating scale is used to evaluate symptoms during exercise testing (6, 19). Cardiovascular, pulmonary, metabolic, and power output measurements are obtained and used to evaluate the severity of disability (table 21.1).

KEY POINT

One of the main pulmonary function tests for COPD is the FEV_1. COPD patients demonstrate a reduced ability to exhale quickly because of obstructed airways. In restrictive lung diseases, lung volumes are often reduced because the ability to expand the lungs is compromised. Exercise testing of patients with lung diseases, with appropriate monitoring of signs (hypoxemia) and symptoms (dyspnea) to assess the severity of the patient's condition, is beneficial.

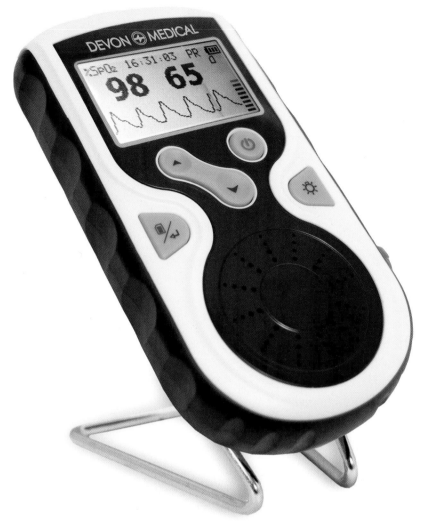

FIGURE 21.3 Portable pulse oximeter used to assess a pulmonary patient's arterial oxygenation. The number on the left of the display shows the percent saturation of hemoglobin in arterial blood (S_aO_2), and the number on the right shows the HR.

Photo courtesy of Devon Medical Products.

TABLE 21.1 Guide to Grading COPD

Grade	Cause of dyspnea	FEV$_1$ (% predicted)	$\dot{V}O_2$max (ml · kg^{-1} · min^{-1})	Exercise $\dot{V}_E$max (L · min^{-1})	Blood gases
1	Fast walking and stair-climbing	>60	>25	Not limiting	Normal P_aCO_2, S_aO_2
2	Walking at normal pace	<60	<25	>50	Normal P_aCO_2, S_aO_2 above 90% at rest and with exercise
3	Slow walking	<40	<15	<50	Normal P_aCO_2, S_aO_2 below 90% with exercise
4	Walking less than one block	<40	<7	<30	Elevated P_aCO_2, S_aO_2 below 90% at rest and with exercise

Table is based on a 40-yr-old man.

Reprinted, by permission, from N.L. Jones et al., 1993, Chronic obstructive respiratory disorders. In *Exercise testing and exercise prescription for special cases*, edited by J.S. Skinner (Baltimore: Lea & Febiger), 229-240.

Typical Exercise Prescription

Given the high prevalence of pulmonary diseases, especially among older adults, fitness professionals can expect to encounter clients who have these conditions in health club and YMCA settings. If a client has severe symptoms of pulmonary disease, the fitness professional should refer the individual to a hospital-based pulmonary rehabilitation program. With a master's degree in exercise physiology, it is possible to get a job in pulmonary rehabilitation, which requires knowledge of the various types of pulmonary diseases, their pathology, and their treatment. Since exercise is recommended for increasing the health and life quality of pulmonary patients, the fitness professional should know how to prescribe exercise for this population.

The goal of a typical pulmonary rehabilitation program is the client's self-care, and to achieve that goal, physicians, nurses, respiratory therapists, exercise specialists, nutritionists, and psychologists are recruited to deal with the various manifestations of the disease (3). The pulmonary patient receives education about ways to deal with the disease, including breathing exercises, ways to approach ADLs at home, and ways to handle work-related problems. The emphasis in most pulmonary rehabilitation programs is on the COPD patient, although patients with restrictive lung disease often participate as well (4, 20). The AACVPR published a detailed description of exercise testing and prescription in its *Guidelines for Pulmonary Rehabilitation Programs* (1).

Aerobic training is usually accomplished with rhythmic, dynamic exercise that uses large muscle groups. Recommended modes are walking, cycling, and swimming (table 21.2). The exercise modes should be enjoyable and improve the ability to perform normal daily activities (11). As with healthy individuals and other clinical populations, the frequency is typically 3 to 5 days · wk^{-1}, with each session lasting at least 30 min. However, assigning appropriate exercise intensities poses a particular problem. Pulmonary patients usually cannot achieve the same peak HRs as healthy individuals of the same age. Thus, computing a THR from a typical percentage of age-predicted HRmax often results in target intensities that are too high. On the other hand, using THR values computed from a typical percentage of measured HRmax underestimates the appropriate training intensity (1, 7).

Various methods can be used to estimate the appropriate exercise intensity for pulmonary patients. Generally, the method of assigning exercise intensity varies with the level of the disability. In patients with mild or moderate impairment, setting the intensity just below the ventilatory

TABLE 21.2 COPD Exercise Prescription

Modes	Goals	Intensity, frequency, duration	Time to goal
Aerobic Large-muscle activities (walking, swimming, cycling)	Increase $\dot{V}O_2$max -Increase lactate threshold and ventilatory threshold -Become less sensitive to dyspnea -Develop more efficient breathing patterns -Facilitate improvements in ADLs	- RPE 11-13/20 (comfortable pace and endurance) -Monitor dyspnea -1-2 sessions, 3-5 days · wk^{-1} -30 min sessions (shorter intermittent exercise sessions may be necessary initially) -Emphasize progression of duration more than intensity	2-3 mo to ensure completion
Strength Free weights Isokinetic/isotonic machines	-Increase maximal number of reps -Increase isokinetic torque/ work Increase lean body mass	-Low resistance, high reps 2-3 days · wk^{-1}	2-3 mo
Flexibility Stretching Tai chi	Increase ROM	3 days · wk^{-1}	Ongoing
Neuromuscular Walking, balance exercise Breathing exercises	Improve gait, posture Improve breathing efficiency		

Reprinted, by permission from C.B. Cooper, 2009, Chronic obstructive pulmonary disease. In *ACSM's exercise management for persons with chronic diseases and disabilities*, 3rd ed. (Champaign, IL: Human Kinetics), 134.

threshold or the point where the person became noticeably dyspneic is appropriate. A **dyspnea rating scale** (table 21.3) should be used to determine the patient's symptoms of shortness of breath. In clients with more severe disability, it is often necessary to let symptoms of dyspnea be the guiding factors (7). Intermittent exercise, interspersed with rest, may be all that the client can tolerate. If the impairment is severe, supplemental oxygen will be needed to maintain S_aO_2 above 90% (13).

Individuals with emphysema should be instructed in pursed-lip breathing, which involves pressing the lips together and exhaling through a small opening in the center of the mouth. This slows the rate of respiration and prevents collapse of small airways, resulting in better oxygenation (4, 12). In some instances, a resistive breathing device may be recommended to train the respiratory muscles at rest.

Upper-body exercise is recommended for pulmonary patients. This exercise can be achieved using modalities that require both arm and leg muscles, such as the Schwinn Airdyne or the rowing ergometer. Additionally, resistance training can be accomplished with dumbbells, machines, or elastic bands. Increasing arm strength and endurance improves the client's ability to perform functional activities and decreases local muscle fatigue (4, 7). Flexibility training (e.g., stretching, tai chi) and balance training may also be incorporated to improve the patient's functional ability (11).

KEY POINT

Pulmonary rehabilitation programs involve many types of health professionals. The primary goals are to educate patients about dealing with their disease and to help them improve their exercise capacity. A health professional in pulmonary rehabilitation must understand the client's medical conditions and physiological limitations. Sensations of dyspnea and pulse oximeter readings are frequently used to determine the appropriate exercise intensity.

TABLE 21.3 Dyspnea Rating Scale

1	Light, barely noticeable
2	Moderate, bothersome
3	Moderately severe, very uncomfortable
4	Most severe or intense dyspnea ever experienced

Reprinted from American College of Sports Medicine 2010.

Medications for Pulmonary Diseases

Bronchodilators relax smooth muscle surrounding airways in the lungs and relieve the symptoms of asthma, bronchitis, and related lung disorders (8, 11). These medications can be taken orally or from an inhaler. The inhalers are generally used for acute asthma episodes, whereas long-term bronchodilation usually is obtained orally. Most of these drugs stimulate the beta-2 receptors that relax bronchial smooth muscle and increase the airway lumen. Because of their beta-adrenergic stimulating effect, these medications can increase HR and BP, although they mostly focus on the smooth muscle found in airways. Some inhaler brand names include Brethaire Inhaler, Alupent, and Maxair. A second class of drugs comprises the methylxanthines, which include Theobid, Aminophyllin, Theo-Dur, and many others. Side effects of this class include tachycardia, arrhythmias, central nervous system stimulation, and risk of seizures. Anticholinergics (Atrovent) make up a third class of bronchodilators. Advair is a relatively new inhaler drug that contains both a bronchodilator and an anti-inflammatory; it is used to prevent asthma attacks and to treat chronic bronchitis and emphysema.

Additional medicines are used to treat common respiratory disorders. These include **decongestants** to dry out the mucous membranes, **antihistamines** to relieve symptoms of seasonal allergies (e.g., hay fever), anti-inflammatory agents, expectorants, and cough medications. Antibiotics are often given to fight off infections (8), which tend to occur if mucous secretions block off the airways.

Diuretics are important in treating cor pulmonale, a condition that occurs in about half of pulmonary patients with severe disease. *Cor pulmonale* is defined as pulmonary hypertension with right ventricular hypertrophy. Because failure of the right ventricle often follows, diuretics may be needed to enhance fluid excretion (10). There are three types of diuretics: thiazide diuretics (e.g., Esidrix), potassium-sparing diuretics (e.g., Aldactone), and loop diuretics (e.g., Lasix) (8).

KEY POINT

Bronchodilators are the most common medications for patients with COPD. Decongestants, antihistamines, anti-inflammatory agents, and antibiotics are often prescribed to treat respiratory disorders. Diuretics are sometimes needed for patients with severe pulmonary disease who also develop heart failure.

STUDY QUESTIONS

1. What is the major problem in COPD, and what are the physiological consequences of severe COPD?

2. What is the major problem in restrictive lung disease, and what are the physiological consequences of severe restrictive lung disease?

3. Define the underlying problems associated with the following subcategories of COPD: asthma, emphysema, bronchitis, and cystic fibrosis.

4. Identify which of the static lung volumes are decreased in people with restrictive lung disease.

5. Describe how the FEV_1 and VC are affected in people with COPD (e.g., asthma).

6. What two physiological variables can be monitored noninvasively via a pulse oximeter?

7. Describe a therapeutic treatment that is available in case a client's SaO_2 falls below 90%.

8. Outline the recommendations for aerobic exercise programming for people with COPD in terms of frequency, intensity, duration, and mode. What are the recommendations for strength training?

9. List five types of medicines used to treat pulmonary disease as well as their physiological effects on the body.

10. Why is upper-body training often recommended for people with pulmonary disease?

CASE STUDIES

You can check your answers by referring to appendix A.

1. A 38-yr-old woman with asthma would like to enter your fitness program. What kinds of questions do you ask her during your screening interview?

2. A 50-yr-old man with a history of smoking a pack of cigarettes a day for the past 25 yr enters a hospital complaining of dyspnea. A chest X-ray shows that his lungs are hyperinflated, and spirometry tests show that his FEV_1 is only half the normal value. What type of pulmonary disease does he have, and what is the logical course of treatment?

3. A middle-aged patient with severe kyphoscoliosis is referred to a pulmonary rehabilitation program. He has restrictive pulmonary disease, demonstrating a vital capacity of only 1.5 L (compared with the normal value of 5.0 L). During a 6 min walk test, he manages to cover 865 ft (264 m), stopping once because of shortness of breath. His S_aO_2 at the end of the test has fallen to 87%. What type of exercise training would you recommend? What other therapies might assist him in completing his exercise sessions?

REFERENCES

1. American Association of Cardiovascular and Pulmonary Rehabilitation (AACVPR). 2004. *Guidelines for pulmonary rehabilitation programs.* 3rd ed. Champaign, IL: Human Kinetics.

2. American College of Sports Medicine (ACSM). 2010. *ACSM's guidelines for exercise testing and prescription.* 8th ed. Baltimore: Lippincott Williams & Wilkins.

3. American Lung Association. 2008. *Lung disease data: 2008.* New York: Author.

4. Barr, R.N. 2001. Pulmonary rehabilitation. In *Essentials of cardiopulmonary physical therapy.* 2nd ed. Ed. E.A. Hillegass and H.S. Sadowsky, 727-751. Philadelphia: Saunders.

5. Berman, L.B., and J.R. Sutton. 1986. Exercise and the pulmonary patient. *Journal of Cardiopulmonary Rehabilitation* 6:52-61.

6. Borg, G.A. 1998. *Borg's perceived exertion and pain scales.* Champaign, IL: Human Kinetics.

7. Brubaker, P.H., L.A. Kaminsky, and M.H. Whaley. 2002. *Coronary artery disease: Essentials of prevention and rehabilitation programs.* Champaign, IL: Human Kinetics.

8. Cahalin, L.P., and H.S. Sadowsky. 2001. Pulmonary medications. In *Essentials of cardiopulmonary physical therapy.* 2nd ed. Ed. E.A. Hillegass and H.S. Sadowsky, 587-607. Philadelphia: Saunders.

9. Clough, P. 2001. Restrictive lung dysfunction. In *Essentials of cardiopulmonary physical therapy.* 2nd ed. Ed. E.A. Hillegass and H.S. Sadowsky, 183-255. Philadelphia: Saunders.

10. Cooper, C.B. 1995. Determining the role of exercise in patients with chronic pulmonary disease. *Medicine and Science in Sports and Exercise* 27:147-157.

11. Cooper, C.B. 2009. Chronic obstructive pulmonary disease. In *ACSM's exercise management for persons with chronic diseases and disabilities*, ed. J.L. Durstine, G. Moore, P. Painter, and S. Roberts, 129-135. Champaign, IL: Human Kinetics.

12. Cooper, C.B., and T.W. Storer. 2010. Exercise prescription in patients with pulmonary disease. In *ACSM's resource manual for guidelines for exercise testing and prescription*. 4th ed. Ed. J.K. Ehrman, 575-599. Baltimore: Lippincott Williams & Wilkins.

13. Davidson, A.C., R. Leach, R.J.D. George, and D.M. Geddes. 1988. Supplemental oxygen and exercise ability in chronic obstructive airways disease. *Thorax* 43:965-971.

14. Davis, P.B. 1991. Cystic fibrosis: A major cause of obstructive airway disease in the young. In *Chronic obstructive pulmonary disease*, ed. N.S. Cheniack, 297-307. Philadelphia: Saunders.

15. Environmental Protection Agency (EPA). 2010. Chronic obstructive pulmonary disease prevalence and mortality. Accessed December 28, 2010, at http://cfpub.epa.gov/eroe/index.cfm?fuseaction=detail.viewInd&lv=list.listByAlpha&r=216638&subtop=381.

16. Garritan, S.L. 1994. Chronic obstructive pulmonary disease. In *Essentials of cardiopulmonary physical therapy*, ed. E.A. Hillegass and H.S. Sadowsky, 257-284. Philadelphia: Saunders.

17. Guyton, A.C., and J.E. Hall. 2010. *Textbook of medical physiology*. 12th ed. Philadelphia: Saunders.

18. Lacroix, V.J. 1999. Exercise-induced asthma. *Physician and Sportsmedicine* 27:75-92.

19. Mahler, D.A., and M.B. Horowitz. 1994. Perception of breathlessness during exercise in patients with respiratory disease. *Medicine and Science in Sports and Exercise* 26:1078-1081.

20. Rundell, K.W., and D.M. Jenkinson. 2002. Exercise-induced bronchospasm in the elite athlete. *Sports Medicine* 32:583-600.

Exercise Programming

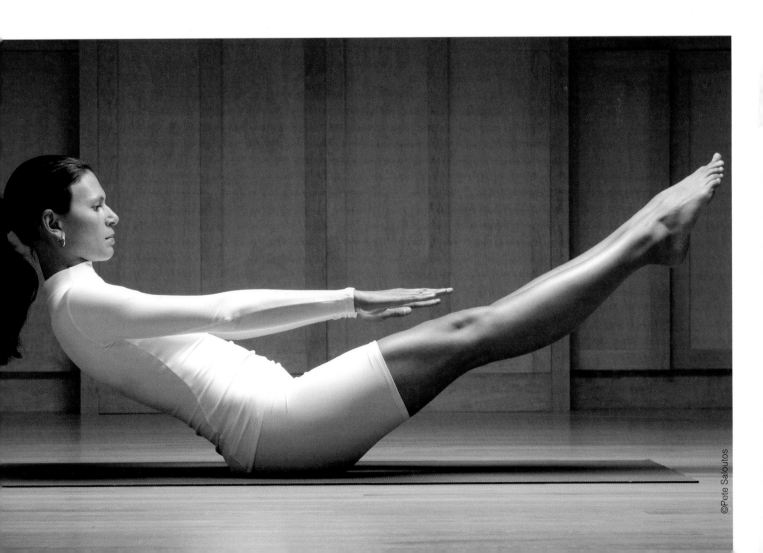

PART VI

The previous parts of this textbook covered assessment and exercise prescription for components of physical fitness for people with a variety of characteristics and health conditions. This section includes other elements needed for a comprehensive and effective fitness program. In chapter 22, we discuss ideas for exercise programming consistent with the latest physical activity guidelines. In chapter 23, we go over ways to help motivate people to adopt and maintain a healthy lifestyle. In chapter 24, we provide an overview of mind–body (mindful) exercises (e.g., yoga, Pilates, tai chi). In chapter 25, we review analysis of the electrocardiogram (ECG) and current medications for cardiovascular problems. Chapter 26 provides information on the prevention and treatment of injuries. Finally, in chapter 27 we describe important legal considerations for fitness professionals.

Exercise Programming for Health and Fitness

OBJECTIVES

The reader will be able to do the following:

1. Describe the differences in the professional competencies needed for exercise programming for diverse populations.

2. Discuss what progression means when a sedentary person begins a physical activity program and when someone transitions from moderate-intensity to vigorous-intensity physical activity.

3. Explain how progression is linked to the risk of adverse events.

4. Describe safety and clothing considerations for walking and jogging programs.

5. Explain the balance between duration and intensity in a typical walking program, and list activities used in walking programs to improve enjoyment and adherence.

6. Outline appropriate walk, jog, walk intervals used at the beginning of a jogging program.

7. Describe exercise recommendations for cycling that improve CRF.

8. List the elements of games that provide effective fitness benefits.

9. Describe the activities done in a swimming pool, other than lap swimming, that can be an effective part of an aerobic exercise program.

10. Provide recommendations for beginners starting group exercise programs.

11. Recommend steps to follow when purchasing exercise equipment.

12. Describe a circuit training program that uses aerobic and resistance training equipment.

The authors wish to thank Margy Wirtz-Henry for her help with updating this chapter.

The purpose of a fitness program must be uppermost in the fitness professional's mind. The fitness professional is trying to help people include physical activity as a vital part of their lives. This assumes that the participants understand what type of physical activity is appropriate, have sufficient skills to achieve satisfaction from the activities, and have the intrinsic motivation to continue to be active for the rest of their lives. Thus, fitness professionals help people increase their physical fitness in ways that are psychologically, mentally, and socially relevant and appealing.

Professional Competency and Exercise Programming

At this point in the text, we have covered a great deal of information about exercise prescription for CRF, strength, body composition, and flexibility for a variety of populations, including children, adults, older adults, those who are overweight or obese, pregnant women, and people with clinical disease. It should be no surprise that the competencies needed to work with some of the latter populations vary greatly.

Since 1980, many organizations have developed certification and education programs to promote exercise programming to address the needs of various populations. One of the earliest to do so was the ACSM. Certification requires the applicant to have a certain knowledge base and to demonstrate specific behaviors. The current major ACSM certification programs include the following:

Health fitness certifications

- ACSM Certified Group Exercise Instructor (GEI)
- ACSM Certified Personal Trainer
- ACSM Certified Health Fitness Specialist

Clinical certifications

- ACSM Certified Clinical Exercise Specialist
- ACSM Registered Clinical Exercise Physiologist

Educational requirements vary from a high school diploma to a master's degree. In addition, the ACSM offers a variety of specialty certifications (go to www.acsm.org and click on Certification for details). ACSM certifications are considered the standard by many professionals in the fields of fitness and cardiac rehabilitation. However, there are a variety of other respected certification programs:

- American Council on Exercise (ACE)—Group Fitness Instructor, Personal Trainer, Lifestyle and Weight Management Consultant, and Advanced Health and Fitness Specialist (www.acefitness.org)

- Aerobics and Fitness Association of America (AFAA)—Personal Trainer and Primary Group Exercise (www.afaa.com)
- National Strength and Conditioning Association (NSCA)—Certified Strength and Conditioning Specialist and Certified Personal Trainer (www.nsca-lift.org)
- National Academy of Sports Medicine (NASM): Certified Personal Trainer (www. nasm.org)

We cannot cover the detail associated with each of these certifications, but we encourage you to get online and check out the differences among these certifications. This recommendation is not just aimed at those interested in a career as a fitness professional but also those going into the allied health professions (e.g., physical therapy) or medicine. Given the limited number of rehabilitation sessions supported by insurance, there needs to be a smooth transition between a rehabilitation program and a fitness program to enable the patient to make a full recovery and achieve a level of physical activity and fitness consistent with good health. Certification programs for unique aspects of exercise leadership are presented later in this chapter. In spite of the wide variety of differences that exist among the various health, fitness, and clinical certifications, there are certain things that all fitness professionals should do, as described next.

Be a Role Model

Fitness professionals should be inspiring role models for their clients. The idea of an overweight, out-of-shape fitness professional is one whose time has passed. A fitness professional must plan activities, evaluate participants' progress, and provide incentives, but the leadership associated with many exercise programs is in the form of subtle value statements that do not require words. When fitness professionals' presence and behaviors demonstrate a healthy lifestyle, it adds much value to their words and programs.

Plan Programs

All programs should have daily, weekly, and monthly plans to provide appropriate activities, meet participants' needs, and reduce the possibility of boredom. This planning allows the fitness professional to judge the usefulness of the activity and encourage systematic modification from one month to the next. If the fitness professional is working with clients who exercise on their own, the need for specific exercise recommendations becomes obvious. The value of the feedback received from these clients depends on the information they were given at the start of their program. The following considerations apply to both group and individual exercise programs.

Establish the Routine of Physical Activity

For clients who are sedentary, the first step in programming is establishing a regular routine of physical activity. In most cases, this means a structured walking program (or equivalent if orthopedic limitations exist) that focuses on the routine of activity. As will be discussed shortly, the program might begin with a short (10 min) bout of activity to realize success and provide a reference point for later modifications. Remember, if a client has been inactive for many years, taking a few weeks to get into the habit of physical activity is not unreasonable.

Vary the Program

Variety should be a cornerstone of every exercise program once the base of regular physical activity has been established. Certain elements appear in every exercise session: a warm-up and stretching, a stimulus phase, and a cool-down. The variety comes from using different exercises in each part of a session, presenting short educational messages to the participants while they are stretching or cooling down, and using games to add spice to routine exercises. The most important thing is to plan the activity sessions far enough in advance to minimize repetition and maximize variety. This is more the case for structured exercise programs than for jogging programs, although variety is helpful for both.

Accommodate Individual Differences

A participant should be able to choose from a variety of activities. A program must address the needs, interests, and limitations of the group being served. The equipment, the activities, and the pace of the class must be considered when planning for younger or older, less fit or very fit, and skilled or unskilled participants (11). Offer people a variety of options: 1 or 5 lb (0.5 or 2 kg) weights, low-impact or high-impact moves, or 1 mi (1.6 km) walks versus 3 mi (4.8 km) jogs. This is obviously more of a challenge when working with a group than one on one with a client, but it is the kind of attention to detail that will increase the chance that all members of the group will be successful.

Maintain Control

The fitness professional must control the exercise session. This is especially true when using games (e.g., indoor soccer), or dance forms of exercise in which the intensity is not as easily controlled as in walking or biking programs. Control implies an ability to modify the session as needed to meet the THR and total work goals of each individual. Some people will have to slow down; others may need encouragement to increase their intensity. The element of control for people who exercise without direct supervision can be provided through written guidelines and verbal instructions about what to do and when to move from one stage to the next. In addition, specific information should be provided about signs or symptoms that indicate inappropriate responses to exercise.

Monitor Progress and Keep Records

Keeping track of participants' responses to exercise sessions reveals their adaptation to that particular session and day-to-day changes overall. This information is important for updating exercise prescriptions and answering specific questions that the participant may raise. Each exercise class should pause regularly to check HR and determine whether people are close to their THRs. Rather than keeping track of a large number of 10 sec THRs, ask each participant to indicate the number of beats over or under the 10 sec goal. This increases the participant's awareness of the THR and indicates how the intensity should be adjusted to stay on target.

The HR response is probably the most objective indicator of adjustment to an exercise session, but do not stop with that. Elicit information about how the participant feels in general, asking about any new pains, aches, or strange sensations. In that regard, the RPE can be used to obtain information about the participant's perception of effort. Record keeping might include a daily attendance check, a weekly weighing, a regular BP check (if appropriate), and a column asking for comments (e.g., THR, any aches or pains). An example of such a form is the Physical Activity Form (see form 22.1). This information allows the fitness professional to make better recommendations about participants' exercise programs and refer them to appropriate professionals if needed. The point is that the fitness professional needs to help the participant to become and remain physically active. See chapter 23 for a variety of motivational strategies that can be used to accomplish that objective.

KEY POINT

The fitness professional must develop relationship-oriented abilities, serve as a role model for others, help clients establish the routine of physical activity, use variety, accommodate differences, control the environment for safety, and monitor and record clients' progress. Asking for participants' HR, RPE, and any unusual responses to the exercise are ways to monitor intensity during an exercise session.

Progression of Activities

A central point made throughout the *2008 Physical Activity Guidelines for Americans* (14) is to use progression when introducing someone to physical activity or helping a client move from moderate-intensity to vigorous-intensity

FORM 22.1   Physical Activity Form

Name_____   Target weight _____   Target HR zone_____

Week	Day	Weight	Resting BP	Resting HR	Exercise HR	RPE	Signs, symptoms, comments
1							
2							
3							
4							

From E.T. Howley and D.L. Thompson, 2012, *Fitness professional's handbook, 6th ed.* (Champaign, IL: Human Kinetics).

activity. This is true for children, adults, older adults, and people with chronic conditions or special needs. Such an approach reduces the risk of adverse events and increases the chance that the client will make a successful transition to a physically active lifestyle. Sedentary people who want to begin a fitness program should follow a logical sequence of activities. Moderate-intensity activities are encouraged for everyone, but a systematic program of activities helps participants increase functional capacity. The following paragraphs summarize our recommendations for accomplishing this progression of activities.

Phase 1: Regular Walking

The first phase for sedentary individuals is to gradually increase the amount of moderate-intensity physical activity in their regular routine. Walking is the most popular activity. The major goal is to increase the amount of physical activity that can be done comfortably, so no emphasis on intensity is necessary at this point. People in this phase start with the distance they can easily walk without pain or fatigue and then gradually increase the distance and pace until they can complete about 30 min of moderate-intensity activity (e.g., 2 mi at 4 mi · hr^{-1}, or 3.2 km at 6.4 km · hr^{-1}) each day. People with orthopedic limitations can substitute

a weight-supported activity such as cycling, rowing, or swimming for walking. Even though some clients may not be able to achieve this 30 min goal, a regular pattern of light physical activity still provides health-related benefits and is better than being sedentary.

Phase 2: Recommended Work Levels for a Change in Fitness

Once phase 1 is accomplished, participants are taught about recommended levels of work for fitness changes (see chapter 11). Again, some clients may not be interested in moving beyond a walking program that they can do most days of the week. That is not an issue since the health-related benefits of physical activity can be realized with a walking program. For those who want to move on to more vigorous activities, a work–relief interval training program is introduced—jogging is the work, and walking is the relief. The participant walks, jogs a few steps, then walks, and so forth. Gradually, jogging covers more distance than walking, until the person can jog continuously for 20 to 30 min at the THR. People interested in cycling and swimming (see later in this chapter) also can use interval training. People interested in group classes should transition from the walking program to the lower-intensity version of the class, if one is available. If a lower-intensity version is not available, the client should communicate with the instructor to get pointers on how to transition into the class.

Phase 3: Variety of Fitness Activities

Once the base of physical activity has been established and the transition to regular vigorous-intensity physical activity has occurred, the client will be able to participate in a wider range of physical activities. Phase 3 is quite individualized and is based on the person's interests. The purpose is to promote continued activity by having people participate in an activity they naturally enjoy. Some people prefer to continue to stretch, walk, and jog; some prefer to exercise alone; and others enjoy working out with other people. Some people like cooperative and relatively low-level competitive activities, and others like the thrill of competition. Some enjoy a variety of movement forms, while others enjoy repeating similar activities. The fitness professional must provide an atmosphere where people feel free to try new things without embarrassment and should allow participants to choose their fitness activities from a variety of options.

Walk, Jog, Run Programs

While walking, the participant keeps at least one foot on the ground at all times. In jogging and running, more muscular force is exerted to propel the body completely off the ground, creating a nonsupport phase. The distinction between jogging and running is not as clearly defined. Some people view speed as being the difference, but no single criterion for speed is commonly accepted. Others distinguish between the two by the intent of the participant—a jogger is simply interested in exercise, whereas a runner trains to achieve performance goals in road races.

General Safety

Safety is an important consideration for all participants, independent of the activity they choose to do. In this context, a variety of safety factors common to both walking and jogging should be mentioned before we discuss how to institute walking and jogging programs.

Footwear

Any comfortable pair of well-supported shoes can be worn for a beginning walking program. Serious walkers and all joggers should invest in appropriate shoes with well-padded heels that are higher than the soles and have fitted heel cups. The shoes should be flexible enough to bend easily. The same kind of socks that will be worn while exercising should be worn during the shoe fitting to ensure a proper fit. Only the serious competitive runner needs racing shoes, which are a lighter weight and offer less cushioning.

Clothing

The weather conditions and activity intensity determine the clothing to be worn. Warm weather dictates light, preferably cotton, loose-fitting clothing. Nothing should be worn that prevents perspiration from reaching the outside air. A brimmed hat should cover the head on hot, sunny days.

In cold weather, walkers and joggers should dress in layers so they can remove or add clothing when necessary. Wool and polypropylene fabrics are good choices for extreme cold, but most joggers tend to overdress. A hat, preferably a wool stocking cap that can be pulled down over the forehead and ears, and gloves or mittens also should be worn. Cotton socks worn as mittens are useful not only to keep hands warm but also to act as wipers for the sniffling nose that often accompanies cold-weather walking and jogging.

Surface

The surface is not as crucial for walkers as it is for joggers, although some walkers (especially those with orthopedic problems) should exercise on a soft surface such as grass or a running track with a shock-absorbent surface. Many people prefer exercising off the track for visual stimulation and interest, but regular jogging on hard surfaces such as concrete or blacktop can lead to stress problems in the ankle, knee, and hip joints and in the low back. Joggers need to observe special precautions when running on the road: Jog facing traffic, assume cars at crossroads do not see joggers, and beware of cracks and curbs. Running cross country usually means running on a softer surface, but joggers must be aware of the uneven terrain and the increased potential for ankle injuries.

Safety Tips

Educate participants to practice the following tips to ensure safety when walking or jogging:

- Move toward the oncoming traffic.
- Yield the right of way to cars.
- Listen to music only while exercising on a quiet street, and always listen for and be aware of traffic.
- Choose well-lighted streets or running tracks on school grounds.
- Walk or jog with a partner if you must exercise at night.

KEY POINT

Walkers and joggers should wear supportive, flexible shoes, and they should wear clothing that accommodates weather conditions and exercise intensity. They should follow the rules of the road and walk or jog in safe areas at safe times.

Walking

The advantages of walking include its convenience, practicality, and naturalness. Walking is an excellent activity, especially for people who are overweight and poorly conditioned and whose joints cannot handle the stresses of jogging. It is the most popular physical activity for adults (3).

As with all exercise programs, the participants begin with a warm-up and perhaps some static stretching. The walk should start at a slow speed and gradually increase to a pace that feels comfortable to the participant. The arms should swing freely, and the trunk should be kept erect with a slight backward pelvic tilt. The feet should point forward at all times. Many walkers have taken to malls, which provide air-conditioned comfort, safety, and a smooth surface and are usually within a short drive.

Walking programs can progress by increasing the distance or the speed. As mentioned previously, the first goal is for participants to accumulate 30 min of moderate-intensity physical activity each day. This is an important milestone and has clear health benefits (see chapter 11). Further, the 30 min can be realized in bouts of 10 min or longer. Participants should gradually increase their distance

until they can easily walk 30 min at a brisk pace on a daily basis. The program in the following sidebar, Walking Program, is graduated and leads to an activity level suitable for beginning a jogging program or participating in other vigorous activities. These stages are not absolute steps to follow in an exact order; clients will vary in their abilities and some will progress faster through the listed stages. Also, some clients may prefer to stay with walking as their only physical activity and increase the duration for each day to 60 min to achieve a level of activity consistent with greater health-related gains, as discussed in chapter 11 (14). A pedometer also can be used to track progress in a walking program (see Research Insight).

How do you make walking interesting for a class of 30 to 40 participants? A fitness professional must emphasize variety to keep interest high in such situations. There are several ways to achieve this:

- Have participants follow the leader up and down steps or slopes, with the walking speed changing from time to time.

- Have the group do line walking on a track—the person at the end of the line must walk faster to

Walking Program

Rules

1. Start at a level that feels comfortable to you.
2. Be aware of new aches or pains.
3. Don't progress to the next level if you are not comfortable.
4. Monitor and record your HR.
5. Walk at least 5 days · wk^{-1}

Stage	Duration	HR	Comments
1	10 min		
2	15 min		
3	20 min		
4	25 min		
5	30 min		
6	35 min		
7	40 min		
8	45 min		
9	50 min		
10	55 min		
11	60 min		

From E.T. Howley and D.L. Thompson, 2012, *Fitness professional's handbook,* 6th ed. (Champaign, IL: Human Kinetics). Reprinted, by permission, from B.D. Franks and E.T. Howley, 1998, *Fitness leader's handbook,* 2nd ed. (Champaign, IL: Human Kinetics), 124.

catch up to the front of the line, which, as a whole, moves at a steady pace. Line walking gives each person an interval-type workout.

- Add a ball to the front of the line, and have participants pass it to the side or overhead until it reaches the end of the line, at which time the last person dribbles to the front and restarts the process.

- Vary the activity used to reach the front of the line, with people skipping, jogging, and so on.

- Vary the length of the line by forming teams, and control the overall pace by balancing the teams and checking the THR.

- Plan a game of tag in a gym or field where all participants must walk, with the leader exerting control by defining the boundaries.

- Establish a distance goal for a 15 wk walking class, such as "We will walk from here to Nashville," for a total of 180 mi (290 km) walked over the 15 wk. Use a large map and pins to monitor each participant's progress from week to week. Award T-shirts or hold a country-western dance (in keeping with the Nashville theme) when everyone finishes. Longer distances can be set as goals along with using the class total of miles walked to focus on group accomplishments.

KEY POINT

Walking programs should begin at a slow speed and gradually increase to a comfortable pace. Distance should be increased gradually until at least 30 min can be walked daily at a brisk pace. The previous list details activities that improve enjoyment and, consequently, adherence to the program.

Jogging

No single factor determines when a person can begin jogging. A person who can walk briskly for 30 min but is unable to reach the THR range should consider a jogging program for additional improvements in CRF and health. A slow to moderate walker whose HR is within the THR zone should increase the distance or speed of walking rather than begin jogging. Also, the ability of the person's joints to withstand the additional stresses of jogging should be considered. Remember, walking may be the first and only activity for many people; it is more important to stay active doing what they like than move to more intense activities just because others choose to do so.

Techniques for jogging are basically the same as those for walking. Jogging requires greater flexion of the knee of the recovery leg, and the arms are bent more at the elbows.

RESEARCH INSIGHT

Most people are familiar with pedometers, devices that can track the number of steps a person takes (see chapter 6). Pedometers have been used successfully in programs aimed at increasing the amount of activity participants do, and popular books have been written about how to help people achieve a physically active lifestyle using these devices (3). What are the characteristics of these successful pedometer-based programs? The answer provides important information for the fitness professionals and allied health professionals who are responsible for increasing their clients' level of physical activity. Bravata et al. (2) did a systematic review of the literature on pedometer-based programs and found that successful programs do the following:

- Set a step goal for each client.
  - First, a baseline is established by having the client wear the pedometer for a week, recording the steps at the end of each day. The average number of steps taken per day is calculated (e.g., 5,500 steps each day).
  - A new step goal is established for each client by adding steps to that baseline (e.g., increase the daily step count by 2,000 over the baseline for a goal of 7,500 steps). The client then has a clear step goal to achieve each day.
- The client keeps a step diary in which the step count is recorded each night. This acts as a motivational device to drive the behavior of walking.
- The records are returned to a fitness professional, who can then interact with the client and help as needed.

Pedometers are simple to use, effective, and worth considering, especially with walking being the most popular activity for adults. There is clear evidence that such programs achieve health-related benefits, and with the newer pedometers capable of storing step data for weeks at a time (that can be downloaded later), the fitness professional's job is made easier.

The arm swing is exaggerated slightly but should still be in the forward and backward direction. The heel makes the first contact with the ground; then the foot immediately rolls forward to the ball of the foot and then to the toes. As speed increases, the landing foot may contact the ground in an almost flat position. Breathing occurs through both the nose and mouth. Common faults of the beginning jogger include breathing with the mouth closed, insufficiently bending the knee during the recovery phase, and swinging the arms across the body.

Many people begin jogging at too high a speed, which results in an inability to continue long enough to accomplish the desired amount of total work and often causes people to dislike jogging. This problem can be prevented by jogging at a speed slow enough to allow conversation and by using work–relief intervals, which for beginners is slow jogging for a few seconds, then walking, then slow jogging, and so forth. Participants should be reassured that they will walk less and jog more as they become more fit. An example of such a progression is shown in the jogging program.

After a person can jog 20 to 40 min (about 2-3 mi, or 3.2-4.8 km) continuously within the THR zone, several jogging programs are available. A person can simply jog 3 or 4 days · wk⁻¹, planning only to exercise at an intensity that will elevate the HR to the training zone for a predetermined minimum length of time (or distance), with the option to go longer (or farther) on days when so desired. Other people do better with a specific program that includes progressive speed and distance goals, even if they do not plan to compete.

As with the walking class mentioned earlier, the fitness professional should include variety in a jogging program, and the same types of modifications cited earlier for the walking program are appropriate. Some communities may have jogging paths with exercise stations along the way to allow people to combine walking or jogging with specific exercises for all parts of the body. In addition, fun runs are held in many communities; the goal of these runs is to finish the distance, and a small prize is usually awarded.

Joggers who are not fast enough to compete successfully in road races may enjoy other competitions, such as predic-

Jogging Program

Rules

1. Complete the walking program before starting this program.
2. Begin each session with walking and stretching.
3. Be aware of new aches and pains.
4. Don't progress to the next level if you are not comfortable doing so.
5. Stay at the low end of your THR zone, and record your HR for each session.
6. Do the program on a work-a-day, rest-a-day basis.

   ○ Stage 1   Jog 10 steps; walk 10 steps. Repeat 5 times and take your HR. Stay within THR zone by increasing or decreasing walking phase. Do 20 to 30 min of activity.

   ○ Stage 2   Jog 20 steps; walk 10 steps. Repeat 5 times and take your HR. Stay within THR zone by increasing or decreasing walking phase. Do 20 to 30 min of activity.

   ○ Stage 3   Jog 30 steps; walk 10 steps. Repeat 5 times and take your HR. Stay within THR zone by increasing or decreasing walking phase. Do 20 to 30 min of activity.

   ○ Stage 4   Jog 1 min; walk 10 steps. Repeat 3 times and take your HR. Stay within THR zone by increasing or decreasing walking phase. Do 20 to 30 min of activity.

   ○ Stage 5   Jog 2 min; walk 10 steps. Repeat 2 times and take your HR. Stay within THR zone by increasing or decreasing walking phase. Do 30 min of activity.

   ○ Stage 6   Jog 1 lap (400 m, or 440 yd) and check your HR. Adjust pace to stay within the THR zone. If HR is still too high, go back to stage 5. Do 6 laps with a brief walk between each.

   ○ Stage 7   Jog 2 laps and check HR. Adjust pace to stay within the THR zone. If HR is still too high, go back to stage 6. Do 6 laps with a brief walk between each.

   ○ Stage 8   Jog 1 mi (1.6 km) and check HR. Adjust pace during the run to stay within THR zone. Do 2 mi (3.2 km).

   ○ Stage 9   Jog 20 to 40 min (2-3 mi [3.2-4.8 km]) continuously. Check HR at the end to ensure that you were within THR zone.

Reprinted, by permission, from B.D. Franks and E.T. Howley, 1998, *Fitness leaders' handbook*, 2nd ed. (Champaign, IL: Human Kinetics), 125.

tion runs, in which speed does not determine the winner. The purpose of a prediction run is to see which joggers come closest to their predicted finishing time, which is declared before the race. A handicapped run requires joggers to declare their previous fastest times for the distance. A percentage (80%-100%) of the time difference between the fastest runner's declared time and each other runner's time is subtracted from the runners' actual finish times. For example, suppose runner A's fastest previous time is 18 min for 3 mi (4.8 km), runner B's is 19 min, and runner C's is 20 min. If 80% of the time difference is used, 48 sec (0.8 times the 60 sec difference between A and B) are subtracted from B's finish time, and 96 sec (0.8 times the 120 sec difference) are subtracted from runner C's finish time. Suppose runner A completes the race in 17:50, runner B in 18:30, and runner C in 20:10. The adjusted finish time for runner A is 17:50 (actual time), for runner B is 17:42 (18:30 − 0:48), and for runner C is 18:34 (20:10 − 0:96). Runner B is the winner. Another method of handicapping a race is to stagger the start according to each jogger's previous best time, with the slowest runner starting first and the fastest beginning last. The first runner over the finish line is the winner. Teams can be formed in which each four-member team, for example, has one runner from each of four groups classified by running speed.

Competitive Running

Almost all communities have road races sponsored by track clubs and service organizations as a means of raising funds, many for worthy purposes. Each entrant pays a registration fee, and most of the races have sex and age divisions, with prizes awarded to the top finishers overall and in each division. Usually every finisher receives an award such as a certificate or T-shirt. The race distances range between 1 mi (1.6 km; often called a *fun run)* and 100 mi (161 km), but the most common are the 5K (3.1 mi) and 10K (6.2 mi). Fitness participants should not be pressured to enter road races, but they should be introduced to the possibility of doing one if the interest is there. The fitness professional should consider entering races with interested participants to help them select a starting spot and establish a pace and to provide encouragement.

KEY POINT

Stages 1 through 5 of the jogging program are appropriate intervals to use at the beginning of a jogging program. Once the program is established, variety can be introduced by jogging on a variety of surfaces, jogging over a variety of terrains, or doing paced or timed workouts leading up to a fun run.

This may help them transition from a jogging group to an individualized jogging program.

Those who train for performance will work at the top of the THR range, 5 or more days · wk^{-1} and for more than 30 to 40 min at a time. Such programs are bound to result in more injuries, and the fitness professional should encourage participants pursuing such goals to have an alternative activity (e.g., swimming, cycling) that they can enjoy while recovering from injuries. See chapter 26 for information on dealing with injuries.

Cycling

Riding a bicycle or stationary exercise cycle is another good fitness activity. Some people who have problems walking, jogging, or playing sports may be able to cycle without difficulty. The cycling program follows the guidelines for improving CRF (see chapter 11). Although bicycles and terrain vary widely, checking THR allows cyclists to adjust the speed so that they work at the appropriate intensity. Generally, cyclists cover 3 to 4 times the distance compared with jogging; a person works up to 3 mi (4.8 km) jogging or 9 to 12 mi (14.5-19.3 km) cycling in each workout. The seat should be comfortable, and its height should be adjusted so that the knee is slightly bent at the bottom of the pedaling stroke. For those who want a challenging indoor cycling program, spinning classes are worth investigating. The cycles are designed to accommodate most people because the handlebars and seat height and their fore–aft positions can be adjusted. The beginner should check in with the instructor and get helpful pointers to avoid doing too much during the first session.

KEY POINT

Cycling is an excellent activity, especially for those who cannot walk or jog due to joint-related problems. In general, participants should cycle 3 to 4 times the distance they would jog for an equivalent caloric expenditure and cardiorespiratory workout.

Games

One of the wonderful characteristics of children that is often lost in adulthood is playfulness. A child does not feel the need to justify spending time playing a game just for fun. One of the attributes that seems to be present in coronary-prone behavior is the inability to appreciate play for its own sake. A good fitness program can provide people with activities that increase both fitness and playfulness.

For games to be an effective part of a fitness program, certain elements must be present:

Cycling Program

Rules

1. Adjust the seat so that it is comfortable.
2. Use either a regular bicycle or a stationary exercise cycle.
3. If you are starting at stage 1, simply get used to riding 1 or 2 mi (1.6-3.2 km). Don't be concerned about time or reaching the lower end of your THR zone.

Stage	Distance in mi (km)	THR (%HRmax)	Time (min)	Frequency (per wk)
1	1-2 (1.6-3.2)	—	—	3
2	1-2 (1.6-3.2)	60	8-12	3
3	3-5 (4.8-8.0)	60	15-25	3
4	6-8 (9.7-12.9)	70	25-35	3
5	6-9 (9.7-14.5)	70	25-35	4
6	10-15 (16.1-24.1)	70	40-60	4
7	10-15 (16.1-24.1)	80	35-50	4-5

Reprinted, by permission, from B.D. Franks and E.T. Howley, 1998, *Fitness leaders' handbook,* 2nd ed. (Champaign, IL: Human Kinetics), 126.

- Competition. Competition is not to be avoided, but little emphasis should be put on winning. The game should not be used to exclude people from participating.

- Cooperation. Having small groups solve problems together to accomplish fitness tasks can be enjoyable and healthy.

- Enjoyment. Enjoyment requires a balance of cooperation and competition, continued participation by everyone, and the chance for everyone to be a winner.

- Inclusion. A key ingredient for a fitness game is including everyone. This may mean modifying the rules.

- Skill. Some fitness games require minimum levels of certain skills that can be taught as part of the fitness program.

- Vigor. The main workout should include games in which all participants are continuously active in the THR range.

Special Considerations

Participants at any fitness level can do the warm-up and cool-down activities of most games. The more vigorous games, however, usually involve high-intensity bursts, stopping, starting, and quickly changing directions. They are not recommended for the early stages of a fitness program. Some additional stretching and easy movements in different directions should be included as part of the warm-up for games. Obviously, the space, number of people, and equipment must be considered in selecting activities. The fitness professional must emphasize safety and should change the rules immediately when the game is not working. A variety of games should be offered so that people with various skill levels can participate. When large groups are involved in activities, the activities should change frequently to maintain interest. In addition to warm-up and cool-down activities, higher and lower intensities should be alternated to prevent undue fatigue. People should be encouraged to go at their own pace, and THR should be checked regularly to ensure that people are within their ranges.

Fitness Games

In general, the level of control in fitness games and activities varies from that associated with circle and line activities to activities with few rules, such as keep-away. Games can involve diverse muscle groups and use the body weight as resistance (see Fitness Games and Activities). Simultaneously, games develop greater balance and coordination, which are not necessarily outcomes of walking, jogging, or exercising with fixed equipment. *The Sport Ball Exercise Handbook* (5), an update of *On the Ball* (4), was written specifically to encourage games in a fitness setting; it should be in every exercise leader's library. *The New Games Book* (12), a classic on the subject, and *Inclusive Games: Movement Fun for Everyone* (9) provide a playful and inclusive approach to games for various numbers of people. In games, as with all activities, the fitness professional needs to include people with disabilities by adapting the activities (13).

KEY POINT

Effective games for fitness are enjoyable, inclusive, vigorous, cooperative, competitive, and skill related.

Aquatic Activities

Aquatic activities can be a major part of an exercise program or can be the needed relief from other exercises, especially during injury. The intensity of the activity can suit the needs of the least and the most fit, from the patient who's just survived an MI to the endurance athlete. HR can be checked at regular intervals to see whether THR has been reached, and a caloric expenditure goal can be achieved, given the high energy requirement of aquatic activities. People with orthopedic problems who cannot run, dance, or play games can exercise in water. The water supports the person's body weight, minimizing problems associated with weight-bearing joints.

Target Heart Rate

One consistent finding is that the maximal HR response to a swimming test is about 18 beats · min^{-1} lower than that found in a maximal treadmill test (linked to the mammalian diving reflex). This suggests that for swimming, THR should be shifted downward (2 beats less for a 10 sec count) to achieve the goal of 60% to 80% $\dot{V}O_2$max associated with an endurance training effect (10).

Progression

Swimming activities can be graded not only by varying the speed of the swim but also by varying the activity. A patient who has just survived an MI and has an extremely low functional capacity will benefit from simply walking through the water. People who have had recent bypass surgery benefit from moving the arms as they walk across the pool. Following are examples of activities that can be used in aquatic exercise programs. Refer to *Water Fitness Lessons Plans and Choreography* (1) for detailed information on aquatic exercise.

Side-of-Pool Activities

A variety of activities can be done while holding onto the side of the pool with one or both hands. These activities range from simply moving the legs to the side, front, or back to practicing a variety of kicks that ultimately can be used while swimming. ROM movements in the pool are a good way to warm up before undertaking the more vigorous activities of walking or jogging across the pool.

Walking and Jogging Across the Pool

A person with a low functional capacity can begin an aquatic program by simply walking across the shallow end of the pool. The water resists the movement while supporting the body weight, reducing the downward load on the ankles, knees, and hips. The arms can be involved by simulating a swimming motion, which increases the ROM of the arms and shoulder girdle. The speed and form of the walk can change as the person becomes accustomed to the activity. The person can take long strides with the head just above the water or can sidestep across the pool.

Fitness Games and Activities

- *Skills and games with balls of various sizes.* The size and type of ball can lead to innovative use—for instance, a cage ball can substitute for a basketball. Examples of other balls include tennis balls, volleyballs, playground balls, basketballs, medicine balls, handballs, softballs, mush balls, and foam balls.

- *Activities with apparatuses.* Examples include hula hoops, Frisbees, paddle rackets, skip ropes, skittles, quoits, surgical tubing, culverts, and play buoys.

- *Chasing games.* Examples include tag, chain tag, fox and geese, and dodgeball.

- *Relays with and without apparatuses.* Examples include running, hopping, rolling, crawling, and dribbling with hands and feet.

- *Stunts and contests.* Examples are dual activities such as balancing stunts, forward rolls, backward rolls, strength moves, push-ups, sit-ups, and limited combat games such as rooster fights and partner sparring.

- *Lead-up games for major sport games.* Examples are soccer, tennis, basketball, volleyball, handball, and football, often with rules adjusted to fit the abilities of the participants.

- *Children's games.* Activities include skittle ball, foursquare, and bounce ball.

Adapted, by permission, from M.D. Giese, 1988, Organization of an exercise session. In *Resource manual for guidelines for exercise testing and prescription,* edited by S.N. Blair et al. (Philadelphia, PA: Lea & Febiger), 244-247.

Last, the person can jog across the pool with the water at chest height. Remember to check whether THR has been achieved.

Flotation Devices

People with limited skill can use flotation devices (e.g., a life jacket or kickboard). The extra resistance of the jacket compensates for the extra buoyancy it provides. The participant should periodically determine whether THR has been reached.

Lap Swimming

Participants must be skilled to substitute swimming for running or cycling. An unskilled swimmer operates at a very high energy cost, even when moving slowly, and may become too fatigued to last the whole workout. But being unskilled at swimming doesn't mean that it should be eliminated as an option in personal fitness programs. A person can learn to swim over several months, gradually adjusting to the exercise. After learning to swim, the person can use swimming as the primary activity, even if using elementary strokes. Increasing the number of exercise activities that people can do increases the chance they will remain active when something interferes with a primary activity.

Lap swimming should be approached the same way as lap running: warming up with stretching activities, starting slowly, taking frequent breaks to check the pulse rate, and gradually increasing the distance. Remember, the caloric cost of swimming compared with the cost of running the same distance is about 4:1. If jogging 1 mi (1.6 km) is a reasonable goal in a physical activity program, then swimming 400 m (0.25 mi) is equivalent in terms of energy expenditure. The sidebar, Swimming Program, describes the stages that could be included in an endurance swimming program, beginning with walking across the pool. All steps assume that a warm-up has preceded the activity and that a cool-down follows.

The stages in the swimming program are not discrete steps that must be followed in a particular order. Two stages can be combined or games can be introduced to make the walk-and-jog and width swims more enjoyable. The goal is to gradually increase the intensity and duration of the aquatic activities.

KEY POINT

Aquatic activities include upright activities (e.g., walking and jogging across the pool, using flotation devices) as well as swimming. Exercises also can be performed while holding onto the side of the pool, such as moving the legs from front to back or practicing a paddle kick.

Swimming Program

Rules

1. Start at a level that is comfortable for you.
2. Don't progress to the next stage if you are not comfortable with the current one.
3. Monitor and record your HR.

   o Stage 1   In chest-deep water, walk across the width of the pool four times and see if you are close to THR. Gradually lengthen the walk until you can do two 10 min walks at THR.

   o Stage 2   In chest-deep water, walk across and jog back. Repeat twice and see if you are close to THR. Gradually lengthen the jogging until you can complete four 5 min jogs at THR.

   o Stage 3   In chest-deep water, walk across and swim back (any stroke). Use a kickboard or flotation device if needed. Repeat this cycle twice and see if you are at THR. Keep up this pattern for 20 to 30 min of activity.

   o Stage 4   In chest-deep water, jog across and swim back (any stroke); repeat and check THR. Gradually shorten the jog and lengthen the swim until four widths can be completed within the THR zone. Accomplish 20 to 30 min of activity per session.

   o Stage 5   Slowly swim 25 yd (22.9 m); rest 20 sec. Slowly swim another 25 yd (22.9 m) and check THR. On the basis of the HR response, change the speed of the swim or the length of the rest to stay within the THR zone. Gradually increase the number of lengths you can swim (e.g., three, then four) before checking THR.

   o Stage 6   Increase the duration of continuous swimming until you can accomplish 20 to 30 min without a rest.

Reprinted, by permission, from B.D. Franks and E.T. Howley, 1998, *Fitness leaders' handbook*, 2nd ed. (Champaign, IL: Human Kinetics), 129.

Group Exercise Classes

Working out with others can be an enjoyable experience, and group exercise classes offer lots of variety to meet individual needs. A person can join a group at a fitness club or exercise at home with videotapes or DVDs.

Advantages

Group exercise classes are enjoyable for many participants, young and old, male and female. Since the mid-1970s, these classes have evolved from aerobic dance classes to a variety of specialized classes that can address everyone's tastes and fitness levels. The inclusion of water, steps, tubing, resistance balls, martial arts, cycling, dance, mind–body activities, and kickboxing provides numerous opportunities for cross-training and learning new techniques. Fortunately, certification and continuing education programs have developed in conjunction with these trends (see later in this chapter).

Getting Motivated

Working out with others is a great way to motivate people to continue exercising. In many cases music is an essential element of the class, and the tempos and rhythms of the songs keep the workout exciting and challenging for participants. The class setting, with familiar instructors and participants, promotes camaraderie and regular participation.

Achieving Target Heart Rate

Group exercise programs can develop all of the fitness components. The recommended frequency, intensity, and total work (see chapter 11) can be achieved when exercising in a group setting and can increase $\dot{V}O_2$max (15). THR can be monitored easily throughout the class, but beginners need to be cautioned about doing too much, too soon. Making a gradual transition into the class is as appropriate as what was stipulated for those making a transition from walking to jogging.

Low Skill Requirement

Many group exercise classes can be adapted to any skill level because no competition is involved; however, there are exceptions and the fitness professional needs to be able to help clients select classes that are consistent with their abilities and goals. Obviously the fitness professional should have some experience with each of these group exercise classes so that client recommendations are based on personal experience rather than simple observation. Most group exercise classes provide participants with an appropriate workout routine within a safe environment (assuming instructors are certified, are experienced, and emphasize safe exercises and good form). Warm-ups are structured to provide low-impact movements and dynamic stretching before the main body of the workout. Gradual progression within each session, as well as from one workout to the next, enhances enjoyment.

Fitness professionals should be familiar with the group exercise programs offered in their community, because some (e.g., Jazzercise, Zumba, Spinning) may require knowledge of dance movements and special equipment (e.g., cycling shorts, proper shoes, supportive undergarments). Fitness professionals should also be aware of the programs that are appropriate for people of various ages, skill levels, and interests.

Adverse Events

Injury is always a potential risk in any fitness program, and group exercise classes are no different. One review found that about 44% of students and 76% of instructors reported injuries resulting from aerobic dance, with the injury rate being 1 injury per 100 hr of activity for students and 0.22 to 1.16 injuries per 100 hr for instructors. The severity of the injuries, however, was such that only once in 1,092 to 4,275 hr of participation did a participant require medical attention (7). For those who want to participate in group exercise classes, a reasonable suggestion is that they do so only after they can walk 2 mi · day^{-1} (3.2 km · day^{-1}) at a moderate intensity without discomfort. They should move from low-intensity, low-impact sessions to more strenuous sessions using THR as a guide. Further, introductory classes to step or other specialized forms of aerobics should be taken to develop the skills needed for participation in the regular classes.

It is not uncommon for people to experience muscle soreness, as well as a variety of acute soft-tissue injuries, because of regular participation in aerobic activities. In addition, evidence shows that chronic conditions may develop because of improper form or simply from doing many repetitions of a specific exercise. These chronic conditions can include the following:

- Chronic shoulder soreness from too many overhead presses
- Elbow or wrist pain from using handheld weights in aerobics classes
- Achilles tendinitis and plantar fasciitis from high-impact forces and improper step techniques
- Low-back problems from exercising with weak abdominal muscles (anterior pelvic tilt) and from improperly stretching
- Knee problems from using a step that is too high

See chapter 26 for advice on how to prevent and deal with acute and chronic problems associated with exercise participation. Here are some suggestions to minimize the risk of injury when participating in group exercise classes.

Participants should do the following:

- Warm up before class with low-impact activity and dynamic stretching; this is especially important for those who are new to group exercise.

- Avoid hyperextension of the neck.

- Avoid forward flexion of the spine unless supported by a bent knee balanced directly over the heel.

- Practice correct standing posture (i.e., pelvis in neutral position, buttocks tight, head and chin up, shoulders back).

- Avoid deep knee bends, and do not squat to where the thighs are below parallel and the knees are over the toes rather than placed properly over the middle of the foot.

- Wear shoes with good cushioning and support that are appropriate for the class.

- Work all muscle groups evenly to achieve a balanced workout.

- Avoid stopping in the middle of a routine, because this can cause venous pooling in the lower legs. If a decrease in intensity is needed, the participant should keep moving with a walk, march, or basic moves.

- Check HR or RPE regularly.

Types of Group Exercise Classes

As mentioned in the introduction of this section, there are a wide variety of group exercise classes, and fitness professionals should have some experience with each before making recommendations to their clients. This exposure to the classes will provide firsthand contact between the fitness professional and the various instructors. The fitness professional will get to know who the best instructors are, which is important information when helping a client make the transition to a group exercise class. The following is a brief list of the categories of group exercise classes (with examples) available in many commercial fitness centers:

- Cardio: boot camp, step, kickboxing, circuit
- Cycling: beginning and advanced spin classes
- Mind–body: Pilates, yoga, tai chi
- Dance: belly dancing, Zumba, Jazzercise, hip-hop
- Water: workout, aerobics
- Muscular strength and endurance: classes focusing on the abs, power, sculpting, and so on

Group Exercise Organizations

Given the wide variety of group exercise classes, it should be no surprise that there are certifications available to support exercise leaders and help maintain quality in the delivery of instruction. Certifications are important credentials for denoting professional stature and for liability concerns (see chapter 27). However, fitness professionals need to be aware of the difference between having a certification and being competent to teach. The latter is achieved by becoming a good student of the class (achieving a high-level skill in the format) and working alongside excellent instructors to learn how to lead others effectively and safely. Here are some examples of the many organizations that certify instructors in group exercise. They also provide educational and professional support materials, and some offer certifications in more than one form of group exercise.

- Aerobics and Fitness Association of America (AFAA) (www.afaa.com)
- American Council on Exercise (ACE) (www.acefitness.org)
- Jazzercise (www.jazzercise.com)
- Spinning (www.spinning.com)
- Zumba Fitness (www.Zumba.com)
- Yoga Alliance (www.yogaalliance.org)

KEY POINT

People should be able to walk 2 mi · day^{-1} (3.2 km · day^{-1}) at a moderate intensity and without discomfort before participating in group exercise classes. There are a wide variety of group exercise classes, and fitness professionals are encouraged to become familiar with each type in order to help clients make the right choice and make a smooth transition into that exercise form. Group exercise leaders should be both certified and competent to teach the class.

Exercise Equipment

Virtually all fitness clubs have a wide variety of exercise equipment such as treadmills, cycle ergometers, elliptical machines, rowers, climbing ergometers, stepping devices, and so on. Equipment can help a participant stay with an exercise program as well as provide feedback about the number of calories used. Participants with orthopedic limitations can choose weight-supported activities (e.g., cycle ergometers). People training for specific performance goals can do so in air-conditioned comfort, although air conditioning may be a problem for participants who plan to engage in races scheduled for hot days. The issue of acclimatization to a hot environment must be addressed for reasons of performance and safety (see chapters 11 and 26).

If a participant plans to buy exercise equipment for home use, the fitness professional can help with the decision by encouraging experimentation with as many types of equipment and brands as possible. Equipment may appear expensive in the short term, but it may be a wise investment in the long run by reducing health care costs. Visit the ACSM website for information on how to select and use a wide variety of exercise equipment (www.acsm.org/Content/NavigationMenu/News/Othermedia/Brochures/Health_and_Fitness_.htm).

Generally, fitness clubs provide a variety of resistance training equipment that can be used as part of an overall workout or as a separate resistance training workout. Chapter 13 offers recommendations for gains in muscular strength and endurance.

KEY POINT

Exercise equipment can add variety to a program and increase the number of muscle groups engaged in a workout. In addition, some devices (e.g., cycles) can provide relief for those who experience joint-related pain or discomfort.

Circuit Training

Circuit training can be an effective exercise program. The point is to maximize the variety of exercise, distribute the work over a larger muscle mass than can be engaged with a single form of exercise, and include exercises for all aspects of a fitness session. Circuits can include the following:

- Moving from one piece of exercise equipment to another with a brief rest accompanying each move. A person might exercise for 5 to 10 min (or 50-100 kcal) on a cycle ergometer, then on a treadmill, then on a rower, then on a bench step, and so on.

- A typical workout for muscular strength and endurance, in which one set is done on a specific machine before moving to the next and the rotation is repeated 2 to 3 times (see chapter 13).

- A circuit set up around the perimeter of a large room with signs describing specific exercises that the participant should do during one trip around the circuit. The circuit could include warm-up activities, flexibility activities, strengthening exercises using body weight as a resistance, and aerobic activities. Beginning, intermediate, and advanced goals specifying the number of repetitions (or duration) can be posted at each station. Include a station to check the THR after the aerobic exercise stations.

Good examples of walk, jog, and run circuits have been in place for the past 30 years. Many communities have set up jogging trails that have signposts along the way indicating specific exercises to do at each stop. They can be found in many cities, and they provide a break in the regular routine of jogging or running while adding flexibility and strengthening exercises.

KEY POINT

Circuit training offers variety and can include exercises in all aspects of fitness (e.g., cardiorespiratory, muscle strength and endurance, flexibility). The preceding list suggests a few circuit training possibilities.

STUDY QUESTIONS

1. What ACSM certification would be appropriate for someone doing exercise testing and prescription of apparently healthy individuals? How about people in a cardiac rehabilitation program?

2. What does *progression* mean when applied to helping a sedentary person become active or helping an active person move from a moderate-intensity program to a vigorous-intensity program?

3. Should all people be encouraged to move from moderate-intensity activity done 5 days · wk^{-1} to a vigorous-intensity program done 3 days · wk^{-1}? Why or why not?

4. Recommend appropriate clothing for someone exercising in the cold.

5. If you are working with someone who is sedentary, should you focus first on increasing the intensity of the walking program or on the duration? Why?

6. Describe how you would use the walk, jog, walk intervals when working with someone who wants to transition from a walking to a jogging program.

7. Who might benefit from a cycling program compared with a walking program?

8. What would you recommend to a sedentary person who wants to do a fitness games program?

9. What kinds of aquatic activities can a client do besides swimming to achieve fitness benefits?

10. If a sedentary client would like to join a group exercise class, what would you recommend that the client accomplish (from a physical activity standpoint) prior to joining that class?

11. Give a brief description of a circuit training program that is designed to achieve both strength and CRF goals.

CASE STUDIES

You can check your answers by referring to appendix A.

1. You are making a presentation to a group of adults who have their own neighborhood walking program. What topics should you address to emphasize safety and comfort?

2. A 50-yr-old woman who has completed your 10 wk moderate-intensity walking class is considering joining a Zumba class at the encouragement of her friends. However, she is a bit ambivalent about it because she likes her current walking program and feels that she can continue to work that into her schedule. How do you advise her?

3. Your 30-yr-old client has been following a moderate-intensity walking program, 5 days · wk^{-1} for 30 min · day^{-1}, for the past 2 mo and would like to shift to a vigorous-intensity exercise program. Her goals are to expend more calories in the same 30 min time period, increase her CRF to a higher level, and be able to participate in a 5K fun run scheduled 3 mo from now. Describe the steps you would take to help her make this transition and realize her goals.

4. A 40-yr-old man has been a regular member of a running club but has developed chronic pain in his knee that his doctor says is arthritis. He wants to stay active doing vigorous-intensity exercise and has come to you for help. What do you advise?

REFERENCES

1. Alexander, C. 2011. *Water fitness lesson plans and choreography.* Champaign, IL: Human Kinetics.

2. Bravata, D.M., C. Smith-Spangler, V. Sundaram, A.L. Gienger, N. Lin, R. Lewis, C.D. Stave, I. Olkin, and J.R. Sirard. 2007. Using pedometers to increase physical activity and improve health - a systematic review. *JAMA.* 298:2296-2304.

3. Fenton, M. and D.R. Bassett, Jr. 2006. *Pedometer walking.* Guilford, CT: Lyons Press.

4. Franklin, B.A., N.B. Oldridge, K.G. Stoedefalke, and W.E. Loechel. 1990. *On the ball.* Carmel, IN: Benchmark Press.

5. Franklin, B.A., N.B. Oldridge, K.G. Stoedefalke, and W.E. Loechel. 2001. *The sport ball exercise handbook.* Monterey, CA: Exercise Science.

6. Franks, B.D., and E.T. Howley. 1998. *Fitness leaders' handbook.* 2nd ed. Champaign, IL: Human Kinetics.

7. Garrick, J.G., and R.K. Requa. 1988. Aerobic dance—A review. *Sports Medicine* 6:169-179.

8. Giese, M.D. 1988. Organization of an exercise session. In *Resource manual guidelines for exercise testing and prescription,* ed. S.N. Blair, P. Painter, R. Pate, L.K. Smith, and C.B. Taylor, 244-247. Philadelphia: Lea & Febiger.

9. Kasser, S.L. 1995. *Inclusive games: Movement fun for everyone.* Champaign, IL: Human Kinetics.

10. Londeree, B.R., and M.I. Moeschberger. 1982. Effect of age and other factors on maximal heart rate. *Research Quarterly for Exercise and Sport* 53:297-304.

11. McSwegin, P.J., and C.L. Pemberton. 1993. Exercise leadership: Key skills and characteristics. In *ACSM's resource manual for guidelines for exercise testing and prescription.* 2nd ed. Ed. J.L. Durstine, A.C. King, P.L. Painter, J.L. Roitman, L.D. Zwiren, and W.L. Kenney, 319-326. Philadelphia: Lea & Febiger.

12. New Games Foundation. 1976. *The new games book.* Garden City, NY: Dolphin Books.

13. Seaman, J. 1999. Physical activity and fitness for persons with disabilities. *PCPFS Research Digest* 3(5).

14. U.S. Department of Health and Human Services (HHS). 2008. *2008 Physcial Activity Guidelines for Americans.* www.health.gov/paguidelines/guidelines/default.aspx.

15. Williford, H.N., M. Scharff-Olson, and D.L. Blessing. 1989. The physiological effects of aerobic dance—A review. *Sports Medicine* 8:335-345.

Behavior Change

Janet Buckworth

The reader will be able to do the following:

1. Describe the transtheoretical model and stages involved in healthy behavior change.

2. Discuss the role of motivation in exercise adoption and adherence and identify behavioral strategies for enhancing motivation.

3. List and describe six strategies that fitness professionals can use to monitor and support behavior change.

4. Describe ways to apply relapse prevention to exercise behavior.

5. Identify effective communication skills useful in motivating and fostering healthy behavior change.

Translating the desire to change a health-related behavior into action is a challenge for most people. They may wish to be more active or to eat a healthier diet but may not have the knowledge, skills, or motivation to make the necessary behavior modifications and stick to them. To help people adopt and maintain a healthier lifestyle, the fitness professional should understand basic principles of behavior change and develop the skills to put those principles into practice.

This chapter begins with a brief description of theoretical models for explaining and predicting human behavior, in particular the transtheoretical model of behavior change (also known as the *stages of change model*). Methods and strategies are presented in the context of behavior change as a process, with suggestions for use based on stages of motivational readiness. For an excellent review of the transtheoretical model applied to exercise, refer to Prochaska and Marcus (20). Factors for fitness professionals to consider as they help participants move through each stage of the model are discussed along with specific strategies for encouraging adoption of and adherence to exercise and other healthy behaviors. Additional strategies and suggestions for interventions can be found in the chapters by Chambliss and King (3) and Whiteley et al. (28) in the ACSM resource manual and in *Motivating People to Be Physically Active* by Marcus and Forsyth (15). The last section in this chapter examines communication skills that fitness professionals should possess in order to motivate participants and foster healthy behavior change.

Transtheoretical Model of Behavior Change

Several theories guide strategies for changing exercise behavior, such as behavior modification, social cognitive theory, self-determination theory, and the transtheoretical model of behavior change (1). Behavior modification theory is based on the assumption that behavior is learned and can be changed by modifying the antecedents (stimuli, cues) and consequences (rewards, punishments). A cue could be a flyer listing the benefits of walking during lunch, and a reward could be a certificate presented to the aerobics participant with the best attendance. Social cognitive theory offers the view that behavior is influenced by the dynamic relationships among the person's characteristics, the environment, and the behavior itself. Someone training for a marathon would be more motivated than a novice fitness walker to exercise outside in the rain, but even the most dedicated marathoner would not run in a lightning storm. Finally, self-determination theory is a theory of motivation that explains human behavior in respect to meeting basic needs (competency, autonomy, and relatedness). People may start exercising to lose weight but later train for a road race because they enjoy a sense of accomplishment from running. Although effective strategies for behavior change have been developed with these and other theories, most theories of behavior treat change as an all-or-none event. In other words, participants go from being sedentary to being regularly active in response to an intervention.

The transtheoretical model presents change as a dynamic process whereby attitudes, decisions, and actions evolve through stages over time. In the late 1970s and early 1980s, Prochaska and DiClemente (19) developed the transtheoretical model of behavior change by observing smokers trying to quit without professional intervention. They discovered that self-changers used specific strategies that varied over time as they tried to decrease or eliminate their high-risk behavior, and they noticed that the self-changers progressed through distinct stages. Although the model was developed to explain how people stop high-risk behaviors, it has been applied with some success to promoting exercise (28). The rest of this chapter highlights the transtheoretical, or stages of change, model and ways this model can be used to help people think about, decide to begin, and continue an active lifestyle.

Concepts

The **transtheoretical model** is a model of intentional behavior modification. Behavior change is a dynamic process that occurs through a series of interrelated stages that are mostly stable but open to change (21). This model emphasizes the individual's motivation, readiness to change, and personal history regarding the target behavior. For example, people who exercised successfully in the past would have more confidence in their ability to exercise again than would people who have been sedentary most of their lives. The problem with most interventions is that they are for people who are prepared to take action (20). According to the transtheoretical model, traditional strategies for participant recruitment will not affect people who are not ready to change. Different strategies must be used to persuade people to consider change and then motivate them to take action. Other approaches will be more effective in supporting adherence to the new behavior.

Components

The transtheoretical model has two key components: stages of change and attitudes, beliefs, and skills for change (21). By evaluating the participant in respect to these factors, the fitness professional can design individually tailored and stage-specific interventions.

Stages of Change

1. *Precontemplation:* In this stage, the individual is not seriously thinking about changing an unhealthy behavior in the next 6 mo or is denying the need to change.

2. *Contemplation:* The individual is seriously thinking about changing an unhealthy behavior within the next 6 mo.

3. *Preparation:* This is a transitional stage in which the individual intends to take action within the next month. Some plans have been made, and the individual tries to determine what to do next.

4. *Action:* This stage is the 6 mo following the overt modification of an unhealthy behavior. Motivation and investment in behavior change are sufficient in this stage, but it is the busiest and least stable stage and has the highest risk of relapse.

5. *Maintenance:* Maintenance begins after the individual has successfully adhered to the healthy behavior for 6 mo. The longer someone stays in maintenance, the lower the risk of relapse.

Attitudes, Beliefs, and Behavioral Skills Hypothesized to Influence Behavior Change

The "how" of behavior change in the transtheoretical model includes attitudes, beliefs, and behavioral skills that are expected to change as someone progresses through the stages. These change elements are self-efficacy, decisional balance, and processes of change.

• *Self-efficacy* is confidence in one's ability to engage in a positive behavior or abstain from an undesired behavior. Expectation of success is important in making the decision to change and in maintaining the new behavior. Types of self-efficacy include confidence to accomplish the elements of a task, which is important when beginning a new behavior, and confidence to overcome personal

and environmental barriers (coping, barrier self-efficacy), which is important for adhering to the behavior.

• *Decisional balance* refers to evaluating and monitoring potential gains (pros, benefits) and losses (cons) arising from any decision. Perceived gains increase and perceived losses decrease in respect to the target behavior as the person moves through the stages of change.

• *Processes of change* are strategies used to change behavior. Experiential or cognitive processes are strategies that involve thoughts, attitudes, and awareness. Behavioral processes involve taking specific actions directed toward yourself or the environment. For example, seeking out information about the best exercise for losing weight is a cognitive process, and creating reminders to register for a water aerobics class is a behavioral process.

Applying the Transtheoretical Model to Exercise

The transtheoretical model is applied to exercise by matching or targeting the appropriate intervention strategy according to the person's physical activity history and readiness for change (21) (see table 23.1). For example, the goal in working with people in the precontemplation stage is to get them to begin thinking about changing their level of physical activity. Discussing information from a fitness test or health risk appraisal followed by education about personal benefits of physical activity is an appropriate strategy for participants in the precontemplation stage. The goal with people in the contemplation stage is to motivate them and help them prepare to take action. They would benefit from learning about the pros of exercise coupled with accurate, easy-to-understand information about how they can start an exercise program or begin to

TABLE 23.1 Intervention Strategies for the Stages of Change

Stage of change	Intervention strategy
Maintenance	Encourage new activities with others, reinforce self-regulatory skills, review and revise goals, introduce cross-training, conduct periodic fitness testing
Action	Identify social support for maintaining exercise, set up stimulus control, teach self-reinforcement, implement self-efficacy enhancement strategies, set goals, teach self-monitoring, employ relapse prevention
Preparation	Conduct psychosocial and fitness assessments, evaluate supports/benefits and barriers/costs, design personalized exercise prescription, set goals, develop behavioral contracts, teach time management skills
Contemplation	Market benefits of exercise, foster self- and environmental reevaluation, provide clear and specific guidelines for starting an exercise program, be a positive role model, identify social support for exercise
Precontemplation	Implement an exercise promotion media campaign, educate about personal benefits of exercise, foster values clarification, conduct health risk appraisals and fitness testing

be more active. Someone in the preparation stage is doing some exercise but realizes that it is not enough and needs help to set up a personalized exercise program. There is awareness of the benefits of exercise, but there are still barriers that must be resolved. Whereas participants in the contemplation stage may not be ready to set goals, those in the preparation stage are ready to set goals and get a personalized exercise prescription.

Participants in the action stage are participating in regular activity, but exercise is not a habit. They are at a high risk of relapsing into a more familiar, inactive lifestyle. Relapse prevention, which is discussed later, can help keep them on track to the maintenance stage. Movement from the action stage to the maintenance stage follows a decrease in the risk of relapse and an increase in self-efficacy. Helpful strategies include periodic reevaluations of goals and updates of plans for coping with life events such as travel, inclement weather, or medical events that can disrupt regular exercise.

KEY POINT

The transtheoretical model addresses the dynamic nature of behavior change. Practitioners apply this model by selecting interventions based on characteristics of the participant, environment, and stage of change. Interventions should match the stage the individual is in and address self-efficacy and perceptions of benefits and costs of exercise (see table 23.1).

Promoting Exercise: Targeting Participants in Early Stages of Change

A variety of strategies and programs can be used to motivate sedentary and low-active individuals to consider becoming more active and adopt regular exercise. These approaches are based on understanding the knowledge, attitudes, beliefs, and behavioral skills that foster adoption of a regular exercise program in the early stages of change. Specific factors related to promoting the adoption of regular exercise are presented next, followed by a review of strategies to market exercise and increase motivation.

Encouraging Exercise: Advancing Precontemplators and Contemplators

People in precontemplation are sedentary and have no plans to start exercising. They may be in this stage because they lack information about the long-term personal conse-

quences of physical inactivity. They also may be demoralized from previous unsuccessful attempts to stick with an exercise program and may have low self-efficacy for exercise. People in the precontemplation stage may feel defensive about their lifestyle because of social pressures to be physically active. They have no personally compelling reasons to change, and the costs of exercising seem to outweigh the benefits. Given these attitudes and beliefs, your clients' perceptions about the benefits of exercise should be strengthened and the costs reduced. Activities to help people develop a personal value for exercise and information about the role of exercise in a healthy lifestyle are useful in moving people to the next stage (15).

Sedentary individuals move to the contemplation stage because of information that is convincing, personal, and timely (16). Contemplators are planning to become more physically active, but they are still ambivalent about changing. For them, the costs of starting to exercise outweigh the perceived benefits. Experiences and information that support the contemplator's desire and motivation to exercise and counter perceived costs and barriers can initiate the move to preparation. Exposure to physically active role models, enhancement of perceived benefits, and strengthening of psychosocial variables such as self-efficacy for exercise are other factors that influence exercise adoption. The cognitive processes of change, such as increasing knowledge about the health benefits of regular exercise and being aware of how one's inactivity affects others, are critical in these early stages of change.

Influencing Exercise Adoption: Successful Planning for the Preparation Stage

People in the preparation stage are doing some exercise, but not enough to meet health and fitness guidelines. The fitness professional's goal is to help them move to the action stage and regular exercise. A thorough assessment of personal, social, and environmental factors that support their current level of activity can be particularly useful. A comprehensive assessment can establish physical fitness, motivation, goals, supports, barriers, and other factors to consider when developing a specific plan for change and implementing strategies. Behavioral strategies come into play more as someone begins to move from the preparation stage. Goal setting, behavioral contracts, and time management training are practical strategies to use with participants in the preparation stage, and information from an assessment will help tailor an intervention to the person's needs and situation.

Personal Influences

Individual characteristics that influence the initiation of exercise include demographics, activity history, past experiences, perception of health status, perception of access to facilities, time, enjoyment of exercise, aptitudes, beliefs, self-motivation, and self-efficacy (26). Higher education, higher income, gender (male), and younger age are positively associated with level of physical activity (26). Exercise history is an important factor in current level of physical activity. Past participation is linked with physical activity in supervised exercise programs and in treatment programs for patients with CHD and obesity (6). Past exercise experience also can influence expectations about exercise and self-efficacy, and high exercise self-efficacy is associated with increased exercise participation.

Motivation is another variable influencing exercise adoption. Motivation depends on expectations for future benefits or outcomes from exercise, such as good health, improved appearance, social outlets, stress management, enjoyment, and opportunities for competition (17). It also varies in degree of self-determination (e.g., autonomy, personal choice)—intrinsic motivation is the most self-determined, whereas extrinsic motivation is motivation based on satisfying others or on the consequences of the behavior. The self-determination theory describes motivation on a continuum from extrinsic to intrinsic and links motivation to seeking to meet basic human needs of competency, autonomy, and relatedness.

Self-motivation for exercise is the ability to continue an exercise program without the benefit of external reinforcement. Participants high in self-motivation are probably good at goal setting, monitoring exercise progress, and self-reinforcement (24) and are high in intrinsic motivation. People with little self-motivation may need more external reinforcement and encouragement (e.g., group activities and social support) to adopt and adhere to exercise, but even people with high intrinsic motivation can benefit from social support.

Perceived behavioral control is significantly correlated with the intention to exercise (9). If participants believe they have more control over the exercise and have choices about when and how to exercise, they are more likely to begin a program. It follows that participants who set their own goals will have a greater chance of success than if goals are assigned to them (14), and they will be more likely to meet the need for autonomy.

Social Influences

Social support involves comfort, assistance, and information provided by individuals or groups. Practical help, such as providing problem-solving tips or a ride to the fitness facility, can result in tangible benefits to the participant, but emotional support also plays a key role. For example, emotional support (encouragement and expressions of care, concern, and sympathy) could be helpful when a participant is emotionally stressed. Other types of emotional support include esteem support (reassurance of worth, expressions

of liking or confidence in the other person), network support (expressions of connection and belonging), and even informational support (information and advice). Exercising with a group can also meet the need for relatedness described by self-determination theory.

Social support for exercise from family, friends, and physicians is usually associated with physical activity (26). Spouses appear to provide a consistent, positive influence on exercise participation; in one study, individuals who joined a fitness center with their spouse had better adherence and lower dropout rates than married individuals who joined without a spouse (27). Group factors may be particularly important for older adults and people who are motivated to exercise primarily for social reinforcement.

RESEARCH INSIGHT

Social support plays a big role in exercise adherence, and most research has assumed that other people have a positive influence on behavior. Gabriele, Walker, Gill, Harber, and Fisher (8) asked 244 young adults about social influence (encouragement *and* constraint), exercise motivation, and exercise behavior. Encouraging social interaction was related to exercise behavior through influencing motivation, but social constraint, which involves expectations or norms that create a sense of obligation or intrusion, was not. Supporting clients to achieve their own exercise goals is more effective than instilling feelings of guilt for not exercising. It seems that we cannot assume that all social influence is helpful for the adoption and maintenance of exercise.

Environmental Influences

Research has shown that social support, environmental prompts, and convenience are factors in exercise adoption (2). Environments that have cues for exercise, easily accessible facilities, and few real or perceived barriers make sustaining an exercise program easier. Posters, e-mails, self-sticking notes, visibly located exercise equipment, and bike and walking paths are examples of environmental cues.

The convenience of exercise is influenced by the sequence, or chain, of behaviors that must be completed for the person to complete each exercise session. The longer and more complicated the behavior chain, the more barriers there are to exercise. For example, there is a greater potential for a break in the link if a person must leave work, drive home, gather up exercise clothes, drive to a facility, park, sign in, and change clothes to walk on a treadmill than if the person walks around the neighborhood first thing in the morning. For many people, exercising in the morning may be easier to stick with than exercising during the day, when numerous demands compete for time.

The primary reason most people give for not exercising is lack of time (2). Time can be a true determinant, a perceived determinant, an indication of poor time management, or a rationalization for the lack of motivation to be active. Flexibility in an exercise program (e.g., classes offered at many times of day and evening, a lunch-hour walking group) can help with actual time problems. Accumulating several shorter bouts of exercise throughout the day may be another effective strategy. The fitness professional can help identify how time is a barrier and then choose appropriate interventions, such as modification of an exercise schedule or referral to a time management class.

Researchers and practitioners recognize that the physical environment powerfully influences the level of physical activity in communities. For example, accessible, attractive, and safe places to walk, bike, or run can make physical activity more appealing and convenient. Certainly, workout facilities that are clean, are well ventilated, and have a good selection of equipment and adequate parking will be more enticing to novice exercisers compared with poorly maintained or managed fitness centers.

RESEARCH INSIGHT

Loops and lollipops is not a snack treat but rather a description of road patterns in neighborhoods characterized by urban sprawl. There is a growing concern that car-friendly environments indicative of sprawl are not good for public health. Ewing, Schmid, Killingsworth, Zlot, and Raudenbush (7) looked at the relationship among sprawl, level of physical activity, and obesity. Using county and metropolitan sprawl indexes and controlling for variables known to influence exercise and obesity, such as age, education, and fruit and vegetable consumption, Ewing and colleagues found small but significant associations between the county sprawl index and minutes walked, obesity, BMI, and hypertension. Greater sprawl in metropolitan areas was also associated with fewer minutes walked.

Marketing and Motivational Strategies for Early Stages of Change

The goal of fitness professionals may be to help people maintain regular exercise, but they may also be called on to promote regular exercise to people who are inconsistently

active (i.e., preparation stage) or have not yet considered starting a fitness program (i.e., precontemplation stage). For example, the primary goal of a media campaign may be to capture the attention of inactive people and motivate them to contemplate beginning an exercise program or another healthy behavior. This might involve putting informational prompts at the point of decision to act, such as hanging catchy posters next to elevators encouraging people to take the stairs (12) (see figure 23.1). Bulletin boards, pamphlets, flyers, and handouts with upbeat information about the benefits of exercise and practical suggestions for increasing physical activity can also catch the attention of potential exercisers. Handing out passes at local restaurants for an aerobics class is a proactive form of recruitment. Fun runs and walks supporting local or national charities may motivate people who primarily want to help the organization to begin thinking about exercise for its own sake. Wellness fairs, health risk appraisals, and fitness testing in communities and at work sites can also prompt contemplation and enhance motivation to become more active.

To increase participation in the early stages of behavior change, the fitness professional's role is to provide education about benefits of being physically active, to describe how to exercise sensibly, and to offer encouragement to follow through with a personal exercise program. Specific strategies to increase adoption and early adherence are recommended (2, 3, 15, 16):

- Ask participants about their exercise history. They may need proper information to dispel myths (e.g., the myth of no pain, no gain) and to develop positive attitudes about exercise.

- Explore ways exercise can benefit them personally. Find out what they think they will get out of

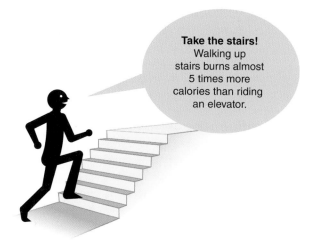

Take the stairs!
Walking up stairs burns almost 5 times more calories than riding an elevator.

FIGURE 23.1 This poster is an example of a point-of-decision prompt to take the stairs.

being physically active and provide information and resources about additional benefits.

- Help participants develop knowledge, attitudes, beliefs, and skills to support the behavior change. In addition to providing information and training in self-management skills, the fitness professional may use cognitive restructuring to identify discouraging thoughts and replace them with positive statements (see Cognitive Restructuring: Reframe Negative Statements Into Positive Statements).

- Bolster the participant's exercise self-efficacy with success-producing learning experiences. There are four sources of information that contribute to self-efficacy beliefs and can be addressed by the fitness professional:

Mastery experiences. These experiences include behavioral rehearsal with proper supervision and positive feedback. The fitness professional can make sure participants have chosen activities that are appropriate for their fitness and skill level so they can experience a sense of accomplishment when they exercise. Practical feedback will also help participants be successful and thus feel more confident. In addition, an increased sense of competency is motivating. We like to do things we are good at!

Verbal persuasion or self-persuasion. Suggesting to people that they can succeed in behaviors they have not been successful in previously and giving specific feedback to help enhance their skills and foster success will promote self-efficacy. The fitness professional can provide verbal encouragement and teach participants positive self-talk.

Modeling. Observing others can serve as a guide to performing a specific behavior. When people see someone successfully doing what they have little confidence to do, they start to expect that they, too, can succeed. The fitness professional can set up situations in which participants see someone like themselves succeed (e.g., post a newspaper story about seniors who now exercise regularly) or watch a peer who has trouble with the task succeed (e.g., point out to a new participant that "Lynette also had difficulty jogging three miles when she first started the program, but after months of hard work, she has now reached her goal!").

Interpretations of physiological and emotional responses. Physiological arousal associated with a behavior can be stressful and contribute to lower self-efficacy for that behavior. The typical increased HR, respiration, and muscle tension that occur during exercise may make novices feel anxious or uncomfortable and less confident. The fitness professional can make sure that participants have information about the normal physiological responses to exercise and know how to interpret their physiological responses accurately.

- Clarify expectations and make sure they are reasonable and realistic. Use guidelines for goal setting to ensure initial successes.

- Identify potential barriers to behavior change and brainstorm with the participant about ways to overcome these barriers. Barriers can be personal (low exercise self-efficacy), physical (past injuries), interpersonal (peer pressure from sedentary friends to engage in sedentary behaviors instead of

Cognitive Restructuring: Reframe Negative Statements Into Positive Statements

Negative Statements

- I'm never going to get in shape.
- I'm fatter than everyone else in the class.
- I've tried to stay with exercise and each time I fail.
- It's just impossible to find time to exercise with my schedule.

Positive Statements

- Change takes time. I didn't get out of shape overnight, and I am making progress bit by bit.
- Everyone has to start somewhere. Other people have worked long and hard to get where they are.
- Every time I begin a new exercise program, I get closer to sticking with it for good.
- I can take a little time for myself to exercise every day because I deserve it. I'm the one in control.

exercising), or environmental (inclement weather or lack of transportation to an exercise facility). For example, one person may want to exercise but does not have access to facilities and another person may think she does not have the willpower to stick with a program. The first person would be helped with a home exercise program, whereas the second would benefit from social support and reconsidering discouraging thoughts.

- Foster motivation to adopt and maintain an exercise program. Set up incentives to exercise. Incentives can be tangible (e.g., T-shirts, certificates, water bottles, recognition on a bulletin board) or intangible (e.g., sense of competence, enjoyment). Tangible incentives are useful early in a program, but intrinsic motivation is associated with better adherence (23). Offer a variety of incentives, but focus on fostering intrinsic motivation, such as a sense of accomplishment or enjoyment. Strategies

KEY POINT

Individual, social, and environmental factors motivate people to move from precontemplation to contemplation of an exercise program and then to actually set up a plan to begin. A variety of strategies can be used, from mass-media campaigns to fitness testing, to motivate people to move from contemplation into the preparation and action stages. Six strategies to facilitate adopting and maintaining exercise are (1) ask participants about exercise history and use what you learn to set up a personalized plan; (2) help participants develop knowledge, attitudes, beliefs, and skills to support behavior change; (3) bolster self-efficacy; (4) involve participants in setting clear and realistic goals; (5) identify and resolve barriers to change; and (6) foster multiple motivators for exercise that have purpose and meaning for participants.

to increase motivation are listed in Motivational Strategies.

Enhancing Adherence: Methods of Behavior Change for Participants in the Action and Maintenance Stages

Various strategies have been discussed to illustrate principles of behavior change and to describe ways to market and motivate exercise. Once a participant has started an exercise program (action stage), the fitness professional plays an important role in monitoring and supporting the establishment and maintenance of regular exercise. For example, the fitness professional and the participant should work together to set goals that are consistent with capabilities, values, resources, and needs. Exercise self-efficacy predicts adoption and maintenance, and it can be increased with mastery experiences. Thus, initial goals should be challenging but certain to be met, which will foster increased exercise self-efficacy. The fitness professional and participant also should evaluate environmental and social supports and barriers and use this information to determine ways that barriers can be managed to promote the new behavior and to enhance coping and barrier self-efficacy.

Assessment

Regardless of the intervention, comprehensive fitness and psychosocial assessments are necessary to select and carry out the appropriate strategies of behavior change for participants in the preparation and early action stages. Reassessment should be conducted periodically to evaluate the effectiveness of the plan.

First, the problem must be identified and defined in behavioral terms. For example, being overweight is not the problem but rather the result of overeating and underexercising. The fitness professional can also help the participant decide what can be realistically changed and what cannot.

Motivational Principles From Self-Determination Theory

Self-determination theory is a theory of human motivation developed by Deci and Ryan in the 1980s that has been applied to promoting exercise (5). According to this theory, humans are naturally inclined toward growth and development and have a set of basic psychological needs that are universal. Motivation to engage in activities results from the fundamental needs for competency, autonomy, and relatedness. Satisfying these three basic psychological needs will foster intrinsic motivation and therefore enhance positive behaviors and mental health as well as the persistence of healthy behavior. Fitness professionals can nurture participants' exercise motivation by setting up exercise tasks to develop a sense of mastery, making sure they have a say in their exercise program, and helping them feel connected to others in the exercise setting.

Motivational Strategies

- Provide positive, practical behavioral feedback.
- Encourage group participation and group support to offer the opportunity for social reinforcement, camaraderie, and commitment.
- Recruit partner and peers to support the behavioral change.
- Make the program enjoyable. Use upbeat, positive music.
- Provide a flexible routine to decrease boredom and increase interest and enjoyment. Consider activities such as games and backpacking as alternatives to traditional exercise modes to provide a variety of exercise options.
- Provide periodic exercise testing to show progress toward goals, increase a sense of competency, and offer an opportunity for positive reinforcement.
- Use strategies for behavioral change, such as personal goal setting, contracts, and self-management, to foster personal control and perceived competency, and emphasize goals that are meaningful to the participant.
- Chart progress on record cards, graphs, or computer programs. Note and record progress daily to give immediate, positive feedback. Encourage self-monitoring.
- Recognize goal achievement in newsletters and bulletin boards. Individual effort increases when that effort is identifiable.
- Set up group or individual competitions.
- Offer lotteries based on individual or group accomplishment of a specific goal. Set a winning criterion (such as the first person to walk a certain distance each week for 5 wk wins) for which the winner is featured in a newsletter or gets money each participant has contributed. An alternative is to set a criterion (e.g., attending 20 of 24 aerobic classes) for participation in a random drawing.
- Organize teams to train for a charity-sponsored fun run or road race.

Next, examine past attempts at behavior change. Find out what worked, what did not, and why. This information will be useful in setting goals and identifying high-risk situations (see the section Relapse Prevention later in this chapter).

Also, find out if initiation of the behavior change is voluntary or recommended by someone else. This will give a sense of the participant's motivation and commitment to change. Participants who are there because a doctor prescribed exercise may need help finding personal reasons for exercising. There are many reasons for beginning an exercise program (e.g., health, weight loss, anxiety reduction), but the initial motivation may not be why someone continues to exercise. Most often, people start exercise to achieve an outcome of exercise or to avoid guilt (extrinsic motivation) rather than for personal enjoyment, expression of creativity, or demonstration of mastery (intrinsic motivation). Extrinsic motivation can be useful to get people started, but research has shown that developing intrinsic motivation for exercise is necessary for long-term maintenance. Ask participants what they expect to get out of exercise and be prepared to pique their interest by presenting additional short- and long-term benefits.

Another useful assessment tool is the decisional balance sheet. The participant lists all short- and long-term consequences, positive and negative, of both changing and not changing the behavior. The participant and the fitness professional then brainstorm ways to avoid or cope with the projected negative consequences of behavior change while also emphasizing and building upon perceived benefits.

Self-Monitoring

Part of the assessment process can be accomplished by self-monitoring, in which the participant records information about the target behavior and also indicates thoughts, feelings, and situations before, during, and after the behavior. The participant can identify the internal and external cues and behavioral consequences that inhibit and prompt exercise. Barriers and supports also become evident with self-monitoring. The fitness professional can help the participant develop strategies to cope with the barriers and use the supports. The chain of behaviors encompassing exercise can also be evaluated and weak links identified. For example, if the participant discovers she always skips her 5:30 a.m. aerobics class when she oversleeps and doesn't have time to pack her workout clothes before she leaves for work, you can suggest that she pack her workout bag the night before. Immediate benefits and reinforcements tailored to individual preferences can also be established at critical links in the chain (e.g., if she packs her workout bag the night before, she can push the snooze button for an extra 10 min of sleep the next morning). Tablets, computer programs, calendars, graphs, and charts can be used for self-monitoring as part of the initial assessment and as a way to record progress. Fitness tracking apps are also available for smartphones and PDAs.

RESEARCH INSIGHT

Achieving the recommendation for 30 min of moderate physical activity each day can be accomplished through the widely advertised walking program of 10,000 steps a day (10). A popular tool for monitoring steps is the pedometer, a device that has been used in several studies to increase the number of steps walked and to help participants become more aware of when and how they can fit physical activity into their day. For example, Croteau (4) used goal setting, pedometers, self-monitoring, and weekly e-mail reminders in a lifestyle intervention to increase walking. After 8 wk, the participants significantly increased daily steps to more than 10,000. Gains were greatest for participants who were obese and for those starting with fewer than 6,000 daily steps.

Goal Setting

The purpose of **goal setting** is to accomplish a specific task in a specific time frame. Goals can be as simple and time limited as making a sandwich for lunch and as complicated and encompassing as earning an advanced degree. Goal setting provides a plan of action that focuses and directs activity and emphasizes a clear link between behavior and outcome.

Effective goal setting has several characteristics:

• Goals should be behavioral, specific, and measurable. Plans are easier to make if the goal is stated in behavioral terms. For example, a goal of walking 4 days $\cdot$ wk^{-1} for 30 to 45 min is easier to implement than a goal to get in shape. Specific, measurable goals make it easier to monitor progress, make adjustments, and know when the goal has been accomplished.

• Goals also must be reasonable and realistic. A goal might be achievable, but personal and situational constraints can make it unrealistic. Losing 2 lb $\cdot$ wk^{-1} (0.9 kg $\cdot$ wk^{-1}) through diet and exercise is reasonable for many people, but it may be almost impossible for the working parent of three who has minimal time for exercise and cooking. Unrealistic goals set the participant up to fail, which

can damage self-efficacy and adherence to the program for behavior change. By using information from the assessment and self-monitoring, the fitness professional can help participants set positive, realistic behavioral goals based on their age, sex, fitness, health, interests, exercise history, skills, and schedule. Both short-term and long-term goals should be included. Short-term goals mobilize effort and direct present actions, but both short- and long-term goals lead to a more effective plan of action (14) (see Characteristics of Effective Goals).

RESEARCH INSIGHT

Goal setting is an essential strategy for exercise behavior change and adherence, and the importance of short-term process goals for fostering intrinsic motivation and adherence was demonstrated by Wilson and Brookfield (29). They conducted a 6 wk intervention based on self-determination theory to examine the impact of goal setting and motivation on adherence. Sixty adult recreational exercisers were randomly assigned to one of three groups: process goal (weekly goals related to behavior, such as maintaining THR or pace), outcome goal (goal to achieve by the end of 6 wk), and no goal (control group). Intrinsic motivation (interest and enjoyment, perceived choice, and pressure and tension [negative indicator]) was measured at the beginning and end of the intervention and 3 mo and 6 mo later. The process-goal group had greater increases in interest and enjoyment and perceived choice and better adherence than the other groups after the intervention and at each follow-up assessment. The outcome-goal group had lower perceived choice and higher pressure and tension than the control group, implying that using only an outcome goal may be detrimental to motivation and success.

Reinforcement

Social **reinforcement** and self-reinforcement are crucial in the action phase, especially because the longer someone has been inactive before starting to exercise, the longer it takes until exercise itself becomes reinforcing. Immediate consequences of exercise can be soreness and fatigue, so external, immediate, positive rewards are necessary for beginners. Monitoring progress is rewarding and can involve charting miles walked after each session or asking for feedback from instructors after a difficult exercise class. Positive reinforcement from others can enhance self-efficacy, especially when feedback comes from people who are important to the participant. Praise is more effective if it is immediate and behaviorally specific (11). "You worked hard in class last week" is not as effective as "You did a great job getting through all the leg lifts today," especially if the participant has been struggling with leg lifts.

Self-reinforcement should involve rewards that are important to the participant. Using special spa soaps and creams only after an aerobic workout and getting tickets to the big game after logging a certain number of miles are rewards that are personalized and self-administered.

Social support can be verbal or tangible, such as transportation to exercise class. It can come from the class instructor, exercise partners, family members, and so on. Significant others must be involved in the exercise plan and educated about the differences between support and nagging. Constructive verbal feedback, praise, encouragement, and positive attention will help a family member stick with exercise, whereas punishing comments, jokes about the person's efforts, and discouraging social comparisons can hinder adherence. Support focuses on what has been accomplished ("You're being consistent in your walking to lose weight. I'm proud of you."), whereas nagging harps on what has not been accomplished ("You should walk faster to lose weight. Why can't you pick up the pace?").

Friends in an exercise program can provide both social support and cues to exercise. They can be positive role models to enhance self-efficacy and part of a buddy system to support the exercise effort. Some participants are more likely to stick with a program if they know someone else is counting on them to be there to work out. Being part of an exercise group can also help participants feel connected to others and support the basic need for relatedness (from self-determination theory).

Behavioral Contracts

Behavioral contracts are written, signed, public agreements to engage in specific goal-directed behaviors, and they have been used effectively to increase exercise adherence (6). Contracts should include clear, realistic objectives and deadlines. Developing a contract engages the participant in a way that is motivating, challenging, and public. The public nature of contracts is especially important because public goals are more likely to be met compared with private or semiprivate goals (14). Having the participant make decisions about the nature of the contract fosters a sense of autonomy and can contribute to intrinsic motivation.

Contracts can be set by individuals or groups. The benefits of a group contract are the feeling it gives participants about not wanting to let others down and the desire to be part of a group. Individual contracts, however, can be tailored to the participant's specific situation and goals.

Consequences of meeting and not meeting the contracted goals should be clear and relevant to the participant. Contingency reinforcement can be set up so that the participant agrees to do a low-preference activity (e.g., squats) before a high-preference activity (e.g., sauna). Material and extrinsic reinforcers may be necessary initially but should become limited as natural reinforcers develop, such as social reinforcement. Inherent benefits of exercise, such as enjoyment and a sense of accomplishment, can foster more

Characteristics of Effective Goals

- Behavioral: Aim for actions, such as lifting weights, rather than outcomes, such as losing weight.
- Flexible: Absolute goals can set someone up for a sense of failure if the goal is not met, whereas planning to jog or cycle 4 to 5 times each week, for instance, allows for options to work around the unexpected.
- Specific: Make the goal absolutely clear. For example, walking 3 mi (4.8 km) without stopping is much more specific than simply working out.
- Measurable: Be able to quantify the goal in miles, minutes, reps, and so on.
- Reasonable: Goals should be practical and achievable—in other words, are they possible?
- Realistic: The outcome should stand a good chance of happening based on the person's circumstances and the amount of effort required.
- Challenging: The goal should be difficult enough to be challenging but not overwhelming.
- Meaningful: The goals should be important to the participant.
- Reward for specific accomplishments: Set up benchmarks with rewards. For example, buy a new music album after completing a yoga course.
- Have a time frame: Establish a time frame for short- and long-term goals.
- Designate the situation: When, where, and under what conditions will the participant engage in the target behavior?

Behavioral Contract

Goal: To walk 10,000 steps each day for a full week   Time frame: By the first week in June

Benefits of meeting the goal: Have more energy, lose weight, take my mind off stress at work, lower my risk for heart disease, and be a better role model for my children.

When I walk 10,000 steps a day for a full week (target behavior), I will go shopping at the outlet mall all day (reward).

To reach my goal, I will do the following:

1. Wear my pedometer every day and record daily steps in my diary.
2. Walk for at least 20 min during my lunch break and 20 min after supper.
3. Take the stairs at work instead of the elevator.
4. Walk around the field during my daughter's soccer practice.

Goal-supporting activities:

1. Keep a spare pair of walking shoes and exercise clothes at work.
2. Ask my husband to walk with me after supper.
3. Tell my friends at work about my plan.
4. Create some upbeat playlists to listen to on my MP3 player while I walk.
5. Use the list of step values for various exercises my fitness instructor gave me so I can add my water aerobics to my daily steps.

Barriers and countermeasures:

1. Forget my pedometer: I will estimate my steps from other days with similar levels of walking and other activities.
2. Snow and ice: I will walk on the treadmill.
3. Fatigue: I will remind myself that a short, brisk walk is better than no walk.

My first short-term goal:

I will wear my pedometer for at least 5 days this week and record my steps each night before I go to sleep. This will help me see how many more steps I have to walk to achieve 10,000 each day.

Signed _____ Date_____

Fitness professional _____ Date_____

This contract will be evaluated every 2 wk:

Date_____ Revisions_____

Date_____ Revisions_____

---

intrinsic motivation and better adherence, as can fostering a sense of autonomy, relatedness, and mastery through the goal-setting process. A sample behavioral contract for a middle-aged woman starting a walking program is shown here.

Relapse Prevention

Over time, most people experience lapses in absolute adherence to an exercise program. The cyclical nature of long-term adherence to behavior change is addressed by the relapse prevention model (25). The relapse prevention model is based on relapses in alcohol abuse, smoking, and drug abuse; the goal is to decrease a high-frequency, undesired behavior. This model is best applied to voluntary behavior. Although exercise is voluntary, the goal is to increase and maintain a low-frequency, desired behavior. Even so, the concepts and techniques of relapse prevention can be used with exercise adherence (13, 25).

Relapse occurs when people who have been exercising regularly or engaging in other positive health behaviors stop the healthy behavior and go back to the old, unhealthy behavior. It is important to understand the concept of

KEY POINT

Assessment is an important first step in the action stage of behavior change. Self-monitoring is useful in determining the antecedents and consequences of the target behavior as well as the potential costs of and barriers to behavior change.

Strategies such as goal setting and behavioral contracts must be tailored to the individual and should be reevaluated regularly during the maintenance stage. Some of the variables that influence exercise maintenance are enjoyment, motivation, convenience, exercise intensity, program flexibility, social support, and skills such as self-regulation and self-reinforcement.

relapse as it applies to exercise because relapse is likely for many people, especially if they don't have many coping skills, such as positive self-talk or good time management. The fitness professional must help participants understand that relapse does not mean failure. Together, they can devise strategies to cope with temporary setbacks in the fitness program and foster an arsenal of coping strategies.

Defining High-Risk Situations

Relapse begins with a **high-risk situation** that challenges an individual's perceived ability to maintain the desired behavioral change. High-risk situations can be bad weather, stress at work, boredom, fatigue, and social situations. A wedding reception with all her favorite foods can be a high-risk situation for a dieter, and weekend guests can challenge a jogger's motivation to keep up with his afternoon runs. Individuals are predisposed to high-risk situations if they have a lifestyle imbalance in which *shoulds* exceed *wants*. This imbalance leads to feelings of deprivation and desires for indulgence. Rationalization, denial, and apparently irrelevant decisions can then occur (13).

Successful coping in a high-risk situation leads to increased self-efficacy and decreased probability of relapse. Not coping or inadequate coping leads to decreased self-efficacy and positive expectations about not maintaining the behavior change (e.g., being able to eat like so-called normal people, having more time to spend with friends). If this leads to an actual slip, the abstinence violation effect (or for exercise, the adherence violation effect) occurs in which participants perceive that they have failed. All-or-none thinking, such as the belief that you cannot skip a weekend of jogging and still be a jogger, makes the participant more susceptible to this effect. Feelings of failure lead to self-blame, lowered self-esteem, guilt, perceived loss of control, increased probability of relapse, and possibly giving up (13).

Fostering Coping Strategies for Exercise

Relapse prevention, as described by Marlatt and Gordon (18), is a method used to identify and deal with high-risk situations. The strategy begins by educating people about the relapse process and enlisting their help as active participants in preventing a relapse. The next step for the fitness professional is determining specific strategies to prevent exercise relapse:

- Identify situations with a high risk of relapse. High-risk situations are those that involve behaviors that are incompatible with exercise, such as eating, drinking, overworking, or smoking. High-risk situations can also involve relocation, medical events, travel, and inclement weather. Personal high-risk situations can be determined from information gathered during assessment and self-monitoring. The fitness professional should help the participant recognize aspects of the exercise behavior itself, such as intensity, time of day, place, people, moods, thoughts, and particular situations, that can threaten exercise adherence.

- Revise plans in order to avoid or cope with high-risk situations. Flexible, short-term goals can be adapted to uncontrollable situational demands. Resetting goals temporarily can decrease the sense of noncompliance and increase a sense of control (e.g., "While my weekend guests are here, I will jog one day in the morning before they get up instead of trying to jog on both Saturday and Sunday afternoons").

- Improve coping responses by referring participants to classes covering techniques related to time management, relaxation, assertiveness, stress management, confidence building, and so on.

- Provide realistic expectations of potential outcomes from not exercising so the behavioral consequences of relapse are placed in proper perspective.

- Encourage participants to expect and plan for potential lapses in an exercise routine. They should plan for some alternative modes of exercise, times of day, places, and so forth. If someone is likely to skip a day of exercise when all the treadmills are in use, suggest the cycle or stair-climber on those days.

- Minimize the tendency to interpret a lapse (e.g., missing one class, not exercising during a business trip) as inevitably leading to a relapse and then defining a relapse as a total failure. Use cognitive restructuring to change the definition of a missed exercise class from "the end of my exercise program" to "a temporary lapse that most exercisers experience."

- Correct a lifestyle imbalance in which *shoulds* outweigh *wants*. Make exercise something participants want to do instead of something they feel they should do. Help them find activities that have purpose and meaning for them. Use positive reinforcement and other strategies to make exercise fun.

KEY POINT

Because missing regular exercise is inevitable for many people, the fitness professional must be prepared to help participants prevent lapses in an exercise routine from ending the exercise program. Strategies such as being flexible in setting and revising goals, realizing that the occasional lapse is just temporary, and building self-confidence and coping skills can help participants deal successfully with a potential relapse.

Health and Fitness Counseling

The fitness professional is called on to provide counseling during assessment, exercise prescription, and ongoing monitoring of exercise programs. More and more professionals are implementing principles of motivational interviewing, such as expressing empathy and fostering self-efficacy in a client-centered, semidirective format (22). Regardless of the approach the fitness professional uses, communication skills are the foundation of effective counseling. Developing good communication skills takes time and focus, so patience is critical to listening and understanding. For additional information, see the excellent chapter on health behavior counseling skills by Whiteley et al. in the ACSM resource manual (28) and the Rollnick et al. text on motivational interviewing in health care (22).

Communication Skills

To be able to communicate well, the fitness professional must be able to listen effectively and respond empathetically. Listening involves being able to accurately discriminate the feeling and meaning of the speaker's message. It is more complicated than simply hearing words. **Communication** occurs at many levels, and thus we should not always assume that what people say is what they mean. The message includes the objective meaning of the words, or the content of the message; however, tone of voice, loudness or softness of speech, speed, and nonverbal behavior can change the meaning of a statement. A participant who smiles, looks you in the eyes, and says, "My program is going really well," is not saying the same thing as a person who mumbles the same words and looks away. To enhance our understanding of the message, we must be able to attend

Putting Responsive Listening Into Practice

Participant: I'm the only one in this class who can't get the new step routines. (The fitness professional should observe the tone of voice, eye contact, and posture.)

Fitness professional: You think the other members of the class catch on before you do. That must be really frustrating. (The fitness professional paraphrased the participant's statement and interpreted probable underlying feelings. Other feelings could be discouragement or a sense of futility or failure. Responding with an offer to teach the participant the steps might not have addressed an underlying lack of confidence. Responsive listening keeps the communications open so the participant can express what kind of help she wants.)

Participant: Yes, I wonder if I can even do aerobics. The steps change faster than I can follow them. (The participant has low self-efficacy for this step aerobics class. The fitness professional now has more information about the problem and can offer a better solution.)

Fitness professional: You doubt this is for you because it is so fast paced, but did you know that many of the people in this class started with Jenny's class? Jenny teaches all the basic routines at a slower pace and focuses on helping everyone learn the steps. (The fitness professional acknowledged the participant's beliefs and provided more information to put her perceptions into another context. She is not the only one who couldn't get the routine without some basic training. A beginners' class could provide mastery experiences to increase the participant's self-efficacy.)

Participant: I've always felt I didn't fit in, but I thought it was just me. Maybe I could try Jenny's step class. (The fitness professional should observe what the participant said and how she said it to see if the information met the underlying need.)

Fitness professional: This class was not the right one for you, but Jenny's class can be a good way for you to learn the steps. We can check the schedule and I can introduce you to Jenny. (The fitness professional paraphrased the participant's statement and offered help rather than telling her what to do. This acknowledges the participant's ability to make choices, promoting her autonomy.)

to the verbal and nonverbal as well as overt and covert messages. The fitness professional should pay attention to facial expressions, body language, and tone of voice in addition to listening to the actual words.

The context of the message, determined by the social and cultural implications of the situation, can create noise that will interfere with sending and receiving the message. Noise is also created by the ideas, experiences, expectations, and prejudices of the speaker and listener. Barriers to communication occur not only in the context of the message but also in the way a listener responds. Ordering, threatening, criticizing, interpreting, interrupting, interrogating, and diverting (often by humor) are responses that shut off understanding and make the speaker feel you do not care. Backing away, looking over your shoulder, and checking your watch are other obvious ways to shut down communication. If you don't have time to talk, be honest about it, but make sure you arrange another time when you won't be distracted and can give the participant the attention she needs and deserves.

Do not automatically assume you understand what a person is saying. We react to a communicated message according to our own perceptions of the nature of the message. Use responsive listening to clarify communication and confirm with the speaker that you comprehend his message. Reflect back what you have heard, and then ask questions and make statements that respond to the feeling and meaning of the message. Responsive listening lets people know you understand what they have expressed, helps build a relationship with them, encourages them to keep talking, and clarifies what they mean.

Characteristics of an Effective Helper

The role of the fitness professional as counselor is to help clients achieve their health-related goals. It is easier to provide this help when the fitness professional responds to the client with empathy, respect, concreteness, genuineness, and confrontation.

- Empathy is an expression of understanding the personal meaning of events and experiences to the participant. It is different from sympathy, which is an attempt to experience another person's feelings. Empathy is also not the same as knowing what the problem is. You may know that John has 28% body fat because he eats fast food every day and does not exercise, but empathy means you have a sense of what it must be like for him to be overweight and inactive, and you are able to communicate your understanding in a nonjudgmental manner. Even if you are not sure you are being empathetic, when the participant perceives that you are trying to understand, he will be encouraged to communicate more about the problem. The additional information will help you empathize more and give you clues to the underlying nature of the problem and how to come up with a more realistic intervention plan. Your

effort to understand also communicates to the participant that you value him as an individual.

- Respect is a feeling of positive regard for the participant. You display warm acceptance of the participant's experiences and place no conditions on your acceptance and warmth. This means not making judgments. It is often hard for the fitness professional to respect a person whose behavior (e.g., smoking, sedentary lifestyle, high-fat diet) shows a lack of self-respect for his body. We must prize the person but not necessarily the behavior. When we respect another person, we help that person develop self-respect.

- Concreteness is the ability to help the participant be specific about feelings and goals she is trying to communicate. Reflective listening enables the participant to become more precise in communicating what he experiences and wants to accomplish, which aids in setting goals.

- Genuineness is being authentic and sincere in a relationship with another person. In a helpful relationship, the counselor is honest and open with the client. Some self-disclosure is appropriate and can help develop trust, but the goal of the relationship is to help the client, not deal with the fitness professional's personal issues.

- Confrontation involves telling the other person that you see things differently from how they are being presented to you. You point out incongruities that are observable facts about which the participant may not be consciously aware. Confrontation should be used only after you have an established relationship, and it should be directed toward the behavior, not the person.

- Other qualities important in effective health counseling are listed in Qualities of an Effective Healthy-Behavior Counselor.

Ethical Considerations

There is an ethical dilemma in promoting healthy behavior change in people who don't want to change. The fitness professional must weigh the importance of persuading people to behave in ways conducive to good health versus the clients' right to do as they please with their own health as long as it does not impinge on the rights of others. Informed consent theoretically gives participants a free choice after they have been given all the information needed to make a decision. If an unhealthy lifestyle is based on ignorance or incorrect information, we should provide the information necessary for an informed choice, not aggravate feelings of guilt or failure. But if someone has chosen an unhealthy lifestyle as a matter of free will, we must accept this informed refusal, although fitness professionals often have difficulty doing so. Thus, an awareness of our own value preferences is essential in helping others set goals. We must consider whose values are to be served by the intervention, the clients' or ours, and we must respect their choices even if we disagree with them.

Qualities of an Effective Healthy-Behavior Counselor

- Knowledgeable
- Supportive
- Model of healthy behavior
- Trustworthy
- Enthusiastic
- Innovative
- Patient
- Sensitive
- Flexible
- Self-aware
- Able to access material resources and services
- Able to generate expectations of success
- Committed to providing timely, specific feedback
- Capable of providing clear, reasonable instructions and plans
- Sensitive to physical barriers to communication while respectful of the physical limits of someone's personal space
- Aware of personal limitations

Confidentiality is another ethical concern for the fitness professional. In addition to client information that is clearly confidential, such as medical records, the fitness professional may become aware of other information the participant wants to keep private. Trustworthiness is an important characteristic of an effective helper and reflects an ethical stand. Participants will trust someone who keeps information confidential, treats them with respect, and keeps the relationship professional.

Also, recognize your limitations and know when to refer your client to a professional therapist. It is the role of the fitness professional to help people change unhealthy behavior, but marital problems, eating disorders, and affective disorders such as depression are a few of the areas that should be handled by someone trained to work with

these issues. We must know our limits and help connect participants with the best resources for handling their unique problems.

KEY POINT

Listening to the actual words and the nonverbal message in context is the foundation of good communication skills. To communicate effectively, the fitness professional should practice reflective listening and empathetic responding. Characteristics of an effective helper include empathy, respect, concreteness, genuineness, and confrontation.

STUDY QUESTIONS

1. What are the five stages of change as applied to exercise? Provide examples of factors fitness professionals must consider in working with clients in each stage.

2. What are the basic human needs according to self-determination theory, and how can participation in a group exercise class help to meet each of these needs?

3. What are strategies fitness professionals can use to target sources of self-efficacy information and to help increase task *and* barrier self-efficacy in a novice exerciser?

4. List the personal, social, and environmental links in a behavioral chain for an overweight woman to participate in a walking program during her lunch hour. Explain how fitness professionals could target the weak links to increase the likelihood of long-term adherence.

5. Discuss and give examples of motivational strategies that could be used with participants who are just starting to exercise regularly and those who have been exercising for at least 6 mo.

6. Describe the elements of successful goal setting and write one long-term and one short-term goal for an older adult who wants to be fit enough to enjoy a vacation at the beach with his grandchildren 4 mo from now.

7. Explain the steps in relapse prevention and why each step is important in helping participants stick with an exercise program and resist relapse.

8. Describe the characteristics of an effective helper and explain how each characteristic is related to good communication skills.

CASE STUDIES

You can check your answers by referring to appendix A.

1. Dana was given a 3 mo membership to your facility by her boyfriend, Mike, who attends aerobics classes regularly. They are going on a backpacking trip to Colorado this summer, and Mike thought you could help her get ready for the physical strain of the trip. She is a self-proclaimed couch potato. She started aerobics classes with Mike last year but got so sore that she stopped after 1 wk. Yesterday, you completed her fitness assessment—Dana is in good health, has 20% body fat, and is slightly below average in aerobic fitness. She said her goal is to be prepared for the trip, and she wants to try aerobics again. However, she confides she is afraid she will disappoint Mike because she is out of shape and doesn't enjoy aerobics. What stage of behavior change is she in, and what strategies could you use to help her?

2. Jack is a middle-aged college English professor who joined the walking club in your facility after you conducted his fitness and psychosocial assessment 3 mo ago. His long-term goal was to walk around the world (in terms of total miles walked), and his progress has been marked on the walkers' promotional map at the front entrance. His office is two blocks from your facility, and he usually walks on your indoor track before he goes home for the day. You notice his mileage has decreased over the past 2 wk, and another walker tells you that Jack said, "I won't make it out of the state thanks to term papers and final exams." What stage of behavior change is he in, and what strategies could you use to help him?

3. Your club has sponsored a 10K race every Thanksgiving for the past 10 yr, and Marty has always placed in the top five of his age group. His brother Jim will be in town this Thanksgiving and they plan to run the 10K together. Marty is determined to beat Jim, so he has been coming into your club at least once a week for the past month to do speed work on the treadmill. However, he's really discouraged by his minor increase in speed and the increased tightness in his legs. When you ask Marty about his training program, you discover that he does no resistance training and rarely stretches, but he has doubled his weekly mileage over the past 4 wk and plans to increase even more to be ready for the race and competition with Jim in 6 wk. What stage is Marty in, and what strategies could you use to help him?

REFERENCES

1. Biddle, S., and C.R. Nigg. 2000. Theories of exercise behavior. *International Journal of Sport Psychology* 31:290-304.

2. Buckworth, J. 2000. Exercise determinants and interventions. *International Journal of Sport Psychology* 2:305-320.

3. Chambliss, H.O., and A.C. King. 2010. Behavioral strategies to enhance physical activity participation. In *ACSM's resource manual for guidelines for exercise testing and prescription*, ed. J.K. Ehrman, 696-708. Baltimore: Williams & Wilkins.

4. Croteau, K.A. 2004. A preliminary study on the impact of a pedometer-based intervention on daily steps. *American Journal of Health Promotion* 18:217-220.

5. Deci, E., and N.D. Ryan. 2008. Self-determination theory: A macrotheory of human motivation, development and health. *Canadian Psychology* 49(3): 182-185. doi: 10.1037/a0012801.

6. Dishman, R.K., and J. Buckworth. 1996. Adherence to physical activity. In *Physical activity and mental health,* ed. W.P. Morgan, 63-80. Washington, DC: Taylor & Francis.

7. Ewing, R., T. Schmid, R. Killingsworth, A. Zlot, and S. Raudenbush. 2003. Relationship between urban sprawl and physical activity, obesity, and morbidity. *American Journal of Health Promotion* 18:47-57.

8. Gabriele, J.M., M.S. Walker, D.L. Gill, K.D. Harber, and E.B. Fisher. 2005. Differentiated roles of social encouragement and social constraint on physical activity behavior. *Annals of Behavioral Medicine* 29:210-215.

9. Hagger, M.S., N.L.D. Chatzisarantis, and S.J.H. Biddle. 2002. A meta-analytic review of the theories of reasoned action and planned behavior in physical activity: Predictive

validity and the contribution of additional variables. *Journal of Sport and Exercise Psychology* 24:3-32.

10. Hultquist, C.N, C. Albright, and D.L. Thompson. 2005. Comparison of walking recommendations in previously inactive women. *Medicine and Science in Sports and Exercise* 37:676-683.

11. King, A.C., J.E. Martin, and C. Castro. 2006. Behavioral strategies to enhance physical activity participation. In *ACSM's resource manual for guidelines for exercise testing and prescription,* ed. L.A. Kaminsky and K.A. Bonzheim, 572-580. Philadelphia: Lippincott Williams & Wilkins.

12. King, A.C., D. Stokols, E. Talen, G.S. Brassington, and R. Killingsworth. 2002. Theoretical approaches to the promotion of physical activity: Forging a transdisciplinary paradigm. *American Journal of Preventive Medicine* 23:15-25.

13. Knapp, D.N. 1988. Behavioral management techniques and exercise promotion. In *Exercise adherence,* ed. R.K. Dishman, 203-236. Champaign, IL: Human Kinetics.

14. Kyllo, L.B., and D.M. Landers. 1995. Goal setting in sport and exercise: A research synthesis to resolve the controversy. *Journal of Sport and Exercise Psychology* 17:117-137.

15. Marcus, B., and L. Forsyth. 2009. *Motivating people to be physically active.* 2nd ed. Champaign, IL: Human Kinetics.

16. Marcus, B.H., P.M. Dubbert, L.H. Forsyth, T.L. McKenzie, E.J. Stone, A.L. Dunn, and S.N. Blair. 2000. Physical activity behavior change: Issues in adoption and maintenance. *Health Psychology* 19:32-41.

17. Markland, D., and L. Hardy. 1993. The exercise motivation inventory: Preliminary development and validity of a measure of individuals' reasons for participation in regular physical exercise. *Personality and Individual Differences* 15:289-296.

18. Marlatt, G.A., and J.R. Gordon. 1985. *Relapse prevention: Maintenance strategies in the treatment of addictive behaviors.* New York: Guilford Press.

19. Prochaska, J.O., and C.C. DiClemente. 1983. Stages and processes of self-change of smoking: Toward an integra-tive model of change. *Journal of Consulting and Clinical Psychology* 51:390-395.

20. Prochaska, J.O., and B.H. Marcus. 1994. The transtheoretical model: Applications to exercise. In *Advances in exercise adherence,* ed. R.K. Dishman, 161-180. Champaign, IL: Human Kinetics.

21. Prochaska, J.O., and W.F. Velicer. 1997. The transtheoretical model of behavior change. *American Journal of Health Promotion* 12:38-48.

22. Rollnick, S., W.R. Miller, and C.C. Butler. 2007. *Motivational interviewing in health care: Helping patients change behavior.* New York: Guilford Press.

23. Ryan, R., C. Frederick, D. Lepes, N. Rubio, and K. Sheldon 1997. Intrinsic motivation and exercise adherence. *International Journal of Sport Psychology* 28:335-354.

24. Sonstroem, R.J. 1988. Psychological models. In *Exercise adherence: Its impact on public health,* ed. R.K. Dishman, 125-153. Champaign, IL: Human Kinetics.

25. Stetson, B.A., A.O. Beacham, S.J. Frommelt, K.N. Boutelle, J.D. Cole, C.H. Ziegler, et al. 2005. Exercise slips in high-risk situations and activity patterns in long-term exercisers: An application of the relapse prevention model. *Annals of Behavioral Medicine* 30(1): 25-35.

26. Trost, S.G., N. Owen, A. Bauman, J.F. Sallis, and W.J. Brown. 2002. Correlates of adults' participation in physical activity: Review and update. *Medicine and Science in Sports and Exercise* 34:1996-2001.

27. Wallace, J.P., J.S. Raglin, and C.A. Jastremski. 1995. Twelve month adherence of adults who joined a fitness program with a spouse vs without a spouse. *Journal of Sports Medicine and Physical Fitness* 35:206-213.

28. Whiteley, J.A., B.A. Lewis, M.A. Napolitano, and B.H. Marcus. 2010. Health behavior counseling. In *ACSM's resource manual for guidelines for exercise testing and prescription*, ed. J.K. Ehrman, 724-734. Baltimore: Williams & Wilkins.

29. Wilson, K., and D. Brookfield. 2009. Effect of goal setting on motivation and adherence in a six-week exercise program. *International Journal of Sport & Exercise Psychology* 7:89-100.

Mindful Exercise for Fitness Professionals

Ralph La Forge

OBJECTIVES

The reader will be able to do the following:

1. Understand the historical origins of two classical mindful exercise traditions and their relevance to modern mindful exercise programming.

2. Describe the essential components common to most mindful exercise programs.

3. Know the tenets of primary forms of classical and modern mindful exercise programs.

4. Be knowledgeable of the research evidence base in support of select mindful exercise modalities and indications for when such programs may be helpful in chronic disease management and prevention.

5. List psychobiological mechanisms responsible for the benefits of mindful exercise and yogic breathing.

6. Become familiar with key resources for further information on both classical and modern mindful exercise.

Mindful exercise (also referred to as *mind–body exercise*) in its most simple form is low- to moderate-intensity physical activity performed with a meditative, proprioceptive, or sensory awareness component. Mindful exercise can also be described simply as physical exercise executed with a profound inward mental focus. The physical activity can be executed with a specific choreographed movement pattern such as in tai chi or can be a free-form pattern as seen in ethnic spiritual dance (e.g., American Indian spiritual dancing). The cognitive component is characteristically nonjudgmental and meditative. The descriptor *mindful* is used here in contrast to the more nebulous *mind–body* because *mindful* more appropriately defines the cognitive process involved. Mindful exercise is not mindfulness meditation; as described here, it incorporates similar mental features but incorporates low-intensity physical exercise. The principal mental feature is awareness without judgment of what is, via direct and immediate kinesthetic experience.

Nearly any form of physical activity can be mindful at some level, but mindful exercise prioritizes the cognitive component as its principal feature. The inward attention is performed with specific focus on breathing and proprioception. Expressed alternatively, mindful exercise combines muscular activity with a sensory awareness of the physical movement or posture (i.e., a self-monitoring of perceived effort). Classical mindful exercises such as hatha yoga and tai chi are attentive to the present moment and are process oriented. This process contrasts with most forms of conventional exercise, in which there is a relative disconnect between the mind and the physical effort of the activity. This disconnect does not necessarily disadvantage conventional aerobic or strength training exercise from their benefits, but for many people this disassociation may obstruct their intention to connect more fully with their body.

From a purely academic perspective, it has been argued that there is no reliable objective means of evaluating the mindful component or its contribution; therefore the psychological benefits are simply a matter of expectancy and perception—which they largely are. Alternatively, it could be argued that few individuals who commit themselves to qigong or yoga are driven by hard scientific justification—they are looking for a real-time contemplative process or relaxation response coupled with some level of muscular work or movement. This consortium of mental and physical processes cannot be precisely measured or well-defined, but it can be experienced and affectively characterized.

Mindful exercise programs can be readily executed at a wide variety of low to moderate exercise intensities and thus are adaptable to a wide range of lower functional capacities. This is an important quality for nonambulatory individuals or those with chronic disease. For example, Iyengar yoga (restorative yoga) can be customized for nearly any age, level of fitness, body type, or chronic disease state. Several blankets under the upper torso during a savasana pose can provide initial support for the lower back when preparing for a bridge pose (back bend; see figure 24.1). This is one example of how including props such as blankets can prepare a participant for a more difficult pose. For someone who is unfamiliar with hatha yoga, the popular triangle pose may appear to be nothing more than a lateral side stretch. However, the yogi's cognition is deeply focused on the simple kinesthesis of the pose and on breath centering. Many will find these attributes beneficial in managing musculoskeletal health concerns, in reducing anxiety and stress-related symptoms, and perhaps most importantly, in improving self-awareness and peace of mind.

This chapter is an overview of both classical and modern mindful exercise. Yoga, tai chi, and qigong are addressed in more depth because they have a much longer heritage and larger research foundation. The information in this chapter is not intended to instruct fitness professionals on how to teach these exercise forms; each requires hundreds of hours of personal exploration and objective feedback

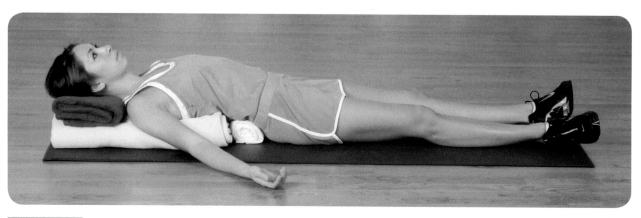

FIGURE 24.1 Supported corpse pose using towels and blankets for back support.

in order for the teacher to attain sufficient instructive skill and knowledge of the tradition. The principal objective is to introduce these forms of contemplative exercise and provide helpful resources.

Origins

The Asian disciplines of yoga and tai chi are at the root of most mindful exercise programs taught today. These two ancient forms integrate mind and body along with an overt sense of spirituality and grounding in nature. At the heart of all meditative practice in Asia is what Indians call *yoga*, a complex system of physical and spiritual disciplines fundamental to a number of Asian religions such as Hinduism and Buddhism. For example, classical yoga, as described in the *Yoga Sutras*, an ancient text of yogic principles attributed to Patanjali, is composed of eight components, or limbs: moral principles, observances, posture, breath control, withdrawal of the senses, concentration, meditation, and pure contemplation (5). Here, *posture* refers to yogic exercises, or *asanas*, that originally were used to prepare for practicing breath control and meditation. In other words, yoga was used as a means to an end, and the end was meditation and spiritual freedom. The physical arm of yoga, hatha yoga, is perhaps the most practiced form of mindful exercise in the West today.

Tai chi has a heritage of nearly 4,000 years and is derived from qigong (also called *chi kung),* which describes the entire tradition of spiritual, martial, and health exercises developed in China. Qigong is the primary Chinese methodology for activating the *medicine within*, or the natural self-healing resource. This ancient practice combines two ideas: Qi is the vital energy of the body, and gong is the skill of working with the qi (also called *chi*). Tai chi, the martial art derivative of qigong, is perhaps best described as a moving meditation. Most of today's mindful exercise programs (see the section Modern Mindful Exercise Programs later in this chapter) are derived from early yoga and qigong practices.

Who, Where, and Why

Nearly anyone can perform mindful exercise because the exercises can be readily adapted to nearly any body type, functional capacity, or health status. This adaptation also depends on the skill and experience of the instructor. Since the early 1990s there has been an explosive growth of mindful exercise programming in yoga and fitness centers, integrated medicine programs, and CVD prevention and rehabilitation programs. These programs often complement or substitute for conventional exercise programs. Fitness professionals should have some understanding, if not at least a limited personal experience, with one or more of these movement forms in order to more fully appreciate their benefits (see Common Benefits of Mindful Exercise).

In recent years, mindful exercise has attracted three principal populations: young and middle-aged adults wishing to improve muscular fitness, flexibility, and stamina; older adults looking for physical activity programs that can be functionally tailored to their aging body and lifestyle; and individuals with stable chronic disease who are seeking a safe and individualized approach to exercise training and rehabilitation. For example, in their recent text, *Integrative Cardiology*, Vogel and Krucoff discuss the clinical indications for qigong and tai chi exercise in CVD management programs, including CHD and heart failure (31). DiBenedetto and colleagues also demonstrated the potential utility of Iyengar yoga in improving ambulation in elderly populations (8). They trained 23 healthy elders with an 8 wk program of gentle Iyengar yoga and demonstrated improved hip extension, increased stride length, and decreased anterior pelvic tilt in the subjects. The common reason these groups cite for seeking mindful exercise, however, is to bring inner tranquility to the mind. Virtually all of the exercise modalities discussed in this chapter can be readily adapted for cardiac, pulmonary, or musculoskeletal rehabilitation in either individualized therapy or therapy in small groups. Several forms of hatha yoga may be difficult to modify for those with chronic disease, such as Bikram yoga (because of the elevated ambient temperature), and

Common Benefits of Mindful Exercise

Reduced state anxiety and mental tension

Improved muscular fitness

Improved muscular flexibility

Improved balance control

Reduced subjective measures of pain and fatigue

Enhanced self-efficacy and mood

Tendency to improve other lifestyle behaviors (e.g., stress control and dietary behavior)

a number of yoga poses, such as full inverted poses, are relatively contraindicated.

Essential Components of Mindful Exercise

The criteria for what constitutes mindful exercise continue to be debated by practitioners and researchers, and a unified set of consensus standards requires more controlled and adequately powered research trials and discussion. For now, mindful exercise should include the following criteria:

- Meditative or contemplative qualities. Mindful exercise includes a self-reflective, present-moment, and nonjudgmental sensory awareness that is process centered rather than strictly goal oriented.
- Proprioceptive awareness. Mindful exercise includes the perception of movement and spatial orientation arising from low to moderate muscular activity.

KEY POINT

Most mindful exercise today is inspired by classical, centuries-old forms such as tai chi and yoga. Mindful exercise has specific features, including meditative, proprioceptive, and breath-centered processes, that distinguish it from most conventional exercise programs. The fitness professional interested in mindful exercise should acquire some understanding of the traditions from which many of the modern forms of mindful exercise have evolved. The central quality of all mindful exercise modalities is its cognitive nature, without which it is merely a physical exercise workout.

- Breath centering. In mindful exercise, cognitive-centering activity is focused on the breath and breath sounds. This breath-centering process includes a variety of breathing techniques as employed in yoga, tai chi, and qigong exercise.
- Anatomic alignment (e.g., of head, spine, trunk, and pelvis) or proper physical form. Disciplining oneself to follow a particular movement pattern or spinal alignment holds true for many forms of mindful exercise, but particularly for hatha yoga, Alexander technique, Pilates, and tai chi. Not all mindful exercise employs a set choreography or disciplined anatomical alignment; exceptions include neuromuscular integrative action (NIA) and expressive ethnic dance exercise (e.g., American Indian and Alaskan spiritual dance).
- Energy centric. The awareness of movement and flow of one's intrinsic energy, vital life force, chi, prana, or other positive energy is common to many classical mindful exercise programs.

The next section describes in detail the most prominent forms of classical mindful exercise.

Yoga

Many modern mindful exercise programs have originated from the Eastern disciplines of yoga and qigong. "The word *yoga* is derived from the Sanskrit root yuj meaning to bind, join, attach and yoke, to direct and concentrate one's attention on, to use and apply. It also means union or communion" (11). The union refers to an integration of mind, body, and spirit.

Yoga historically refers to the physical and spiritual disciplines fundamental to Buddhist, Jainist, and Hindu religious practices throughout Asia. There are at least

Factors Determining the Response to Hatha Yoga

Level of mental focus or kinesthetic focus

Position of the asana (e.g., head down or head up)

Duration of the asana

Level of difficulty of the asana

Pose sequence

Duration of entire pose sequence or yoga session

Breathing technique

Skill level of the student (i.e., years of yoga experience)

Anthropometric characteristics of the student (e.g., BMI, body structure, musculoskeletal health)

eight branches of yoga, but for many people in the West, *yoga* means hatha yoga. We must differentiate the all-encompassing practice of *yoga* from participation in hatha yoga classes such as those taught in yoga centers and fitness centers in the United States. Hatha yoga may or may not include spiritual, moral, and related yogic lifestyle behaviors. It is the physical aspect of the yoga discipline but also includes breathing and meditation. Hatha yoga includes a vast repertoire of physical postures, or *asanas*, that are performed while seated, kneeling, standing, or lying prone or supine on the floor. Traditionally, hatha yoga poses are used to ready the mind for meditation. Their Western names of some of the more popular asanas include corpse pose, cobra, triangle, bridge, warrior, downward or upward facing dog, and the sun salutation (a sequence of nine poses; see figure 24.2). The popular sun salutation is the core of a vinyasa-style yoga practice (*vinyasa* means a sequence of poses). This series of poses is done in succession so that one pose flows into the next. The pace of the flow and how long the poses are held vary considerably, but the movement is coordinated with the breath. The purpose of the sun salutation is to warm up the body for more intense asanas.

The factors determining the response to hatha yoga are shown in Factors Determining the Response to Hatha Yoga. The participant accrues optimal benefits from a hatha yoga training program when the teacher specifically emphasizes each of these variables in a graduated and safe manner.

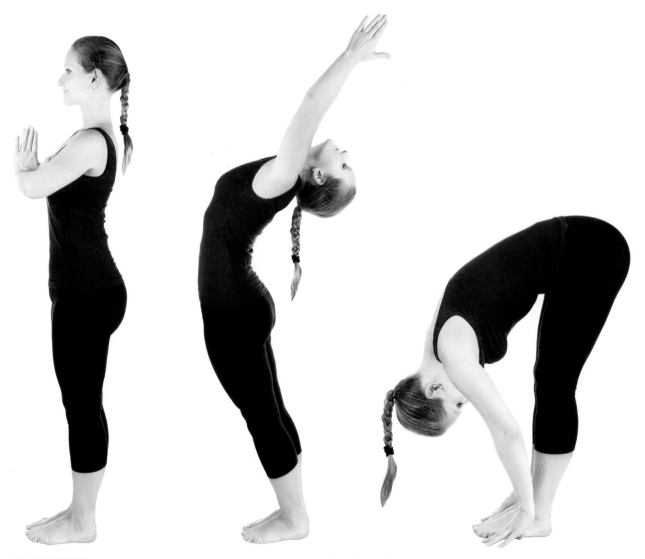

FIGURE 24.2 Nine poses of the sun salutation sequence. *(continued)*

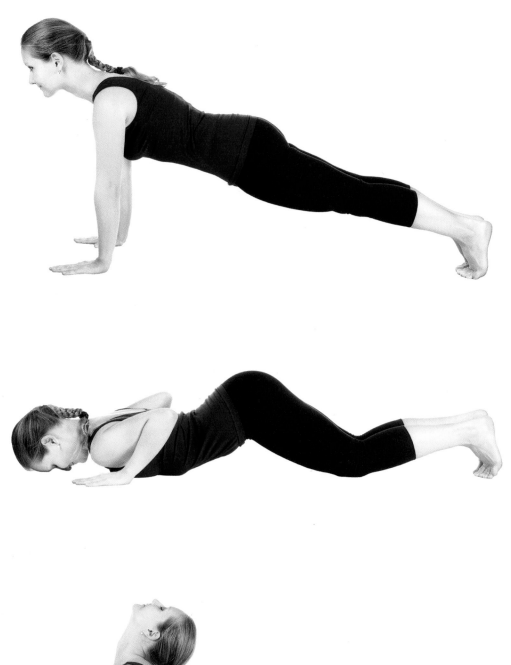

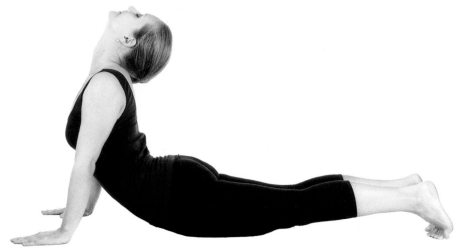

FIGURE 24.2 *(continued)* Nine poses of the sun salutation sequence. *(continued)*

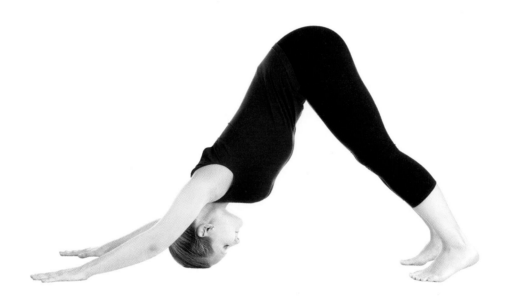

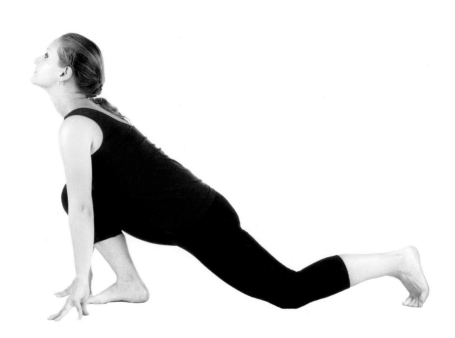

FIGURE 24.2 *(continued)* Nine poses of the sun salutation sequence. *(continued)*

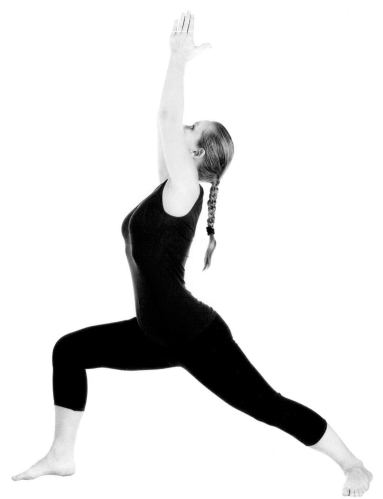

FIGURE 24.2 *(continued)* Nine poses of the sun salutation sequence.
© byheaven/fotolia.com

Popular hatha yoga styles in the West are shown in the sidebar Popular Hatha Yoga Styles. The principal challenge of nearly all styles is to become proficient at handling increasingly greater resistance (i.e., complexity and difficulty) in the various postures and breathing patterns while maintaining a homeostasis of mind and body—or the simultaneous quieting of thoughts and relaxing of body tension. The stamina and discipline required to attain the proper mental state and near-perfect stance and alignment can take many years to master. It is this mental and physical discipline that draws many to hatha yoga, since this process can establish a template for other healthy lifestyle changes (e.g., regular meditation, healthier diet). Finally, it is paramount that yogic breathing, of which there are many techniques, be executed in synchrony with each pose during the asana. It may be difficult for fitness professionals to

rationalize any breath holding because they are taught not to do this during resistance exercise (and for good reason). That said, the breath is held for brief periods of time with some forms of asana work (e.g., breath suspensions and retentions). Restorative yoga may be the safest and most productive starting point for those just learning yogic breathing and poses.

Does Yoga Practice Meet Current Exercise Guidelines?

A number of studies have evaluated whether the cardiovascular and energy cost of yoga meet ACSM and AHA guidelines to promote and maintain health in healthy adults. Marshall Hagins and coworkers at Long Island University evaluated the cardiovascular and metabolic cost of yoga

Popular Hatha Yoga Styles

- **Iyengar yoga.** Iyengar yoga was originally developed by B.K.S. Iyengar, who systematized over 200 classical asanas (poses), from very simple to very difficult. Iyengar yoga emphasizes precise anatomical alignment, which over the years has refined the therapeutic aspects of yoga. Iyengar also emphasizes breathing (pranayama).

- **Restorative yoga.** This style of hatha yoga derives from the Iyengar yoga tradition and is perhaps most appropriate for those who are just embarking on a yoga program because it uses props (blankets, pillows, lumbar and neck rolls, bolsters) and elementary but progressive poses.

- **Ashtanga yoga.** This vigorous, more athletic style of yoga synchronizes a progressive series of postures with a specific breathing method (ujjayi pranayama). The asanas are sequenced in groups of poses ranging from moderate to very difficult. The sequence pace and pose difficulty often characterize ashtanga as power yoga.

- **Anusara yoga.** Founded by John Friend of Shenandoah, Texas, this form of hatha yoga closely resembles Iyengar and stresses three focus points: attitude, alignment, and action. Participants are taught to be cognizant of their key power center, or focal point (the point at which most of the body weight or musculoskeletal force is placed during an asana).

- **Viniyoga.** This is a softer and more individualized method of hatha yoga. It carefully integrates the flow of breath with movement of the spine. It is also known for therapeutic application of the classical asanas.

- **Vinyasa yoga.** Although this style of hatha yoga does not have a specific text or philosophy, it is a form that combines many asanas into a flowing series of poses. The word *vinyasa* means "breath-synchronized movement," and this technique is integrated into a sequence of asanas where the student moves from one pose to the next on an inhalation or exhalation. Vinyasa can be combined with ashtanga or Iyengar asanas to create one dynamic session.

- **Kripalu yoga.** This is a three-level style of hatha yoga customized to the needs of Western students. It blends the physical postures of hatha yoga with the contemplative meditation of raja yoga.

- **Integral yoga.** This is another gentle yoga form that gently stretches, strengthens, and calms the body and mind. It includes comfortable postures, deep relaxation, and breathing practices. It significantly emphasizes diet and is employed across the United States in Dr. Dean Ornish's programs for heart disease reversal.

- **Bikram yoga.** Bikram yoga is a vigorous 90 min series of 26 poses designed to warm and stretch muscles, ligaments, and tendons in a particular sequence. Bikram classes are taught in a heated room, usually between 90 and 105 °F (32-41 °C).

- **Kundalini yoga.** Also called the *yoga of awareness*, each class usually entails spine and flexibility warm-up, specific asana sequences commensurate with one's coiled-up energy, and relaxation. Each asana symbolizes life habits, emotion, and a specific associated breath.

- **Sivananda yoga.** This is a style of classical yoga with traditional poses, breathing exercises, and relaxation. It teaches 12 postures that constitute the sun salutation and can be readily adapted to beginners or those who have low functional capacities.

- **Ananda yoga.** This is a relatively gentle, nonathletic style of hatha yoga. A unique feature of this system is that participants use silent affirmations while performing the asanas.

A key point for fitness professionals, especially exercise physiologists unfamiliar with yoga, is that there are many forms and styles of hatha yoga. Depending on the asana difficulty and sequence, the energy expenditure of a given yoga session can vary from 150 to 600 kcal.

(50 min of sun salutations and standing poses) compared with several treadmill walking speeds in 20 intermediate to advanced yoga practitioners, mean age 31.4 yr (10). Mean values across the entire yoga session were as follows: $\dot{V}O_2$ = 0.6 L · kg^{-1} · min^{-1}, HR = 93.2 beats · min, %HRmax = 49.4%, METs = 2.5, and energy expenditure = 3.2 kcal · min^{-1}. They concluded that the metabolic costs of yoga averaged across an entire session represent low levels of physical activity, are similar to walking on a treadmill at 2 mi · hr^{-1} (3.2 km · hr^{-1}), and do not meet ACSM and AHA recommendations for levels of physical activity for improving or maintaining health or CRF.

Other studies have confirmed these findings that the standard yoga sequences generate cardiorespiratory and energy costs that are at best at the low end of the moderate-intensity range and most often fall in the low-intensity range (4, 6, 22). These studies represent the metabolic and cardiorespiratory costs of a standard set of 6 to 10 yoga asanas (e.g., sun salutation); however, there are over 700 yoga asanas. The inclusion of more difficult yoga asanas, which are practiced in many intermediate and advanced yoga programs, can generate significant total energy costs up to 400 or more kcal per session, falling in the moderate and even high-moderate range of intensity. For this reason it would be a mistake to stereotype the practice of yoga as any one level of energy expenditure.

Hatha yoga should be characterized by the form and style as well as by beginning, intermediate, and advanced levels. It is also important to understand that the low-moderate intensity of many yoga sessions does not preclude other established health-related outcomes, including increased HR variability, lower plasma glucose, and improved subjective measures of fatigue, pain, and sleep in apparently healthy and ill populations (25).

KEY POINT

Hatha yoga combines yogic breathing with yoga exercise in a very logical way. Whenever a yoga movement expands your chest or abdomen, you inhale. Conversely, when a movement compresses your chest or abdomen, you exhale.

Yogic Breathing (Pranayama)

In the yogic and qigong traditions, breathing functions as an intermediary between mind and body. Breath centering stands as an independent method of reducing mental tension and promoting relaxation in the short term and psychological well-being in the long term. There are many yogic breathing techniques, but the simplest is often the most beneficial. Simply focusing on the breath and breath sounds is often sufficient to calm the mind. Herbert Benson's classic book and technique *The Relaxation Response* is an excellent example of this integration of breath awareness and meditation (2).

Yogic breathing is the practice of voluntary breath control, consisting of conscious inhalation, retention, and exhalation of the breath, and is often practiced in conjunction with both meditation and yoga asanas. Breathing is done through the nose during both inhalation and exhalation. Each breath is intentionally slow and deep with an even distribution, or smoothness, of effort. In its simplest

Comparative Energy Cost of Mindful Exercise Programs

When recommending a mindful exercise modality to inexperienced clients, it may be helpful to start with forms requiring lower energy expenditure, such as qigong or restorative yoga.

The following are approximate energy costs of mindful exercise modalities.

Level I (≤3 METs)

Yogic breathing exercise, restorative yoga asanas, some viniyoga and Iyengar yoga sequences, tai chi chih, most qigong exercises, beginner Pilates mat exercise

Level II (3-5 METs)

Vinyasa asana sequences, select Bikram yoga asana sequences, tai chi chuan, intermediate Pilates mat exercise, intermediate NIA exercise sequences

Level III (≥6 METs)

Select ashtanga and Bikram asana sequences, advanced tai chi chuan, NIA, advanced Pilates mat exercise, some American Indian dance routines

These are average estimated energy requirements. Some yoga sessions are 60 to 75 min and therefore can generate substantial energy expenditures. This figure is not based on actual comparative energy expenditure studies but is an approximation based on overall movement dynamics and case studies. Individual fitness, style proficiency and familiarity, and body mass all play roles in the energy expenditure of each exercise form.

form, yogic breathing is diaphragmatic, nasal, deep, smooth, even, quiet, and free of pauses (see Simple Yogic Cleansing Breath).

In addition to reduced stress and mental tension, cardiovascular benefits result from yogic breathing. For example, Prakash (21) demonstrated that 10 subjects who had frequent premature ventricular contractions (PVCs) experienced a 50% reduction of PVCs after controlled deep yogic breathing at 6 breaths · min⁻¹ (21). One of the mechanisms responsible for the mental quiescence experienced with yogic breathing is its stimulation of the parasympathetic nervous system. When fully stimulated by adequate yogic inspiration and expiration, mechanical receptors in pulmonary tissue (i.e., alveoli) activate parasympathetic nerves, which transiently reduces mental tension and increases a relaxation response (20) (see figure 24.3). Acute reductions in BP also have resulted from yogic breathing training (19).

To explain how these breathing strategies work in health and disease, Jerath recently reviewed the most plausible neurobiologic pathways by which yogic breathing acts as a therapeutic tool for treating a variety of autonomic nervous system disorders as well as reducing mental tension (13). Jerath proposed that in voluntary slow breathing, particularly during inspiration, stretching of lung tissue produces inhibitory signals by action of slowly adapting stretch receptors and hyperpolarization current by action of fibroblasts. This synchronizes neural elements in the heart, lungs, limbic system, and cerebral cortex, which, at least theoretically, describes a common physiological mechanism underlying yogic breathing therapy.

Yoga Instructor Standards

When choosing a yoga teacher, fitness instructors may wish to seek those with significant teaching experience. The Yoga Alliance's Registered Yoga Teachers (RYTs) registry is one such resource of experienced teachers (http://yogaalliance.org/content/search). RYTs have significant teaching experience—at least 2 yr and 1,000 hr for an RYT 200 and at least 4 yr and 2,000 hr for an RYT 500. The 200 and 500 designations relate to the number of approved training contact hours the registered yoga teacher has completed. The 200 and 500 training hours include training from the following curriculum categories:

- Technique and practice (asanas, pranayamas, meditation)
- Teaching methodology (demonstration, observation, instruction)
- Anatomy and physiology (human anatomy and physiology, energy anatomy)
- Yoga philosophy (yoga history, lifestyle, ethics)
- Practicum (practice teaching, feedback, assisting students)

Continuing Education

RYTs must complete continuing education hours every 3 yr to maintain their registration and continue to grow their yoga knowledge and teaching skills. Continuing education consists of both teaching hours (45) and training hours (30).

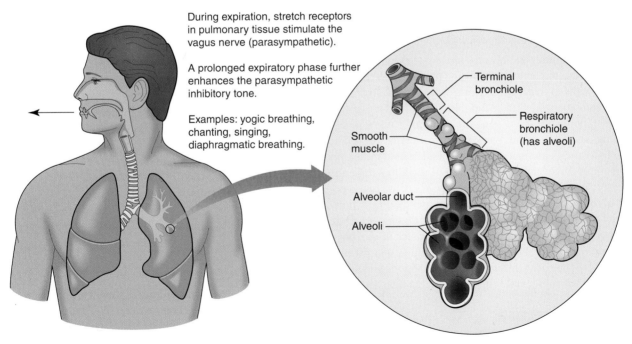

During expiration, stretch receptors in pulmonary tissue stimulate the vagus nerve (parasympathetic).

A prolonged expiratory phase further enhances the parasympathetic inhibitory tone.

Examples: yogic breathing, chanting, singing, diaphragmatic breathing.

Terminal bronchiole

Respiratory bronchiole (has alveoli)

Smooth muscle

Alveolar duct

Alveoli

FIGURE 24.3 Yogic breathing and the parasympathetic nervous system.

Simple Yogic Cleansing Breath

1. Sit quietly and comfortably.

2. Breathe normally.

3. Exhale forcefully and then begin to inhale deeply. When the lungs are completely full, exhale through the nose. Assist this exhalation by contracting the abdominal muscles.

4. Let the abdominal muscles relax completely as the air begins to come back in through the nose.

5. Fill the lungs again, and exhale through the nose quickly once again with the aid of the abdominal muscles. (If the exhalation is complete, you will find that the act of breathing in again is quite sudden and automatic, establishing a rhythm.)

6. Do this inhale–exhale pattern 4 to 6 times.

7. Repeat this cycle once or twice.

KEY POINT

It is important for the fitness professional to understand the origin and practice of yoga, which involves spiritual, meditation, and moral disciplines, versus just the physical practice of hatha yoga asanas. There are many styles of hatha yoga, ranging from the softer restorative yoga to the vigorous ashtanga style. To receive the greatest benefits from hatha yoga, participants must integrate appropriate asanas, yogic breathing, and meditative processes. Hatha yoga can improve muscular strength and flexibility and become a path for improved living habits, including stress reduction.

Qigong Exercise and Tai Chi

Possibly the simplest and the most practiced mindful exercise is qigong exercise. *Qigong* (pronounced "chee gung") refers to Chinese mental and physical exercises that cultivate the *qi (chi)*. Qigong originates from Daoism and is often associated with healing, longevity, and enlightenment. The word *qigong* is a combination of two Chinese characters. The second, *gong*, refers to work or merit. The *qi*, however, is more complex; it is understood to be ever changing and ever flowing, a force at work in nature and society as well as in the human body. There are two types of qigong: internal and external. Internal qigong is practiced to promote self-healing. External qigong is a form of psychic therapy that involves the transfer of qi from a qigong master to another person. Tai chi is one form of internal qigong. The difference between qigong and tai chi is somewhat subtle and is discussed in the next section.

Qigong Exercise

Qigong involves controlled breathing, soft and flowing movements, and calm and careful focus. Although these exercises are ancient, traceable to texts found in Han-period tombs from 2,000 years ago, the term itself is relatively recent, not seen before the Ming period (1368-1644). Furthermore, before 1900, knowledge and dissemination of such exercises extended to the relative few who received training through traditional lineage holders. Only in the 1980s was qigong popularized to become the widespread exercise it is today.

Qigong exercise, also known as *Chinese health exercise,* dates back more than 3,000 years. Qigong movements require very low energy expenditure, usually between 2 and 4 METs, and include standing, seated, and supine positions. For this reason, qigong exercise is perfectly suited to older people and people who have disabilities. There are thousands of forms of qigong practice that have developed throughout China by many teachers during various historic periods. All qigong practice is based on balance, relaxation, breathing, and good posture. Some styles are named after animals whose movements they imitate (e.g., dragon, swan, crane, snake, wild goose, animal frolics). Qigong culture holds that inhaling brings positive qi into your body and usually accompanies an opening movement (i.e., arms opening away from the body) while exhaling releases the negative qi and accompanies a closing movement (i.e., arms back to the body). Taiji qigong, or tai chi qigong (particularly tai chi chuan), is ideal as preparation for high-intensity conditioning exercise or as a cool-down. Taiji qigong consists of 18 movements taken from the tai chi and qigong forms. It is recommended that this series be practiced once or twice a day for 15 to 20 min. Numerous published studies, mostly with small subject numbers, have found many health benefits of qigong exercise (12).

Tai Chi

Tai chi (shorthand for tai chi chuan) is one form of the more ancient qigong. Tai chi chuan is a complex martial arts choreography of over 100 flowing graceful movements that can be practiced for health, meditation, and self-defense. Tai chi is a form of qigong, but not all qigong exercise is tai chi.

Some qigong exercises are done while sitting or lying, but all tai chi exercises involve moving and standing. Some of the numerous styles of tai chi chuan are listed in the sidebar Forms of Tai Chi. Each form emphasizes a particular aspect, such as breathing, generating power, or relaxing. Some styles have a short form, which may be more adaptable to people with disabilities. In tai chi, students are taught to allow the practice to evolve into a free-flowing exercise such that the movements and breathing become one unified energy (qi) flow. Tai chi chih, developed by American Justin Stone, is a simpler form of tai chi chuan and consists of a series of 20 movements and 1 ending pose (28). Qigong exercise, described earlier, involves an even simpler set of movements than its martial arts relative, tai chi.

> We are very logical and intellectual in the West. But when we try to fit Tai Chi Chih (or tai chi) in to a neat definition, or hold on to our own personal ideas about it, we miss its essence. Trying to categorize it is like three blind men describing an elephant while each holds on to a different part of it. Tai Chi Chih is at one personal and impersonal, physical and ethereal. It is not an exercise, and yet it is the best "exercise" you can do. Unlike exercise, though, it will not tire you.
>
> Carmen Brocklehurst, 1997
> From Stone, *Tai Chi Chih*, 1997

Tai chi and qigong have a rich research-based tradition backed by more than 5,000 published papers in international medical and sport science journals, although most of these studies are not controlled, statistically powered trials (www.qigonginstitute.org/html/database.php). Perhaps the most current and comprehensive single review of the clinical utility and benefits of tai chi interventions, including research outcomes, is that by Zhu, Guan, and Yang. (32). After evaluating 25 reviews of tai chi research, they concluded that this form of mindful exercise requires no equipment and little space, and it can be practiced anytime, anywhere, and by older adults and individuals with chronic diseases. Zhu and his colleagues also advise that since short forms (e.g., 10 or 24 forms) have been shown to have benefits that are similar to longer forms, beginners should start with simple, short forms first.

KEY POINT

The ancient qigong and tai chi practices have inspired many modern mindful exercise programs. The calming and introspective qualities of qigong and tai chi rank among the highest of the mindful exercise modalities seen in the West today. Qigong and tai chi are best suited for those who are older, those who are less ambulatory with lower functional capacity, and those who wish to improve balance and coordination. Patient populations ideally suited for qigong and tai chi are cardiopulmonary rehabilitation patients, especially those in early phases following MI or cardiovascular intervention procedures; hypertensive patients; and patients with stress-related disorders.

Research-Supported Medical Benefits of Qigong and Tai Chi

Reduced asthma-related symptoms (bronchospasm)

Increased cerebral blood flow

Increased cardiopulmonary function

Increased cardiorespiratory endurance

Reduced pain in patients with chronic pain

Reduced mental tension and state anxiety

Reduced BP

Increased functional capacity

Reduced falls in seniors

Increased bone density

Improved cognitive performance

Improved immunocompetence

Reduced blood coagulation

Improved sexual function

Reduced risk of stroke

Adapted from Jahnke et.al., 2010; Zhu, Guan, and Yang 2010.

Forms of Tai Chi

- **Original Chen form.** The original Chen style (old form) is thought to be the template from which the more recent Wu, Yang, and Sung forms descended. Chen form is generally characterized by lower stances, constant twisting, varying speeds, and soft and more intense movements with power expression.

- **Yang style.** The Yang style is the most widely practiced form of tai chi in the West today. The original Yang long form consists of 108 movements; however, the yang 24 short form is a popular modification practiced today.

- **Chang style.** The Chang style is a relatively new style of tai chi developed by Chang Tung Sheng in the 1930s. The Chang style consists of more than 100 movements and is based on modifications to the Yang long form.

- **Wu style.** The Wu style is an easier form of tai chi with smaller steps. Its movements, which involve less twisting, impose less stress on the legs and knees. The condensed Wu style includes 36 postures.

- **Sun style.** The Sun style combines elements of the Wu and Yang styles. It is characterized by very energetic steps.

- **Mulan quan style.** This is a modern form based in traditional tai chi movement and wushu (Chinese martial arts). However, it adds aspects of Chinese folk dance and gymnastics for an expressive movement process.

Modern Mindful Exercise Programs

Since the early 1980s, numerous forms and styles of mindful exercise have evolved from qigong, tai chi, and yoga, including NIA, Gyrotonics, chi ball, walking meditation, E-Motion, Brain Gym, yogarobics, Yogilates, aqua tai chi, yo chi, ChiRunning, labyrinth walking, ChiWalking, Flow Motion, mind–body circuit exercise, and many ethnic dance routines. Asian martial arts (e.g., aikido, karate, taekwondo, kempo, judo) also share many of the characteristics of early classical forms such as tai chi. Pilates, the Alexander technique, the Feldenkrais method, and various modern hatha yoga styles have likewise matured as respected mindful exercise and rehabilitative methods as their techniques have been largely standardized over the last three decades.

Pilates

According to the Pilates Method Alliance (PMA), in 2006, approximately 9 million Americans practiced Pilates and there were approximately 13,000 Pilates instructors in the United States, although many of these are not certified by the PMA or any of the several other Pilates organizations. As of 2010 there is no one nationally recognized Pilates instructor certification. However, the PMA, along with a number of Pilates schools and companies, has created a national exam and is working toward greater standardization of teaching practices.

The Pilates method was developed by J.H. Pilates in the early 20th century. Pilates is an orderly system of slow, controlled, distinct movements that demand a profound internal cognitive focus. This method is essentially divided into two modalities: floor or mat work and work on the resistance equipment that Pilates developed (e.g., the Universal Reformer). Mat work is taught in either a group or a private setting, whereas work on the equipment is generally learned one on one or in small groups. Pilates is essentially a movement reeducation in which the student learns to overcome faulty compensatory movement patterns. These inefficient movement patterns are broken down into components using a Reformer machine (there are also other machines such as the Trapeze Table), which employs a series of levers and springs and changes the body's orientation to gravity (see figure 24.4). Pilates exercises facilitate more efficient movement by allowing the student to be in a position that minimizes undesirable muscle activity that can cause early fatigue and injury. Pilates equipment adapts to many human anatomic variations and can be adjusted such that similar movement sequencing can be applied to a variety of body types and limb and torso lengths.

Pilates is advantageous for those who desire low-impact exercise to improve posture, flexibility, and functionality. Technique varies among Pilates training programs, most of which assert advantages over conventional strength and muscle reeducation training, although there is little controlled research support for this assertion.

The main features of the Pilates method are mental concentration, fluid muscular contraction, breathing, alignment, and relaxation. In this sense, Pilates incorporates an intense mindful aspect. The ultimate goal is to decompress the joints (especially the spine) and uniformly develop the body. Perhaps the most acclaimed benefit of Pilates train-

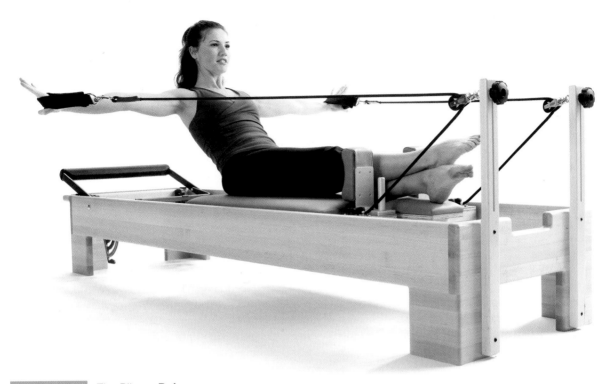

FIGURE 24.4 The Pilates Reformer.

Photo courtesy of Balance Body. Available: http://www.pilates.com/BBAPP/V/store/pilates-reformers.html

ing is improved core strength, or lumbar stabilization and motor control, which has been promoted as a preventive and performance-enhancing regimen. In essence, core strengthening describes the muscular control required around the lumbar spine to maintain functional stability (see chapter 14).

A somewhat dated but seminal scientific introduction to Pilates was published by Anderson and Specter (1) in 2000 and should help anyone unfamiliar with Pilates to gain a better understanding of its application in rehabilitation medicine. Segal and colleagues (27) published one of the first studies quantifying improvements in flexibility (fingertip-to-floor distance) with Pilates after 6 mo of Pilates mat exercise. More recently, scientific reports of improvements in objective measures of core strength through Pilates training appear to be increasing. For example, three recent, reasonably well-controlled studies have demonstrated the utility of using adaptive Pilates exercises for low-back pain (7, 9, 26). All three demonstrated improvements in disability scores, pain indices, and low-back function. These findings are promising; however, there is no evidence that Pilates exercise is superior to lumbar stabilization exercises or massage therapy in the treatment of low-back problems. Four out of five North Americans experience low-back problems at least once in their lifetime (18). Kloubec recently demonstrated statistically significant increases in abdominal endurance, hamstring flexibility, and upper-body muscular endurance

in 25 subjects after 12 wk of Pilates training compared with a 25-subject control group (15).

In a 2007 review of published Pilates research trials, Bernardo found that most trials are still statistically underpowered with small subject numbers (3). However, this review also found that there is cautious support for the effectiveness of Pilates in improving flexibility, abdominal and lumbopelvic stability, and muscular activity, primarily due to a lack of sound research methodology surrounding each study. The increasing number of research studies on Pilates in the coming years should help separate claims from validated outcomes.

Alexander Technique

The Alexander technique, established by Frederick Matthias Alexander in the late 19th century, teaches the transformation of neuromuscular habits by helping an individual focus on sensory experiences. It is a simple and practical method for improving ease and freedom of movement, balance, support, and coordination. It corrects unconscious habits of posture and movement, which may be precursors to injuries. This method is useful for individuals with disc trouble, sciatica, low-back pain, whiplash injury, shoulder and arm pain, neck pain, or arthritis and athletes who wish to move with greater ease and coordination. The Alexander technique is taught one on one or in small groups by a certified Alexander teacher. Little and colleagues recently demonstrated significantly lower disability scores and less

Typical First Session in Alexander Technique

During the first lesson, your teacher will observe your posture and movement patterns. The teacher will also supplement the visual information by using her hands, gently placing them on your neck, shoulders, back, and so on. The teacher uses her hands in order to get more refined information about your patterns of breathing and moving. The teacher will ask you to perform some simple movements—perhaps walking, standing up, or sitting down in a chair—while she keeps her hands in easy contact with your body. At the same time the teacher's hands gather information, they also convey information to you, gently guiding your body to encourage a release of restrictive muscular tension. In early stages of Alexander training, pupils are usually urged to come for lessons fairly frequently, perhaps 2 or 3 days · wk^{-1} (23).

back pain in 144 patients with chronic and recurrent back pain after as few as six Alexander lessons with registered Alexander teachers (17).

Fitness professionals are encouraged to become familiar with referring participants to an Alexander teacher when advising them on improving faulty biomechanical habits or exercise performance, especially competitive performance, through more efficient postures and movement patterns. There are several thousand Alexander teachers worldwide. Most are members of one or more professional societies, and most of these societies publish both a written and an online list of teachers. See also www.alexandertechnique. com/teacher/ for a teacher list by country and state.

Feldenkrais Method

The Feldenkrais method was developed by the Russian Moshé Feldenkrais (1904-1984) and consists of two interrelated, somatically based educational methods. The first, awareness through movement (ATM), is a verbally directed technique designed for group work. The second, functional integration (FI), is a nonverbal manual contact technique designed for people desiring more individualized attention. ATM incorporates active movements, imagery, and other forms of directed attention. These are gentle, nonstrenuous exercises that reeducate the nervous system and emphasize learning how to learn from the individual's own kinesthetic feedback.

Feldenkrais applications include pain management, sport performance improvement, performing arts improvement, stress relief, and confidence building. Activities that require significant coordination are prime examples of where the Feldenkrais method can be helpful (e.g., competitive running, golf, skiing, kayaking, rowing, horseback riding, hatha yoga). Sessions are taught individually or in small groups with the practitioner gently touching or moving the student to facilitate awareness and vitality. Similar to the Alexander technique, Feldenkrais teachings emphasize thinking rather than doing. A typical session might begin with the teacher observing movements associated with a specific sport or activity. The Feldenkrais teacher would systematically place his hands on the student to see which muscles were working, which ones

weren't working, and which ones were not disengaging. From this the teacher can evaluate movement patterns and habits interfering with other movements. The ATM or FI method (a sequence of gentle reeducation movements) is then introduced and supervised. Two recently published benefits of the Feldenkrais method are increasing balance and reducing falls in seniors. Ullmann demonstrated favorable and significant improvements in balance and reduced fear of falling in a group of 25 seniors (average age = 75 yr) compared with a control group (30).

The Feldenkrais Educational Foundation of North America publishes a list of Feldenkrais teachers and is an excellent resource of professional publications on the Feldenkrais method. Additionally, the Feldenkrais Guild, accessed through the Feldenkrais Foundation, is the arm of the foundation that upholds teacher standards of practice, public education, and professional development.

Neuromuscular Integrative Action

NIA was created by Debbie and Carlos Rosas in 1983. It is a composite of Eastern and Western mind–body exercise and has grown in popularity in many health clubs and fitness centers throughout the United States. It combines dance movements and moderately intense martial arts moves infused with subtle mindful techniques designed to heighten body awareness and what NIA professionals call *sensory IQ*. NIA is generally performed in bare feet and, through music and movement, each NIA session is "uniquely crafted to both calm and invigorate" (24).

NIA classes blend concepts from tai chi, yoga, martial arts, Feldenkrais, and ethnic and modern dance. The technique is based on a process termed *the body's way* and incorporates 9 movement energies, 13 principles, and 52 basic moves. Beginners and highly fit athletes alike can adapt NIA to meet their needs by choosing from three intensity levels. Unlike other mindful exercise programs, NIA also includes a moderate aerobic component to address cardiorespiratory endurance. The aerobic segment fosters creativity and spontaneity rather than requiring strict adherence to standard movement patterns. Participants are taught to move with self-expression and to couple movement tempo with their emotion. NIA trainings include a systematic approach to developing technique proficiency. Similar to the traditional martial arts model, the NIA training series includes several progressive belt levels, with the black belt representing the highest level of mastery. Each belt addresses five core competency areas (movement, music, anatomy, science, and philosophy) while exploring the 13 NIA principles; however, the green belt is dedicated solely to the craft of teaching.

KEY POINT

Modern styles of mindful exercise have grown markedly in popularity over the last two decades. Benefits of these programs depend on the energy expenditure, physical work, breathing technique, and mindful processes involved. Pilates in particular has grown in popularity to become a means to improve posture and core strength, although more controlled research is needed to support its utility in fitness and rehabilitation. The fitness professional should become knowledgeable about the Alexander technique and Feldenkrais method, two relatively simple techniques that address important deficiencies in skeletal mechanics, breathing, and anatomical alignment.

Mindful Exercise Outcomes

Monitoring mindful exercise training responses and outcome measures is not as straightforward as monitoring them in conventional exercise training. For example, during and after a 10 wk aerobics class you could show a measurable trend and objectively demonstrate improved aerobic capacity from a number of field or laboratory exercise capacity tests. Assessing the benefits of a 10 wk hatha yoga or tai chi program may also require cognitive or affective outcome measures, considering that much of the response is psychobiological. A number of indications that are helpful in evaluating the outcomes of mindful exercise programs, including affective responses, are listed in Mindful Exercise Outcome Measures.

Psychobiological Nature of Mindful Exercise

Mindful exercise induces relaxation from within by relaxing the muscles, slowing breathing, and, most importantly, calming the mind. Published scientific evidence shows that hypertension, insulin resistance, anxiety disorders, pain, CVD risk factors, and depression all favorably respond to regular participation in mindful exercise, particularly tai chi, qigong exercise, and hatha yoga. Many of the extolled benefits of mindful exercise still lack objective research support. Quality published research on mindful exercise outcomes is progressing slowly; most research published thus far uses small subject numbers, is statistically underpowered, or suffers from inadequate controls. For example, Kirkwood et al. recently reviewed the existing research for hatha yoga and anxiety and found only eight studies that were reasonably well designed (14). Together these studies showed an encouraging trend for hatha yoga to reduce anxiety, although it was not possible to say that yoga was clearly effective in treating anxiety.

Another research issue is adequately measuring the muscular strength gained. For example, if hatha yoga or Pilates was the primary intervention, is it valid to measure strength gains with 1RM on a weight machine? There are no yoga, Pilates, or tai chi ergometers that specifically replicate the exercise mechanics associated with these modalities. Still, it is reasonable to assume that the core benefits of mindful exercise programs are increased balance, muscular strength, and flexibility as well as real-time relaxation and mental quiescence.

Mindful Exercise Outcome Measures

- Quality-of-life measures (e.g., SF-8, SF-12 quality-of-life scale instruments)
- Measures of physical mobility in ADLs and physical function (e.g., Functional Status Questionnaire, Kela Coordination test)
- Flexibility and muscular strength measures that closely replicate the training program
- Resting and ambulatory BP
- Forced expiratory volume in 1 sec (i.e., FEV_1, an appropriate pulmonary measure for mindful exercise programs that focuses on breath work)
- Measures of balance control (e.g., Berg Balance Scale, standing balance test, Tinetti Balance Scale)
- Mood and affect measures (e.g., state anxiety measures, Profile of Mood States)
- Pain or symptom measures (e.g., visual analog scale)
- Disability measures (e.g., Oswestry Disability Index, Roland Morris Disability Questionnaire)
- Spirituality measures (e.g., Spirituality Index of Well-Being, INSPIRIT, Serenity Scales)

Much has been written about the psychobiological mechanisms responsible for the affective responses and mood alterations observed with meditation and mindful exercise. This issue is somewhat complicated by the fact that muscular exercise is conjoined with meditative activity such that our bodies have combined metabolic and cognitive mechanisms. The actual mechanism is likely a synergy of biological transactions, including genetic, environmental, acute, and adaptive neurobiologic processes, not unlike that comprehensively reviewed by the author in 1995 (16). The following are putative mechanisms that play a role in mindful exercise programs that have significant physical, breathing, and cognitive components (16, 29):

- Psychological changes—expectancy (Rosenthal effect) and special attention (Hawthorne effect)
- Cortical and hemispheric lateralization changes in the brain
- Deactivation of the hypothalamic pituitary adrenal axis, resulting in reduced catecholamine production (see figure 24.5)
- Central endorphinergic changes, or acute endorphin changes in the brain that act on neurotransmission
- Respiration-induced affective changes (e.g., pulmonary parasympathetic stimulation) (see figure 24.3)
- Musculoskeletal neural endocrine mechanisms, in which ascending neural pathways carry sensory information from the muscles and joints to a variety of thalamic and cortical structures of the brain that affect mood and cognition
- Thermic neuroendocrine affective changes induced by mindful exercise programs taught in high temperatures, as experienced with Bikram yoga

KEY POINT

The benefits of mindful exercise can be measured by objective changes in quality of life, life stress, and stress-related symptoms. Depending on the type of mindful exercise, changes in muscular strength and flexibility have been difficult to quantify because many mindful exercise routines are largely nonstandardized and there is a lack of objective musculoskeletal fitness assessment tools that quantify strength changes (e.g., evaluating strength gains due to hatha yoga). There remains a need to develop and validate measures of muscular fitness outcomes for mindful exercise, particularly Pilates. The mechanisms responsible for the affective changes observed with mindful exercise are complex and overlap with similar responses and mechanisms observed with conventional aerobic and strength training. One attribute of mindful exercise is that positive affective changes can occur at much lower energy expenditures with less risk of injury or undue cardiovascular stress.

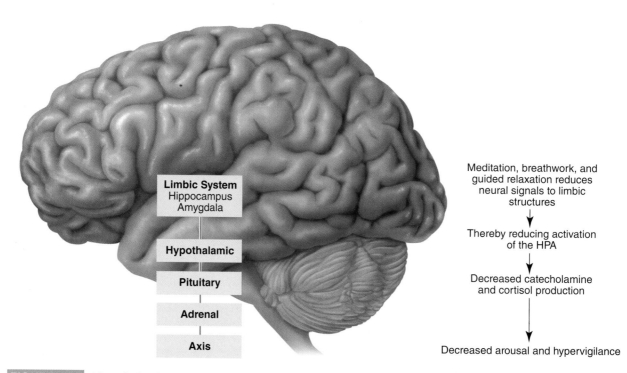

Limbic System
Hippocampus
Amygdala

Hypothalamic

Pituitary

Adrenal

Axis

Meditation, breathwork, and guided relaxation reduces neural signals to limbic structures

↓

Thereby reducing activation of the HPA

↓

Decreased catecholamine and cortisol production

↓

Decreased arousal and hypervigilance

FIGURE 24.5 Hypothalamic, pituitary, and adrenal mechanisms involved in meditation and mindful exercise. CRH = corticotrophin-releasing hormone; ACTH = adrenal corticotropic hormone.

Mindful Exercise Training Resources

There are many training and certification programs for prospective tai chi, qigong, Pilates, NIA, and yoga teachers. Unlike some certification programs (e.g., ACSM, ACE), most of the mindful instructor certification programs do not follow a standardized set of practice guidelines that cover a core curriculum such as exercise, preexercise assessment, program implementation, and exercise safety. This is not to imply that well-planned and professionally conducted hatha yoga and tai chi teacher training programs do not exist, however. In the case of the classical forms (hatha yoga and tai chi), standardizing practice guidelines will be difficult because some of these traditions steadfastly adhere to ethnic heritages and ancient teachings in an effort to maintain a purity and respect for the tradition. For yoga, however, the Yoga Alliance has excelled in establishing teacher standards across many yoga training programs. This organization maintains a national registry of yoga teachers and schools that meet its recommended educational standards, and it strongly encourages the inclusion of core competencies. Select continuing education and training resources for mindful exercise include the following:

- Alexander Technique International: www.ati-net.com/contact.php
- Alexander Technique online resource: www.alexandertechnique.com/research.htm
- ChiRunning and ChiWalking instructor training: www.chirunning.com
- Directory of qigong teachers and therapists: www.qigonginstitute.org/listing/directory.php
- Feldenkrais Educational Foundation of North America: www.feldenkrais.com
- International Association of Yoga Therapists: www.iayt.org
- Tai Chi Chih Association: www.taichichihassociation.org
- Kripalu Center for Yoga and Health: www.kripalu.org
- National Qigong Association (United States): http://nqa.org/
- Pilates Method Alliance: www.pilatesmethodalliance.org
- Nia training: www.nianow.com/training
- Qigong Institute: www.qigonginstitute.org
- YogaFit International: www.yogafit.com
- Yoga for the West Teacher Training Course by Mara Carrico: 760-942-4244
- Yoga Alliance: http://yogaalliance.org/

STUDY QUESTIONS

1. What characterizes mindful exercise in contrast to conventional aerobic and resistance exercise programs?

2. How does yogic breathing therapy reduce stress and benefit the cardiovascular system?

3. How might the elements of mindful exercise be integrated with a conventional aerobic and resistance training class?

4. What are the benefits of including tai chi and qigong exercise in fitness programming?

5. What outcome measures would you use at baseline, serially, and at the conclusion of a 10 wk, 4 times · wk^{-1}, tai chi training program for deconditioned but apparently healthy adults—particularly if you wanted to demonstrate improvement in balance?

CASE STUDIES

You can check your answers by referring to appendix A.

1. You are referred a competitive college-aged 10,000 m runner who wants to improve his running form, particularly during the sprint phase of a race (i.e., the last 200 m). Aside from specific resistance and running training, what mindful activity could you advise that may help his sprint technique?

2. A 54-yr-old gentleman with type 2 diabetes has clearance from his physician to embark upon a moderate-level strength training program. His diabetes is well controlled. His BMI is 32 and he has chronic mild-moderate low-back pain. His goals are to improve overall strength and flexibility, lose about 20 lb (9 kg) of body weight, and reduce the magnitude and frequency of his low-back pain. What are some options for mindful exercise for this client, particularly with regard to his low-back pain?

3. You are asked to lead a beginning exercise class for a group of relatively functional seniors (65-75 yr of age), with a particular emphasis on improving balance. Many in this group have some level of fear of falling, and this particular component of your program should be emphasized.

REFERENCES

1. Anderson R., and D. Specter. 2000. Introduction to Pilates-based rehabilitation. *Orthopaedic Physical Therapy Clinics of North America* 9:395-410.

2. Benson, H., and M.Z. Klipper. 1975. *The relaxation response.* New York: Morrow.

3. Bernardo, LM. 2007. The effectiveness of Pilates training in healthy adults: An appraisal of the research literature. *Journal of Bodywork & Movement Therapies* 11:106-110.

4. Boehde, D., and J. Porcari. 2005. Does yoga really do the body good? *ACE Fitness Matters* Sept/Oct.

5. Bryant, E.F. 2009. *The yoga sutras of Patanjali: A new edition, translation, and commentary.* New York: North Point Press.

6. Clay, C.C., L.K. Lloyd, J.L. Walker, K.R. Sharp, and R.B. Pankey. 2005. The metabolic cost of hatha yoga. *Journal of Strength and Conditioning Research* 19:604-610.

7. Curnow, D., et al. 2009. Altered motor control, posture and the Pilates method of exercise prescription. *Journal of Body Movement Therapy* 13:104-111.

8. DiBenedetto, M., K.E. Innes, A. Taylor, P.F. Rodeheaver, J.A. Boxer, H.J. Wright, and D.C. Kerrigan. 2005. Effect of a gentle Iyengar yoga program on gait in the elderly: An exploratory study. *Archives of Physical Medicine and Rehabilitation* 86:1830.

9. Donzelli, S., et al. 2006. Two different techniques in the rehabilitation treatment of low back pain: A randomized controlled trial. *Eura Medicophys* 42(3): 205-210.

10. Hagins, M., et.al. 2007. Does practicing hatha yoga satisfy recommendations for intensity of physical activity which improves and maintains health and cardiovascular fitness? *BMC Complementary and Alternative Medicine* 7:40-49.

11. Iyengar, B.K.S. 1977. *Light on yoga: Yoga dipika.* New York: Schocken Books.

12. Jahnke, R., L. Larkey, C. Rogers, et al. 2010. A comprehensive review of health benefits of qigong and tai chi. *American Journal of Health Promotion* 24:e1-e25.

13. Jerath, R., J.W. Edry, V.A. Barnes, and V. Jerath. 2006. Physiology of long pranayamic breathing: Neural respiratory elements may provide a mechanism that explains how slow deep breathing shifts the autonomic nervous system. *Medical Hypotheses* 67(3): 566-571.

14. Kirkwood, G., H. Rampes, V. Tuffrey, J. Richardson, and K. Pilkington. 2005. Yoga for anxiety: A systematic review of the research evidence. *British Journal of Sports Medicine* 39:884-889.

15. Kloubec, J.A. 2010. Pilates for improvement of muscle endurance, flexibility, balance, and posture. *Journal of Strength and Conditioning Research* 24:661-667.

16. La Forge, R. 1995. Exercise-associated mood alterations: A review of interactive neurobiological mechanisms. *Medicine, Exercise, Nutrition and Health* 4:17-32.

17. Little, P., F. Webley, M. Evans, et al. 2008. Randomised controlled trial of Alexander Technique lessons, exercise, and massage (ATEAM) for chronic and recurrent back pain. *British Journal of Sports Medicine* 42(12): 965-968.

18. Luo, X., et.al. 2004. Estimates and patterns of direct health care expenditures among individuals with back pain in the United States. *Spine* 29:79-860.

19. Murrgesan, R., N. Govindarajulu, and T.K. Bera. 2000. Effect of yogic practices on the management of hypertension. *Indian Journal of Physiological Pharmacology* 44:207-210.

20. Pal, G.K., and S. Velkumary. 2004. Effect of short-term practice of breathing exercises on autonomic functions in normal human volunteers. *Indian Journal of Medical Research* 120:115-121.

21. Prakash, E.S. 2005. Effect of deep breathing at six breaths per minute on the frequency of premature ventricular complexes. *International Journal of Cardiology.* doi: 10.1016/j.ijcard.2005.05.075.

22. Ray, U.S., A. Pathak, & O.S. Tomer. 2010. Hatha yoga practices: Energy expenditure, respiratory changes and intensity of exercise. *Evidence-Based Complementary and Alternative Medicine* June: 1-12.

23. Rickover, R.M. 1988. *Fitness without stress: A guide to the Alexander technique.* Portland, OR: Metamorphous Press.

24. Rosas, D., and C. Rosas. 2005. *The NIA technique.* New York: Broadway Books.

25. Ross, A., & S. Thomas. 2010. The health benefits of yoga and exercise: A review of comparison studies. *Journal of Complementary and Alternative Medicine* 16:3-12.

26. Rydeard, R., et al. 2006. Pilates-based therapeutic exercise: Effect on subjects with nonspecific chronic low-back pain and functional disability—a randomized trial. *Journal of Orthopaedic and Sports Physical Therapy* 36:472-484.

27. Segal, N.A., J. Hein, and J.R. Basford. 2004. The effects of Pilates training on flexibility and body composition: An observational study. *Archives of Physical Medicine and Rehabilitation* 85:1977-1981.

28. Stone, J. 2004. *T'ai chi chih: Joy through movement.* Boston: Good Karma.

29. Tsang, H.W., and F.M. Fung. 2008. A review on neurobiological and psychological mechanisms underlying the anti-depressive effect of qigong exercise. *Journal of Health Psychology* 13:857-863.

30. Ullmann, G., H.G. Williams, J. Hussey, J.L. Durstine, and B.A. McClenaghan. 2010. Effects of Feldenkrais exercises on balance, mobility, balance confidence, and gait performance in community-dwelling adults age 65 and older. Journal of Complementary and Alternative Medicine 16(1): 97-105.

31. Vogel, J.H.K., and M.K. Krucoff. 2007. *Integrative cardiology: Complementary and alternative medicine for the heart.* New York: McGraw-Hill.

32. Zhu, W., S. Guan, and Y. Yang. 2010. Clinical implications of tai chi interventions: A review. *American Journal of Lifestyle Medicine* 4:418-432.

Exercise Related to ECG and Medications

David R. Bassett, Jr.

OBJECTIVES

The reader will be able to do the following:

1. Describe the basic anatomy of the heart.

2. Describe the basic electrophysiology of the heart.

3. Define *electrocardiogram (ECG)* and identify the standard settings for paper speed and amplitude.

4. Identify the basic electrocardiographic complexes and calculate HR from ECG rhythm strips.

5. Describe the types of atrioventricular conduction defects and their probable effect on a subject's exercise response.

6. Identify the normal and abnormal cardiac rhythms and predict the probable effect of the abnormal rhythms on exercise performance.

7. Describe electrocardiographic signs and biochemical markers of a heart attack.

8. List the common categories of prescription medications used to treat CVD, some examples of each category, and the probable effect of these medications on exercise performance.

This chapter provides background information on the heart, ECG analysis, and cardiovascular medications and how these factors affect exercise testing and prescription in the basically healthy population. This chapter is not intended to be a complete guide to ECG interpretation and cardiovascular medications; there are several excellent texts on these topics (4, 7, 9, 10).

Structure of the Heart

The heart is a muscular organ composed of four chambers: the right atrium, right ventricle, left atrium, and left ventricle (see figure 25.1). The flow of blood through the heart is directed by pressure differences and valves between the chambers. Venous blood from the body is returned to the heart by the inferior and superior vena cava, which empty into the right atrium. From the right atrium, blood passes through the **tricuspid valve** into the right ventricle. The right ventricle pumps blood through the **pulmonary valve** into the pulmonary arteries leading to the lungs. In the lungs, blood gives up carbon dioxide and picks up oxygen. The oxygen-rich blood is returned to the heart via the pulmonary veins emptying into the left atrium. From the left atrium, blood passes through the **mitral valve** into the left ventricle. The left ventricle pumps oxygenated blood past the **aortic valve** into the aorta and coronary arteries and to the rest of the body. The left ventricle, which generates more pressure than the right ventricle, is thicker.

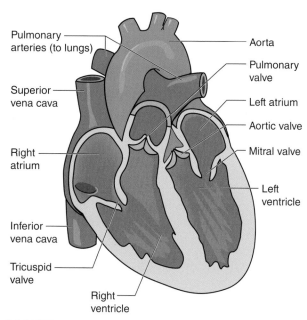

Pulmonary arteries (to lungs)
Aorta
Pulmonary valve
Superior vena cava
Left atrium
Aortic valve
Mitral valve
Right atrium
Left ventricle
Inferior vena cava
Tricuspid valve
Right ventricle

FIGURE 25.1 The chambers and valves of the heart.

Reprinted from J.E. Donnelly, 1990, *Living anatomy,* 2nd ed. (Champaign, IL: Human Kinetics), 199. By permission of J.E. Donnelly.

Coronary Arteries

The heart muscle, or **myocardium**, does not receive a significant amount of oxygen directly from blood in the atria or ventricles. Oxygenated blood is supplied to the myocardium via the **coronary arteries**, which lie on the surface of the heart. There are two coronary artery systems (the right and left coronary arteries), which branch off the aorta at the coronary sinus. The left main coronary artery follows a course between the left atria and the pulmonary artery and branches off into the left anterior descending and left circumflex arteries (figure 25.2). The left anterior descending artery follows a path along the anterior surface of the heart and lies over the interventricular septum, which separates the right and left ventricles. The left circumflex artery follows the groove between the left atrium and left ventricle on the anterior and lateral surface of the heart. The right coronary artery follows the groove that separates the atria and ventricles around the posterior surface of the heart and forms the posterior descending artery. Numerous smaller arteries split off the major arteries, becoming smaller and smaller and finally forming the capillaries in the muscle cells of the heart, where gas exchange occurs. A major obstruction in any of these coronary arteries results in **myocardial ischemia**, or reduced blood flow to the myocardium and decreased ability of the heart to pump blood. If the coronary arteries become blocked and the heart muscle does not receive oxygen, then a portion of the heart muscle might die, which is known as a **myocardial infarction (MI)**, or heart attack.

Coronary Veins

Venous drainage of the right ventricle occurs via the anterior cardiac vein, which normally has two or three major branches and eventually empties into the right atrium. The venous drainage of the left ventricle occurs primarily through the anterior interventricular vein, which roughly follows the same path as the left anterior descending artery, eventually forming the coronary sinus and emptying into the right atrium.

Oxygen Use by the Heart

The myocardium is well adapted to use oxygen to generate ATP. Approximately 40% of the volume of a myocardial muscle cell is composed of mitochondria, the cellular organelle responsible for producing ATP with oxygen. The oxygen consumption of the heart in a resting person is about 8 to 10 ml · min⁻¹ per 100 g of myocardium; in comparison, the total resting oxygen consumption for the body is about 0.35 ml · min⁻¹ per 100 g of body mass (5). Myocardial oxygen consumption can increase six- to sevenfold during heavy exercise in adults, whereas in

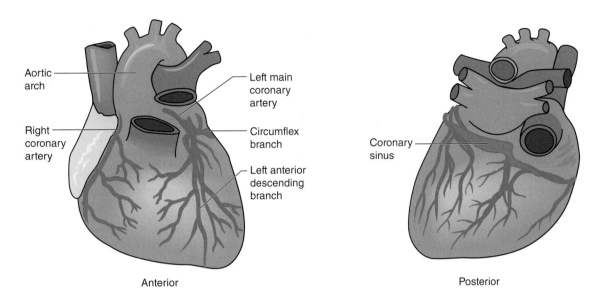

FIGURE 25.2 Coronary blood vessels.

Aortic arch

Left main coronary artery

Right coronary artery

Circumflex branch

Left anterior descending branch

Anterior

Coronary sinus

Posterior

Reprinted from J.E. Donnelly, 1990, *Living anatomy*, 2nd ed. (Champaign, IL: Human Kinetics), 202. By permission of J.E. Donnelly.

young people the total body oxygen consumption can easily increase 12 to 15 times. Heart muscle has a limited capacity to produce energy via anaerobic pathways and depends on the delivery of oxygen to the mitochondria to produce ATP. At rest, the whole body extracts only about 25% of the oxygen present in each 100 ml of arterial blood, and the body can meet an increased need for oxygen by simply extracting more from the blood. In contrast, the heart extracts about 75% of the oxygen available in the arterial blood. Consequently, an increase in the oxygen needs of the heart must be met by delivering more blood via the coronary arteries. An adequate oxygen supply to the heart is needed not only to allow the heart to pump blood but also to maintain normal electrical activity, which is covered in the next section.

KEY POINT

The heart is a muscular organ composed of four chambers: the right atrium, the right ventricle, the left atrium, and the left ventricle. The coronary arteries supply the heart muscle (myocardium) with blood, and the heart meets increasing oxygen demands by increasing blood flow.

Electrophysiology of the Heart

The electrical activity of the heart leads to mechanical activity (contraction), which causes the blood to be pumped. At rest, the insides of the myocardial cells are negatively charged and the exteriors are positively charged. This charge difference is due to the fact that the cell membrane is selectively permeable, and the concentrations of certain ions (Na^+, K^+, Ca^{++}, Cl^-) differ inside and outside of the cells. When the cells are depolarized (stimulated), the insides of the cells become positively charged and the exteriors become negatively charged. Depolarization occurs as positively charged Na^+ ions enter the cells. If a recording electrode is placed on the chest so that the wave of depolarization spreads toward the electrode, the ECG records a positive (upward) deflection. If the wave of depolarization spreads away from the recording electrode, a negative (downward) deflection occurs. When the myocardial muscle cell is completely polarized or depolarized, the ECG does not record any electrical potential but shows a flat baseline, known as the *isoelectric line*. After depolarization, the myocardial cell undergoes repolarization to return to its resting electrical state. During repolarization, positively charged K^+ ions leave the cells. The steps leading from rest (complete polarization) to complete stimulation (complete depolarization) back to rest (repolarization) are shown in figure 25.3.

Conduction System of the Heart

The **sinoatrial (SA) node** is the normal pacemaker of the heart and is located in the right atrium near the superior vena cava (figure 25.4). The pacemaker cells in the SA node can depolarize on their own, without any input from the brain. This occurs because the slow movement of

1 Completely polarized

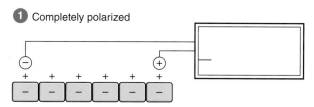

The myocardial cells shown on the left are at rest and are completely polarized. Because both of the recording electrodes are surrounded by positive charges, there is no voltage difference between them and the electrocardiogram shown on the right records the isoelectric line (0 mV).

2 Partially depolarized

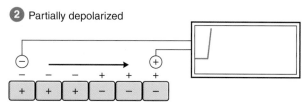

The process of depolarization (positive charges inside the cell and negative charges outside) is spreading from left to right. Because the electrode on the right is surrounded by positive charges, the ECG records a positive deflection. The amplitude of the deflection is proportional to the mass of the myocardium undergoing depolarization.

3 Completely depolarized

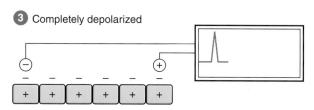

Depolarization is now complete, and both electrodes are surrounded by negative charges. Because there is no voltage difference between electrodes, the ECG is now recording 0 mV, or the isoelectric potential.

FIGURE 25.3 Steps in an electrocardiographic cycle.

4 Partially repolarized

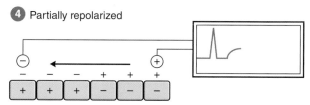

Repolarization has started from the right and is moving to the left. The ECG shows a positive (upward) deflection, because the right-hand electrode is surrounded by positive charges. Note that repolarization occurs in the opposite direction from depolarization in the human heart, and this is the reason the depolarization and repolarization complexes are both normally positive. If repolarization had started on the left and moved to the right, the ECG deflection would have been negative.

5 Completely repolarized

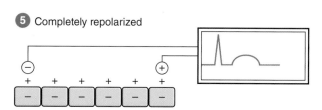

The muscle cells are now completely repolarized, or in the resting state, and the ECG records the isoelectric line. The myocardial cells are now ready to be depolarized again.

ions across the cell membrane causes it to creep up to the threshold, and then an action potential occurs. Depolarization spreads from the SA node across the atria and results in the P wave (see the section Basic Electrocardiographic Complexes). There are three tracts within the atria that conduct depolarization to the **atrioventricular (AV) node**. Impulses travel from the SA node through the atrial muscle and conduction tracts and enter the AV node, where conduction slows to allow the atrial contraction to empty blood into the ventricles before the start of ventricular contraction. The **bundle of His** is the conduction pathway that connects the AV node with **bundle branches** in the ventricles. The right bundle branch splits off the bundle of His and forms ever-smaller branches that serve the right ventricle. The left bundle splits into two major branches

that serve the thicker left ventricle. **Purkinje fibers** are the terminal branches of the bundle branches and form the link between the specialized conductive tissue and the muscle fibers. Small electrical junctions between adjacent cardiac muscle cells, known as **intercalated discs**, allow the electrical impulses to pass from cell to cell. The intercalated discs allow for simultaneous contraction of the ventricular muscle fibers, which is needed for effective pumping of the heart.

Interpreting the ECG

This section on analyzing the ECG may appear to go beyond what a fitness professional needs to know about the topic; the physician is the person to judge whether an

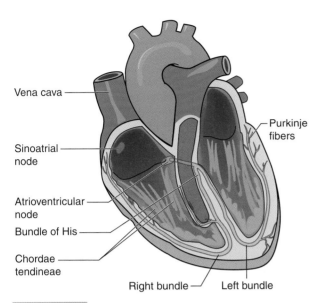

FIGURE 25.4 Electrical conduction system of the heart. These are the normal pathways used to ensure the rhythmic contraction and relaxation of the heart chambers.

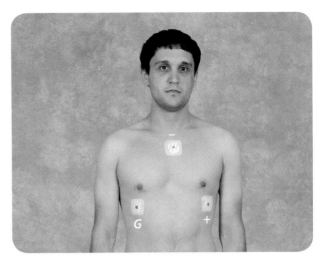

FIGURE 25.5 Lead placement for CM5: (−) negative electrode, (+) electrode, and (G) ground.

KEY POINT

The electrical impulse originates in the SA node, located in the right atrium. From there the electrical impulse spreads to the AV node, the bundle of His, the left and right bundle branches, and the Purkinje fibers. Waves of depolarization then spread from cell to cell throughout the ventricular muscle. Any restriction in blood flow to the myocardium could upset the electrical activity of the heart or damage the myocardium.

ECG response is normal. However, the fitness professional must be aware of the basic ECG interpretation to communicate with the physician, program director, and clinical exercise specialist.

Systematically evaluating the ECG allows the examiner to determine the HR, rhythm, and conduction pathways and to search for signs of ischemia or infarction. Physicians normally evaluate a 12-lead ECG, but for our purposes a single ECG lead is adequate. A commonly used single ECG lead for exercise testing is the CM5 (see figure 25.5), which looks similar to lead V5 on a 12-lead ECG. A 12-lead ECG allows a cardiologist to look at the heart from 12 different views. (Six limb leads provide views of the heart from various angles in the frontal plane of the body, and six precordial leads provide views of the heart from various angles in the transverse plane of the body.) These 12 leads are made up of various combinations of 10 electrodes. The 12-lead ECG contains much more information than a single ECG lead, and it allows a more detailed picture

of the heart's electrical activity. A detailed discussion of 12-lead ECG electrode placement and interpretation is beyond the scope of this chapter. For further information, consult the texts by Dubin (9) or Stein (18).

Defining the ECG

The **electrocardiogram (ECG)** is a graphic recording of the heart's electrical activity. As waves of depolarization travel through the heart, electrical currents spread to the tissues surrounding the heart and then travel throughout the body. If recording electrodes are placed on the skin, small voltage differences between various regions of the body can be detected. Thus, the electrocardiograph is a sensitive voltmeter that records the electrical activity of the heart.

Time and Voltage

ECG paper markings are standardized to allow measurement of time intervals and voltages. Time is measured on the horizontal axis, and the paper normally moves at 25 mm · sec⁻¹. Most ECG machines can run at 50 or 25 mm · sec⁻¹, so one must know the paper speed when measuring the duration of ECG complexes (see the section Basic Electrocardiographic Complexes). ECG paper is marked with a repeating grid (see figure 25.6). Major grid lines are 5 mm apart, and at a paper speed of 25 mm · sec⁻¹, 5 mm correspond to 0.20 sec. Minor lines are 1 mm apart, and at a paper speed of 25 mm · sec⁻¹, 1 mm equals 0.04 sec. Voltage is measured on the vertical axis, and the standard calibration factor is normally 0.1 millivolt (mV) per millimeter of deflection. Most ECG machines can be adjusted to reduce this factor by 50% or to double it. You must know the voltage calibration before evaluating an ECG. All ECG measurements in this chapter refer to a paper speed of 25 mm · sec⁻¹ and a voltage calibration of 0.1 mV · mm⁻¹.

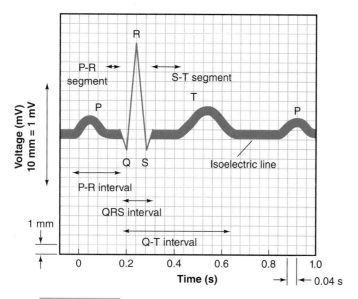

FIGURE 25.6 ECG complex with time and voltage scales.

Adapted, by permission, from M.J. Goldman, 1982, *Principles of clinical electrocardiography,* 11th ed. (Los Altos, CA: Appleton & Lange), 25. ©The McGraw-Hill Companies.

KEY POINT

The pattern of electrical activity across the heart is called the *electrocardiogram (ECG)*. The ECG is recorded with an electrocardiograph, and it provides information about the rhythm of the heart. The ECG paper speed is normally 25 mm · sec⁻¹, and at this speed each 1 mm mark represents 0.04 sec. The standard calibration factor is normally 0.1 mV per millimeter of deflection.

Basic Electrocardiographic Complexes

The **P wave** is the graphic representation of atrial depolarization. The normal P wave lasts less than 0.12 sec and has an amplitude of 0.25 mV or less. The T_a wave is the result of atrial repolarization. It is not normally seen, because it occurs during ventricular depolarization and the larger electrical forces generated by the ventricles hide the T_a wave. The **Q wave** is the first downward deflection after the P wave, and it signals the start of ventricular depolarization. The **R wave** is a positive deflection following the Q wave; it results from ventricular depolarization. If there is more than one R wave in a single complex, the second occurrence is called *R′.* The **S wave** is a negative deflection preceded by Q or R waves, and it is also the result of ventricular depolarization. Collectively, the Q, R, and S waves are referred to as the **QRS complex.** The **T wave** follows this complex, and it results from ventricular repolarization.

Electrocardiograph Intervals

The **R-R interval** is the time between successive R waves. When the heart rhythm is regular, the duration of an R-R interval can be used to determine the HR (beats · min⁻¹). If the heart rhythm is irregular, the R-R interval varies and HR must be determined from the number of R waves in a 6 sec time interval (see figure 25.7).

The PP interval is the time between two successive atrial depolarizations. The **PR interval** is measured from the start of the P wave to the beginning of the QRS complex. The interval is called *PR* even if the first deflection after the P wave is a Q wave. Thus, the PR interval includes the time periods corresponding to atrial depolarization and the delay in the electrical impulse at the AV node. The upper limit for the normal PR interval is 0.20 sec, or 5 small blocks on the grid of the ECG paper.

The width of the QRS complex depends on the time for depolarization of the ventricles. A normal QRS complex lasts less than 0.10 sec, or 2.5 small blocks on the ECG paper. The **QT interval** is measured from the start of the QRS complex to the end of the T wave and corresponds to the duration of ventricular systole.

Segments and Junctions

The **PR segment** is measured from the end of the P wave to the beginning of the QRS complex. This segment forms the isoelectric line, or baseline, from which ST segment deviations are measured. The **J point** is the point at which the S wave ends and the ST segment begins. The **ST segment** is formed by the isoelectric line between the QRS complex and the T wave. During an exercise test this segment is examined closely for depression or elevation, which may indicate the development of myocardial ischemia or perhaps MI. A description of the process for determining MI and myocardial ischemia can be found later in this chapter. ST segment deviation usually is measured 60 or 80 ms after the J point.

KEY POINT

The P wave signifies atrial depolarization, the QRS complex signifies ventricular depolarization, and the T wave signifies ventricular repolarization. If the rhythm is regular, HR can be determined by dividing 1,500 by the number of millimeters between successive R waves. HR also can be determined by starting with an R wave that falls on a thick black line and counting off the next six black lines as 300, 150, 100, 75, 60, and 50 and determining at which corresponding number the next R wave occurs. If the rhythm is irregular, HR can be determined by counting the number of R-R intervals in a 6 sec ECG strip and multiplying by 10.

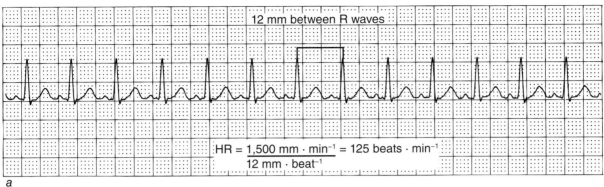

12 mm between R waves

$$HR = \frac{1,500 \text{ mm} \cdot \text{min}^{-1}}{12 \text{ mm} \cdot \text{beat}^{-1}} = 125 \text{ beats} \cdot \text{min}^{-1}$$

a

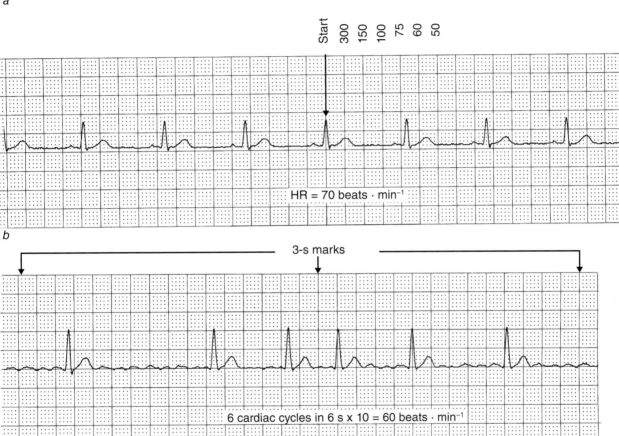

Start 300 150 100 75 60 50

HR = 70 beats · min⁻¹

b

3-s marks

6 cardiac cycles in 6 s x 10 = 60 beats · min⁻¹

c

FIGURE 25.7 Three methods of determining HR from the ECG. *(a)* An approximate HR (beats · min⁻¹) can be determined by dividing 1,500 (60 sec at 25 mm · sec⁻¹) by the number of millimeters between adjacent R waves. *(b)* A second method is to begin with an R wave that falls on a thick black line. As you move to the right, count off the next six black lines as 300, 150, 100, 75, 60, and 50 (memorize these numbers). If the next R wave falls on one of these lines, the corresponding number indicates the HR. If the next R wave falls in between two thick black lines, you can estimate the HR by interpolation. *(c)* A third method is commonly used when the HR is irregular. With this method, you count the number of complete R-R intervals in a 6 sec ECG strip and multiply by 10.

Heart Rhythms

The ECG provides vital information about heart rhythms. Abnormalities in the electrical activity of the heart can be diagnosed from the ECG.

Sinus Rhythm

Sinus rhythm is the normal rhythm of the heart (see figure 25.8). The HR is 60 to 100 beats · min⁻¹ and the pacemaker is the sinus node.

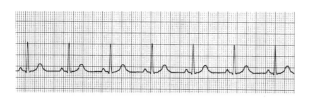

FIGURE 25.8 Normal sinus rhythm. In this example, the HR is 71 beats · min⁻¹.

Sinus Bradycardia

The HR in **sinus bradycardia** is less than 60 beats · min⁻¹ (see figure 25.9). This is a normal rhythm, and it is often seen in conditioned subjects and patients taking beta-blockers.

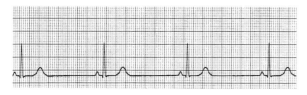

FIGURE 25.9 Sinus bradycardia. In this example, the HR is 35 beats · min⁻¹.

Sinus Tachycardia

Sinus tachycardia (HR >100 beats · min⁻¹) is normally seen during moderate and heavy exercise (see figure 25.10). Thus, exercise-induced sinus tachycardia is perfectly normal. Resting sinus tachycardia may be seen in deconditioned people or in patients who are apprehensive before exercise testing. In these heart rhythms, the SA node still functions as the pacemaker.

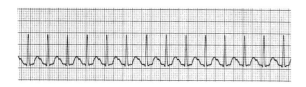

FIGURE 25.10 Sinus tachycardia. In this example, the HR is 143 beats · min⁻¹.

KEY POINT

If the SA node is pacing the heart and the HR is between 60 and 100 beats · min⁻¹, the heart is in normal sinus rhythm. Bradycardia is an HR less than 60 beats · min⁻¹, while tachycardia is an HR greater than 100 beats · min⁻¹ (normally seen during moderate and heavy exercise).

Atrioventricular Conduction Disturbances

Atrioventricular conduction disturbances refer to a blockage of the electrical impulse at the AV node. The blockage may be either partial or complete.

First-Degree AV Block

When the PR interval exceeds 0.20 sec and all P waves result in ventricular depolarization, a **first-degree AV block** exists (see figure 25.11). Causes of a first-degree AV block include medications such as digitalis and quinidine, infections, and vagal stimulation.

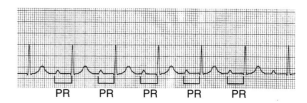

FIGURE 25.11 First-degree AV block. PR marks the prolonged PR interval (0.28 sec in this example).

Second-Degree AV Block

The distinguishing feature of **second-degree AV block** is that some but not all P waves result in ventricular depolarization. There are two types of second-degree AV blocks: Mobitz type I and Mobitz type II. **Mobitz type I AV block,** or Wenckebach AV block, is characterized by a PR interval that progressively lengthens until an atrial depolarization fails to initiate a ventricular depolarization and the QRS complex is skipped (see figure 25.12). This conduction disturbance is seen most commonly after an MI. The site of the block is within the AV node and is probably the result of reversible ischemia.

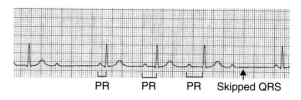

FIGURE 25.12 Mobitz type I (Wenckebach) AV block. The PR interval gradually lengthens until finally a QRS complex is skipped.

Mobitz type II AV block is the more serious of the second-degree AV blocks, and it is characterized by atrial depolarization occasionally not resulting in ventricular depolarization, even though PR intervals remain constant (i.e., do not lengthen; see figure 25.13). The site of the block is beyond the bundle of His, and it is usually the result of irreversible ischemia of the interventricular conduction system.

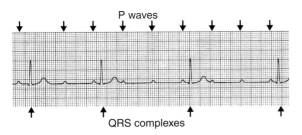

FIGURE 25.13 Mobitz type II AV block. Occasionally, and without lengthening of the PR interval, QRS complexes are skipped.

Third-Degree AV Block

Third-degree AV block is present when the ventricles contract independently of the atria (see figure 25.14). The PR interval varies and follows no regular pattern. The ventricular pacemaker may be the AV node, the bundle of His, Purkinje fibers, or the ventricular muscle, and it almost always results in a slow ventricular rate of fewer than 50 beats · min⁻¹.

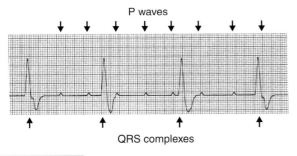

FIGURE 25.14 Third-degree AV block. There is no relationship between the atrial rate (e.g., 94 beats · min⁻¹) and the ventricular rate (e.g., 36 beats · min⁻¹), indicating complete blockage of the AV node.

Arrhythmias

An arrhythmia is an irregular heartbeat. Arrhythmias often arise when the myocardium becomes hyperexcitable because of a lack of blood flow or the use of stimulants.

Sinus Arrhythmia

Sinus arrhythmia is a sinus rhythm in which the R-R interval varies by more than 10% from beat to beat. In sinus arrhythmia, a P wave precedes each QRS complex, but the QRS complexes are unevenly spaced. Sinus arrhythmia is seen often in highly trained subjects and occasionally in patients taking beta-adrenergic blocking medications. The rhythm may be associated with respiration because HR increases with inspiration and decreases with expiration.

Premature Atrial Contraction

In **premature atrial contractions**, the rhythm is irregular and the R-R interval is short between a normal sinus beat and the premature beat (see figure 25.15). The premature beat originates somewhere other than the sinus node and is known as an **ectopic focus** (an irritable spot on the myocardium that depolarizes on its own). An ectopic focus often is caused by stimulants (e.g., caffeine), antihistamines, diet pills, cold medications (e.g., ephedrine), and nicotine. Premature atrial contractions may be seen before exercise testing in apprehensive subjects.

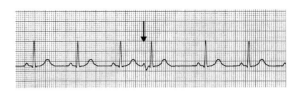

FIGURE 25.15 Premature atrial contraction. The arrow indicates a premature, diphasic P wave coming from an ectopic focus in the atria.

Atrial Flutter

During **atrial flutter**, the atrial rate is from 200 to 350 beats · min⁻¹, whereas the ventricular response is 60 to 160 beats · min⁻¹. The atrial rhythm is usually irregular, whereas the ventricular rhythm is either regular or irregular. The pacemaker site during atrial flutter is not the SA node but an ectopic focus, so normal P waves are not present. F waves, resembling a sawtooth pattern, may be seen (see figure 25.16). The causes of atrial flutter include increased sympathetic drive, hypoxia, and CHF.

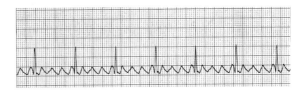

FIGURE 25.16 Atrial flutter. The atrial rate is 200 to 350 beats · min⁻¹ (300 beats · min⁻¹ in this example), but the ventricular rate is much slower.

Atrial Fibrillation

During **atrial fibrillation**, the atrial rate is 400 to 700 beats · min⁻¹, while the ventricular rate is usually 60 to

467

160 beats · min⁻¹ and irregular. Multiple pacemaker sites are present in the atria, and P waves cannot be discerned (see figure 25.17). The significance of atrial fibrillation in exercise testing and training lies in its effect on ventricular function. During atrial fibrillation, the atria and ventricles are not coordinated, and the ability of the left ventricle to maintain an adequate cardiac output may be impaired. The causes of atrial fibrillation are essentially the same as those for atrial flutter.

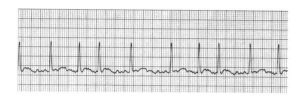

FIGURE 25.17 Atrial fibrillation. A jagged baseline and irregularly spaced QRS complexes are seen.

Premature Junctional Contractions

A **premature junctional contraction (PJC)** results when an ectopic pacemaker in the AV junctional area depolarizes the ventricles. Inverted P waves frequently accompany PJCs as the atrial depolarization proceeds in an abnormal direction (see figure 25.18). This characteristic of PJCs may distinguish them from premature atrial contractions, which frequently have diphasic P waves. If these two conditions cannot be distinguished, the more general term *premature supraventricular contraction* may be used to indicate an ectopic focus above the ventricles.

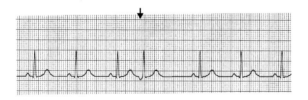

FIGURE 25.18 Premature junctional contraction (PJC). The arrow indicates a premature, inverted P wave coming from the AV node.

If the nodal tissue remains in the refractory phase after a PJC, then normally conducted waves of depolarization initiated from the sinus node will not pass into the ventricles and a compensatory pause will develop. PJCs usually result in a QRS complex of normal duration, or they may slightly prolong the QRS complex. They may be caused by catecholamine-type medications, increased parasympathetic tone on the AV node, or damage to the AV node. PJCs are of little consequence, unless they occur frequently (more than 4 to 6 PJCs · min⁻¹) or compromise ventricular function (9).

Although supraventricular arrhythmias may concern fitness professionals and patients, Ellestad (10) found that exercise-induced supraventricular arrhythmias do not seem to compromise the long-term prognosis of patients with CAD. The significance of the supraventricular arrhythmias lies in the uncoupling of the atria and ventricles and in the resulting effect on the ability of the ventricles to maintain an adequate cardiac output. Recurrent atrial fibrillation may have little effect on the exercise response of a person with good left ventricular function, but it may cause significant symptoms in a person with poor ventricular function. Another problem with chronic atrial fibrillation is that the blood in the atria may clot and lead to a stroke because there is no concerted pumping action with atrial fibrillation.

Premature Ventricular Contractions

Premature ventricular contractions (PVCs) result from an ectopic focus in the His-Purkinje system, which initiates a ventricular contraction. PVCs have a QRS complex that is wide (>0.12 sec) and irregularly shaped (see figure 25.19). They often result in the ventricles being in the refractory phase of depolarization when the normal sinus depolarization wave reaches the ventricle, and a compensatory pause develops. PVCs are among the most common arrhythmias seen with exercise testing and training in patients with CAD. If PVCs have the same shape, they originate from the same site (ectopic focus) and are called *unifocal*. Multiple-shape PVCs that originate from multiple sites in the ventricles are called *multifocal* and are much more serious than unifocal PVCs. The rhythm of normal contractions alternating with PVCs is called *bigeminy*; if every third contraction is a PVC, the rhythm is called *trigeminy*. Three or more consecutive PVCs are known as **ventricular tachycardia**. If a single PVC falls on the descending portion of the T wave, the ventricles may be thrown into fibrillation. PVCs adversely affect the prognosis of patients with CAD; generally, the more complex the PVC, the more serious the problem. Ellestad (10) showed that the combination of ST segment depression and PVCs increases the incidence of future cardiac events.

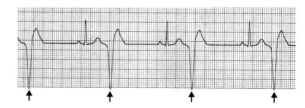

FIGURE 25.19 Premature ventricular contractions (PVCs). The arrows indicate PVCs coming from a single ectopic focus in the ventricles (unifocal PVCs).

If a PVC occurs during pulse counting, patients may report that the heart skipped a beat and may undercount their HR. They should be instructed to not increase the exercise intensity in an attempt to keep the HR in the target zone as a result of skipped beats. They should immediately reduce the exercise intensity and should report the appearance or increase of skipped beats to the fitness professional and physician.

Ventricular Tachycardia

Ventricular tachycardia is present whenever three or more consecutive PVCs occur (see figure 25.20). This situation is an extremely dangerous arrhythmia that may lead to ventricular fibrillation. The HR is usually 100 to 220 beats · min⁻¹, and the heart may be unable to maintain adequate cardiac output during ventricular tachycardia. Ventricular tachycardia may be caused by the same factors that initiate PVCs, and it requires immediate medical attention.

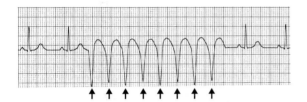

FIGURE 25.20 Ventricular tachycardia. A succession of three or more PVCs in a row is seen.

Ventricular Fibrillation

Ventricular fibrillation is a life-threatening rhythm. It requires immediate CPR until a defibrillator can be used to restore a coordinated ventricular contraction; otherwise, death will result. A fibrillating heart contracts in an unorganized, quivering manner, and the heart is unable to maintain significant cardiac output. P waves and QRS complexes are not discernible; instead the electrical pattern is a fibrillatory wave (see figure 25.21).

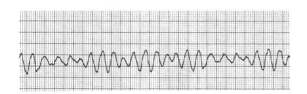

FIGURE 25.21 Ventricular fibrillation. When there are no discernible P waves or QRS complexes, the heart contracts in a disorganized, quivering manner.

Automated External Defibrillators

Defibrillators are devices used to treat ventricular fibrillation. They send a momentary electrical shock to the heart, often causing the heart to return to its normal rhythm. Recent technology has permitted the development of por-

> **KEY POINT**
>
> The ECG can be used to detect disturbances in the electrical conducting system of the heart, such as first-, second-, or third-degree AV block. The ECG can also indicate arrhythmias (abnormal heart rhythms), including sinus arrhythmia, premature beats, tachycardia, flutter, and fibrillation. Abnormal rhythms may limit exercise performance by decreasing cardiac output. In the case of severe arrhythmias, the fitness professional should terminate the exercise session and obtain immediate medical assistance.

table, battery-powered devices called *automated external defibrillators*, or AEDs. The operator applies two surface electrodes to the person's chest. These electrodes are connected to the AED, which has software that is capable of determining the person's heart rhythm. If ventricular fibrillation is detected, the AED gives a command to stand clear and then signals the operator to deliver a shock by pushing a button. Police, fitness professionals, flight attendants, and even laypeople are receiving AED training by organizations such as the AHA and the American Red Cross. Research studies have shown that using AEDs hastens response time and greatly improves chances of survival (3).

Myocardial Ischemia

Myocardial ischemia is a lack of oxygen in the myocardium attributable to inadequate blood flow. Obstruction of the coronary arteries is the most common cause of myocardial ischemia. A coronary artery is significantly obstructed if more than 50% of its diameter is occluded. A 50% reduction in diameter equals a loss of 75% of the arterial **lumen** (12). An obstructed coronary artery may supply an adequate blood flow at rest, but it will probably be unable to provide enough blood and oxygen during increased demand such as during exercise. Ischemia often, but not always, results in angina pectoris.

Angina pectoris is pain or discomfort caused by temporary, reversible ischemia of the myocardium that does not result in death or infarction of heart muscle. The pain often is located in the center of the chest, but it also may occur in the neck, jaw, or shoulders or may radiate into the arms and hands. Angina pectoris tends to be reproducible; patients often report anginal symptoms at roughly the same level of exertion. During exercise, patients experiencing anginal discomfort may deny pain, but on further questioning, they will admit to the sensation of burning, tightness, pressure, or heaviness in the chest or arms. Patients frequently confuse angina pectoris with musculoskeletal pain and with the discomfort resulting from the sternal incision of coronary artery bypass surgery. Anginal pain generally does not alter with movements of the trunk or arms, whereas such movement may decrease or increase musculoskeletal pain. Discomfort is probably not angina if the pain changes in quality or intensity when you press on the affected area (12).

Myocardial ischemia may cause **ST segment depression** on the ECG during an exercise test. ST segment depression usually occurs at a relatively constant double product. The double product equals HR · SBP, and it is a good estimate of the amount of work the heart is doing. Three types of ST segment depression are recognized: upsloping, horizontal, and downsloping (figure 25.22). Ellestad (10) has shown that the prognostic implications of upsloping and horizontal ST segment depression are roughly similar. Downsloping ST segment depression, however, affects survival more adversely.

ST segment elevation also may occur during exercise testing. ST segment elevation during an exercise test usually indicates an **aneurysm**, or a weakened area of noncontracting myocardium or scar tissue.

Myocardial Infarction

If the myocardium is deprived of oxygen for a sufficient length of time, a portion of the myocardium dies; this partial death is known as a myocardial infarction (MI). Pain is the hallmark symptom of an MI. It is often very similar to anginal pain, only more severe, and may be described as a heavy feeling, a squeezing in the chest, or a burning sensation. Other symptoms that may accompany an MI are nausea, sweating, and shortness of breath.

ST segment elevation is often the first ECG sign of an acute MI. Later, pronounced Q waves and T wave inversion may appear in certain leads. Over time, the ST segment changes subside and the T wave returns to normal (see figure 25.23) (18). Other clinical signs of an acute MI include elevations in cardiac muscle enzymes (serum lactate dehydrogenase and creatine phosphokinase), which leak into the blood after the myocardium is damaged (12).

The Framingham Heart Study demonstrated that up to 25% of MIs may be silent infarctions, meaning that the infarction does not cause sufficient symptoms for the person to seek medical attention (13). These silent infarctions may be recognized later during routine ECG examinations by the presence of significant Q waves in certain leads.

Patients with CAD should be instructed how to differentiate anginal attacks from possible MIs. If an anginal attack occurs, the patient should stop the activity, if any, that precipitated the discomfort and should take a nitroglycerin (NTG) tablet under the tongue. If the anginal discomfort persists after 5 min, the patient takes a second sublingual NTG tablet. This procedure is repeated, if needed, one more time. If the pain persists 5 min after the third NTG tablet, the patient should seek immediate medical attention (4).

KEY POINT

Inadequate blood flow to the myocardium often, but not always, results in symptoms of chest pain (angina pectoris). ST segment depression or elevation on the ECG can indicate inadequate blood flow (ischemia). Significant Q waves on the ECG can indicate that a portion of the heart muscle has died (MI).

Cardiovascular Medications

A variety of medications are used to treat people with heart disease. Some control BP, whereas others control HR or rhythm, and still others affect the force of contraction of the ventricles. Other drugs the fitness professional will likely encounter include medications to control blood glucose concentrations, medications for patients with hyperlipidemia to control abnormal blood lipid levels, and bronchodilators for individuals with asthma. Fitness

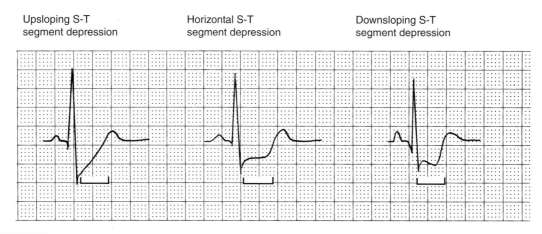

Upsloping S-T segment depression   Horizontal S-T segment depression   Downsloping S-T segment depression

FIGURE 25.22 ST segment depression.

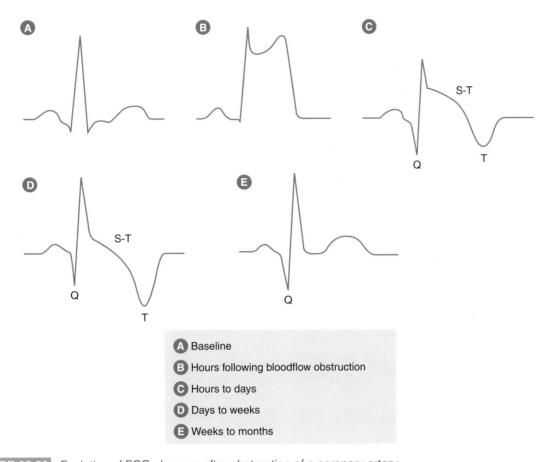

FIGURE 25.23 Evolution of ECG changes after obstruction of a coronary artery.

Reprinted, by permission, from E. Stein, 1992, *Rapid analysis of electrocardiograms*, 2nd ed. (Philadelphia, PA: Lea & Febiger), 150.

professionals do not prescribe medications or deal on a day-to-day basis with patients taking these medications, but they do encounter participants taking some of them. This section summarizes the major classes of drugs, describes how they affect the exercise HR response, and indicates possible side effects.

Beta-Adrenergic Blockers

Beta-adrenergic blocking medications (beta-blockers) are commonly prescribed for patients with CAD or with hypertension and occasionally for patients with migraine headaches. They compete with epinephrine and norepinephrine for the limited number of **beta-adrenergic receptors**. Beta-blockers are generally used to reduce the HR and the vigor of myocardial contraction, thus lowering the oxygen requirement of the heart. Because these medications influence submaximal and maximal HR, they have a profound effect on exercise prescription. Subjects should be tested while on beta-blockers if they will be training while taking them. All beta-blockers lower HR at rest and particularly during exercise, as seen in figure 25.24.

Two types of beta-adrenergic receptors are recognized: beta-1 and beta-2. Beta-1 receptors are found mainly in

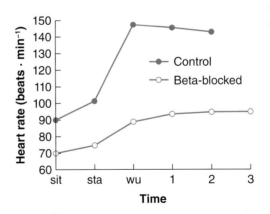

FIGURE 25.24 HR before and after beta-blockade (2 days of 40 mg of Inderal per day) in an apprehensive patient undergoing treadmill testing. Sit = sitting; sta = standing; wu = warming up at 1.0 mi · hr⁻¹ (1.6 km · hr⁻¹), 0% grade. Min 1 and 2 are 2.0 mi · hr⁻¹ (3.2 km · hr⁻¹), 0% grade. Min 3 is 2.0 mi · hr⁻¹ (3.2 km · hr⁻¹) and 3.5% grade.

the heart, and beta-2 receptors are located primarily in the smooth muscle in the lungs, arterioles, intestine, uterus, and bladder. Some beta-blockers selectively block the beta-1

471

receptors in the heart. The beta-1-selective (cardioselective) blockers include Sectral, Tenormin, Brevibloc, and Lopressor. Other beta-blockers are less selective and act on both the beta-1 and beta-2 receptors. These nonselective beta-blockers include Inderal, Corgard, Visken, and Blocadren. An undesirable side effect of the nonselective beta-blockers is contraction of the smooth muscle surrounding the airways in the lungs and reduction of the airway lumens, which increases the work of breathing. This side effect can result in labored breathing, shortness of breath, and other asthma-like symptoms.

Indications for using beta-blockers include hypertension, angina pectoris, and supraventricular arrhythmias. In addition, as previously mentioned, some beta-blockers are used to treat migraine headaches. Nonselective beta-blocking medications are not recommended for patients with asthma, bronchitis, or similar lung problems. Beta-blocking medications may also blunt some of the symptoms of hypoglycemia in people with insulin-dependent diabetes, an undesirable side effect (4).

Using Inderal and presumably other beta-blocking medications does not invalidate the THR (target HR) method of prescribing exercise intensity. Hossack, Bruce, and Clark (11) showed that the regression equations relating %HRmax to %$\dot{V}O_2$max are similar in beta-adrenergic-blocked and nonblocked patients with CAD. Thus, the THR method of exercise prescription is assumed valid if the measured HRmax is determined while the patient is on beta-blocking medications.

Because beta-blockers lower HRmax, their use invalidates estimating THR by taking 70% to 85% of age-adjusted, predicted HRmax (predicted HRmax = 220 − age). For example, a 40-yr-old individual has a predicted HRmax of about 180, with an estimated 70% to 85% THR of 126 to 153 beats · min^{-1}. If this individual takes a beta-blocker, HRmax could easily drop to 150 beats · min^{-1}. If the estimated THR of 126 to 153 beats · min^{-1} is used for training, this participant may be training at HRmax. HRmax must be measured to calculate an appropriate THR for anyone taking beta-blockers, and this measurement should be repeated after any change in beta-blocking medicines.

There has been some question as to whether beta-blocking medicines reduce or block the effectiveness of endurance training. In general, work capacity and endurance training are impaired more after nonselective beta-blockade than after beta-1-blockade (19). Ades and coworkers (1) examined the effects of endurance training in 30 adults with hypertension taking a placebo, metoprolol (a beta-1-selective blocker), or propranolol (a nonselective beta-blocker). $\dot{V}O_2$max increased 24% in the placebo group and 8% in the metoprolol group but did not increase in the propranolol group. Pavia and colleagues (17) found that chronic use of a beta-1-selective blocker (metoprolol) in postmyocardial patients did not interfere with the typi-

cal effects of endurance training. They observed similar increases in $\dot{V}O_2$peak in patients taking metoprolol and in those who were not on beta-blockers.

Nitrates

The **nitrates** exist in several forms, including patches, ointments, long-acting tablets, and sublingual tablets, and they are used to prevent or stop attacks of angina pectoris. Nitrates are produced from amyl nitrate (a volatile agent), which is rendered nonexplosive by adding an inert chemical such as lactose. Nitrate preparations relax venous smooth muscle, which reduces venous return and the quantity of blood the heart has to pump. Arterial smooth muscle is also relaxed, although to a lesser degree than venous smooth muscle, thus lowering the peripheral vascular resistance against which the heart has to pump. Both actions help reduce the work and oxygen requirement of the heart. Many patients use NTG (nitroglycerine) on a 24 hr basis with ointment or patches. Patients may take longer-acting tablet forms of NTG (Isordil, Sorbitrate, Dilatrate-SR) before beginning activities that are likely to provoke anginal attacks, whereas sublingual tablets (Nitrostat) are used to treat acute anginal episodes. Headaches, dizziness, and hypotension are the main side effects of NTG (4). Beta-adrenergic-blocking medications may potentiate the hypotensive actions of NTG.

Calcium Channel Blockers (Calcium Antagonists)

The **calcium channel blockers** currently include verapamil (Isoptin), nifedipine (Procardia), and diltiazem (Cardizem). These drugs interfere with the slow calcium currents that occur during depolarization in cardiac and vascular smooth muscle. Verapamil is used primarily to treat atrial and ventricular arrhythmias, whereas nifedipine and diltiazem are used to treat exertional angina and variant angina pectoris, or angina pectoris attacks that occur at rest (4).

The effects of calcium channel blockers on exercise prescription and training have been studied. Chang and Hossack (6) showed that the regression equations relating %HRmax and %$\dot{V}O_2$max are the same in patients taking diltiazem and in unmedicated patients. Isoptin and Procardia are assumed not to alter the relationship between %HRmax and %$\dot{V}O_2$max. Calcium antagonists are not thought to adversely affect endurance training in healthy subjects or in patients with CAD (15). MacGowan and coworkers (16) showed that verapamil does not diminish training responses in healthy, young subjects.

Antiarrhythmic Medications

Common **antiarrhythmics** include Pronestyl, Norpace, Cardioquin, Quinaglute, Tambocor, Sectral, Cordarone, Tonocard, and the digitalis preparations. The beta-blocking medications also are used to treat some types of arrhythmias. With the exception of the beta-blockers, these medications have little influence on the HR response to exercise; in fact, the reduction in arrhythmias may improve work capacity.

Digitalis Preparations

The **digitalis** medications are used to increase the vigor of myocardial contractions (contractility) and treat atrial flutter and fibrillation (4). In individuals with poor ventricular function, the increased contractility resulting from digitalis preparations may increase work capacity. Digitalis medications are marketed under several trade names, including Lanoxin, Lanoxicaps, and Digitek. Cardiac side effects of the digitalis group include PVCs, Wenckebach AV block, and atrial tachycardia. Digitalis drugs can cause false-positive tests for CHD due to ST segment depression during exercise testing (9). The side effects of digitalis drugs can be potentiated by quinidine sulfate.

Antihypertensives

Antihypertensives can be divided into five groups according to the mechanism of action. Drugs in the first group, *diuretics*, work by increasing the excretion of electrolytes and water. These drugs include Lasix, Diamox, Diuril, Esidrix, Enduron, HydroDIURIL, and many others. This group is often used as the first treatment for hypertension. Side effects include hypokalemia, or low blood levels of potassium. Hypokalemia can induce arrhythmias and is a potentially serious problem. Diuretic-induced hypokalemia often can be prevented by consuming more citrus fruits, which are high in potassium. If dietary sources of potassium prove to be ineffective, a prescription potassium supplement (K-Tab, Kay Ceil, or Slow-K) can be used (4). Alternatively, a potassium-sparing diuretic (Midamor, Aldactone, Dyrenium) can be prescribed.

The second group of antihypertensive medications comprises the *antiadrenergic agents*. These include drugs that act at the level of the central nervous system, such as clonidine (Catapres) and methyldopa (Aldomet), and they reduce sympathetic outflow from the brain. This group also includes drugs that act principally on alpha-adrenergic receptors to lower peripheral vascular resistance, such as prazosin (Minipress). In addition, this group includes drugs that block beta-adrenergic receptors (see previous section) to decrease cardiac output, renin release, and sympathetic outflow from the brain.

In an important side effect, the diuretics and beta-blockers elevate triglyceride and cholesterol levels and impair glucose and insulin metabolism. Thus, although they effectively lower BP and reduce the incidence of stroke and severe kidney disease, they have a less-than-predicted effect on preventing heart attacks.

Vasodilators make up the third group of antihypertensive medications. These medications decrease BP by relaxing vascular smooth muscle. Some of the brand names in this category are Apresoline, Vasodilan, and Loniten. Their side effects include hypotension, dizziness, and tachycardia. The active chemical in Loniten is also marketed under the name *Rogaine* as a topical solution for stimulating hair growth in male-pattern baldness. Rogaine has little or no antihypertensive effect.

Antihypertensive medications in the fourth group work through the renin-angiotensin system. These drugs lower BP by inhibiting angiotensin-converting enzyme (ACE), which converts angiotensin I to angiotensin II. They are called *ACE inhibitors* for that reason. Some of the brand names in this category are Vasotec, Zestril, and Capoten. ACE inhibitors are expensive and may produce a dry cough in 5% to 10% of patients. They decrease left ventricular hypertrophy, reduce proteinuria in diabetic patients, and maintain blood lipid levels.

The fifth group of antihypertensive medications includes the *calcium antagonists* (calcium channel blockers; see the section Calcium Channel Blockers). As with the ACE inhibitors, drugs in this class do not adversely affect lipid, glucose, and insulin metabolism.

Lipid-Lowering Medications

The lipid-lowering medications (Questran and Colestid; Pravachol, Zocor, and Lescol; Lopid and Atromid-S; and nicotinic acid) lower cholesterol and triglycerides in individuals who are unable to adequately control lipids through diet and exercise. These lipid-lowering medications are unlikely to have any substantial effects on exercise testing or training. Patients taking these medications need to be closely monitored by their physician because of potential toxic effects on the liver. Some lipid-lowering agents (Lopid, Atromid-S) can potentiate anticoagulants and make participants more susceptible to bruising.

Anticoagulants

The **anticoagulants** delay blood clotting and are used to prevent strokes and heart attacks in those who are at risk for those conditions. Oral anticoagulants include Dicumarol, Coumadin, and Plavix. These medications are unlikely to directly affect exercise testing or training, but they do increase the risk of bruising. Aspirin and some other medications (e.g., nonsteroidal anti-inflammatory drugs such as Motrin, Advil, and Nuprin) can potentiate anticoagulants and increase the risk of bruising with minimal trauma.

Nicotine Gums and Patches

Nicotine gums and patches are used as smoking substitutes for people who are trying to stop smoking. With **nicotine gum**, the nicotine is absorbed through the oral mucosa, providing sufficient plasma nicotine concentrations to curb the craving to smoke. Nicotine gums are marketed under the names Nicotinell and Nicorette. With transdermal nicotine patches, the nicotine is absorbed through the skin. Nicotine may affect the exercise response, particularly if a person chews nicotine gum but also continues to smoke. Nicotine may increase HR and BP as well as the incidence of cardiac arrhythmias (2).

Bronchodilators

The **bronchodilators** relax smooth muscle surrounding airways in the lungs and relieve the symptoms of asthma, bronchitis, and related lung disorders. These medications can be taken orally or from an inhaler. The inhalers are generally used for acute asthma episodes, whereas long-term bronchodilation is usually obtained with oral preparations. Most of these drugs stimulate the beta-2 receptors that relax bronchial smooth muscle and increase the airway lumen. Because of their beta-adrenergic stimulating effect, they can increase HR and BP, although most of their effect is on the smooth muscle found in airways. Some of the inhaler brand names include Advair, Ventolin, Alupent, and Maxair. The oral bronchodilators include Theobid, Aminophylline, Theo-Dur, and many others (4).

Oral Antiglycemic Agents

A substantial number of obese participants in fitness programs have hyperglycemia, or elevated levels of blood glucose. In this condition the pancreas is able to produce insulin, but it is unable to produce sufficient quantities to maintain normal blood glucose control. This condition is called *type 2 diabetes* or *non-insulin-dependent diabetes mellitus*, and it often can be controlled with **oral antiglycemic agents**. The oral antiglycemic medications stimulate the pancreas to secrete more insulin, which facilitates tissue uptake of glucose. The stimulating action of the oral antiglycemic medications requires a functioning pancreas. Brand names include DiaBeta, Diabinese, Glucotrol, Micronase, Orinase, and Tolinase. These drugs are in the sulfonylurea class (4). Recently, a new type of oral antiglycemic drug has become available (Glucophage, in the metformin class). Metformin reduces insulin resistance, thereby lowering blood sugar. A serious side effect of these drugs is hypoglycemia, or low blood sugar. Hypoglycemia is potentially dangerous, and the fitness professional should be cognizant of any changes in alertness and orientation in patients taking any medication that can lower plasma glucose concentrations.

Insulin-dependent diabetes mellitus, or type 1 diabetes, is a more serious disorder of carbohydrate metabolism. It is characterized by an absence of insulin and requires frequent insulin injections. Insulin cannot be taken orally because it is a protein and would be inactivated by the digestive process. When working with an insulin-dependent diabetic, the fitness professional should be aware of the possibility of hypoglycemia. Signs of hypoglycemia include bizarre behavior and slurred speech. When individuals with insulin-dependent diabetes mellitus are exercising, it is a good idea to have a source of sugar readily available in the event of a hypoglycemic episode. See chapter 20 for additional details on diabetes.

Depressants

Tranquilizers reduce anxiety. Minor tranquilizers may lower HR and BP by controlling anxiety, but otherwise the exercise response is not affected. With major tranquilizers, HR may increase while BP either drops or remains unchanged (2). **Alcohol** is a depressant that can affect the exercise test by impairing motor coordination, balance, and reaction times. Chronic alcohol consumption tends to elevate resting and exercise BP. The acute effects of alcohol ingestion on the exercise response have been examined. During brief maximal exercise, small to moderate doses of alcohol do not affect oxygen uptake, SV, ejection fraction, cardiac output, arteriovenous oxygen difference, and peak lactate concentration (20). However, higher doses (blood alcohol content = 0.20 mg $\cdot$ dl^{-1}) may impair myocardial function, as shown by a 6% decrease in ejection fraction (14). Alcohol intake can provoke arrhythmias at rest and during exercise.

KEY POINT

Medications are prescribed for a variety of reasons, including high BP, abnormal heart rhythms, elevated blood lipids, asthma, and other medical concerns. Appendix D summarizes the common categories of prescription medicines for cardiovascular and related diseases, lists some members of each category, and describes their effects on exercise performance.

STUDY QUESTIONS

1. Draw a picture of the heart, and label the four heart chambers, the four heart valves, the pulmonary artery, and the aorta.

2. Name the coronary arteries, and identify what region of the myocardium they supply blood to.

3. Draw the major components of the heart's electrical conducting system, and label the SA node, AV node, bundle of His, left and right bundle branches, and Purkinje fibers.

4. Define the term *electrocardiogram* (ECG) and give the standard settings for paper speed and amplitude.

5. Identify the electrical event in the heart that corresponds to the P wave, PR segment, QRS complex, and T wave of the ECG.

6. If an individual in normal sinus rhythm has 20 mm between two adjacent R waves, what is the HR? If an individual in atrial fibrillation has 11 complete cardiac cycles in a 6 sec strip, what is the HR?

7. Define the following conduction abnormalities: first-degree AV block, second-degree AV block (Mobitz type I and type II), third-degree AV block.

8. Examine the ECGs in this chapter and point out abnormalities of HR, conduction defects, and arrhythmias.

9. What are the clinical signs (both electrocardiographic signs and plasma markers) associated with an MI (i.e., heart attack). What are the symptoms of a heart attack?

10. List the general categories of cardiovascular medicines and describe their physiological effects on the body.

CASE STUDIES

You can check your answers by referring to appendix A.

1. The following ECG tracing (see case study figure 25.1) was obtained on a 38-yr-old female before she took a GXT on the treadmill.
    a. Determine the HR (beats · min^{-1}) and the durations of the PR interval, QRS complex, and QT interval (in seconds).
    b. What condition does she have?
    c. What factors might cause this condition?

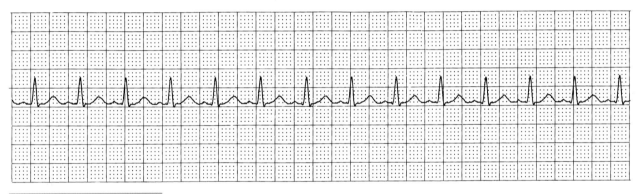

CASE STUDY FIGURE 25.1

2. A 21-yr-old male college student who was taking a cold medication containing ephedrine showed the following ECG tracing at rest (see case study figure 25.2).
    a. What type of arrhythmia does he have?
    b. What is the ventricular rate?

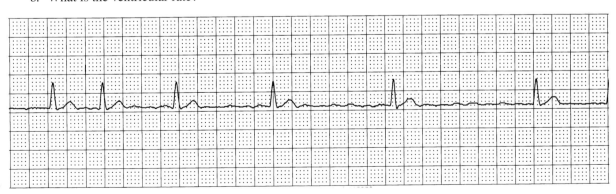

CASE STUDY FIGURE 25.2

3. A 57-yr-old participant in your exercise program showed the following ECG tracing (see case study figure 25.3) while she was exercising at 3.5 mi · hr⁻¹ on a 6% grade on the treadmill.

   a. What ECG abnormality is shown?

   b. What action should be taken?

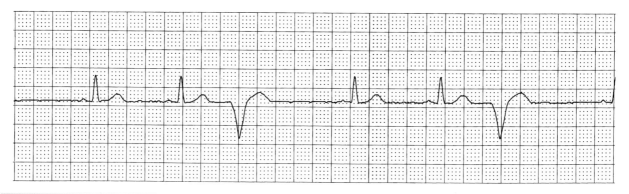

CASE STUDY FIGURE 25.3

4. An apparently healthy 55-yr-old male is referred to your facility for an exercise program and brings with him the results of his most recent exercise test. You notice that the participant was taking Coumadin and Inderal when he took his exercise test. Since the test, his physician has stopped the Inderal. What effect, if any, would this change in medication have on the exercise prescription? (See appendix D)

5. A participant in your exercise program has been taking a beta-blocking medication for several years without experiencing any significant side effects. He was recently given a prescription for Isordil and now reports that he often becomes dizzy upon standing suddenly. Could this be related to his medication? If so, why? (See appendix D)

REFERENCES

1. Ades, P.A., P.G. Gunter, W.L. Meyer, T.C. Gibson, J. Maddalena, and T. Orfeo. 1990. Cardiac and skeletal muscle adaptations to training in systemic hypertension and effect of beta blockade (metoprolol or propranolol). *American Journal of Cardiology* 166(5): 591-596.

2. American College of Sports Medicine (ACSM). 2010. *Guidelines for exercise testing and prescription.* 8th ed. Baltimore: Lippincott Williams & Wilkins.

3. American College of Sports Medicine (ACSM) and American Heart Association (AHA). 2002. Joint position statement: Automated external defibrillators in health/fitness facilities. *Medicine and Science in Sports and Exercise* 34(3): 561-564.

4. American Hospital Formulary Service. 2010. *Drug information 2010.* Bethesda, MD: American Society of Hospital Pharmacists.

5. Berne, R.M., and M.N. Levy. 2001. *Cardiovascular physiology.* 8th ed. St. Louis: Mosby.

6. Chang, K., and K.F. Hossack. 1982. Effect of diltiazem on heart rate responses and respiratory variables during exercise: Implications for exercise prescription and cardiac rehabilitation. *Journal of Cardiac Rehabilitation* 2:326-332.

7. Conover, M.B. 1996. *Understanding electrocardiography.* 7th ed. St. Louis: Mosby.

8. Donnelly, J.E. 1990. *Living anatomy.* 2nd ed. Champaign, IL: Human Kinetics.

9. Dubin, D. 2000. *Rapid interpretation of EKGs.* 6th ed. Tampa: Cover.

10. Ellestad, M.H. 2003 *Stress testing: Principles and practice.* 5th ed. New York: Oxford University Press.

11. Hossack, K.F., R.A. Bruce, and L.J. Clark. 1980. Influence of propranolol on exercise prescription of training heart rates. *Cardiology* 65:47-58.

12. Hurst, J.W. 1994. *Diagnostic atlas of the heart.* Philadelphia: Lippincott-Raven.

13. Kannel, W.B., and R.D. Abbot. 1984. Incidence and prognosis of unrecognized myocardial infarction. *New England Journal of Medicine* 311:1144-1147.

14. Kelbaek, H., T. Gjorup, S. Floistrup, O. Hartling, N. Christensen, and J. Godtfredsen. 1985. Acute effects of alcohol on left ventricular function in healthy subjects at rest and during upright exercise. *American Journal of Cardiology* 55:164-167.

15. Kinderman, W. 1987. Calcium antagonists and exercise performance. *Sports Medicine* 4(3): 177-193.

16. MacGowan, G.A., D. O'Callaghan, and J.H. Horgan. 1992. The effects of verapamil on training in patients with ischemic heart disease. *Chest* 101(2): 411-415.

17. Pavia, L., G. Orlando, J. Myers, M. Maestri, and C. Rusconi. 1995. The effect of beta-blockade therapy on the response to exercise training in postmyocardial infarction patients. *Clinical Cardiology* 18(12): 716-720.

18. Stein, E. 2000. *Rapid analysis of electrocardiograms: A self study program.* 3rd ed. Philadelphia: Lea & Febiger.

19. Tesch, P.A. 1985. Exercise performance and beta-blockade. *Sports Medicine* 2(6): 389-412.

20. Williams, M.H. 1991. Alcohol, marijuana and beta blockers. In *Perspectives in exercise science and sports medicine: Vol. 4. Ergogenics: Enhancement of performance in exercise and sport,* ed. D.R. Lamb and M.H. Williams, 331-372. Dubuque, IA: Brown & Benchmark.

Injury Prevention and Treatment

Sue Carver

The reader will be able to do the following:

1. Describe ways to minimize injury risk and prevent the transmission of bloodborne pathogens.

2. Describe the signs and symptoms of soft-tissue injuries (sprains, strains, contusions, and heel bruises), how to initially treat injuries, and when to use heat in long-term treatment.

3. Identify signs, symptoms, and proper treatment for bone injuries, wounds, and common skin irritations.

4. Describe the causes of heat-related disorders, how to prevent heat illness, and how to treat a heat-related emergency. Provide guidelines for fluid replacement before and after exercise.

5. Explain the causes of cold-related disorders; how to prevent frostnip, superficial and deep frostbite, and hypothermia; and how to treat a cold-related emergency.

6. Distinguish between the signs and symptoms of diabetic coma and those of insulin shock and describe the proper treatment for each.

7. Identify common cardiovascular and pulmonary complications resulting from exercise participation.

8. Identify the signs, symptoms, and management of common orthopedic problems; classify injuries as mild, moderate, and severe; and recommend appropriate modification of exercise programs when injury occurs.

9. Describe procedures to check vital signs.

10. Describe artificial respiration and cardiopulmonary techniques for adults.

The fitness professional must be prepared to safely handle an emergency medical situation. This chapter discusses injury prevention, injury recognition, and common treatment approaches as well as planning for and handling medical emergencies.

Preventing Injuries

Although there are inherent risks associated with participating in physical activity, the benefits far outweigh the risks. The human body is designed for motion. Without use, organs shut down, muscles atrophy, bones become weak, posture becomes dysfunctional, and physical abilities are limited. Most people are not aware of the gradual deterioration of their systems and the loss of function that occurs with a sedentary lifestyle. The price of inactivity may include joint and muscle stiffness, weakness, loss of balance, obesity, loss of normal spinal curves, and poor posture.

Through fitness activities and movement, however, all the major systems of the body can be energized. Mental function may be improved when circulation is increased (22). Regular physical activity reverses some of the neurocognitive decline that occurs with aging, and the prevalence of dementia is reduced in people who are active on a regular basis (32). Increasing respiratory rate stimulates the ability of the lungs to expand and increases the mobility of the rib cage while delivering greater oxygen to the tissues. The increased oxygenation of tissues helps to improve energy levels. Bones, ligaments, and muscles are stimulated to increase in strength, providing increased joint stability and reduced risk of fractures. An increase in metabolic rate improves the burning of calories, reducing the risk for obesity. Physical activity also improves insulin sensitivity and, along with diet modification, may help prevent or correct type 2 diabetes and other chronic disease processes. In middle age, 10% of muscle mass is lost per decade unless strength training is continued into later years. In addition, the ability to move and function is linked to self-esteem and confidence.

Injury risk is reduced by better balance in muscle length and muscle strength, proper posture, and proper function of joints. For those who have sustained an injury, exercise aimed at rebalancing dysfunctional structures while working the body as a closely integrated unit can promote recovery of function (22). As presented in chapter 1, there is a dose–response relationship between physical activity and physical fitness and the risk of CVD and CAD.

Increasing physical activity and fitness levels beyond the minimum recommended amounts has been shown to provide additional health benefits. In other words, more is better (up to a point; see Adverse Events in chapter 1). Likewise, there is an inverse relationship between physi-

cal fitness and type 2 diabetes, obesity, colon cancer, all causes of mortality, and independent living and quality of life among older adults (1).

The fitness professional should be aware of inherent risks associated with activity and control factors that increase the risk of injury. Advanced planning, training in injury recognition and emergency care, adequate equipment and facilities, and counseling in activity selection all help reduce the possibility of injury. The following is a brief discussion of factors contributing to injury and steps that can be taken to reduce injury risk (4-14, 16-18, 21, 24-25, 27, 31, 36).

Controlling Injury Risk

Injury risk in competitive athletic events is controlled by game rules. In exercise programs where games are used for aerobic activity, injury risk may be reduced by controlling the tempo of the activity or by modifying existing rules to enhance participant safety (e.g., limiting body contact, using a softer ball).

The fitness professional should encourage participants to seek professional advice regarding the selection and fitting of exercise equipment. The equipment most commonly used—and most widely abused—is footwear. Inadequately protecting the foot is a major contributor to a variety of leg and low-back problems. Improperly maintained exercise equipment and facilities also contribute to higher overall injury risk.

In this age of concern over bloodborne pathogens such as the **human immunodeficiency virus (HIV)** and **hepatitis B virus (HBV)**, precautions should be taken to protect both the participant and the fitness professional. Open cuts should be covered, and clothing that is saturated with blood should be changed. Necessary supplies should be available to care safely for an open wound, including protective gloves, biohazard containers, antiseptic solution, dressings, disinfectant, and a sharps container if applicable. Participants should be instructed to report all wounds immediately. The fitness professional should know **universal precaution** guidelines for managing acute blood exposure as well as appropriate cleaning and disposal policies for contaminated areas (21).

Contributing Factors to Injury

Activity implies movement, and with increased movement comes a corresponding increase in the risk of injury. In fitness programs, the incidence of injury increases when the frequency of the exercise sessions increases and when the intensity of the exercise is maintained at the high end of the THR zone (figure 26.1). The risk of injury is also heightened by faster movements, as found in competitive activities; by quick changes in direction, as found in fitness games; and by increased focus on smaller muscle groups.

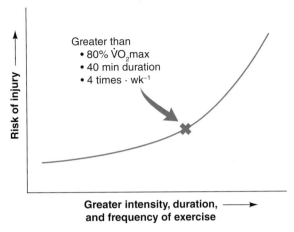

Greater than
• 80% $\dot{V}O_2$max
• 40 min duration
• 4 times · wk^{-1}

Greater intensity, duration, and frequency of exercise

FIGURE 26.1 Risk of injury increases with too much activity.

Environmental conditions such as pollution or poor weather can also increase the risk associated with physical activity. Lack of adaptation to the environment, as well as lack of education in prevention, recognition, and treatment of problems associated with these extreme environments, can lead to devastating results.

Age, sex, and body structure influence the risk of injury. In general, the very young and the very old are at the greatest risk, and older people usually require longer recovery times. Because of differences in body structure and strength, females are often more susceptible to injury in coed activities and games requiring quick changes of direction or body contact. For both males and females, a lack or imbalance of muscle strength, a lack of joint flexibility, and poor CRF increase the chance of injury. Obese participants may not only have low CRF but also excess weight that additionally stresses weight-bearing joints. Participants with specific medical problems such as asthma, diabetes, or known allergic reactions may need special attention to avoid potentially serious complications.

KEY POINT

The fitness professional should be aware of inherent risks associated with activity and minimize risk by planning in advance, using proper equipment and facilities, educating participants regarding injury recognition and care, evaluating participants to determine fitness needs or special health problems that may need monitoring, and giving clear guidelines for graduating activity. The fitness professional should follow universal precautions and use appropriate gloves, biohazard containers, sharps containers, and disinfectant to reduce the spread of bloodborne pathogens.

Reducing Injury Risk

Screening participants can help reduce injury risk before they begin any physical activity program. The screening should highlight the major areas that increase health risk, assist the participant in recognizing problems, and alert the fitness professional to potential problems that could occur in an exercise session (e.g., asthma attack, diabetic shock). Proper planning for emergency situations lowers overall risk. People who cannot be properly supervised or given adequate care for their physical problems should be referred to a program or facility that can provide the needed services. Policies to handle such referrals and all major emergency situations should be written and communicated to all fitness professionals in a fitness center.

A major factor in reducing the risk associated with physical activity is the design and implementation of an exercise program. The program can focus on problems encountered in the preliminary tests, which might include the following:

• Flexibility measures
• Assessment of body composition
• Evaluation of muscular strength, power, and endurance
• Posture assessment
• CRF evaluation

The way the fitness professional conducts the exercise program has a major bearing on the risk of injury to the participant. To highlight this point, figure 26.2 contrasts the "train, don't strain" fitness goal with the "train hard, train smart" performance goal. It is necessary to educate participants about the proper intensity of the exercise session (i.e., to stay in the THR zone) and how to recognize the signs and symptoms of overuse in order to reduce injury risk. The fitness professional should emphasize that the entire program and individual sessions are graduated so the participant will avoid doing too much too soon. This precaution is especially true for people who have not been involved in a regular exercise program and who tend to overestimate their abilities. Overexertion can lead to chronic overuse injuries, extreme muscle soreness, and undue fatigue.

In educating participants about the signs and symptoms of overuse, the fitness professional should distinguish between simple muscle soreness and injury. Muscle soreness tends to peak 24 to 48 hr following exercise and dissipates with use and time. The signs and symptoms of injury include the following:

• Exquisite point tenderness
• Pain that persists even when the body part is at rest
• Joint pain

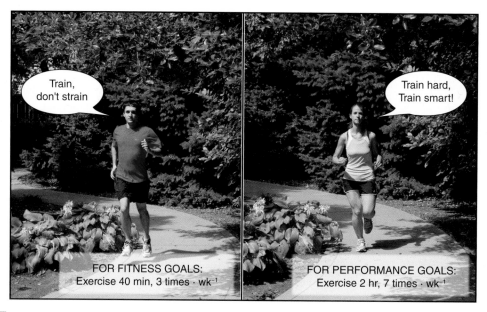

FIGURE 26.2 Fitness training versus performance training.

- Pain that does not go away after warming up
- Swelling or discoloration
- Increased pain with weight-bearing activities or with active movement
- Changes in normal bodily functions

Injury Treatment

Treating an injury depends on the type and severity of the injury. This section describes approaches to take with injuries that are common to fitness programs and sports (3, 4, 7-10, 12-15, 18-21, 23-25, 28-30).

Treating Soft-Tissue Injuries

Sprains (overstretching or tearing of **ligaments**) and strains (overstretching or tearing of muscle or **tendon**) are common injuries associated with adult fitness programs. Most significant injuries to joint structures or to soft tissue require protection, rest, and the immediate application of ice, compression, and elevation (known by the acronym *PRICE*). Figure 26.3 reinforces the **PRICE** concept. Usually, a wet wrap is applied first to give compression. Start distal to the injury and wrap toward the heart. Compression should be firm but not tight. When a joint is involved, apply a wet compression wrap and surround the entire area with ice. Secure with another elastic wrap. If the injury involves a contusion (bruise) or strain to a muscle belly, put the muscle on mild stretch before applying a wet compression bandage and ice. If possible, elevate the injured part above heart level to minimize the effect of gravity and

KEY POINT

When soft tissues are injured, proper assessment and initial treatment can reduce the possibility of further trauma and can aid in the healing process (see table 26.1). Protection, rest, ice, compression, and elevation (PRICE) are the important steps for immediate care of most musculoskeletal and joint injuries. Heat is often used with chronic inflammatory conditions or general muscle soreness; it should be applied in the later stages of an acute injury only when the risk of bleeding into tissues is minimal.

reduce bleeding into tissues. With any injury, shock is a possibility, and the fitness professional should be prepared to handle this situation.

In most cases, the participant should be instructed to continue applying ice from 24 to 72 hr, depending on the severity of the injury. Ice causes vasoconstriction of the blood vessels, thus helping to control bleeding into tissues. Ice also reduces the sensation of pain. Standard treatment times with ice are 15 to 20 min, with reapplication hourly or when pain is experienced. If the possibility of bleeding into the tissues still exists and ice is not being used, the compression bandage should be in place to minimize swelling. Using ice or compression at bedtime is not necessary unless pain interferes with sleep. If this occurs, applying ice frequently (every 1-2 hr) may help control the pain. Physician referral is recommended in cases of moderate or severe injury.

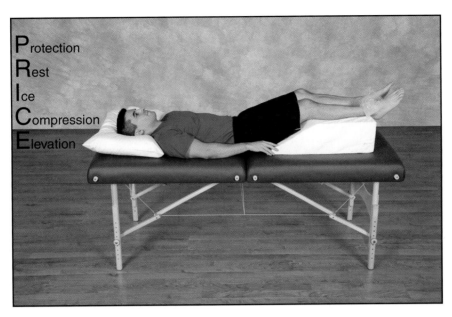

FIGURE 26.3 The PRICE method for treating sprains and strains.

TABLE 26.1 Soft-Tissue Injuries and Their Treatment

Injury	Signs and symptoms	Immediate care

Sprain—stretching or tearing of ligamentous tissue
Strain—overstretching or tearing of muscle or tendon
Contusion—impact force that results in bleeding into the underlying tissues; bruising
	1st degree—mild injury resulting in overstretching or minor tearing of tissue; limited ROM, minimal point tenderness, no swelling
	2nd degree—moderate injury resulting in partial tearing of tissue; limited function, point tenderness and probable muscle spasm, painful ROM, swelling or discoloration (probable if immediate first-aid care is not given)
	3rd degree—severe tearing or rupture of tissue; exquisite point tenderness, immediate loss of function, swelling and muscle spasm likely to be present with discoloration appearing later, possible palpable deformity
		Protection, rest, ice, compression, and elevation (PRICE).
		Usual treatment time:
		   15 to 20 min ice bag
		   5 to 7 min ice cup or ice slush
		How often:
		   Moderate and severe—every hour, or when pain is experienced
		   Less severe—as symptoms necessitate
		Continue with ice treatments at least 24 to 72 hr, depending on the severity of the injury.
		Refer to physician if function is impaired.
		Mild to moderate strains—gradual stretching to the point of discomfort is recommended.

Heel bruise (stone bruise)—sudden abnormal force to heel area that results in trauma to underlying tissues		PRICE Pad for comfort when weight bearing is resumed.

Information from references 2-3, 13-18, 20, 24, 26, 28, 29, 40.

An injured participant may want to apply heat sooner than is warranted. Heat usually is applied in the later stages of an acute injury, when the risk of bleeding into tissues is minimal. In contrast, heat is a common treatment for chronic inflammatory conditions as well as generalized muscle soreness. Heat causes vasodilation of the blood vessels and reduces muscle spasm. Standard treatment time for using a moist heat pack is 15 to 20 min. When in doubt about which mode of treatment to use, ice is the safer choice. Table 26.1 outlines common soft-tissue injuries, signs and symptoms, and immediate care.

Treating Fractures

Fractures, or injury to bone, should be suspected if there is exquisite point tenderness over a bone, visual or palpable deformity, or referred pain to an area of bone upon percussion or vibrational stress. X-rays should be taken if a fracture is suspected. If deformity is present, do not push the bone back into place; instead, splint and refer to a physician. Table 26.2 gives additional procedures to follow when treating a fracture.

Treating Wounds and Other Skin Disorders

Wounds are also common injuries associated with activity programs. The major concern with an open wound is bleeding. Once bleeding is controlled, further care can be given. This may consist of protecting the wound from infection, covering the wound with a bandage, treating the participant for shock, or referring the participant immediately to a physician for suturing. In minor cases, a thorough cleansing and application of a sterile dressing may be all that is needed. The fitness professional should use safety measures to prevent risk from exposure to blood.

Internal bleeding is a very serious condition; the fitness professional should treat for shock and obtain medical assistance immediately.

Shearing and pressure forces are attributable to poorly fitting shoes and socks, poorly conditioned or sensitive skin, and incorrect foot biomechanics that lead to friction and compression injuries of the foot. Hand calluses and other skin irritations can develop from friction during activities that require frequent gripping (e.g., of a tennis racket or a bat) or rubbing of body parts against each other or another object (as is frequently the case in gymnastics or wrestling, for example).

Table 26.3 outlines guidelines for immediate care of wounds. Table 26.4 discusses care of common skin irritations. The fitness professional should use universal precautions in treating an open wound. Protective gloves should be worn when handling potentially infectious materials. Proper disposal of infectious materials and decontamination of infected areas should be a routine policy.

> ## KEY POINT
>
> The steps for dealing with simple and compound fractures, wounds and excessive bleeding, and other skin disorders are listed in tables 26.2, 26.3, and 26.4.

TABLE 26.2 Fractures and Their Treatment

Injury	Signs and symptoms	Immediate care
Fracture—disruption of bone with or without loss of continuity or external exposure, ranging from periosteal irritation to complete separation of bony parts **Simple**—bone fracture without external exposure **Compound**—bone fracture with external exposure	Acute: Direct trauma to bone resulting in disruption of continuity and immediate disability; deformity or bony deviation; swelling, pain, palpable tenderness, referred pain Crepitus, false joint, discoloration (usually becomes apparent later)	Acute: Control bleeding—elevation, pressure points, direct pressure. Treat for shock. If an open fracture, control bleeding, apply sterile dressing, and prevent further disruption and infection; do not move bones back into place. Control swelling with pressure and ice, if wound is closed. Splint above and below the joint and apply traction if necessary. Protect body part from further injury. Refer to physician.
	Chronic: Low-grade inflammatory process causing proliferation of fibroblasts and generalized connective-tissue scarring; progressively worsening pain until present all the time; direct point tenderness	Chronic: Rest and apply heat. Refer to physician.

Information from references 2, 3, 9, 14, 15, 26, 28-29.

TABLE 26.3 Wounds and Their Treatment

Injury	Signs and symptoms	Immediate care
Incision—cutting of skin resulting in an open wound with cleanly cut edges and exposure of underlying tissues	Smooth edges that may bleed freely Signs of infection (see Laceration)	Clean wound with soap and water, moving away from injury site. Minor cuts can be closed with butterfly bandages. Apply a sterile dressing. Refer to a physician if wound needs suturing (e.g., facial cuts and large or deep wounds) or signs of infection are present.
Laceration—tearing of skin resulting in an open wound with jagged edges and exposure of underlying tissues	Jagged edges that may bleed freely Signs of infection: redness; swelling; increase in skin temperature; tender, swollen, and painful lymph glands; mild fever; headache	Soak in antiseptic solution such as hydrogen peroxide to loosen foreign material. Clean with antiseptic soap and water using sterile technique and moving away from the injury site. Apply sterile dressing. Instruct person to seek medical attention if signs of infection are recognized. Usually refer to a physician; a tetanus shot or sutures may be needed. If injury is extensive, control bleeding, cover with thick sterile bandages, and treat for shock. Refer to a physician.
Puncture—direct penetration of tissues by a pointed object	Small opening that may bleed freely Signs of infection (see Laceration)	If object is embedded deeply: Protect body part and refer to physician for removal and care. Treat for shock. Clean around wound, moving away from injury site. Allow wound to bleed freely to minimize risk of infection. Apply sterile dressing. Puncture wounds are usually referred to a physician; tetanus shot may be needed. Instruct person to seek medical attention if signs of infection are present.
Abrasion—scraping of tissues resulting in removal of outermost layers of skin and exposure of numerous capillaries	Superficial, reddish, irregular surface Oozing or weeping from underlying capillaries May contain dirt, debris, or bacteria embedded in tissue	Debride and flush with antiseptic solution such as hydrogen peroxide; then cleanse with soap and water. Apply petroleum-based antiseptic agent to keep wound moist and allow healing to take place from the deeper layers. Cover with nonadherent gauze. Instruct person to seek medical help if signs of infection are recognized.
Excessive bleeding—internal or external bleeding that results in massive loss of circulating blood volumes; often results in shock and can lead to death	External hemorrhage 1. Arterial Color: bright red Flow: spurts, bleeding usually profuse 2. Venous Color: dark red Flow: steady, oozing	Elevate affected part above heart. Put direct pressure over the wound, using a sterile compress if possible. Apply a pressure dressing. Use pressure points. Treat for shock. Refer to a physician.

(continued)

TABLE 26.3 *(continued)*

Injury	Signs and symptoms	Immediate care
Internal bleeding— bleeding within deep structures of the body (chest, abdominal, or pelvic cavity) and bleeding of organs contained within these cavities	Generally, no external signs, except when an individual coughs up blood or finds blood in the urine or feces or experiences the following: Restlessness Thirst Faintness Anxiety Cold, clammy skin Dizziness Rapid, weak, irregular pulse Significant BP fall	Treat for shock. Refer to hospital immediately. Don't give water or food.
Shock caused by bleeding	Restlessness Anxiety Weak, rapid pulse Cold, clammy, skin temperature; profuse sweating Pale skin color, later cyanotic Shallow, labored respiration Dull eyes Dilated pupils Thirsty Nausea and possible vomiting Marked BP fall	Maintain an open airway. Control bleeding. Elevate lower extremities approximately 12 in. (31 cm) (exceptions: heart problems, head injury, or breathing difficulty—place in comfortable position, usually semireclining, unless spinal injury is suspected, in which case do not move). Splint any fractures. Maintain normal body temperature. Avoid further trauma. Monitor vital signs and record at regular intervals (every 5 min or so). Do not feed or give any liquids.

Information from references 2-3, 9-11, 13-19, 21, 26-28, 36, 39.

Environmental Concerns

The environment can play a detrimental role in the development of serious medical issues. Breathing problems, dangerous changes in HR and BP, and a decline in mental clarity and the ability to focus can result from extreme weather conditions. In addition, pollution can be a major factor in performance and safety, particularly in urban areas, where pollution from factories and motor vehicles may be more prevalent.

People who are affected by asthma or who have allergies could have extreme reactions to exercising outdoors, particularly when pollen counts or pollution levels are high. Extreme hot or cold temperatures, wind, or precipitation can prove deadly in some instances. This section examines these issues and discusses ways to minimize risk to participants.

Pollution

Fitness professionals must take into consideration the general health of the population they are working with and the environmental conditions that prevail. Although pollution can occur in any environment, air pollution is generally more of a concern in urban areas. (37) Awareness of environmental conditions such as weather, humidity level and temperature, pollution index, and pollen count is needed in order to determine appropriate times and places for activity. People with asthma, severe allergies, or other breathing problems may be severely affected by pollutants or allergens in the air. High concentrations of pollutants can affect health and performance. Breathing may become more difficult because of a decreased capacity to transport oxygen to the tissues or an increase in lung resistance. Burning eyes and burning lungs may alter the perception of effort. Small particles of pollutants can cause a lung

TABLE 26.4 Skin Irritations and Their Treatment

Skin irritation	Signs and symptoms	Immediate care
Blister—collection of serum just below the superficial layer of skin	Defined area of fluid accumulation under skin Feels hot Painful to touch	Prevent by engaging in heavy activity slowly and toughening skin with astringents (tannic acid or salt water). Stop activity if friction area develops, apply ice, and cover irritation with friction-proofing material or donut pad. Prevent contamination of torn blister; clean with soap and water. Refer to physician if signs of infection are present.
Callus—markedly thickened area of skin, usually over an area of pressure	Visible and excessive callus formation: May be painful May have cracks or fissures May become infected May develop blisters	Prevent excessive callus formation by using an emery callus file. Take measures to reduce friction by wearing properly fitted shoes and socks, using powder or lubricant, and correcting abnormal biomechanical foot faults with orthotics. Protect susceptible areas by using special protective devices such as gloves, tape, or pad. Prevent infection by keeping callus trimmed and using lubricant to prevent cracks and tears in callus.
Corns **Hard corn**—thickening of skin on toes **Soft corn**—circular area of thickened, white, macerated skin between toes and proximal head of phalanges	Local pain Inflammation and thickening of soft tissue Generally seen on top of toes and associated with hammer toes Pain and inflammation	Prevent by wearing properly fitted shoes or fitting with orthotics if cause is due to abnormal foot biomechanics. Control moisture accumulation by keeping skin dry between toes. Separate toes with cotton or lamb's wool.
Ingrown toenail—leading side edge of toenail grows into soft tissue	Severe inflammation, pain, and infection	Apply hot antiseptic soaks for 20 min, 2 to 3 times daily, at 110 to 120 °F (43.4-48.9 °C). When toenail is pliable, insert wisp of cotton under leading edge of toenail and lift from soft tissue beneath. Refer to physician or podiatrist if signs of infection are present.
Intertrigo—chafing due to excessive rubbing of body parts in combination with perspiration	Pain, inflammation, burning, itching, moistness, cracking, lesion	Cleanse frequently. Use medicated drying powder.
Plantar wart—viral infection on foot leading to localized overgrowth of skin; can be confused with callus	Distinct edge with central core Sometimes appears to be growing inward; small black dot in center surrounded by clearer callus area Excessive thickening of skin	Use donut to take pressure off wart. Keep callus area around wart filed down (do not file down wart). See physician or podiatrist for cure or removal.

Information from references 13-17, 18-19, 26, 28, 34, 36, 39.

infection that could pass through the epithelium into the circulation. And fine-particle pollution can cause a rise in BP and compromise a person with preexisting CVD. (32)

Training or exercising should not be scheduled during times of peak pollution. Participants should be advised if there is a high index for certain allergens. The air quality index (AQI), regulated by the Clean Air Act, measures the quality of the air for five major pollutants. See chapter 11 for information about the AQI and values and recommendations for participation.

KEY POINT

A high pollution index or extreme pollen counts can compromise the performance and health of participants. The fitness professional must be aware of environmental conditions and the sensitivities of the people they are training. Activities should be scheduled during times and places where the participants are unlikely to be affected.

Heat-Related Problems

Heat illness can strike anyone. Poor physical condition, although a contributing factor, is not the primary cause; even the most highly conditioned athlete can experience a heat-related disorder. Exercise and the environment can place large heat loads on the body. Environmental heat loads stimulate sweat production because **evaporation** of sweat is the major mechanism for cooling the body. As a result, large amounts of water may be lost during physical activity, causing an increase in the core body temperature, or **hyperthermia**. If too much water is lost, circulatory collapse and death can occur. The following information outlines methods of recognizing dehydration (excessive loss of body fluids) and preventing heat illness. A water loss up to 3% of body weight is considered safe. A 3% to 5% loss is considered borderline, and more than a 5% loss is considered serious. Water loss can be monitored by weighing participants before and after activity. People who are outside the 3% range from one workout to the next may have an increased risk of heat injury and should be monitored carefully if they are allowed to participate.

The practical experience of military and athletic teams working in the heat and humidity has led to guidelines for preventing heat injury. Applying these guidelines to adult fitness programs will enhance participants' enjoyment and safety. Participants should do the following to prevent heat injury:

- Acclimatize to heat and humidity by gradually increasing training intensity and duration over 7 to 10 days.

- Hydrate before activity and frequently during activity.

- Decrease the intensity of exercise if the temperature or humidity is high; use THR as a guide.

- Monitor weight loss by weighing before and after workouts. Consume fluids if more than 3% of body weight is lost during activity. Minimize participation until weight is within the 3% range.

- Consume a high carbohydrate meal, which has high water content and helps to maintain fluid balance.

- Wear appropriate clothing for hot or humid weather conditions. Expose as much skin surface as possible.

Further precautions include wearing light-colored clothing, because lighter colors do not retain as much heat as darker colors, and wearing cotton materials that absorb sweat and allow evaporation to occur. Certain synthetic clothing and materials with paint screens do not absorb sweat and should be avoided.

Participants should be educated to recognize symptoms of overexertion: nausea or vomiting, extreme breathlessness, dizziness, unusual fatigue, muscle cramping, and headache. Symptoms related to heat illness include hair standing on end on the chest or upper arms, body chills, headache or throbbing pressure, nausea, vomiting, labored breathing, dry lips, extreme cotton mouth, faintness (heat syncope), muscle cramping (heat cramps), and cessation of sweating. Heat rash can also be a symptom and is attributable to inflamed sweat glands. It usually occurs in children who have sweated profusely. If these symptoms are present, the risk for developing heat exhaustion or heatstroke rises dramatically, and participants should stop activity and get into the shade. In addition, participants should be instructed to ask for help if they are disoriented or if the symptoms are severe. The fitness professional should provide fluids and encourage everyone to drink.

People who experience heatstroke may sustain permanent damage to their thermoregulatory system. People who do not have efficient cooling mechanisms are susceptible to heat injury, as are people who take medications such as antihistamines or diuretics, consume high quantities of salt in their diet or salt tablets, or drink alcohol in large quantities (particularly before activity). Furthermore, people who participate in physical activity while experiencing fever could elevate their body temperature to dangerous levels. Table 26.5 outlines the various stages of heat illness, the signs and symptoms associated with each, and guidelines for immediate care.

Be aware of environmental factors such as relative humidity and temperature. The relative humidity can be calculated by measuring dry-bulb and wet-bulb atmospheric temperatures (see chapter 11) using a sling psychrometer. As mentioned earlier, evaporation of sweat is a primary means to lose heat during exercise. This fluid loss must be replaced to minimize health risk and maximize safe and enjoyable participation in an exercise program. For most participants in CRF programs, thirst is an adequate indicator of when to hydrate. Generally, replacing fluids as they are used is the best way to meet the demands of the body. When extreme sweating or dry atmospheric conditions are present, however, the thirst mechanism may not keep up with the need for fluid intake.

Normal daily fluid intake for the sedentary person is between 60 and 80 oz (1.8-2.4 L). The actual fluid requirement depends on too many factors to establish a single recommendation for maintaining hydration. However, drinking 8 to 10 oz (240-300 ml) of fluid before heavy exercise, in addition to drinking frequently during activity, helps prevent heat illness.

TABLE 26.5 Heat-Related Problems and Their Treatment

Heat illness	Signs and symptoms	Immediate care
Heat cramps—spasmodic muscular contractions caused by exertion in extreme heat	Muscle cramping (calf is common location) Multiple cramping (very serious)	Isolated cramps: Apply pressure to the cramp and release, stretch muscle slowly and gently, and apply gentle massage and ice. Hydrate by drinking lots of water. Multiple cramps: Danger of heatstroke; treat as heat exhaustion.
Heat exhaustion—collapse with or without loss of consciousness, suffered in conditions of heat and high humidity, largely resulting from the loss of fluid and salt by sweating	Profuse sweating Cold, clammy skin Normal or slightly elevated temperature Pale Dizzy Weak, rapid pulse Shallow breathing Nausea Headache Loss of consciousness Thirst	Move person out of the sun to a well-ventilated area. Place in shock position, with feet elevated 12 to 18 in. (31-46 cm); prevent heat loss or gain. Gently massage the extremities. Apply gentle ROM movement to the extremities. Force consumption of fluids. Reassure the person. Monitor body temperature and other vital signs. Refer to a physician.
Heatstroke—final stage of heat exhaustion in which the thermoregulatory system shuts down to conserve depleted fluid levels	Generally no perspiration Dry skin Very hot Temperature as high as 106 °F (41.1 °C) Skin color bright red or flushed (dark-pigmented people will have ashen skin) Rapid, strong pulse Labored breathing Change in behavior Unresponsive	Treat as extreme medical emergency. Transport to hospital quickly. Remove as much clothing as possible without exposing the person. Cool quickly, starting at the head and continuing down the body; use any means possible (fan, hose down, pack in ice). Wrap in cold, wet sheets for transport. Treat for shock; if breathing is labored, place in semireclining position.
Heat syncope—fainting or excessive loss of strength because of excessive heat	Headache Nausea	Normal intake of fluids.

Information from references 2-3, 13-17, 33-36, 38-40.

Salt and other minerals may be lost during prolonged exercise, particularly during hot and humid weather. Even so, using **salt tablets** is not recommended unless accompanied by a large intake of water. Water with a 0.1% to 0.2% salt solution may be given to people with high water loss. Consuming more salt at mealtimes and a high intake of water throughout the day, however, generally meets the body's need for sodium and fluid replacement.

Most **electrolyte** drinks are diluted solutions of glucose, salt, and other minerals, with added artificial flavoring. Some brands also contain as much as 200 to 300 kcal in 1 qt (946 ml) of solution. Other than sodium, the minerals provided by an electrolyte solution do not provide much benefit. When sweating is profuse, large amounts of electrolyte solution may serve the same function as a diluted salt solution. In cases of mild to moderate sweating, the normal intake of salt in food adequately replaces sodium. The main advantage of using a flavored solution is that the person might drink more than if ingesting plain water or a salt solution. However, considering the prices of commercially prepared electrolyte solutions, plain water or homemade solutions, such as the one presented here, are much more economical.

Homemade Electrolyte Solution

1 qt (946 ml) water

1/3 tsp. (5 ml) salt

0.5 to 1.5 tbsp. (7-22 ml) sugar for flavoring

Fluids at a temperature of 5 to 15 °C (41-59 °F) are absorbed faster than fluids at other temperatures.

KEY POINT

Inefficient body cooling mechanisms, certain medications, high intake of salt or alcohol, and exercising with a fever or in high heat and humidity may cause heat-related disorders. Heat illness is potentially deadly, and the fitness professional must be aware of ways to prevent it and must be able to recognize the signs of heat illness and take action (see table 26.5). Proper hydration, evaluated through a weight chart, is a good first step in prevention. Provide water before, during, and after activity to prevent dehydration.

Cold-Related Problems

Exercising in cold, windy weather can cause problems if certain precautions are not taken. Considerable heat loss can occur through convective heat loss from the skin and evaporation of skin moisture. Hypothermia occurs when body heat is lost at a faster rate than it is produced and core body temperature drops below 35 °C (95 °F). Peripheral blood vessels in cold areas constrict, which conserves body heat but increases the risk of frostbite. Exercising in cold, rainy weather can compound the problem by increasing the rate of evaporation. Windchill is another factor that must be taken into account. A high windchill factor can result in severe loss of body heat even when the air temperature is above freezing (see chapter 11). Additionally, body temperature drops even more quickly in cold water than in air of the same temperature. Cold-related problems are preventable if participants follow these precautions:

- Avoid exercising outdoors in extreme cold and wind.
- Layer clothing and remove layers as needed to avoid sweating.
- Warm up before exercise and avoid bouts of inactivity.
- Stay dry.
- Cover the face, nose, ears, fingers, and head (a great deal of heat is lost when the head is exposed).
- Avoid swimming or exercising in cold water, particularly when the surrounding air temperature is low.

Table 26.6 describes how to recognize and treat cold-related problems.

KEY POINT

Exercising in cold, rainy weather or when the windchill factor is high, as well as exercising in cold water, may lead to cold-related disorders. Precautionary measures such as avoiding exposure to extreme cold, wearing removable layers, warming up before activity, remaining constantly active, and understanding the effect of windchill on air temperature can help prevent cold-related problems. See table 26.6 for specific advice on how to treat cold-related problems.

Medical Concerns

Some people have controlled medical conditions that might be aggravated by exercise. In addition, it is important to recognize major cardiovascular and respiratory problems. This section summarizes common medical concerns.

Diabetic Reactions

The fitness professional should be familiar with the signs and symptoms of diabetic coma and insulin shock (see table 26.7). When an emergency arises and a person with diabetes is conscious, she is usually able to name the problem. If she cannot tell you the problem, then ask

TABLE 26.6 Cold-Related Problems and Their Treatment

Cold-related problems	Signs and symptoms	Immediate care
Deep frostbite—freezing of deep tissue, including muscle and bone	Hard, cold, numb, pale, or white area Permanent tissue damage may be sustained	Protect body part. Remove jewelry from injured part. Remove from further cold exposure. Handle gently. Refer to a physician. Rapid rewarming is necessary.
Frostnip—freezing of tips of extremities such as ears, nose, or fingers, involving only the surface of the skin	Skin firm and cold Burning, itching, local redness Skin may peel or blister in a day or two	Rewarm by applying firm pressure over the affected area, blowing warm air over the area, submerging in warm water 100 to 105 °F (37.8-40.6 °C), and holding frostnip area against body.
Superficial frostbite—freezing of skin layers and subcutaneous tissue	Pale, waxy, cold skin Purple coloring Following rewarming there may be swelling and superficial blisters Stinging, burning, and aching may be present for several days or weeks	Remove from cold. Rewarm area.
Hypothermia—core body temperature drops below 95 °F (35.0 °C)	Shivering Impairment of neuromuscular function Decreased ability to make decisions Muscle rigidity Hypotension Shock Death	Treat as a medical emergency. Remove from cold. Treat for shock. Immediately transport to hospital.

Information from references 2-3, 13-17, 33-36, 38-39.

when food was last eaten and whether insulin was taken that day. If the person has eaten but has not taken insulin, then she is probably going into a diabetic coma, a condition in which there is too little insulin to fully metabolize the carbohydrate consumed (hyperglycemia). If the person has taken insulin but has not eaten, then she is probably experiencing insulin shock, a condition in which there is too much insulin or not enough carbohydrate to balance the insulin intake (hypoglycemia).

If the person lapses into unconsciousness, check for a medical-alert identification tag to try to identify the problem. If you don't know whether the person is suffering from diabetic coma or insulin shock, give sugar. Brain damage or death can occur quickly if insulin shock is left untreated; it is a far more critical state than diabetic coma. If the problem is insulin shock, the person should respond within 1 to 2 min; at that point you should transport the person to a hospital as quickly as possible. If the individual is in a diabetic coma, there is little chance of seriously worsening the condition by giving sugar. Several hours of fluid and insulin therapy under a physician's direction will

be needed. Table 26.7 outlines the diabetic reactions, their signs and symptoms, and their immediate care.

KEY POINT

Diabetic coma results from extreme hyperglycemia, whereas insulin shock is attributable to extreme hypoglycemia.

Cardiovascular and Pulmonary Complications

Cardiovascular complications can occur with injury because of decreased circulating blood volumes, as may occur with bleeding, hyperthermia or hypothermia, shock, or heart attack. The fitness professional should be able to recognize and deal with potential complications such as **tachycardia** (excessively rapid heartbeat), **bradycardia** (abnormally slow heartbeat), **hypertension** (high BP), and **hypotension** (low BP).

TABLE 26.7 Diabetic Reactions and Their Treatment

Diabetic reaction	Signs and symptoms	Immediate care
Diabetic coma/hyperglycemia—loss of consciousness caused by too little insulin	Headache Confused Disoriented Stuporous Nauseated Coma Flushed, dry skin Cherry red lids Decreased body temperature Sweet, fruity breath odor Vomiting Abdominal pain Air hunger Rapid, weak, thready pulse Normal or slightly low BP Unconsciousness	Call for medical assistance. Little can be done unless insulin is at hand. If medical assistance is not quickly available, 1. treat as shock, 2. administer fluids in large amounts by mouth if person is conscious, 3. maintain an open airway, 4. turn the head to the side to prevent aspirating vomitus, and 5. do not give sugar, carbohydrate, or fat in any form. Recovery—gradual improvement over 6 to 12 hr. Fluid and insulin therapy should be directed by a physician.
Insulin shock/hypoglycemia—anxiety, excitement, perspiration, delirium, or coma caused by too much insulin or not enough carbohydrate to balance insulin intake	Pale skin (dark-pigmented people will appear ashen) Moist and clammy skin; cold sweat Normal or rapid and bounding pulse Normal or slightly elevated BP Normal or shallow and slow breathing Weakness on one side of body No odor of acetone on breath Intense hunger Possible double vision Unusual behavior—confused, aggressive, lethargic Fainting, seizure, coma, or unconsciousness	Administer sugar as quickly as possible (e.g., orange juice, candy). If person is unconscious, place sugar granules under the tongue. If person is unconscious or recovery is slow, call for medical assistance. Recovery—generally quick (1-2 min). Refer to a physician if still unconscious or recovery is slow.

Information from references 2-3, 13-17, 24, 26.

Pulmonary complications may be observed more readily. **Apnea**, or temporary cessation of breathing, can be caused by an obstructed airway, allergic reaction, drowning, or intrathoracic injury. Dyspnea, or labored breathing, can be caused by hyperventilation, asthma, and chest or lung injury. **Tachypnea**, excessively rapid breathing, may be a sign of overexertion, shock, or hyperventilation. The fitness professional should feel comfortable assessing circulation and respiration and should have the knowledge and skills to perform appropriate emergency procedures.

Common respiratory disorders include hyperventilation, asthma, and airway obstruction. Hyperventilation can occur with heavy exhalation or rapid breathing, resulting in breathing out too much carbon dioxide (CO_2) and thereby reducing CO_2 levels in the blood. Low CO_2 levels may cause dizziness, faintness, chest pains, and tingling in the feet and hands. Reassuring the person in a calm manner, encouraging a slower breathing rate, and helping the person breathe into a paper bag or into hands cupped over the nose and mouth will help restore CO_2 levels.

Asthma is a condition in which the smooth muscles of the bronchial tubes go into spasm; edema and inflammation of the mucous lining are triggered by exercise, changes in barometric pressure or temperature, virus, emotional stress, and noxious odors. The affected person may appear anxious, pale, and sweaty; may cough or wheeze; and may seem short of breath. Hyperventilation may occur, resulting in dizziness, and, because of mucous secretions, the person may frequently try to clear the throat.

The fitness professional should be prepared to handle an asthma attack. Generally, people with asthma know how to care for themselves and carry medication. Individuals with exercise-induced asthma are often prescribed medication to take before activity. Encourage people with asthma to drink water, and promote relaxation and breathing exercises. Remove any known irritants from the environment if possible. If bronchial spasm is excessive, seek medical attention.

Airway obstruction can occur when a foreign object or the tongue blocks the airway. If breathing is labored but the person is coughing forcefully, stay with him and encourage continued coughing. If, however, the person is unsuccessful in expelling the object or the airway becomes totally blocked, have someone call for an ambulance and begin the **Heimlich maneuver** (abdominal thrusts). In an unconscious person, visually checking the airway passage and removing a seen object with the fingers or using the Heimlich maneuver for an unseen object may dislodge a known obstruction. Generally, moving the lower jaw forward or tilting the head and lifting the chin will open an airway blocked by the tongue. **Rescue breathing** should be performed if the person has stopped breathing and repositioning the head does not change the status.

Respiratory shock, a condition in which the lungs are unable to supply enough oxygen to the circulating blood, can result in a medical emergency. Signs and symptoms include restlessness and anxiety; cool, clammy skin; weak, rapid pulse; profuse sweating, rapid, shallow breathing; decreased BP; and changes in personality (including disinterest, irritability, and excitement). In the later stages, paleness of skin or cyanosis may be evident, and the patient may complain of extreme thirst, feel nauseated, or vomit. Fainting may occur.

Treatment includes maintaining body heat and elevating feet and legs 12 to 18 in. (31-46 cm). If head or neck injury is suspected, protect the involved area and raise the head and shoulders by placing a pillow or rolled-up blanket underneath the person. Keep the individual warm, reassure her, and seek medical attention. Employ CPR techniques (discussed later in this chapter).

KEY POINT

Common cardiovascular complications from exercise include excessively rapid or abnormally slow heartbeat and high or low BP. Pulmonary complications include temporary cessation of breathing, labored breathing, and airway obstruction.

Common Orthopedic Problems

Many injuries that are commonly referred to an orthopedic physician for diagnosis and treatment result from overuse or irritation of a chronic musculoskeletal problem. In most instances, the injuries do not immediately incapacitate the participant, and it may be weeks or months after the onset of pain before the participant seeks medical consultation. By this time, the inflammation is severe and generally prevents normal function of the part involved. In many cases, a severe injury can be avoided if proper care is initiated early. Table 26.8 outlines common orthopedic problems, their causes, their signs and symptoms, and general treatment guidelines.

Shin Splints

Shin splint is a catchall expression used to describe a variety of conditions of the lower leg. The term is often used to define any pain located between the knee and the ankle (usually anterior medial and lateral). Diagnosis of shin splints should be limited to conditions involving inflammation of the musculotendinous unit caused by overexertion of muscles during weight-bearing activity. A more specific diagnosis is preferred over the general term *shin splint*. In any event, the physician must rule out the following conditions: stress fracture, metabolic or vascular disorder, **compartment syndrome**, and muscular strain. Physical complaints often accompanying shin splint pain include the following:

- A dull ache in the lower leg after workouts
- Decreased performance and work output because of pain
- Soft-tissue pain
- Mild swelling along the area of inflammation
- Slight temperature elevation at the site of inflammation
- Pain when moving the foot up and down

People with shin splints usually have no history of trauma. The symptoms start gradually and progress if activity is not reduced. The following is the usual symptomatic treatment:

- Rest in the acute stage; reduce weight-bearing activity.
- In mild cases brought on by overuse, decrease or modify activity for a few days (e.g., choose swimming or cycling workouts instead of running).
- Apply heat or ice before activity; use ice after activity. Heat treatments may consist of applying moist heat packs for 15 to 20 min or using a whirlpool. The temperature of the whirlpool water should be approximately 100 to 106 °F (37.8-41.1 °C). Treatment time is usually 15 to 20 min. Ice treatment may consist of applying an ice bag for 15 to 20 min or applying ice massage or ice slush for 5 to 7 min.

TABLE 26.8 Common Orthopedic Problems and Their Treatment

Injury	Common causes	Signs and symptoms	Treatment
Inflammatory reactions **Bursitis—** inflammation of bursa (sac between a muscle and bone that is filled with fluid, facilitates motion, provides padding, and helps to prevent abnormal function) **Capsulitis—**inflammation of joint capsule **Epicondylitis—** inflammation of muscles or tendons attached to epicondyles of humerus **Myositis—**inflammation of voluntary muscle **Plantar fasciitis—** inflammation of connective tissue spanning bottom of foot **Tendinitis—**inflammation of tendon (band of tough, inelastic, fibrous tissue that connects muscle to bone) **Tenosynovitis—** inflammation of tendinous sheath **Synovitis—**inflammation of synovial membrane	Overuse Improper joint mechanics Improper technique Pathology Trauma Infection	Redness Swelling Pain Increased skin temperature over area of inflammation Tenderness Involuntary muscle guarding	Ice and rest in the acute stages. If chronic, use heat before exercise or activity, followed by ice after activity. Massage. Perform muscle-stretching exercises. Correct cause of problem. If correction of cause and symptomatic treatment do not relieve symptoms, refer to physician; anti-inflammatory medication is usually prescribed. If disease process or infection is suspected, refer to physician immediately.
Tennis elbow—inflammation of musculotendinous unit of elbow extensors where they attach on outer aspect of elbow (lateral epicondylitis)	Faulty backhand mechanics, such as leading with elbow, using improper grip, dropping racket head, or using topspin backhand with whipping motion Improper grip size (usually too small) Racket strung too tightly Hitting off center, particularly if using wet, heavy balls Overuse of forearm supinators, wrist extensors, and finger extensors	Pain directly over outer aspect of elbow in region of common extensor origin Swelling Increased skin temperature over area of inflammation Pain on extension of middle finger against resistance with elbow extended Pain upon racket gripping and extension of wrist	Ice and rest in the acute stages. If chronic, use heat before exercise or activity, followed by ice after activity. Apply deep friction massage at elbow. Perform strengthening and stretching exercises for wrist extensors. Correct cause of problem: 1. Use proper techniques. 2. Use proper grip size (when racket is gripped, there should be room for one finger to fit in gap between thumb and fingers). 3. Use racket that is strung at proper tension (usually 50-55 lb, or 22.7-25.0 kg. 4. Avoid stiff rackets that vibrate easily. Keep elbow warm, particularly in cold weather. Use counterforce brace (circular band placed just below elbow to reduce stress at origin of extensors). If correction of cause and symptomatic treatment do not relieve symptoms, refer to physician; anti-inflammatory medication is usually prescribed.

Injury	Common causes	Signs and symptoms	Treatment
Mechanical low-back pain— pain that results from poor body mechanics, inflexibility of certain muscle groups, or muscular weakness	Tight low-back musculature Tight hamstrings Poor posture or postural habits Weak trunk musculature, particularly abdominal muscles Differences in leg length due to structural or functional problem Structural abnormality Obesity	Generalized low-back pain, usually aggravated by activity that accentuates the curve in low back (e.g., hill running) Muscle spasm Palpable tenderness limited to musculature and not located directly over spine Possible difference in pelvic height or other signs that indicate possible leg-length discrepancy Muscle tightness, particularly of hamstrings, hip flexors, and low back	Refer anyone with acute onset of low-back pain or any signs of nerve impingement to physician for evaluation and X-ray. Rule out structural abnormalities such as spondylolisthesis, ruptured disc, fracture, neoplasm, or possible segmental instability before instituting general exercise program. Further diagnostic procedures may be warranted. Symptomatic treatment consists of ice application and referral to physician in acute cases. Chronic cases are generally treated with moist heat to reduce muscle spasm and ice after activity. Correct the causes of low-back pain: 1. Stretch tight muscles. 2. Strengthen weak muscles. 3. Thoroughly warm up before activity and cool down following activity. 4. Correct leg-length differences. 5. Emphasize correct postural positions. 6. If possible, correct or compensate for structural abnormality (e.g., orthotics for biomechanical problem; heel lift for true leg-length deficit).

Information from references 13, 16-18, 29.

Treatment should begin at the first sign of pain. If pain is extreme, the participant should see a doctor. Determining and treating the cause, in addition to symptomatic treatment, are necessary to prevent recurrence. Table 26.9 cites the major causes for shin splints as well as the signs and symptoms and steps that can be taken to prevent the onset or recurrence of lower-leg pain.

Exercise Modification

Most orthopedic injuries can be classified as mild, moderate, or severe. When in doubt, conservative treatment is recommended. Any injury that results in acute pain or affects performance and any injury in which the person hears or feels a pop at the time of injury should be referred to a physician. If conservative measures fail to improve the condition within a reasonable time (2-4 wk), physician consultation is again recommended.

Other conditions may call for modifying the exercise program. The participant may be obese or arthritic or may have a history of musculoskeletal problems. Exercise in a pool is often employed with such participants since warm water is therapeutic, supports the body weight, and generally allows for a greater range of movement. In any case, the activity should suit the condition. Anyone who requires exercise modification should be monitored closely. Table 26.10 summarizes the general guidelines for classifying injuries and offers suggestions for modifying activity.

TABLE 26.9 Shin Splint Syndrome

Injury	Common causes	Signs and symptoms	Treatment
Shin splints—inflammatory reaction of musculotendinous unit, caused by overexertion of muscles during weight-bearing activity (following conditions must be ruled out: stress fracture, metabolic or vascular disorder, compartment syndrome, muscular strain)	Fallen metatarsal arch Weak longitudinal arch Muscular imbalance Poor leg, ankle, and foot flexibility Improper running surface Improper running shoes Overuse Biomechanical problems or structural abnormalities Improper running or skills technique Training in poor weather	Lower longitudinal arch on one side in comparison to opposite side Tenderness in arch area Abnormal wear patterns of shoes Prominent callus in metatarsal region	Keep callus filed down. Wear a metatarsal arch pad. Conduct strengthening exercises for toe flexors. Wear longitudinal arch tape for support. Wear arch supports. Conduct strengthening exercises for the dorsiflexors and inverters. Exercise to increase ROM. Avoid hard surfaces. Avoid changing from one surface to another. Select shoes that absorb shock well; be sure that shoes are properly fitted. Be flexible about changing training program if there are signs that a great deal of physical stress is occurring. Encourage year-round conditioning. Always warm up properly. Refer to podiatrist or other professional specializing in foot care; orthotics may be indicated. Design special training program to allow for individual differences (e.g., increase intensity of workouts and reduce duration). Correct technique. Perform specific stretching or strengthening exercises as well as technique work. Use common sense when training in cold or inclement weather. Dress properly to maintain warmth. Warm up and cool down properly.
Stress fracture—bone defect that occurs because of overstress to weight-bearing bones, which accelerates rate of remodeling; inability of bone to meet demands of stress results in loss of continuity in bone and periosteal irritation **Tibial stress fractures—**more common in people with high arches in feet **Fibula stress fractures—**more common in pronators	Overuse or abrupt change in training program Change in running surface Change in running gait	Referred pain to fracture site when percussion test is used (e.g., hitting the heel may cause pain at site of tibial stress fracture) Pain usually localized to one spot and exquisitely tender to palpation Pain generally present all of the time but increases with weight-bearing activity; no lessening of pain after warm-up	Refer to physician. X-rays should be obtained. Usually no crack is detected in the bone. A cloudy area becomes visible when the callus begins to form. Often this does not show up until 2 to 6 wk after onset of pain. Early detection can usually be made through bone scan or thermogram. If stress fracture is suspected but not diagnosed, treat as stress fracture. Running and other high-stress, weight-bearing activities should not be allowed until fracture has healed and bone is no longer tender to palpation. Tibial stress fractures usually take 8 to 10 wk to heal; fibula stress fractures take approximately 6 wk. When acute symptoms have subsided, bicycling and swimming activities can usually be initiated to maintain CRF. This should be cleared with supervising physician. If a specific cause is attributed to the development of stress fracture, steps should be taken to correct the cause.

Information from references 4, 8-9, 13-19, 23-29, 33, 35.

TABLE 26.10 Injury Classification Criteria and Exercise Modifications

Criteria	Modifications
Mild injury Performance is not affected. Pain is experienced only after athletic activity. Generally, no tenderness is felt on palpation. No or minimal swelling is present. No discoloration is apparent.	Reduce activity level, modify activity to take stress off the injured part, treat symptomatically, and gradually return to full activity.
Moderate injury Performance is mildly affected or not affected at all. Pain is experienced before and after athletic activity. Mild tenderness is felt on palpation. Mild swelling may be present. Some discoloration may be present.	Rest the injured part, modify activity to take stress off the injured part, treat symptomatically, and gradually return to full activity.
Severe injury Pain is experienced before, during, and after activity. Performance is definitely affected because of pain. Movement is limited because of pain. Moderate to severe point tenderness is felt on palpation. Swelling is most likely present. Discoloration may be present.	Rest completely and see a physician.

From Arnheim 1987.

Cardiopulmonary Resuscitation and Emergency Procedures

All fitness professionals should be well versed in **cardiopulmonary resuscitation (CPR)** techniques. (Courses are generally available through the AHA and American Red Cross.) In an emergency situation there is little time to think, and most reactions occur automatically. Having a plan of action and routinely practicing the plan help to ensure that proper **emergency procedures** are followed in these situations (2-17).

Basic Emergency Plan

First, *be prepared*. Carry a cell phone, or make sure a phone is available for use during the exercise class and know where the phone is located. If a phone is not available, have an alternative emergency plan in mind. The fitness professional should identify the **emergency medical system (EMS)** and services (e.g., ambulance, hospital, doctor) that are to be used and keep a phone list in a convenient location. Decide who is to phone for medical help in an emergency, and make sure that person knows how to direct help to the location of the injured person. All necessary medical information (e.g., release forms, medical history forms) should be readily available, and all emergency equipment and supplies (e.g., stretcher, emergency kit and supplies, AED, splints, ice, inhaler, money for phone call, blanket, spine board) should be easily accessible. The equipment should be checked periodically to ensure that it is in proper working order, and the supplies should be up to date. And, of course, know where the fire alarms and fire exits are located.

Remain calm to reassure the injured person and help prevent the onset of shock. Clear thinking allows for sound judgment and proper execution of rehearsed plans. In most instances, speed is not necessary. Cases of extreme breathing difficulty, stopped breathing or circulation, choking, severe bleeding, shock, head or neck injury, heat illness, and internal injury are exceptions and require urgent action. Otherwise, careful evaluation and a deliberate plan of action are desirable. The fitness professional should have a system for evaluating and dealing with life-threatening situations. All procedures should be conducted calmly and professionally.

Determine the history of the injury from direct observation of what happened, the injured person's account of what happened, or a witness's account of the injury. If the injured person is unconscious or semiconscious and no cause is determined, check for a medical-alert identification tag.

Check vital signs (HR, breathing, BP, and bleeding) to determine the seriousness of the situation. This evaluation will identify a course of action.

Checking Vital Signs

The following paragraphs describe vital signs and how to monitor each. Important vital signs to check include pulse, color, body temperature, mobility, and BP.

- Check HR. Use light finger pressure over an artery to monitor pulse rate. The most common sites for checking HR are the carotid, brachial, radial, and femoral pulses. If there is no pulse and the person is unconscious, begin CPR. The average HR for an adult is between 60 and 100 beats · min^{-1}.

- Assess color. For light-pigmented people, if skin, fingernail beds, lips, sclera of eyes, and mucous membranes are red or flushed, heatstroke, high BP, carbon monoxide poisoning, fever, and sunburn are possible. If the person is pale or ashen, changes in skin color could be attributable to shock, fright, insufficient circulation, heat exhaustion, insulin shock, or a heart attack. If the person is bluish, the poor oxygenation of the blood could be the result of airway obstruction, respiratory insufficiency, heart failure, or some poisonings. For dark-pigmented people, assess the nail beds, the inside of the lips, the mouth, and the tongue. Pink is the normal color for these; a bluish cast suggests shock. A grayish cast suggests shock from **hemorrhage**. A red flush at the tips of the ears suggests fever.

- Take body temperature. Normal body temperature is 98.6 °F (37.0 °C). Record temperature with a thermometer placed under the tongue (for 3 min); in the axilla, or armpit (10 min); or in the rectum (1 min). Cool, clammy, damp skin suggests shock or heat exhaustion; cool, dry skin indicates exposure to cold air; and hot, dry skin suggests fever or heatstroke.

- Check mobility. Inability to move (paralysis) suggests injury or illness of the spinal cord or brain.

- Take blood pressure. BP usually is taken at the brachial artery with a BP cuff and sphygmomanometer. The following results will help determine the problem:

  - Normal BP—<120 mmHg systolic and <80 mmHg diastolic

  - Severe hemorrhage, heart attack—marked decrease in BP (20-30 mmHg)

  - Damage or rupture of vessels in the arterial circuit—abnormally high BP (>150 SBP/>90 DBP)

  - Brain damage—increase in SBP with a stable or falling DBP

  - Heart ailment—decrease in SBP with an increase in DBP

Questions to Determine Action

Ask the following questions to help determine a course of action for treating injured participants.

- Is the person conscious? If not, a head, neck, or back injury is possible. If you are unsure why the individual is unconscious, check for a medical-alert identification tag. Assess airway, breathing, and circulation. Do not use ammonia capsules to arouse the person; the person may jerk the head backward in response, causing additional injury. If breathing has stopped and the person is in a prone position, logroll them as carefully as possible, keeping the head, neck, and spine in the same relative position, to begin CPR.

If the person is unconscious but breathing, protect against further injury. Do not move the person unless their life is in danger. Wait for medical assistance to arrive. Systematically evaluate the entire body and perform necessary first-aid procedures.

- Is the person breathing? If not, establish an airway and administer artificial respiration. Summon medical help. The following information will aid in determining why the person has stopped breathing.

  - Normal respiration—20 breaths · min^{-1}

  - Respiration in well-trained people—6 to 8 breaths · min^{-1}

  - Shock—rapid, shallow respiration

  - Airway obstruction, heart disease, pulmonary disease—deep, gasping, labored breathing

  - Lung damage—frothy sputum with blood at the nose and mouth, accompanied by coughing

  - Diabetic acidosis—alcoholic or sweet, fruity odor to breath

  - Cessation of breathing—abdomen and chest movement and airflow at nose and mouth have ceased

- Is the person bleeding profusely? If so, control bleeding by elevating the body part, applying direct pressure over the wound or at **pressure points**, and, as a last resort, putting on a tourniquet. A tourniquet should only be used in life-threatening situations in which risking a limb is a reasonable action to save a life. Treat for shock.

- Is there evidence of a head injury? Head injury is indicated by a history of a blow to the head or a fall on the head, deformity of the skull, loss of consciousness, clear or straw-colored fluid coming from the nose or ears, unequal pupil size, dizziness, loss of memory, and nausea. Prevent any unnecessary movement. If it is necessary to move the person, use a stretcher and keep the head elevated. If the person is unconscious, assume there is also a neck injury. Summon medical help immediately. The following information will help determine the reason for head injury:

  - Drug abuse or nervous system disorder—constricted pupils

  - Unconscious, cardiac arrest—dilated pupils

  - Head injury—pupils of unequal size

  - Disease, poisoning, drug overdose, injury—pupils do not react to light

  - Death—pupils widely dilated and unresponsive to light

- Is there evidence of a neck or back injury? The history of the injury may provide a clue. Other indications of a possible neck or back injury include pain directly over the spine, burning or tingling in the extremities, and loss of muscle function or strength in the extremities. When in doubt, assume there is a neck or back injury. The following information will aid in determining the injury:

- Probable injury of spinal cord—numbness or tingling in the extremities
- Occlusion of a main artery—severe pain in the extremity, with loss of cutaneous sensation
- Hysteria, violent shock, excessive drug or alcohol use—no pain

KEY POINT

When an exercise participant is injured, check for consciousness, breathing, and bleeding as well as head, neck, or back injuries. Take a pulse, temperature, and BP reading according to the guidelines in the previous section.

Rescue Breathing, Cardiopulmonary Resuscitation, and Automated External Defibrillators

Cardiac arrest is the single leading cause of death in the United States, leading to more than 350,000 deaths each year. An abnormal, chaotic heart rhythm known as *ventricular fibrillation* (see chapter 25) keeps the heart from filling with blood. When started early enough, CPR can keep oxygen flowing to the brain, but it cannot correct or restore a normal heartbeat. Shocking the heart with an electrical impulse often restores the sinus rhythm. The sooner the shock is delivered, the greater the chance of survival. The AED allows rescuers with limited experience and training to defibrillate a heart, and it has significantly increased the survival rate of people experiencing MI.

In another situation, the participant may stop breathing and not be undergoing cardiac arrest. In this case, rescue breathing (RB) helps restore breathing, but pulse should also be checked to ensure that the heart is pumping blood throughout the body. A pulse may be faint or undetectable and the rescuer may believe that the person requires both CPR and the AED or just one or the other. If no pulse is found, CPR should be started until the AED is available. The AED allows the rescuer to prepare to shock but has a safety device to ensure that a shock is not delivered unless needed. The fitness professional should be trained and prepared to use CPR, RB, and the AED to restore breathing and blood flow in a potentially fatal situation involving a participant. The following discussion outlines the steps the AHA teaches for RB, CPR, and AED use. The

fitness professional should review current recommended techniques (4).

If a participant appears to have stopped breathing, RB should be initiated. If the fitness professional finds that breathing has stopped and there is no pulse, the AED (if available) should be used or CPR should be started immediately. Recent recommendations include using hands-only CPR for an adult who has suddenly collapsed. First, find someone to call 911 or else make the call to report the emergency. Then, start compressions at a rate of 100 per minute. You do not have to stop the compressions to give breaths. This is only recommended for adults and only when the collapse is observed; however, when in doubt or insecure about providing mouth-to-mouth resuscitation, giving compressions is better than doing nothing. The compressions will allow blood to be circulated, likely preventing the death of vital organs. (5) Although the following steps for RB and CPR techniques are for adults only, the fitness professional should review current recommended techniques for all age categories (adults, children, and infants). The following is a list of steps to use in rescuing an unconscious person:

1. Check the scene for safety and to help determine probable cause for collapse.

2. Check the person for injuries and responsiveness as well as for any additional clues about the cause of collapse.

3. Determine responsiveness by gently shaking or tapping the person and asking if he is OK.

4. If you are alone and the person is unresponsive, immediately call for help, get any needed supplies and the AED if close by, and determine whether the person should be moved before you begin the rescue attempt. If there are other people around, instruct one bystander to call for help and another to get needed supplies and the AED, and cautiously move the person if safety dictates moving. Then begin the rescue attempt, following basic precautions for preventing disease transmission.

5. Look, listen, and feel for breathing. If the person is not breathing, move her to a faceup position while supporting the head and neck. Reposition the neck by using a head tilt and chin lift or jaw thrust and then reassess. If the person is still not breathing, pinch the nose shut, cover the mouth with yours, and give two slow breaths. Then assess circulation by sliding the index and middle finger of one hand into the groove at the side of his neck closest to you. Take no more than 10 sec to check the carotid pulse.

6. If there is a pulse but the person is still not breathing, initiate RB at a rate of 1 breath every 5 to 6 sec. Recheck for signs of circulation and breathing every 2 min.

7. If there is no breathing but circulation is still present, continue RB.

8. If there is no breathing or pulse, begin using the AED and CPR. If the AED is not readily available, begin CPR and continue until the AED arrives.

9. If CPR is initiated, place two fingers above the xiphoid process at the lower end of the sternal notch, place the heel of one hand above the two fingers in the middle of the sternum, and place the second hand on top. Interlace fingers and lift off the chest wall. With your shoulders positioned over your hands, compress the chest 1.5 to 2 in. (3.8-5.1 cm). Give 30 compressions and 2 RBs at a rate of 100 compressions · min^{-1} for an adult. Continue for 5 cycles or 2 min and recheck for signs of circulation. If there is no circulation, continue CPR, checking circulation every few minutes. If the AED is ready to use, recheck the pulse, and if you find no pulse, follow the steps as outlined by the manufacturer. The following guidelines are a typical protocol for using an AED.

10. Turn on the AED. Do not use the AED near alcohol or any other flammable material, in a moving vehicle, on a person lying on a conductive surface, or in water.

   - Use caution when using an AED on a person who weighs less than 55 lb (24.9 kg) or is younger than 8 yr old. Try 5 cycles or 2 min of CPR before using the AED.

   - Use children's pads and a child's shock dosage if available. If using adult pads, the pads should not touch.

   - Do not use cellular phones within 6 ft (1.8 m) of the AED.

   - To use the defibrillator, perform the following steps:

     1. Wipe the person's chest dry.

     2. Remove any metal on or around the person, including a bra with underwire and clothing with metal hooks.

     3. Remove any patches on the chest, such as a transdermal medication patch, with a gloved hand.

4. Attach the pads as instructed, one to the upper right of the chest and the other on the lower left side.

5. Plug the electrode into the AED. Follow the instructions as the computerized voice runs you through the various steps in using the AED.

6. Be ready to analyze the person's heart rhythm.

7. Make sure no one is touching the person, and advise others to stand clear. Push the analyze button.

8. The AED will analyze the rhythm and will instruct to shock or to begin CPR.

9. If a shock is advised, anyone near the scene should be instructed to stand back; deliver the shock by pushing the shock button.

10. The AED will analyze the rhythm again.

11. If the AED advises that no shock is needed, check the pulse again. If there is no pulse, begin CPR until the AED reanalyzes.

If a second rescuer is available and the initial rescuer gets tired, the second rescuer can prepare the AED (if available) for use or can take over CPR at the end of a cycle of 30 compressions. Two-person CPR is conducted in a cycle of 15 compressions and 2 breaths at a rate of 100 compressions · min^{-1}.

Emergencies are difficult to predict. Therefore, everyone of qualifying age should go through basic life-saving training through a reputable organization such as the AHA or Red Cross and maintain current certification. Because recommendations may change based on current research, it is important to learn correct techniques to avoid unnecessary injuries to the victim and to have optimal outcomes.

KEY POINT

Fitness professionals should update their training regularly to keep informed about the latest technology for dealing with emergency situations.

STUDY QUESTIONS

1. Name three precautions to take when dealing with bloodborne pathogens.

2. What is the difference between a sprain and a strain?

3. What does the acronym *PRICE* stand for?

4. When should internal bleeding be suspected?

5. List five actions to take when shock is suspected.

6. What percentage of weight loss during an exercise session is considered serious?

7. Which is the more serious condition, insulin shock or diabetic coma?

8. What condition affects the smooth muscle of the bronchial tubes, causing them to spasm?

9. List five vital signs that can be monitored when an emergency occurs.

10. A chaotic heart rhythm is known as _____.

CASE STUDIES

You can check your answers by referring to appendix A.

1. You are instructing an aerobics class when a participant collapses. On approaching the participant, you note that her breathing is shallow and slow and her skin color is pale, moist, and clammy. She is conscious but not alert, reports double vision and an intense hunger, and is wearing a medical-alert tag.

   a. What illness do you suspect?

   b. What questions do you ask?

   c. What action should you take?

2. You are leading an aerobics class and a participant collapses. You observe that the participant's skin is dry and red, breathing is labored, and pulse is rapid and strong. No trauma was experienced.

   a. What heat-related illness should be suspected?

   b. What is the immediate care?

   c. What emergency planning should be in effect?

3. You have a new participant who is breathing rapidly, is complaining of tingling in his feet and hands, and is experiencing dizziness and chest pains following an aerobic exercise program.

   a. What is the most likely cause of the symptoms?

   b. What other conditions need to be ruled out?

   c. What procedures can you perform to further assess and treat the condition?

4. You are running outside with one of your clients when suddenly she starts coughing and displaying obvious difficulty with breathing. It is hot and humid and there is a haze in the air.

   a. What problem do you suspect?

   b. What action should you take?

5. You have a participant complaining about anterior lateral shin pain. There is no history of trauma.

   a. What injury do you suspect?

   b. What other conditions need to be ruled out?

   c. What symptoms would you expect to find with the initial injury you suspected?

REFERENCES

1. American College of Sports Medicine (ACSM). 2010. *ACSM's guidelines for exercise testing and prescription.* 8th ed. Philadelphia: Wolters Kluwer/Lippincott Williams and Wilkins.

2. American Academy of Orthopedic Surgeons (AAOS). 1977. *Emergency care and transportation of the sick and injured.* 2nd ed. Menasha, WI: Banta.

3. American Academy of Orthopedic Surgeons (AAOS). 1998. *Emergency care and transportation of the sick and injured.* 7th ed. Sudbury, MA: Jones and Bartlett.

4. American Medical Association (AMA). 1966. *Standard nomenclature of athletic injuries.* Chicago: Author.

5. American Heart Association (AHA). 2006. *Heartsaver AED student workbook.* Dallas, AHA.

6. American Heart Association (AHA). 2005. *BLS for Healthcare Providers.* Dallas, AHA .

7. American Red Cross. 1993. *Adult CPR.* St. Louis: Mosby.

8. American Red Cross. 1993. *Community CPR.* St. Louis: Mosby.

9. American Red Cross. 1993. *Community first aid and safety.* St. Louis: Mosby.

10. American Red Cross. 1993. *Emergency response.* St. Louis: Mosby.

11. American Red Cross. 1993. *Preventing disease transmission.* St. Louis: Mosby.

12. American Red Cross. 2001. *First aid/CPR/AED program: Participant's booklet.* San Bruno, CA: Author.

13. Arnheim, D.D. 1987. *Essentials of athletic training.* St. Louis: Times Mirror/Mosby.

14. Arnheim, D.D., and W.E. Prentice. 2002. *Essentials of athletic training.* Boston: McGraw-Hill.

15. Arnheim, D.D., and W.E. Prentice. 1993. *Principles of athletic training.* 8th ed. St. Louis: Mosby.

16. Arnheim, D.D. 1989. *Modern principles of athletic training.* St. Louis: Times Mirror/Mosby.

17. Arnheim, D.D., and W.E. Prentice. 1993. *Principles of athletic training.* St. Louis: Mosby.

18. Bloomfield, J., P.A. Fricker, and K.P. Fitch, eds. 1992. *Textbook of science and medicine in sport.* Champaign, IL: Human Kinetics.

19. Booher, J.M., and G.A. Thibadeau. 1994. *Athletic injury assessment.* 3rd ed. St. Louis: Mosby.

20. Burke, E.R., and J.R. Berning. 1996. *Training nutrition: The diet and nutrition guide for peak performance.* Traverse City, MI: Cooper.

21. Department of Labor, Occupational Safety and Health Administration (OSHA). 1991. Occupational exposure to bloodborne pathogens: Final rule. *Federal Register* [Online], 56(235): 1-36. Available: www.osha.gov (Bloodborne Pathogens 29CFR 1910.1030, March 1992.) [July 10, 2002].

22. Egoscue, P., with R. Gittines. 1998. Pain free: A revolutionary method for stopping chronic pain. New York: Bantam Books.

23. Fahey, T.D. 1986. *Athletic training.* Mountain View, CA: Mayfield.

24. Franks, B.D., and E.T. Howley. 1989. *Fitness facts: The healthy living handbook.* Champaign, IL: Human Kinetics.

25. Franks, B.D., and E.T. Howley. 1989. *Fitness leaders' handbook.* Champaign, IL: Human Kinetics.

26. Henderson, J. 1973. *Emergency medical guide.* 3rd ed. St. Louis: Mosby.

27. Hillman, S.K. 2000. *Introduction to athletic training.* Champaign, IL: Human Kinetics.

28. Klafs, C.E., and D.D. Arnheim. 1977. *Modern principles of athletic training.* St. Louis: Mosby.

29. Morris, A.F. 1984. *Sports medicine: Prevention of athletic injuries.* Dubuque, IA: Brown.

30. Nieman, D.C. 1990. *Fitness and sports medicine: An introduction.* Palo Alto, CA: Bull.

31. Pfeiffer, R.P., and B.C. Pfeiffer. 1995. *Concepts of athletic training.* Boston: Jones & Bartlett.

32. Rahl, R.L. 2010. *Physical activity and health guidelines: Recommendations for various ages, fitness levels, and conditions from 57 authoritative sources.* Champaign, IL: Human Kinetics.

33. Rankin, J.M., and C.D. Ingersoll. 1995. *Athletic training management: Concepts and applications.* St. Louis: Mosby.

34. Rankin, J.M., and C.D. Ingersoll. 2001. *Athletic training management: Concepts and applications.* 2nd ed. Boston: McGraw-Hill.

35. Reid, D. 1992. *Sports injury assessment and rehabilitation.* New York: Churchill Livingstone.

36. Ritter, M.A., and M.J. Albohm. 1987. *Your inquiry: A commonsense guide to sports injuries.* Indianapolis: Benchmark Press.

37. Socha, T. 2007. Air pollution causes and effects. http://healthandenergy.com

38. Scribner, K., and E. Burke, eds. 1978. *Relevant topics in athletic training.* New York: Mouvement.

39. Thygerson, A.L. 1987. *First aid and emergency care workbook.* Boston: Jones & Bartlett.

40. Torg, J.S., P.R. Welsh, and R.J. Shepard. 1990. *Current therapy in sports medicine.* St. Louis: Mosby.

Legal Considerations

JoAnn M. Eickhoff-Shemek

The reader will be able to do the following:

1. Describe why it is essential that fitness professionals develop knowledge, skills, and abilities in the area of legal liability and risk management.

2. Distinguish injuries due to inherent risks, negligence, and product liability.

3. Develop a basic understanding of the law and legal system.

4. Understand the fault basis of tort liability.

5. Define *ordinary negligence* and *gross negligence.*

6. Describe the four elements of negligence that a plaintiff must prove.

7. Explain the primary assumption-of-risk and waiver defenses.

8. Identify the four essential elements of a valid contract.

9. Discuss how courts determine duty in negligence cases.

10. Define *risk management* and describe the four steps in the risk management process.

11. Develop risk management strategies that will help minimize legal liability in the areas of personnel, preactivity screening, fitness testing and prescription, instruction and supervision, equipment and facilities, and emergency action plans (EAPs).

12. Understand the many legal issues that can arise in negligence cases.

As presented in chapter 1, many physiological and psychological health benefits are associated with regular physical activity. Although these benefits outweigh the risks, it is important to understand that risks (e.g., heart attacks, fractured bones, cuts that cause bleeding) do occur, and many individuals become injured (and sometimes die) each year while participating in physical activity. Unfortunately, in today's litigious society, injured participants do not hesitate to file a negligence claim or lawsuit against fitness professionals and their employers. To help minimize injuries and subsequent litigation, it is essential that fitness professionals learn the laws that pertain to the field and how to apply the laws to their daily practices. Recent studies show poor adherence by fitness facilities to laws and safety standards and guidelines published by professional organizations (23). This poor adherence is most likely due to a lack of education among fitness professionals. Therefore, the purpose of this chapter is to help fitness professionals gain basic knowledge, skills, and abilities in this area.

Tables 27.1 and 27.2 demonstrate the frequency of injuries that occur with participation in physical activities and the types of injuries that have occurred in cases involving negligence lawsuits against fitness professionals and facilities. The data in table 27.1 reflect estimates from actual injuries reported to the National Electronic Injury Surveillance System (NEISS), a system in which hospital

emergency departments record the frequencies and types of injuries they treat. Interestingly, these estimates increased by 41%, 19%, and 23% from 2007 to 2009 for exercise, weightlifting equipment, and exercise equipment, respectively. Table 27.2 lists the names of selected negligence lawsuits and the type of injury the plaintiff (injured party) suffered. These cases are described later in this chapter.

Although most of the injuries listed in table 27.2 would be considered serious, other types of injuries also can result in costly claims and lawsuits. The Association Insurance Group conducted a 12 yr study (1995-2007) of **liability** claims involving both minor and major injuries occurring in fitness facilities, and table 27.3 lists the top five most frequent types of claims and the average cost (23).

Member malfunction claims include injuries where participants hurt themselves (e.g., smashing fingers when racking weights, dropping a weight on their foot, straining a muscle). The equipment malfunctions claims reflect injuries resulting primarily from poor maintenance of the equipment (e.g., seats falling off spin bikes, exercise balls that burst, and cable failure on selectorized machines). The average claim value includes the amount paid to the injured party as well as defense and others costs.

KEY POINT

Several studies have demonstrated that participation in fitness activities and programs can lead to all types of injuries—minor, major, and even death. It also is well established that these injuries can lead to legal claims and lawsuits against fitness professionals and their employers. To help minimize injuries and subsequent litigation, it is essential that fitness professionals learn the laws that pertain to the field and how to properly apply them to their practices.

Causes of Injuries and Negligence

There are many causes of injuries in fitness facilities and programs. The most common are due to inherent risks, negligence, and product liability. **Inherent risks** are those that happen simply as a result of participation in physical activity—they are no one's fault and are inherent in (or inseparable from) the activity. Almost everyone who has participated in physical activity or sport has experienced an injury due to inherent risks. Injuries caused by **negligence** are due to fault—the fault of a participant (e.g., the participant is careless while lifting weights) or of a fitness professional or facility (e.g., the failure to properly instruct and supervise participants, inspect and maintain exercise

TABLE 27.1 National Electronic Injury Surveillance System Data, 2007 to 2009

Type of injury	Year	Total number of injuries*
Exercise (includes activities without equipment, such as aerobics, stretching, jogging, and running)	2009	210,360
	2008	173,555
	2007	149,080
Weightlifting equipment	2009	86,307
	2008	79,027
	2007	72,369
Exercise equipment (excludes weightlifting and gymnastics equipment)	2009	55,578
	2008	50,869
	2007	45,351

*The total number of injuries presented in the table reflects estimates based on data obtained from U.S. hospital emergency departments across the country through the National Electronic Injury Surveillance System (NEISS). Retrieved October 8, 2010, from www.cpsc.gov/LIBRARY/neiss.html.

TABLE 27.2   Types of Injuries Leading to Negligence Lawsuits Against Fitness Professionals and Facilities

Type of injury	Negligence lawsuit
Stroke resulting in death	*Capati v. Crunch Fitness International, Inc., et al.* (9, 10)
Fractured ankle requiring surgical insertion of pins	*Santana v. Women's Workout and Weight Loss Centers, Inc.* (43)
Acute renal failure due to rhabdomyolysis	*Guthrie v. Crouser* (27)
Serious neck injury requiring five-level fusion of spine	*Sanford v. Vision Quest Sport and Fitness* (42)
Heart attack	*Rostai v. Neste Enterprises* (40)
Severe head injury resulting in death	*Xu v. Gay* (53)
Fractured ankle and crushed foot	*Thomas v. Sport City, Inc.* (49)
Serious and permanent injuries to mouth and lips	*Alack v. Vic Tanny International of Missouri, Inc.* (4)
Serious neck and back pain	*Goynias v. Spa Health Clubs, Inc.* (26)
Heart attack resulting in death	*Hicks v. Bally Total Fitness Corp.* (31)

TABLE 27.3   Frequent Injury Claims Occurring in Fitness Facilities (23)

	Number of claims	Average claim value
Member malfunction	388	$8,902
Premises liability (tripping and falling)	350	$18,554
Equipment malfunction	339	$17,063
Slips and falls in wet areas	252	$12,478
Treadmill	233	$8,933

equipment, and carry out emergency procedures). Injuries also can be caused by **product liability** (e.g., defects in exercise equipment for which the manufacturer can be held liable if they cause injury).

This chapter focuses on negligence, the major legal concern facing all fitness professionals and facilities. Negligence is failing to do something that a reasonable, prudent professional would do or doing something that a reasonable, prudent professional would not have done under the same or similar circumstances. (23). In other words, negligence can be an act of omission (failure to perform) or commission (improper performance). Unfortunately, negligence lawsuits against fitness professionals and facilities continue to increase (1), which reflects negatively upon the profession. However, this problem

can be addressed—professionals can learn about their many legal duties toward their participants and take steps to adhere to these duties, which will lead to fewer injuries and subsequent negligence claims and lawsuits. To begin this learning process, the next section provides an overview of the law and legal system.

KEY POINT

The most common causes of injuries in fitness programs are inherent risks, negligence, and product liability. Of these, negligence is the major legal concern facing fitness professionals. Negligence is the failure to do something that a reasonable, prudent professional would do or doing something that a reasonable, prudent professional would not have done under the same or similar circumstances.

The Law and Legal System

This section describes primary and secondary sources of law, criminal versus civil law, trial and appellate courts, tort law, and contract law. It also covers certain federal laws applicable to the fitness profession.

Primary and Secondary Sources of Law

In the United States, the law is created from the three branches of government at both the federal and state levels:

statutory law from the legislative branch, administrative law from the executive branch, and case law from the judiciary branch. **Statutory law** is enacted through the legislative process. Examples of federal statutes are the Americans with Disabilities Act (ADA) and the Health Insurance Portability and Accountability Act (HIPAA). Examples of state statutes include statutes such as the unauthorized practice of medicine or other allied (or licensed) health professions, Good Samaritan statutes, and statutes that require fitness facilities to have an AED. **Administrative law** is formed by numerous administrative agencies that exist at both the federal and state levels. At the federal level, these include the Food and Drug Administration (FDA), Internal Revenue Service (IRS), and Occupational Safety and Health Administration (OSHA). These agencies enact rules and regulations, investigate potential violations, and have the power to impose sanctions (e.g., fines) for any violations. **Case law** is derived from written court opinions and is sometimes referred to as *common law*. Courts often rely on the written opinions from previous cases to help form an opinion for a current case in which the facts are the same or similar to a previous case. The terms *precedent* and *stare decisis* (to stand by that which is decided) reflect this legal doctrine. Not all litigation results in precedent; most negligence cases are settled out of court and therefore never go to trial.

In addition to these three primary sources of law (statutory, administrative, and case law), there are many secondary sources of law, including books, treatises (e.g., the *Restatement of the Law of Torts*), and law review journals. Secondary sources do not reflect the law, but they are helpful to find primary sources of law or to explain a specific area of law. Both primary and secondary sources of law can be found using electronic legal databases such as LexisNexis Academic and Westlaw Campus, often available to students and faculty members through university libraries.

KEY POINT

The law is created from the three branches of government at both the federal and state levels: statutory law from the legislative branch, administrative law from the executive branch, and case law from the judiciary branch. Statutory law is enacted through the legislative process, administrative law is formed by numerous administrative agencies, and case law is derived from written court opinions.

Criminal Law Versus Civil Law

The law also can be categorized into criminal law and civil law. If someone violates a statute, the government can bring criminal charges against that person—the defendant.

If the defendant is found guilty, she may have to pay a fine, perform community service, be placed on probation, or be sentenced to prison (23). It must be shown that the defendant was guilty beyond a reasonable doubt, meaning she was 100% guilty of the crime. Fitness professionals could face criminal charges for violating state statutes such as assault and battery, theft, and the unauthorized practice of medicine.

Civil law addresses noncriminal matters and deals primarily with civil disputes between individuals, businesses, organizations, and government agencies (23). For example, if a member of a fitness facility is injured while working out in the facility, he could sue the facility for negligence—a civil claim. In this example, the injured member is referred to as the **plaintiff** and the fitness facility is referred to as the **defendant**. The plaintiff in a civil lawsuit has the burden of proof, so he must prove that the defendant was liable for the injury by the preponderance of the evidence— meaning it was more likely than not (51% or greater) that the negligent conduct of the defendant caused the harm to the plaintiff. Note that the term *liable* is used in civil law rather than the term *guilty*, which is used in criminal law. In civil claims such as negligence, the plaintiff seeks monetary damages from the defendant to compensate for the injury (e.g., medical expenses, lost wages).

Trial Courts and Appellate Courts

The U.S. court system is made up of trial and appellate courts at the federal, state, and local levels. Trial courts, the lowest courts, are the first to carry out the legal proceedings. At the end of the trial, the judge or a jury renders a decision in favor of one of the parties. Within a given time frame, the losing party can appeal the trial court's decision to a higher court—an appellate court. Appellate courts are made up of an odd number of judges who review the evidence and proceedings of the trial court. An appellate court has several options when forming its opinion about a case. It can remand it (send it back to trial with instructions), reverse it (disagree with the trial court's decision), affirm it (agree with the trial court's decision), or modify the trial court's decision (23). There are intermediate and supreme (highest) appellate courts at the state and federal levels.

Tort Law and Contract Law

Although there are many types of substantive law, tort law and contract law are most relevant to the fitness field. "A tort can be defined as conduct that amounts to a legal wrong that also causes harm on which the courts can impose civil liability" (23, p. 30), and a contract "is an agreement that can be enforceable in court" and is most often "formed when two (or more) parties exchange binding promises" (23, p. 37). The elements of both tort law and contract law are described next, along with their applications to the fitness field.

Tort Law

Tort law can be classified into three levels of fault, as shown in figure 27.1: intentional, negligence, and strict liability. Intentional torts involve conduct that requires the intent to cause harm to another. Examples are assault, battery, false imprisonment, defamation of character, and invasion of privacy. Although uncommon in fitness facilities, this type of behavior can occur among fitness staff members and participants. Many times this type of conduct also can be considered a crime (violation of a statute) and so the wrongdoer can face both civil claims and criminal charges.

Of the three levels of fault, negligence is the most common in the fitness field and can involve both gross negligence (also referred to as *reckless, willful,* or *wanton conduct*) and ordinary negligence. An example of gross negligence would be when a piece of exercise equipment is broken down and fitness staff members do not take any precautions (e.g., posting warning signs) to prevent participants from using it. Gross negligence usually requires prior knowledge of a risk or danger that is clearly foreseeable and then doing little or nothing to minimize that risk. Ordinary negligence is considered careless conduct as defined earlier—the failure to do something (omission) that a reasonable, prudent professional would do or doing something that a reasonable, prudent professional would not have done (commission) given the same or similar circumstances (e.g., the failure to provide proper instruction or maintenance of exercise equipment).

Various forms of strict liability also exist in the fitness field. Two of these are product liability and vicarious liability. Product liability involves some type of defect in the product (e.g., design defect, manufacturing defect, or marketing defect such as inadequate instructions or warnings). For example, if a plaintiff could show that her injury was due to the manufacturer's defective design of the equipment, then the manufacturer could be held strictly liable for the injury. Product liability is based on public policy (i.e., judicial determination of what is in the best interest of society) rather than fault such as intentional or negligent wrongdoing (23).

Vicarious liability is imposed upon employers even if the employer has not been negligent. Under the legal doctrine of **respondeat superior**, employers can be held strictly liable for harm to third parties (e.g., fitness participants) caused by negligent acts of their employees while performing their jobs (11). It is common in negligence lawsuits for the plaintiff to name several defendants in the case; for example, it may have been the personal trainer who committed the negligent act, but the plaintiff can name the trainer, his manager, and the owner of the facility as defendants who all could be potentially liable for the plaintiff's injury.

KEY POINT

Tort law involves three levels of fault: intentional, or conduct that requires the intent to cause harm to another; negligence, or careless conduct that causes harm to another (ordinary negligence) and reckless conduct that causes harm to another (gross negligence); and strict liability, such as product liability and vicarious liability. Vicarious liability occurs when employers (e.g., fitness facility managers and owners) are held liable for the negligent acts of their employees through a legal doctrine called *respondeat superior.*

Four Elements to Prove Negligence   In a negligence lawsuit, the plaintiff has to prove the following four elements (18):

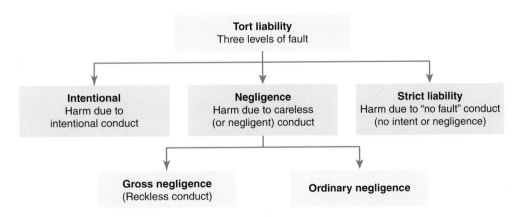

FIGURE 27.1   Fault basis of tort liability.

Reprinted, by permission, from J. Eickhoff-Shemek et al., 2009, *Risk management for health/fitness professionals: Legal issues and strategies* (Baltimore, MD: Lippincott Williams & Wilkins).

- Duty—the defendant owed a duty (or standard of care) to the plaintiff.
- Breach of duty—the defendant failed to carry out the duty.
- Causation—the breach of duty was the cause of the harm.
- Harm and damages—harm occurred to the plaintiff, resulting in damages (losses) to the plaintiff (e.g., medical expenses, lost wages).

It is important to realize that courts (judges) determine the first element of duty—not attorneys, juries, plaintiffs, or defendants. The approaches that courts use to determine duty are discussed later. The plaintiff then has to prove that the defendant breached her duty. Therefore, the conduct of the defendant becomes a key factor in determining whether or not there was a breach of duty. If the conduct was consistent with the duty owed, even if the plaintiff was seriously hurt or died, it will be difficult for the plaintiff to prevail with his suit. However, if the defendant's conduct was inconsistent with the duty owed, it will be easier for the plaintiff to show that the defendant breached her duty.

To determine if the breach of duty was the cause of the injury, courts often use the "but for" test: "But for the defendant's negligent conduct, would the injury have occurred?" (38). Sometimes injuries are caused by reasons other than the conduct of the defendant, such as inherent causes or the plaintiff's own negligence. There must be a link between the breach of duty and the cause (sometimes referred to as *proximate cause*) of the injury. If the plaintiff can show that the breach of duty caused harm to him (physical or emotional injury or damage to his property), monetary damages can be awarded to compensate for the harm. In ordinary negligence cases, these are called *compensatory damages* and can be both economic, such as medical expenses and lost wages, and noneconomic, such as pain, suffering, and loss of consortium (e.g., loss of companionship of a loved one). In gross negligence cases, plaintiffs usually seek compensatory damages as well as punitive damages (additional damages to punish the defendant for reckless conduct).

Defenses Against Negligence Defendants involved in negligence lawsuits have various defenses they can use to refute (or defend) the negligent claims made against them. The best defense always is to carry out legal duties properly. If the plaintiff cannot prove that the defendant breached a duty, it will be difficult for the plaintiff to win the negligence lawsuit and recover any damages. Two additional defenses, the primary-assumption-of-risk defense and the waiver defense, are discussed next.

Primary assumption of risk is a defense often used by defendants in negligence cases. As discussed, injuries are sometimes due to inherent causes. Primary assumption of risk is a legal theory in which plaintiffs are generally not allowed to seek damages for an injury that was due to inherent risks. However, in order for defendants to successfully use this defense, the following three elements must be met: "(a) The risk must be inherent to the activity, (b) the participant must voluntarily agree to participate, and (c) the participant must know, understand, and appreciate the inherent risk" (23, p. 35).

In determining whether the injury was due to an inherent risk, courts will examine the nature of the activity and the experience of the plaintiff. For example, in *Rutnik v. Colonie Center Court Club, Inc.* (41), a man died from a cardiac arrest while participating in a racquetball tournament. The estate of the decedent sued the club for negligence, claiming they failed to carry out certain duties such as emergency procedures. Using primary assumption of risk, the defendants claimed the decedent assumed the risk of a heart attack and, therefore, they were not liable. The appellate court agreed with the defendants, stating "relieving an owner . . . of a sporting facility from liability for the inherent risk of engaging in sports is justified when the consenting participant is aware of the risks, has an appreciation of the nature of the risks, and voluntarily assumes the risk" (p. 452). The court also stated that because the decedent was an experienced racquetball player who had played in many previous tournaments, he must have known and appreciated the risk of cardiac arrest while participating in this strenuous sport. The court found no negligence on part of the club, that is, they carried out emergency procedures properly. In this case, the primary assumption of risk defense protected the defendants from any liability.

In another case, *Corrigan v. Musclemakers, Inc.* (14), the primary assumption of risk defense did not protect the defendants from liability. In this case, a personal trainer placed a woman on a treadmill during her first training session, gave her little or no instruction on how to use the treadmill, and then left her unattended. After a short while, she began to drift back on the belt of the treadmill. She tried to walk faster but instead was thrown from the treadmill, which resulted in her fracturing her ankle. Prior to this incident, she had never been in a fitness facility or on a treadmill. She filed a negligence lawsuit against the defendants (the trainer and the facility), claiming the trainer failed to ensure that she understood how to use the treadmill (i.e., failed to provide proper instruction and supervision). The appellate court stated that the "doctrine of primary assumption of risk . . . may be applied in cases where there is an elevated risk of danger typically in sporting and recreational events" (p. 145), but the doctrine was not applicable in this case because fitness activities like exercising on a treadmill are not the same as sporting activities. In addition, the court ruled that the risks associated with using the treadmill were not known, understood, and appreciated by the plaintiff, a novice exerciser and treadmill user. Therefore, the plaintiff's injury was not due to inherent causes but most likely due to the negligence of the trainer and thus primary assumption of risk was not an effective defense for negligence.

Strengthening the Primary Assumption of Risk Defense
Informing participants of the inherent risks associated with physical activity *may* help to strengthen the primary-assumption-of-risk defense. Often, a section that informs an individual of inherent risks (minor, major, and even death) is included in protective legal documents such as waivers, informed consents, express assumptions of risk, and agreements to participate. Examples of these documents and a description of the legal protection they each provide can be found elsewhere (15, 23, 30). The following text describing inherent risks is taken from an **informed consent** that would be read and signed by a participant prior to fitness testing:

> I understand and have been informed that there exists the possibility of adverse changes during the actual test. I have been informed that these changes could include abnormal blood pressure, fainting, disorders of heart rhythm, stroke, and very rare instances of heart attack or even death. Every effort, I have been told, will be made to minimize these occurrences by preliminary examination and by precautions and observations taken during the test. I have also been informed that emergency equipment and personnel are readily available to deal with these unusual situations should they occur. I understand that there is a risk of injury, heart attack, stroke, or even death as a result of my performance of this test, but knowing those risks, it is my desire to proceed to take the test as herein indicated. (30, p. 468).

A **waiver** (or prospective release) is a defense based upon contract law. A waiver, signed by an individual before participation, contains an **exculpatory clause** such as the following that was included in the waiver in *Randas v. YMCA of Metropolitan Los Angeles* (37):

> THE UNDERSIGNED HEREBY RELEASES, WAIVES, DISCHARGES AND COVENANTS NOT TO SUE the YMCA, its directors, officers, employees, and agents (hereinafter referred to as "releases") from all liability to the undersigned, his personal representatives, assigns, heirs, and next of kin for any loss or damage, and any claim or demands therefore on account of injury to the person or property or resulting in death of the undersigned, whether *caused by the negligence of the releases* or otherwise while the undersigned is in, upon, or about the premises or any facilities or equipment therein [emphasis added]. (p. 165)

The exculpatory clause in this case was effective because it absolved (protected) the defendant YMCA from its own negligence. Without this waiver, the YMCA may have been found liable for its negligent conduct that caused the injury to the plaintiff. Therefore, when a person signs a waiver, she gives up (waives) her civil right to recover any damages due to the ordinary negligence of the defendant. Waivers do not protect defendants against gross negligence or intentional acts.

In order for the waiver to be effective and enforceable, it must be written and administered properly. It is also important to realize that the validity and enforceability of a waiver varies significantly from state to state. For example, in some states, the language used in the exculpatory clause must be very explicit in order for it to be enforceable. In addition, waivers are not enforceable in some states such as Virginia because they are against public policy. Many other factors also need to be considered when preparing an effective waiver; see *Waivers and Releases of Liability* for more information (15). Because of the many differences in the requirements for waivers among states, fitness professionals should never adopt a waiver they find in a book or some other source—it must be reviewed and edited by a competent lawyer prior to use.

KEY POINT

Two defenses often used by defendants in negligence cases are primary assumption of risk and waivers. Primary assumption of risk is effective for injuries due to inherent causes if the plaintiff knows, understands, and appreciates the inherent risks and voluntarily assumes those risks. The waiver defense can protect (absolve) defendants of their own negligence if the exculpatory clause within the waiver document is valid and enforceable based on state law. Because waiver law is quite complex and can vary significantly from state to state, fitness professionals must have a competent lawyer approve any waiver prior to use.

Contract Law

Contracts are commonly used in the fitness field. Examples include waivers, informed consents, employment contracts for employees and independent contractors, membership contracts, and purchase and lease agreements. In order for a contract to be valid and legally enforceable, it must meet the following four elements (13):

1. *Agreement.* An agreement to form a contract includes an *offer* and an *acceptance.*

2. *Consideration.* Any promises made by the parties to the contract must be supported by legally sufficient and bargained-for consideration.

3. *Contractual capacity.* Both parties entering into the contract must have contractual capacity to do so.

4. *Legality.* The purpose of the contract must be to accomplish some goal that is legal and not against public policy.

An agreement occurs when a fitness facility offers a membership to an individual and he accepts. The consideration is the money promised to the fitness facility paid by the member in exchange for programs and services promised by the facility to the member. Contractual capacity means that both parties must be capable and competent to form a contract. For example, minors (children under the age of 18) do not have contractual capacity; only adults can sign contracts such as waivers and informed consents. *Legality* refers to the terms within a contract—they must be legal. For instance, exculpatory clauses in waivers are against public policy in some states and therefore do not meet the legality requirement.

A valid contract meets all four elements. An unenforceable contract is one that violates a statute or law (13). For example, some contracts must be in writing (e.g., contracts involving the sale of goods of $500 or more) and if they are not, they will likely be rendered unenforceable. If one party fails to meets its contractual obligations, it might be considered a breach of contract and the breaching party may be required by a court to pay compensatory damages to the other party.

Federal Laws Applicable to the Fitness Profession

Although there are a variety of federal laws that fitness professionals should be aware of, this section focuses on three major ones: the ADA, OSHA's Bloodborne Pathogens Standard, and the HIPAA Privacy Rule and Final Nondiscrimination Rules.

The ADA (Americans with Disabilities Act), a federal statute, was enacted in 1990. The purpose of this law is to prohibit discrimination against people with disabilities. According to the ADA, a person with a disability has a physical or mental impairment that substantially limits one or more major life activities, has a record of such impairment, and is regarded as having such impairment (2). The ADA contains five titles, and two of these, Title I and Title III, pertain to fitness facilities. Title I, Employment, prohibits discrimination in employment procedures for private employers with 15 or more employees (3). These employers must provide reasonable accommodations for disabled employees. A reasonable accommodation is something that will help the employee to perform her job without creating an undue burden (significant difficulty or expense) to the employer.

Title III, Public Accommodations and Services Operated by Private Entities, requires that privately owned or operated places of public accommodation provide access for individuals with disabilities and make reasonable accommodations with regard to programs and services. There are 12 categories of places of public accommodation according to Title III, and the 12th category is "places of exercise or recreation" (2). Therefore, fitness facilities not only need to address architectural barriers (e.g., ramps for stairs) but also provide programs and services for people with disabilities. Again, the ADA requires a reasonable accommodation with regard to the provision of programs and services—meaning facilities do not need to purchase expensive, specialized exercise equipment, but they do need to provide appropriate programs and services to people with disabilities. This may require fitness facilities to have staff members who are qualified to conduct health and fitness assessments and design exercise prescriptions for people with disabilities. One credential that fitness professionals should consider in this regard is the Certified Inclusive Fitness Trainer certification established by ACSM and the National Center on Physical Activity and Disability (NCPAD). See the NCPAD website (www.ncpad.org) for more information on this certification as well as other helpful information, including the NCPAD free electronic newsletter to which fitness professionals can subscribe.

OSHA's Bloodborne Pathogens Standard is an administrative law that became effective in March 1992. Exposure to bloodborne pathogens (BBPs) such as HIV and HBV can lead to serious illness and death. The major goal of OSHA's BBP Standard is to reduce or eliminate occupational exposure to these pathogens that can be transmitted via blood or other potentially infectious materials (OPIM). It specifically applies to employers whose employees could come in contact with blood or OPIM while performing their jobs (e.g., fitness staff members who would be responsible for carrying out first aid). There are numerous requirements of this law (6), including the establishment of a written exposure control plan (ECP) that describes the job classifications where the occupational exposure occurs as well as how and when the provisions within the law will be implemented. To assist with the development and implementation of the many provisions within this complex law, fitness professionals can contact their regional OHSA office. A list of these offices is available at www.osha.gov./html/oshdir.html. Each regional office has a BBP coordinator.

The HIPAA Privacy Rule, a federal statute, mandates that an individual's private health information be protected. This law became effective on April 14, 2001, and required all covered entities to become compliant with it by April 14, 2003 (5). Covered entities include those who provide health care services such as health insurance plans and health care providers. It is likely that most fitness facilities would not be considered a covered entity, but some health promotion and disease prevention programs may be (5). However, it may be wise for fitness facilities to adopt provisions that this law requires with regard to protected health information (PHI)—all individually identifiable health information—because even if this law does not apply, there may be state privacy laws that do apply with regard to PHI. In addition, many professional organizations in the fitness field recommend in their ethical statements that individual health and fitness data be kept confidential. Fitness professionals should consider how they can go about developing and implementing procedures in their facilities that reflect the following HIPAA-related definitions when handling PHI by paper, electronically, or orally:

- *Privacy:* The right of an individual to enjoy freedom from intrusion or observation, the right to maintain control over certain personal information, and the right to expect health care providers to respect the individual's rights.
- *Confidentiality:* The practice of permitting only certain authorized individuals to access information, with the understanding that they will disclose it only to other authorized people.
- *Security:* The physical, technical, and administrative safeguards used to control access and protect information from accidental or intentional disclosure to unauthorized people and from alteration or destruction to maintain the integrity of the information (5).

These provisions also apply when fitness professionals want to obtain medical information (e.g., stress test results) from a participant's physician. The participant must first sign a **medical release** granting permission for the physician to release that information. An example of a HIPAA-compliant medical release is available elsewhere (23).

Another HIPPA federal statute, the HIPAA Final Nondiscrimination Rules, became effective on February 12, 2007, and applies to employer-sponsored wellness programs that provide incentives linked with the health plan (e.g., premium discounts, rebates, lower deductibles) for employees who achieve a predetermined health standard,

such as a BMI under $25 \text{ kg} \cdot \text{m}^{-2}$, cholesterol below 200 mg $\cdot \text{dl}^{-1}$, and so on. For these types of standard-based wellness programs, this HIPAA law provides five requirements that must be met. However, the five requirements are not necessary for wellness programs that provide incentives linked with the health plan for participation or completion in a behavior-change program. A description of the five requirements and specific examples of how to apply them for standard-based programs are available elsewhere (24, 34).

Determining Duty in Negligence Cases

As mentioned, courts (i.e., judges) determine duty in negligence cases. One of the first things courts consider when determining duty is the relationship that is formed between the plaintiff and defendant. Most courts will classify the relationship between fitness professionals and their participants (e.g., members, clients, patients, athletes) as an *inherent relationship*. When an inherent relationship is formed, professionals have a legal duty to provide reasonably safe facilities and programs for their participants. This involves taking precautions (developing and implementing risk management strategies, as discussed later) that will help prevent foreseeable injury risks. Injury risks—minor, major, and even death—are all foreseeable risks that can occur in fitness facilities and programs. Two ways in which inherent relationships are commonly formed in the fitness field are through the professional standard of care and through a special relationship between a person on land (e.g., fitness participant) and a landowner or occupier (e.g., owner or manager of a fitness facility).

Professional Standard of Care

As stated, negligence is the failure to do something that a reasonable, prudent professional would do or doing something that a reasonable, prudent professional would not have done under the same or similar circumstances. Therefore, the action (omission or commission) or conduct of the professional is a critical factor that courts will investigate to determine whether or not the professional's conduct was commensurate with the standard of care (or duty) that was owed to the plaintiff. According to the *Restatement of the Law (Third) of Torts*, "If an actor has skills or knowledge that exceed those possessed by most others, these skills and knowledge are circumstances to be taken into account in determining whether the actor behaved as a reasonably careful person" (39, p. 18). Because fitness professionals possess special knowledge, skills, and abilities, they are not only required to exercise reasonable care but also a level of care that would be consistent with the knowledge, skills, and abilities expected of fitness professionals.

KEY POINT

Federal laws that fitness professionals should be familiar with are the ADA, Bloodborne Pathogens Standard, and HIPAA Privacy Rule and Final Nondiscrimination Rules. With the assistance of legal counsel, fitness professionals need to develop and implement procedures that reflect the requirements within these laws.

According to van der Smissen, "If one accepts responsibility for giving leadership to an activity or providing a service, one's performance is measured against the standard of care of a qualified professional **for that situation**" (51, p. 40) The term *qualified professional* in this context means a professional who provides a standard of care that a prudent (competent) professional would provide. In negligence cases, courts will investigate the credentials (e.g., degrees, certifications) but also, more importantly, the competence of the professional, that is, what he did (or did not do) given the situation. The phrase "for that situation" in the van der Smissen quote means that "the professional standard of care is situation-determined—the nature of the activity, the participants, and the environmental conditions" (51, p. 40). For example, if a fitness professional is teaching a prenatal exercise class, she must be aware of the skills and abilities needed by pregnant women to safely participate in the program (nature of the activity). In addition, the professional must be aware of any factors related to exercise and pregnancy that might impose increased risks and then know

KEY POINT

It is important for fitness professionals to understand that it is likely they will be held to the professional standard of care in a negligence case against them. This will involve the court investigating the conduct of the professional. If the conduct is consistent with the standard of care, it will be difficult for the plaintiff (injured participant) to prove that the defendant (fitness professional) breached his duty. However, if the conduct is inconsistent with the standard of care, it will be easier for the plaintiff to prove that the defendant breached his duty, which could lead to the defendant being liable for the plaintiff's injury.

how to minimize those risks to the participants. Regarding environmental conditions, the professional must be aware of any conditions (e.g., heat, humidity, slippery floor surfaces) and take steps to minimize those risks.

Published Standards of Practice

In recent years, numerous standards of practice (e.g., standards, guidelines, position papers) have been published by both professional organizations (e.g., ACSM, NSCA, YMCA) and independent organizations such as the American Society for Testing and Materials (ASTM) and Consumer Products Safety Commission (CPSC). According to Herbert and Herbert (30), these published standards of practice reflect "benchmark behaviors or actions that are universally exhibited by properly trained and experienced professionals" (pp. 80-81) and should be viewed "as the threshold or minimal acceptable level of service owed to a client, patient, or participant" (pp. 205-206).

It is important for fitness processionals to be aware of and to implement the behaviors and actions reflected in published standards of practice because of the potential legal impact they can have (see figure 27.2). Expert witnesses, who educate the court as to the duty the defendant owed to the plaintiff in professional negligence cases, often introduce published standards of practice in their expert testimony as evidence of the standard of care owed to the plaintiff. Courts often allow these published standards of practice as admissible evidence to help determine duty, as demonstrated in *Elledge v. Richland/Lexington School District Five* (25).

In this case, a 9-yr-old girl was playing on modified monkey bars on her school's playground when her foot slipped, resulting in a fall that trapped her right leg between the bars. She suffered a severe spiral-type fracture in her femur that damaged the growth plate. Prior to this injury, the principal of the school had the monkey bars modified

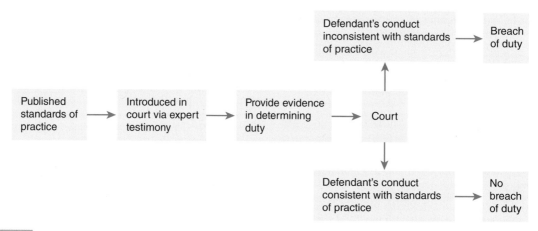

FIGURE 27.2 Example of the potential legal impact of published standards of practice.

Reprinted with permission from J. Eickhoff-Shemek and Kendall/Hunt Publishing Company. Standards of practice. In: *Law for Recreation and Sport Managers*, 5th ed., 2010.

by a playground equipment salesperson, who was not trained or licensed as an engineer to modify monkey bars. The mother of the child sued the school district, claiming that it was negligent because it deviated from the accepted standard of care (i.e., the modification of the monkey bars did not meet the standards published by ASTM and the guidelines published by CPSC for playground equipment). The trial court excluded the evidence presented by an expert witness that clearly showed that the district did not adhere to industry standards, and it ruled in favor of the school district. Upon appeal, the mother claimed that the trial court erred in excluding the evidence, arguing that such evidence was relevant to establish the appropriate standard of care. The appellate court (an intermediate appellate court) stated the following:

> Safety standards promulgated by government or industry organizations in particular are relevant to the standard of care for negligence. . . . Courts have become increasingly appreciative of the value of national safety codes and other guidelines issued by governmental and voluntary associations to assist in applying the standard of care in negligence cases. . . . A safety code ordinarily represents a consensus of opinion . . . and is not introduced as substantive law but most often as illustrative evidence of safety practices or rules generally prevailing in the industry that provides support for expert testimony concerning the proper standard of care. (25, pp. 477-478)

Given this reasoning, the appellate court reversed the ruling of the trial court. The case was further appealed to the South Carolina Supreme Court, which upheld the intermediate appellate court's ruling.

Because of the proliferation of standards of practice published by professional and independent organizations in recent years, it is difficult to include all of them in this chapter. Therefore, in the section, Strategies to Minimize Legal Liability, only selected standards of practice published by the ASTM and ACSM (48, 50) are included as examples. According to ACSM (48), *standards* are minimum requirements that fitness facilities must meet and *guidelines* are recommendations to improve the quality of services.

It is often difficult for fitness professionals to know which published standards of practice to follow, especially when inconsistencies exist among them, such as how each defines terms such as *standards* and *guidelines*, as well as the fact that specific actions provided vary quite a bit among the publications. Therefore, "it is best . . . to adhere to all published standards and guidelines. In the event of inconsistency or conflict . . . follow those that are the most authoritative or safety-oriented in their approach, regardless of how they are defined and/or stated" (23, p. 53).

Special Relationship: Person on Land and Landowner or Occupier

A type of special relationship is formed between a person on land and a landowner or occupier. The duty owed to a person entering the land of a landowner or occupier depends on the circumstances surrounding the person's entry, as defined in *Duncan v. World Wide Health Studios* (19):

> (1) A *trespasser* is one who enters the premises without the permission of the occupier. . . .
>
> (2) A *licensee* is one who enters the premises with the occupier's express or implied permission, but only for his own purposes which are unconnected with the occupant's interests. . . .
>
> (3) An *invitee* is a person who goes on the premises with the express or implied invitation of the occupant . . . for their mutual advantage. (p. 837)

The level of duty owed to each type of person varies. For example, the duty owed to the trespasser is to refrain from willful or wanton conduct that could harm him, whereas the duty owed to the licensee is to warn her of any dangers of which the occupier is aware. Invitees are owed the highest level of duty—a duty to maintain the premises in a reasonably safe condition, which requires inspection as well as warning or correction of any dangers.

The plaintiff in the *Duncan* case, a guest of the health club, was injured while using a leg press. After defining each of the three relationships between a person and landowner or occupier, the court determined that the plaintiff was an invitee because he was "in the position of one who may confer a future benefit upon the defendant" (19, p. 838). Therefore, the health club had a duty to inspect its premises to make them safe to visit as well as to inspect the leg press to help ensure its safe use. There was no evidence that the club breached these duties and therefore it was not liable for the plaintiff's injury. His injury was due to his misuse of the machine, that is, his own negligence or carelessness. Because virtually all participants of fitness facilities would be classified as invitees, fitness professionals need to carry out the following legal duties:

1. Inspect the premises both inside and outside, including all equipment and facilities, on a regular basis.
2. Upon inspection of any reasonable dangerous conditions, it is necessary to warn the invitee of the danger (e.g., post signage) or correct the condition.

Risk Management

Risk management is a broad term that reflects an overall goal of many organizations—to reduce accidental losses to help prevent slowed growth, reduced profits, and general interruption of operations (28). Liability losses (claims and lawsuits due to negligence) are one type of these accidental losses. Because this chapter focuses on legal liability in fitness programs and facilities, **risk management** in this context is defined as "a proactive administrative process that will help minimize liability losses for health/fitness professionals and the organizations they represent" (23, p. 9).

There are four steps to the risk management process (23). When assessing legal liability exposures (situations that can lead to injuries or the violation of any laws) in step 1, fitness professionals need to become aware of the many laws and published standards of practice that are applicable to the field. To assist in this step, as well as steps 2 through 4, it is recommended that every fitness facility have a risk management advisory committee that is made up of experts (e.g., legal, medical, and insurance) who work with the professional fitness staff members in developing a comprehensive risk management plan for the facility. Because the law is often complex and varies among jurisdictions, it is essential that fitness professionals utilize their risk management experts when making the many decisions involved in the four-step risk management process.

Step 2 involves the development of three types of risk management strategies that should reflect the laws and published standards of practice identified in step 1: *loss-prevention strategies* (i.e., strategies that help prevent injuries from occurring in the first place, such as providing proper instruction and supervision), *loss-reduction strategies* (i.e., strategies that help decrease the severity of an injury once it does occur, such as carrying out proper emergency procedures), and strategies that utilize a *contractual transfer of risks* (e.g., a waiver transfers the liability risks back to the participant who signed it and the liability insurance provider pays for the damages up to the limits of the policy when a defendant is found liable for negligence).

Step 3 involves the implementation of the risk management plan. Once the risk management strategies are developed as written policies and procedures for staff members to follow (step 2), they can be organized into a risk management policy and procedures manual (RMPPM). The policies and procedures should be presented in an organized fashion within the manual, divided into sections such as preactivity screening, equipment inspection and maintenance, EAP, and so on. Another component of step 3 is staff training. Staff training is essential so that staff members learn how to carry out the policies and procedures properly. New employees should receive training upon hiring, and there should also be regular in-service trainings throughout the year. An example of an in-service training would be training that includes a review and rehearsal of the EAP. EAP training should occur at least four times per year.

Step 4, evaluation of the risk management plan, includes two types of evaluation—formative and summative. Formative is ongoing and conducted throughout the year. For example, after every injury, an evaluation as to whether or not the EAP was carried out properly should be conducted. If it was not carried out properly, retraining of staff members may be needed. Summative evaluation involves a formal, annual review of the entire risk management plan. Laws often change, as do published standards of practice, and therefore the risk management advisory committee and fitness professionals will need to revise and update certain policies and procedures in the RMPPM and then retrain staff members on the changes. For more information on these four important risk management steps, see *Risk Management for Health/Fitness Professionals: Legal Issues and Strategies* (23).

Strategies to Minimize Legal Liability

This part of the chapter includes six sections: (1) personnel, (2) preactivity screening, (3) fitness testing and prescription, (4) instruction and supervision, (5) equipment and facility, and (6) EAPs. For each section, selected standards of practice published in *ACSM's Health/Fitness Facility Standards and Guidelines* (48) are provided, followed by important risk management strategies that will help minimize legal liability. By no means do these strategies reflect all of the legal liability exposures that exist.

Personnel

A variety of legal issues can arise with regard to personnel in fitness facilities and programs. This section focuses on hiring qualified and competent employees; incorporating proper procedures in the hiring, training, and supervision of employees; purchasing both general and professional liability insurance; and working with independent contractors.

Selected ACSM Standards Related to Personnel "The health/fitness professionals who have supervisory responsibility and oversight responsibility for the physical activity programs and the staff who administer them shall have an appropriate level of professional education, work experience, and/or certification. Examples of health/fitness professionals who serve in a supervisory role include the fitness director, group exercise director, aquatics director, and program director." (48, p. 32).

"The health/fitness and healthcare professionals who serve in counseling, instruction, and physical activity supervision roles for the facility shall have an appropriate level of professional education, work experience, and/or certification. The primary professional staff and independent contractors who serve in these roles are fitness instructors, group exercise instructors, lifestyle counselors, and personal trainers" (48, p. 33).

ACSM (48) also provides recommendations regarding the education, certification, and experience needed for professionals serving in supervisory roles as well as instructional roles. For example, those serving in a supervisory role such as fitness director should have a 4 yr degree in fitness, exercise science, or a related field; fitness instructor or personal trainer, or health/fitness specialist certification from a nationally recognized and accredited certifying organization; and 3 yr experience.

Strategy 1: Hire qualified and competent employees

Fitness professionals who serve in a supervisory role (e.g., manager, owner, fitness director, group exercise coordinator) need to hire qualified and competent employees. It is important to realize that a qualified professional (one who possesses certain credentials) is not necessarily competent to carry out her legal duties (i.e., knows how to apply safe and effective principles of exercise to meet the specific needs of a participant).

A variety of efforts to address the issue of qualified and competent professionals have been made in the field, including voluntary or self-regulated efforts, such as the accreditation of certifications through independent agencies such as the National Commission for Certifying Agencies (NCCA), as well as government-regulated efforts, such as legislative bills proposing licensure in various states. However, many unnecessary injuries and subsequent negligence claims and lawsuits continue to occur in the field.

Although many in the field believe that the accreditation of certifications through the NCCA and similar agencies enhances safety and minimizes legal liability, there are no formal education requirements prior to sitting for the accredited exams. Therefore, it is possible that these individuals may be considered qualified by employers because they possess the certification credential, but they may not be competent if they have not received any formal educational experiences that included coursework and evaluation of their practical skills (i.e., their ability to apply safe and effective principles of exercise).

In contrast, many of the licensure proposals have required formal education; for instance, the New Jersey proposal to license personal trainers and group exercise leaders requires 200 hr in the classroom and a 50 hr internship or an associate's degree in health and fitness (29). For more on licensure issues, see a three-part article published in *ACSM's Health and Fitness Journal* (20-22). Whether the field remains self-regulated or is regulated by the government in the future, the provision of well-designed formal education programs that prepare both qualified and competent fitness professionals is one of the most important risk management strategies that will help minimize injuries and subsequent litigation in the field. Formal education programs to prepare quality personal trainers and group exercise leaders have been described elsewhere (7, 8, 16, 17).

Strategy 2: Hire, train, and supervise employees properly

Fitness professionals who serve in a supervisory role have a duty to use reasonable care in the hiring, training, and supervising of their employees. To prevent claims of negligent hiring, it is necessary to hire qualified and competent employees, as demonstrated in *Seigneur v. National Fitness Institute, Inc.* (45). In *Seigneur*, the plaintiff, who was injured while using a weight machine during an initial evaluation, claimed that the facility breached its duty to her "by negligently hiring . . . a defendant employee who . . . lacked sufficient training, experience, certification and/or other qualifications and knowledge to properly . . . direct and guide [her] in lifting weights and in the use of the weight equipment" (p. 277).

Fitness facilities also have been sued for negligent hiring because they did not conduct criminal background checks before hiring employees (23, 33). Generally, employers would not be held liable under the legal principle of *respondeat superior* for an employee who conducts a criminal act (e.g., sexual assault) while on the job because the criminal act would not be within the scope of employment. However, employers do have a responsibility to conduct criminal background checks prior to hiring employees who will be working with vulnerable populations (e.g., children, elderly, people with disabilities), as well as those who work closely with clients, such as massage therapists and personal fitness trainers. In addition, employers have a responsibility to supervise employees serving in these roles. If a fitness supervisor (or any staff member) observes or is made aware of any inappropriate behavior by another staff member or participant, proper steps based on consultation from legal counsel need to take place in a timely fashion.

The failure to train employees also is a common negligence claim against fitness facilities, as demonstrated by the following claims made in *Chai v. Sports & Fitness Clubs of America, Inc.* (12, p. 55-56):

- Negligently failed to have personnel adequately trained to recognize cardiac arrest and to subsequently start CPR
- Negligently failed to have employees adequately trained in the use and operation of an automated external defibrillator
- Negligently failed to require sufficient training of staff members designated to train the member

These claims demonstrate the importance of staff training as a risk management strategy. Staff members who are well trained are more likely to carry out their legal duties properly compared with those who receive little or no training.

Strategy 3: Purchase proper liability insurance coverage

If a fitness professional and facility are found liable for negligence, liability insurance will pay for the damages up to the limits of the policy, thus protecting the financial assets of the professional and the facility. Most fitness facilities provide general liability insurance coverage for their employees through a commercial general liability (CGL) policy. This type of liability insurance protects fitness professionals and facilities from ordinary negligence, but not professional negligence. The need for professional liability insurance coverage is demonstrated in *York Insurance Company v. Houston Wellness Center, Inc.* (54).

The plaintiff in *York* claimed that she was injured due to improper instruction given by an employee on how to use an exercise machine. The fitness club contended that their liability insurance provider had a duty to defend and indemnify the club in this negligence case. However, the insurance company claimed they did not have this duty because of a clause in the CGL policy that stated that "this insurance does not apply to 'bodily injury' . . . arising out of the . . . failure to render any service, treatment, advice, or instruction relating to the physical fitness . . . or physical training programs" (54, pp. 904-905). A court ruling agreed with the insurance company. The facility had a CGL policy that specifically excluded professional services such as providing fitness instruction. If they had also purchased professional liability insurance coverage for their professional staff members, the outcome of this case probably would have been different. Fitness professionals should have both general and professional liability insurance policies and should be sure the policies cover all the programs and services they provide. As a member of a professional organization, fitness professionals can usually purchase professional liability insurance through a low-cost group plan. For example, ACSM has a group plan through the Forrest T. Jones & Company (www.ftj.com/acsm). It is also important to realize that general and professional liability insurance policies do not cover acts that would be considered gross negligence or intentional.

Strategy 4: Have procedures in place for independent contractors

Fitness facilities often hire independent contractors to provide various services. Several legal implications are involved when hiring independent contractors (23); this discussion will focus on a few of these. First, based on IRS tax law, employers do not have a lot of behavioral control over independent contractors. Therefore, it is essential that they hire only qualified and competent independent contractors. Second, all independent contractors should sign a written contract that specifies the responsibilities of both parties, including a clause in which the independent contractor must provide proof of having both general and professional liability insurance (the fitness facility's liability insurance coverage does not cover independent contractors—only employees). Third, it is critical that independent contractors do not appear to be employees by their actions or what they wear.

For example, they should not wear a shirt with the facility logo on it but perhaps a badge indicating that they are an independent contractor. This is because if they are deemed to be *ostensible agents*, employers could be liable for their negligent acts the same as they would be for employees under the legal principle of *respondeat superior* (23). It is also wise for fitness facilities to inform participants in a membership contract or signage that some services are provided by independent contractors.

KEY POINT

Many injuries (and subsequent litigation) that occur in the field are due to the negligent conduct of staff members. Therefore, it is essential to hire both qualified and competent staff members as well as provide them with proper training and supervision. Additional risk management strategies associated with personnel include conducting criminal background checks before hiring certain staff members, purchasing adequate general and professional liability insurance to cover all programs and services provided by employees, and having several procedures in place when hiring independent contractors.

Preactivity Screening

Recent research has shown that many fitness facilities, as well personal trainers, are not conducting preactivity screening procedures (46, 47). The failure to conduct such procedures has been a claim in several negligence cases against fitness facilities, especially when there has been a serious injury (e.g., heart attack) or death (23), such as in *Rostai v. Neste Enterprises* (40). During his first personal fitness training session, Rostai, a 46-yr-old, overweight, and inactive male, allegedly suffered a heart attack toward the end of his 60 min session. In his negligence lawsuit against the trainer and the health club, Rostai claimed that the trainer knew he was overweight and was not physically fit but aggressively trained him in his first workout, even though he complained several times during the workout that he needed a break. Rostai claimed that the defendant owed him a duty to investigate his health history, physical condition, and cardiac risk factors. The trainer and the club were not liable in this case because the court ruled that Rostai assumed the risks, even though the trainer was negligent. The court indicated that the trainer and club would only have been liable if the conduct of the trainer was intentional or reckless. Most courts would probably disagree with this ruling because the assumption-of-risk defense is usually only effective in protecting defendants for injuries due to inherent causes, not negligence.

Selected ACSM Standards Related to Pre-activity Screening

"Facility operators shall offer a general pre-activity screening tool (e.g., Par-Q) and/or specific pre-activity screening tool (e.g., health risk appraisal [HRA], health history questionnaire [HHQ]) to all new members and prospective users" (48, p. 2). (See chapter 2 for more information on screening.)

"All specific pre-activity screening tools (e.g., HRA, HHQ) shall be reviewed and interpreted by qualified staff (e.g., a qualified health/fitness professional or healthcare professional), and the results of the review and interpretation shall be retained on file by the facility for a period of at least one year from the time the tool was reviewed and interpreted" (48, p. 4).

"If a facility operator becomes aware that a member, user, or prospective member has a known cardiovascular, metabolic, or pulmonary disease, or two or more major cardiovascular disease risk factors, or any other self-disclosed medical concern, that individual shall be advised to consult with a qualified healthcare provider before beginning a physical activity program" (48, p. 5).

Strategy 1: Select preactivity screening devices for self-guided and professionally guided programs

With the assistance of the risk management committee, preactivity procedures need to be established for participants in self-guided and professionally guided programs. According to *ACSM's Guidelines for Exercise Testing and Prescription* (50), self-guided programs are guided by the participant with little or no input or supervision from a fitness professional, whereas professionally guided programs are guided by a fitness professional with academic training and practical knowledge, skills, and abilities (KSAs) in assessment, design, and supervision. For self-guided programs, participants would likely complete a device such as the PAR-Q, and then on their own they would follow the recommendations on the device with regard to seeking medical consultation prior to participation in physical activity. Some fitness facilities may decide to have participants obtain medical clearance, for example, if they indicate *yes* to one or more of the questions on the PAR-Q.

Fitness professionals involved in professionally guided programs may want to consider using the Preactivity Screening Questionnaire (PASQ). Forms such as an HRA or HHQ may or may not contain the criteria necessary to classify participants into low, moderate, and high risk categories as established by ACSM (50). The PASQ meets the ACSM screening criteria for professionally guided programs and has been successfully used at the University of South Florida with both students and employees. This form and related documents (e.g., detailed interpretive guidelines that describe how the PASQ meets the screening criteria) are available upon request from the author of this chapter (eickhoff@usf.edu).

Strategy 2: Have only qualified fitness professionals interpret data from screening devices used in professionally guided programs

To comply with the ACSM standards of practice (48, 50), only qualified fitness professionals (e.g., those with academic training) should interpret data from screening devices used in professionally guided programs. Anyone who attempts to carry out this interpretation and is not qualified to do so may be practicing outside her scope of practice (discussed later). They also would likely not possess the necessary KSAs to meet the professional standard of care needed to properly conduct the interpretation process, because the professional standard of care is determined from situation-based factors, as described previously.

Strategy 3: Develop procedures for medical clearance for professionally guided programs

When using a screening device in professionally guided programs to classify individuals into low, moderate, or high risk categories, the fitness professional can follow the guidelines in *ACSM's Guidelines for Exercise Testing and Prescription* to determine whether or not medical examination and exercise testing are recommended prior to initiation of exercise training (see chapter 2). Most fitness professionals would interpret *medical examination and exercise testing* in this context to mean medical clearance. The participant's physician then would decide the need for a medical examination and what it would entail, such as a diagnostic or clinical GXT.

> ### KEY POINT
>
> Preactivity screening is essential to help ensure the safety of participants. Risk management strategies include selecting and using appropriate screening devices for both self-guided and professionally guided programs as well as having only qualified professionals interpret data from professionally guided screening devices and make decisions regarding the need for medical clearance.

Fitness Testing and Prescription

This section focuses on health-related fitness testing and prescription (commonly conducted in fitness facilities) versus clinical exercise testing and prescription (conducted in clinical settings for diagnostic purposes). Conducting fitness testing and prescription procedures requires the necessary KSAs in order to carry out these procedures safely. According to *ACSM's Guidelines for Exercise Testing and Prescription* (50), testing procedures include (a) completing preactivity screening procedures as described previously, (b) selecting protocols that safely meet the needs of each individual and proper interpretation of test results, (c) inspecting and calibrating fitness testing equipment, (d) having emergency procedures in place, (e) providing instructions and administering informed consent, and (f) observing participants for any signs and symptoms of overexertion during and after the testing. For fitness prescription, procedures include (a) designing a safe and effective prescription based on the individual's health and fitness needs and (b) prescribing within one's **scope of practice**, or activities in which a fitness professional engages when carrying out his practice that are within the boundaries or limitations of his education, training, experience, and certifications (23).

Practicing outside one's scope of practice can lead to civil claims such as negligence because the fitness professional would likely not possess the necessary KSAs to meet the professional standard of care, and it could also lead to criminal charges for crossing the line into a licensed profession (e.g., practicing medicine or dietetics without a license). There is little case law involving negligent conduct among fitness professionals while performing health-related fitness testing. However, ample case law exists with regard to fitness prescription, and therefore

the risk management strategies presented next will focus on this issue.

Selected ACSM Standards Related to Fitness Testing and Prescription In addition to ACSM standards previously listed under personnel, there are guidelines in *ACSM's Health/Fitness Facility Standards and Guidelines* (48) that address the qualifications of fitness professionals who provide fitness prescription services for individuals with special needs.

Strategy 1: Develop scope-of-practice guidelines for fitness professionals who conduct fitness testing and prescription The scope-of-practice descriptions are provided by ACSM. These can be useful for fitness supervisors when establishing scope-of-practice guidelines for their fitness staff.

Based on the ACSM scope-of-practice descriptions, Certified Personal Trainers should not be conducting fitness testing and prescription, but they can lead exercise and provide exercise recommendations for healthy populations and those with medical clearance. The scope of practice for the Health Fitness Specialist includes conducting fitness

Scope-of-Practice Descriptions

ACSM Certified Personal Trainer*

The ACSM Certified Personal Trainer (CPT) is a fitness professional who develops and implements an individualized approach to exercise leadership in healthy populations and those individuals with medical clearance to exercise.

Using a variety of teaching techniques, the ACSM Certified Personal Trainer is proficient in the following:

- Leading and demonstrating safe and effective methods of exercise by applying the fundamental principles of exercise science
- Writing appropriate exercise recommendations
- Motivating individuals to begin and continue with their healthy behaviors

ACSM Certified Health Fitness Specialist**

The ACSM Certified Health Fitness Specialist (HFS) is a degreed health and fitness professional qualified to pursue a career in university, corporate, commercial, hospital, and community settings. The Health Fitness Specialist is skilled in the following:

- Conducting risk stratification
- Conducting physical fitness assessments and interpreting results
- Constructing appropriate exercise prescriptions for healthy adults and individuals with controlled conditions released for independent physical activity
- Motivating apparently healthy individuals with medically controlled diseases to adopt and maintain healthy lifestyle behaviors
- Motivating individuals to begin and continue with their healthy behaviors

*www.acsm.org/Content/NavigationMenu/Certification/GetCertified/CertifiedPersonalTrainer/ACSM_Certified_Pers1.htm#CPT_Scope_of_Practice

**www.acsm.org/Content/NavigationMenu/Certification/GetCertified/HealthFitnessInstructor/ACSM_Health_Fitness1.htm#HFI_Scope_of_Practice

testing and prescription for healthy individuals as well as those with medically controlled diseases who have medical clearance.

The following cases, *Guthrie v. Crouser* (27) and *Makris v. Scandinavian Health Spa, Inc.* (32) demonstrate the importance for fitness professionals to have the necessary KSAs to design safe and effective prescriptions based on the participant's needs and to prescribe exercise within their scope of practice. In *Guthrie*, the plaintiff complained to her trainer that the exercise program he designed for her was too rigorous and painful, but he assured her that the exercises would not cause her any harm and they would help her reach her goals. She continued with the exercise program, but after a few days she was unable to perform any activity due to extreme muscle soreness. After her physician examined her, she was sent immediately to the hospital emergency room and diagnosed with acute renal failure due to rhabdomyolysis. In her lawsuit, the plaintiff brought several claims against the defendant, including negligence, intentional infliction of emotional distress, fraud in the inducement (i.e., the trainer intentionally misrepresented himself to be a certified trainer but was not), and gross negligence. The plaintiff won this case but the jury only awarded $80.00 in damages with interest and costs (27).

While using the leg press machine, the plaintiff in *Makris* informed her trainer that she felt a sharp pain in her neck that radiated down her arm. The trainer told her the pain was due to upper-body weakness and would subside as she got stronger. The trainer had her continue with the exercises despite complaints of intense pain. Later, an MRI revealed she had three herniated cervical disks. She filed a personal injury lawsuit against the defendants (the trainer, Scandinavian Health Spa, and Bally's Total Fitness Corporation) alleging they rendered negligent training, monitoring, instruction, supervision, and advice. It appears that the trainer did not possess the necessary KSAs for training clients. The trainer was not able to distinguish types of pain (i.e., general pain or discomfort associated with training versus pain associated with a possible medical condition). In addition, it appears that the trainer diagnosed the pain—stating it was due to upper-body weakness—and treated the pain by having her continue to perform the exercise to increase her strength. Fitness professionals need to understand that diagnosing and treating medical conditions is outside their scope of practice and they risk violating state statutes such as practicing medicine without a license. An appellate court in this case indicated that the defendant was negligent and remanded (sent back) the case to the trial court for further proceedings.

Strategy 2: Use a medical liaison (or advisory committee) and resources regarding fitness testing and prescription programs for people who have risk factors or medical conditions

Because almost all fitness facilities serve individuals with risk factors or medical conditions, it is important to have a medical liaison or advisory committee that can help establish guidelines and protocols for fitness professionals to follow when testing and prescribing fitness programs for these participants. This can help enhance the safety of these individuals. In addition, fitness professionals should use published resources such as *ACSM's Exercise Management for Persons with Chronic Diseases and Disabilities* and *Physical Activity Guidelines: Recommendations for Various Ages, Fitness Levels, and Conditions from 57 Authoritative Sources*, both published by Human Kinetics, as well as refer to the many chapters in this text addressing these topics.

Strategy 3: Develop scope-of-practice guidelines for staff members who provide nutrition advice

Because fitness professionals often provide nutrition advice, it is essential that the advice they provide does not cross over into the licensed practice of dietetics (44). To establish scope-of-practice guidelines in this area, it may be wise to use the following, as stated in an Ohio statute, which describes the types of general nonmedical nutrition information that can be provided by unlicensed nutrition educators (35):

1. Principles of good nutrition and food preparation
2. Foods to be included in the normal daily diet
3. Essential nutrients needed by the body
4. Recommended amounts of the essential nutrients
5. Actions of nutrients on the body
6. Effects of deficiencies or excesses of nutrients
7. Food and supplements that are good sources of essential nutrients

Two cases, the *Ohio Board of Dietetics v. Brown* (36) and *Capati v. Crunch Fitness International, Inc.* (9, 10) are good examples of individuals practicing outside their scope of practice with regard to nutritional advice. In the first case, the defendant performed nutritional assessments and recommended nutritional supplements to individuals for the purpose of treating specific complaints and ailments. The court ruled that the defendant was not licensed to practice dietetics in the state of Ohio and was engaged in the practice of dietetics as defined by the Ohio statute. In *Capati*, a personal trainer recommended his client take a variety of over-the-counter nutritional and dietary supplements, including some that contained ephedra. The client also was taking prescribed medications for hypertension, but the trainer did not advise his client that there may be negative health consequences for her to take the supplements while on hypertension medication. While exercising at the club, she became ill, lost consciousness, and later died at the hospital from a stroke. This case was settled out of court, with the defendants (trainer and the club) liable for $1,750,000 of the total settlement amount of over $4,000,000.

KEY POINT

A variety of risk management strategies can be developed and implemented to help minimize liability associated with fitness testing and prescription. Perhaps the most important strategies involve establishing written scope-of-practice guidelines that describe the qualifications that staff members need in order to carry out fitness testing and prescription activities, especially for participants with risk factors and medical conditions. Practicing outside one's scope of practice can lead to civil claims such as negligence and criminal charges such as practicing medicine or dietetics without a license.

Instruction and Supervision

A variety of legal liability exposures exist involving instruction and supervision. According to Betty van der Smissen, the "lack of or inadequate supervision is the most common allegation of negligence" (52, p. 163). She also states that there is an inherent duty to supervise, meaning that fitness professionals have a duty to supervise participants who are engaged in activities that are sponsored by them—in other words, virtually all programs and services offered by fitness facilities. She also describes three types of supervision: specific, general, and transitional. *Specific supervision* occurs when a supervisor is directly with an individual or small group in an instructional format, such as a personal fitness trainer or group exercise leader. *General supervision* occurs when a supervisor has responsibility for overseeing activities going on in a facility, such as a fitness floor supervisor. Finally, *transitional supervision* occurs when a supervisor changes from general to specific supervision while supervising an area, such as a fitness floor supervisor who provides individual instruction to a participant on how to use a piece of exercise equipment and then transitions back to general supervision of the area.

Selected ACSM Standards Related to Instruction and Supervision

"Once a new member or prospective user has completed a pre-activity screening process, facility operators shall then offer the new member or prospective user a general orientation to the facility" (48, p. 10).

"Facilities shall provide a means by which members and users who are engaged in a physical activity program within the facility can obtain assistance and/or guidance with their physical activity program" (48, p.11).

"A facility that offers youth services or programs shall provide evidence that it complies with all applicable state and local laws and regulations pertaining to their supervision" (48, p. 40).

Strategy 1: Provide a general orientation to the fitness facility and equipment for all new participants

Providing new participants with an orientation is an important risk management strategy that should focus on fitness safety. For example, the orientation should include information on how to properly use the exercise equipment and any facilities such as swimming pools and saunas. Participants should be informed of posted policies and signage as they go through the orientation. In addition, they should receive information on principles of safe exercise as well as the programs and services offered that might best meet their needs.

An excellent case that demonstrates the importance of providing instruction on the proper and safe use of exercise equipment is *Thomas v. Sport City, Inc.* (49). The plaintiff was injured while using a hack squat machine at the defendant's facility. He thought he had properly engaged the hook to secure the weights, but he had not and the rack of weights (180 lbs [81.6 kg]) fell, fracturing his ankle and crushing his foot. Thomas claimed that Sport City failed to instruct and supervise him on the proper use of the hack squat machine, but the court ruled that he did know how to use the machine. He testified that he was an experienced, sophisticated user of the machine and that if he had properly secured the hook, the carriage would not have fallen. Therefore, the failure of the club to instruct and supervise was not the cause of the plaintiff's injury, but his own carelessness (negligence) was. The club was not found negligent in this case. However, the following statement made by the court with regard to a duty to instruct is important for fitness professionals: "Members of health clubs are owed a duty of reasonable care to protect them from injury on the premises," and "this duty includes a general responsibility to ensure that their members know how to use gym equipment" (p. 1157), and the failure to instruct or supervise the plaintiff on proper use of the machine would normally be a breach of duty because the machine could easily cause injury.

Strategy 2: Provide fitness staff supervision during all operating hours

Fitness facilities should have continual staff supervision during all operational hours. There should be a designated manager on duty at all times who has overall responsibility for any situation that might come up, such as a medical emergency. Fitness facilities should have a job description for fitness professionals who serve in this important role as well as train them to properly handle any number of situations that might arise in a facility. If situations are handled properly and in a timely fashion, there is less potential for liability problems to arise.

Strategy 3: Conduct job performance appraisals of all fitness staff members

In addition to providing training of fitness staff members as discussed earlier, fitness professionals who serve in supervisory roles also should conduct regular job performance appraisals that include direct observation and evaluation of the conduct (actions) of staff members. After a performance appraisal, fitness supervisors should discuss the results of the appraisal with the staff member and design an action plan to address any areas in which the staff member needs improvement, especially those areas that focus on participant safety. More on performance appraisals is available elsewhere (23), as is a sample performance appraisal tool for group exercise leaders. In cases discussed previously (e.g., *Corrigan* and *Rostai*) as well as the following cases, it is likely that the injuries that occurred to the plaintiffs would not have occurred if the fitness professionals had been trained well and their job performance had been evaluated by a qualified fitness supervisor.

In *Santana v. Women's Workout and Weight Loss Centers, Inc.* (43), the plaintiff was participating in a modified step aerobics class when she fell and fractured her ankle, requiring surgical insertion of pins. She claimed the defendant was negligent because the activity (step aerobics combined with upper-body strengthening exercises using an exercise band) was unreasonably difficult and dangerous. An expert witness testified that the simultaneous activities created an inherently dangerous situation, which increased the risks over and above those that were inherent. In other words, the instructor's conduct did not meet the standard of care and was negligent. The defendants claimed that the plaintiff assumed the risks, which should bar her lawsuit against them. The court ruled that "defendants have a duty to use due care not to increase the risks to a participant over and above those inherent in the sport" (p. 26). The *Santana* court also distinguished sport and exercise when deciding that the primary assumption of risk defense did not protect the defendant from liability. The court stated that sports, by their nature, inherently create extreme risks of injuries due to physical contact between participants and competition aimed at scoring points, racing against time, or accomplishing feats of speed and strength, whereas exercise programs, such as a step aerobics class, are meant to enhance health and fitness and therefore should not be designed to create extreme risks of injury.

In *Sanford v. Vision Quest Sport and Fitness* (42), the plaintiff was seriously injured when her personal fitness trainer walked away and stopped spotting her while performing a bench press. She could not control the weights on the bar, causing the bar to come down onto her neck, which resulted in a serious injury requiring a five-level fusion of her cervical spine. Prior to the incident, she had informed her trainer that she was fatigued from her extensive cardio workout, but he continued to have her exercise with increased weight and repetitions. In her lawsuit, she made the following negligent claims against the defendants (the trainer and Vision Quest Sport and Fitness): (a) misrepresentation (the trainer was not certified as he represented himself), (b) failure to evaluate and supervise the plaintiff,

(c) failure to monitor the plaintiff, and (d) abandonment of the plaintiff. The outcome of this case is pending.

Unfortunately, there are many more negligence cases where personal trainers, like those in *Guthrie*, *Rostai*, and *Sanford*, have pushed their clients beyond their limits, resulting in serious injuries. These trainers either did not know or did not know how to apply important exercise principles such as progression and overload. This improper training of clients is most likely due to trainers not having adequate formal education and the failure of fitness supervisors to observe, evaluate, and correct the conduct of their personal trainers.

Strategy 4: Provide proper supervision of all youth programs All youth programs should be adequately supervised by responsible and well-trained individuals. As mentioned previously, employees and volunteers who serve in these roles should have criminal background checks prior to hiring. Proper supervision also involves preactivity screening procedures as well as having children and their parents or legal guardian sign an *agreement to participate* (15, 23, 30) that not only informs them of the inherent risks associated with the activity or sport but also informs them of the rules and policies they need to follow for safe participation.

KEY POINT

The failure to provide proper instruction and supervision reflects common negligence claims made by plaintiffs. To help minimize these types of claims, fitness professionals can provide an orientation that shows new participants how to properly use the equipment and facility, evaluate the job performance of staff members who provide instruction (including direct observation and feedback of their teaching behavior) to help ensure they are providing safe and effective programs, and make sure all programs and services are properly supervised at all times.

Equipment and Facility

Fitness professionals have numerous legal duties in this area, but this section focuses on installation and maintenance of exercise equipment, facility access, inspection of premises, and signage. For more information on facilities, fitness professionals should refer to one of the most authoritative and comprehensive resources, *Facility Design and Management for Health, Fitness, Physical Activity, Recreation, and Sports Facility Development*, published by Sagamore.

Negligence claims and lawsuits against fitness professionals and facilities are quite common in this area, but sometimes the plaintiff is also negligent (e.g., misuses the equipment, as described in *Thomas v. Sport City, Inc.*), and sometimes the manufacturer may be held strictly liable (i.e., product liability) for a defect in the equipment design, manufacturing, or warnings. For example, in the *Thomas* case, the plaintiff claimed that there was a design defect in the hack squat machine, but he was unable to prove that there was a design defect, so the manufacturer was not held liable for his injury.

ACSM (48) has one facility equipment standard related to providing proper safety equipment in aquatic and pool facilities. It does not include any standards related to exercise equipment, but it does have a few guidelines, including having a preventive maintenance schedule for equipment, a system in place to remove broken or damaged equipment, and a sufficient quantity and quality of equipment. The following standards relate to the fitness facility.

Selected ACSM Standards Related to Equipment and Facility

"Facilities shall have an operational system in place that monitors, either manually or technologically, the presence and identity of all individuals (e.g., members and users) who enter into and participate in the activities, programs, and services of the facility" (48, p. 40).

"Facility operators shall post proper caution, danger, and warning signage in conspicuous locations where facility staff know, or should know, that existing conditions and situations warrant such signage" (48, p. 68).

"All cautionary, danger, and warning signage shall have the required signal icon, signal word, signal color, and layout as specified in ASTM F1749" (48, p. 70).

Strategy 1: Install exercise equipment properly

Manufacturers of exercise equipment publish an owner's manual for each piece of equipment. Fitness professionals need to follow the information provided in these manuals, including specifications related to installation, spacing, user safety precautions, warning and caution signage, cleaning, inspections, and maintenance. Other published standards of practice might also apply; for instance, the ASTM standard titled Standard Specification for Motorized Treadmills, F2115, requires 39 in. (99 cm) of space behind treadmills and 19.7 in. (50 cm) on each side of the treadmill.

The importance of proper treadmill spacing was a key issue in *Xu v. Gay* (53). In this case, Ning Yan died from a severe head injury after falling off a treadmill at a fitness facility. The treadmill only had 2.5 ft (76 cm) clearance behind it. An expert witness for the plaintiff testified that there should be a minimum of 5 ft (152 cm) behind treadmills in order to meet the industry's standard of care for safe distance. He did not indicate which industry standards he was referring to, but he stated they were voluntary. The court stated that the "defendant's ignorance of and failure to implement the standards . . . establish a case of ordinary negligence" (p. 171).

Strategy 2: Maintain exercise equipment properly

As determined from a 12 yr study of liability claims conducted by the Association Insurance Group, poor maintenance of exercise equipment was one of the most common claims. It is important that fitness professionals properly maintain their exercise equipment based on the specifications provided in the owner's manual for each piece of equipment. This includes equipment such as exercise balls and resistance tubing. *Alack v. Vic Tanny International of Missouri, Inc.* (4) is an excellent case to demonstrate why this is so important from a legal perspective. While the plaintiff was using an upright rowing machine, the handle of the machine disengaged, causing serious and permanent injuries to his mouth and lips. The plaintiff claimed that his injury was due to Vic Tanny's negligence because they did not ensure that the clevis pin was in place. Testimony showed that Vic Tanny did not conduct regular inspections to make sure that the clevis pin was in place, and there was no doubt in the judge's mind that the defendant was negligent. Although the plaintiff had signed a waiver in this case, the court found the waiver to be unenforceable because the exculpatory clause was ambiguous and inconspicuous within the membership agreement. Therefore, Vic Tanny was liable for damages of $17,000 in medical expenses.

Strategy 3: Have a system in place to monitor facility access

The main purpose of this strategy is to help ensure that only authorized participants have access to the facility. It also helps to protect participants from anyone entering the facility who might commit crimes such as sexual assault and theft. Most facilities use computerized monitoring systems in which members have an identification card that is scanned upon entry.

Strategy 4: Conduct regular inspections of the premises

Because participants would be classified as invitees, there is a legal duty to (a) regularly inspect the premises, both inside and outside, including all equipment

KEY POINT

Fitness professionals have many legal duties related to exercise equipment and the fitness facility. These include installing and maintaining exercise equipment according to the manufacturer's specifications in the owner's manual as well as inspecting the facility premises both inside and outside. Given the duty owed to invitees (participants), any dangerous condition found upon inspection must be corrected or a warning must be posted. Fitness professionals also should have a system in place that monitors facility access and includes the posting of signage as required by the ASTM.

and facilities, and (b) upon inspection of any reasonable dangerous conditions, warn the invitee of the danger (e.g., post signage) or correct the condition. For example, if inspection of an exercise machine reveals that it is not functioning properly, there is a duty to warn of the danger (e.g., post a sign on the machine), repair the machine, or remove it from use.

The duty to inspect is demonstrated in *Goynias v. Spa Health Clubs, Inc.* (26). The plaintiff in this case was injured from a fall on a wet, slippery floor in the locker area. The court stated: "A property owner is required to exercise reasonable care to provide for the safety of all lawful visitors on his property. . . . [This] includes the duty to exercise ordinary care to keep the premises in a reasonably safe condition and to warn the invitee of hidden perils or unsafe conditions that can be ascertained by reasonable inspection and supervision" (p. 555).

Strategy 5: Post signage throughout the facility

There are a variety of signage requirements for fitness facilities. To discuss all of these is beyond the scope of this chapter, but two of these requirements include warning labels that need to be placed on exercise equipment and a facility safety sign that needs to be posted in the exercise equipment area. Requirements for warnings labels and the safety sign are published in ASTM's Standard Specification for Fitness Equipment and Fitness Facility Safety Signage and Labels, F1749. The facility safety sign is shown in figure 27.3. This ASTM publication also provides classifications for danger, warning, and caution to indicate the relative seriousness of a potential hazard.

Emergency Action Plans

All of the risk management strategies presented thus far focus on preventing injuries from occurring in the first place—they are loss-prevention strategies. This section will address loss-reduction strategies—actions that need to take place to mitigate a medical emergency once it has occurred. Numerous negligence cases have occurred because fitness professionals did not carry out proper emergency procedures. Unfortunately, negligence claims and lawsuits continue to occur in this area, even though published standards of practice requiring facilities to have an emergency action plan (EAP) have existed for nearly two decades. A variety of factors need to be considered when developing an EAP, as reflected in the following risk management strategies. It is best to designate a professional fitness staff member to serve as the facility's EAP coordinator and to have a medical liaison or advisor who can be directly involved with this effort.

Selected ACSM Standards Related to Emergency Action Plans

"Facility operators must have written emergency response policies and procedures, which shall be reviewed regularly and physically rehearsed at least twice annually. These policies shall enable staff to respond to basic first-aid situations and emergency events in an appropriate and timely manner" (48, pp. 18).

"In addition to complying with all applicable federal, state, and local requirements relating to automated external defibrillators (AEDs), all facilities (i.e., staffed and unstaffed) shall have as part of their written emergency response policies and procedures a public access defibrillation (PAD) program in accordance with generally accepted practice" (48, p. 21).

"Health/fitness and healthcare professionals engaged in pre-activity screening or prescribing, instructing, monitoring, or supervising of physical activity programs for facility members and users shall have current automated external defibrillation and cardiopulmonary resuscitation (AED and CPR) certification from an organization qualified to provide such certification. A certification should include a practical examination" (48, p. 35).

Strategy 1: Prepare a written emergency action plan

Fitness professionals clearly have a legal duty to render aid to a participant who becomes injured while participating in programs and services provided

---

White letters on a Safety Green background ↓

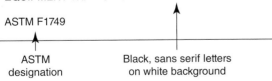

BE ALERT!

THE FITNESS EQUIPMENT IN THIS FACILITY PRESENTS HAZARDS WHICH, IF NOT AVOIDED, COULD CAUSE SERIOUS INJURY OR DEATH.

PRIOR TO USING THE EQUIPMENT, READ THE WARNING LABELS AND INSTRUCTION PLACECARDS AFFIXED TO EACH MACHINE.

IF YOU ARE UNSURE OF HOW TO USE A MACHINE, SEEK THE ASSISTANCE OF OUR FLOOR PERSONNEL. WE WILL BE HAPPY TO INSTRUCT YOU ON HOW TO USE THE EQUIPMENT PROPERLY.

IMMEDIATELY REPORT ANY PIECE OF EQUIPMENT THAT IS NOT FUNCTIONING PROPERLY TO OUR FLOOR PERSONNEL SO THAT IT MAY BE EVALUATED AND SERVICED PROMPTLY.

DO NOT ATTEMPT TO USE OR FIX ANY PIECE OF EQUIPMENT THAT IS NOT FUNCTIONING PROPERLY.

ASTM F1749

ASTM designation ↑   Black, sans serif letters on white background ↑

FIGURE 27.3 Example of facility safety sign to be posted in the equipment room.

Reprinted, with permission, from F1749-09 Standard Specification for Fitness Equipment and Fitness Facility Safety Signage and Labels, copyright ASTM International, 100 Barr Harbor Drive, West Conshohocken, PA 19428.

by the fitness facility. Because of this legal duty, every fitness facility should have a written EAP. Sometimes, fitness professionals believe that Good Samaritan statutes protect fitness professionals while on the job, but they do not. These statutes are designed to protect individuals who voluntarily render aid to someone in need, such as providing first aid to someone while shopping in a store. The written EAP should contain several components, including (a) the job description of the manager on duty who has the overall responsibility of an emergency when it occurs; (b) descriptions of responsibilities of other staff members who are first responders or who should assist in other ways; (c) contingency plans for minor, major, and life-threatening injuries; (d) internal and external (e.g., EMS) communication procedures; and (e) inspection and maintenance procedures for first-aid kits and AEDs. Additional components are reflected in the following risk management strategies.

Strategy 2: Ensure the written emergency action plan includes procedures for having and using an automated external defibrillator

In recent years, the failure to have and use an AED has been a common claim in negligence lawsuits filed against fitness facilities when someone has suffered a cardiac arrest while participating in fitness activities. For example, in a 2008 case, *Hicks v. Bally Total Fitness Corp.* (31), Hicks suffered a sudden cardiac arrest while exercising at the facility. No Bally employee began CPR, nor did any employee use an AED, but EMS was called. About 12 min after the call, paramedics from the EMS unit applied the first electric shock using their defibrillator. Their attempts to resuscitate Mr. Hicks were unsuccessful and he died at the hospital about 10 days later. In her wrongful death actions, Gloria Hicks, the wife of the decedent, filed the following claims: (a) breach of express warranty (Bally had pledged and warranted to its members that in the event of a medical emergency it would respond in a timely manner and that it would also abide by ACSM guidelines), (b) negligence (Bally failed to properly respond to Mr. Hicks' cardiac arrest and failed to have an AED and staff trained in its use), and (c) gross negligence (Bally knew for at least 8 yr prior to Mr. Hicks' death that cardiac arrest killed at least 36 members each year in their facilities and, therefore, their failure to take action to help prevent this known, foreseeable risk was considered reckless conduct). The outcome of this case is pending.

Fitness professionals also need to be aware of AED statutes that have already been passed in several states that require fitness facilities to have an AED and to have staff members certified and trained on its use. It is likely that more states will propose similar legislation.

Strategy 3: Have qualified staff members who are trained to carry out the emergency action plan

Fitness staff members who have responsibilities to carry out the EAP should maintain current first aid, CPR,

and AED certifications. It is also a good idea to have a staff member, perhaps the EAP coordinator, be a certified instructor in these areas who can provide recertification classes for staff members. In addition, it is critical that the EAP is reviewed and rehearsed by staff members at least four times a year, as recommended by ACSM (48).

Strategy 4: Establish postemergency procedures

In addition to proper completion of an incident report form (see figure 27.4) after every medical emergency, the manager on duty should gather and record any evidence, such as photographs of any equipment and conditions involved in the incident and interviews with witnesses who can describe the what, how, why, when, and where of the incident. The evidence gathered may be helpful in defending future negligence lawsuits against staff members and the facility. In addition, after an incident, especially a serious one, a copy of the incident report should be sent to the facility's legal counsel and insurance carrier.

KEY POINT

Numerous negligence cases against fitness facilities have occurred for failing to have or properly carry out an EAP. A variety of factors need to be considered when preparing a well-thought-out and effective EAP. To assist with this important risk management strategy, it is recommended that each facility designate a professional staff member as the EAP coordinator and have a medical liaison or advisor who can be directly involved with this effort. Once the EAP is written, staff members should attend in-service trainings that include drills at least four times a year to help ensure the plan will be properly carried out in the event of an emergency.

Conclusion

This chapter has covered various legal issues to help educate fitness professionals about their major legal duties and how they can carry out these duties through the development and implementation of risk management strategies. By no means has this chapter covered all of the legal issues relevant to the fitness field. It would be best for students and professionals in the field to have an entire academic course in order to receive a more thorough exposure to legal issues than what can be covered in this chapter. This final section includes one additional but important risk management strategy—record keeping and documentation of evidence—as well as two topics that summarize major concepts discussed throughout the chapter: risk management as a management function, and the risk management pyramid.

HEALTH, FITNESS & RACQUET SPORTS CLUB INCIDENT REPORT
[COMPLETE FOR ALL INCIDENTS AND REPORT IMMEDIATELY – PLEASE PRINT]

Date

Month   Day   Year   Time of Accident
A.M.
P.M.

Club Member
☐ Yes
☐ No

Club Name

Club Location

Injured Person

FIRST   (M.I.)   LAST   AGE

NUMBER AND STREET

CITY   STATE   ZIP

BUSINESS PHONE   HOME PHONE

HOSPITAL OR FIRST AID SQUAD NOTIFIED
☐ Yes   ☐ No

NAME:_____

TIME OF INITIAL CALL: _____

TIMES OF FOLLOW-UP CALLS: 1. _____
2._____3._____4. _____

TIME OF ARRIVAL: _____

TIME OF DEPARTURE: _____

TAKEN TO HOSPITAL? _____

NAME OF FIRST AID ATTENDANT: _____

DESCRIPTION OF ACCIDENT:

CHECK ITEMS THAT APPLY TO INJURED PERSON:

BLEEDING INJURY: ☐ YES ☐ NO   **OTHER VISIBLE INJURY:** ☐ YES ☐ NO

NO VISIBLE INJURY, BUT COMPLAINT OF PAIN: ☐ YES ☐ NO

IF EYE INJURY, WEARING EYEGUARDS? ☐ YES ☐ NO

DESCRIBE EXACT INJURY SUSTAINED:

_____

_____

_____

DESCRIBE FIRST AID ADMINSTERED BY CLUB:

_____

_____

_____

First Witness	**Second Witness**
FIRST (M.I.) LAST	FIRST (M.I.) LAST
NUMBER AND STREET	NUMBER AND STREET
CITY STATE ZIP	CITY STATE ZIP
BUSINESS PHONE HOME PHONE	BUSINESS PHONE HOME PHONE
DESCRIPTION OF ACCIDENT BY WITNESS:	DESCRIPTION OF ACCIDENT BY WITNESS:
_____	_____
_____	_____
_____	_____
SIGNATURE:	SIGNATURE:

FIGURE 27.4   Incident report from Creative Agency Group. *(continued)*

HEALTH, FITNESS & RACQUET SPORTS CLUB INCIDENT REPORT
[continued]

NAME OF CLUB PERSONNEL WHO INSPECTED THE SCENE:

POSITION

DATE OF INSPECTION:

CONDITIONS FOUND: _____

_____

_____

ACTION TAKEN, IF PRACTICAL, TO AVOID RECURRENCE: _____

_____

Description of Place of Accident

☐ INTERIOR ☐ EXTERIOR ☐ WALKING AREA ☐ PLAYING SURFACE ☐ LOCKER ROOM

☐ PHY. FITNESS ROOM ☐ OTHER: _____

CONDITIONS: ☐ DRY ☐ WET ☐ SMOOTH ☐ EVEN SURFACE ☐ SLIPPERY

FOREIGN SUBSTANCE? ☐ YES ☐ NO   IF 'YES', DESCRIPTION: _____

_____

IF INJURY TOOK PLACE OUTSIDE CLUB BUILDING, CHECK APPROPRIATE ITEMS:

WEATHER CONDITION: ☐ DRY ☐ RAIN ☐ SNOW ☐ ICE ☐ DAY ☐ NIGHT LIGHTING CONDITIONS:_____

IMPORTANT: IF INJURY TOOK PLACE ON A COURT, PROVIDE NAME, ADDRESS AND TELEPHONE NUMBER OF THOSE INDIVIDUALS WHO USED OR RENTED THE COURT DURING THE PRIOR HOUR.

_____

_____

_____

ADDITIONAL COMMENTS

_____

_____

DID POLICE INVESTIGATE?   NAME AND RANK OF OFFICER   DEPARTMENT   PHONE NUMBER
☐ YES   ☐ NO

_____

SUBMITTED BY: SIGNATURE: TELEPHONE: DATE / TIME

_____

This information is for reporting purposes only. The information provided is the responsibility of the insured and/or club.

CREATIVE AGENCY GROUP

FIGURE 27.4 *(continued)* Incident report from Creative Agency Group.

Reprinted, by permission, from Creative Agency Group.

Record Keeping and Documentation of Evidence

Reference to various documents (e.g., waivers, informed consents) was made throughout this chapter. It is important to store these types of documents in a secure place because they can provide valuable evidence in the event of a claim or lawsuit. For example, if the fitness facility has retained a copy of the waiver signed by a member, it will provide evidence that can help protect the facility if that member ever files a negligence lawsuit against the facility. Other record keeping can help provide evidence that a fitness facility and its staff members properly carried out their legal duties. For example, if a facility kept records documenting proper maintenance of exercise equipment, it will be difficult for a plaintiff to prove that the facility failed to carry out this duty. If a plaintiff cannot prove that a defendant breached her duty, it will be difficult for the plaintiff to prevail in a negligence lawsuit. It also is important to have duplicate copies of records (written or electronic) stored at another location in case the original is lost or destroyed. Fitness professionals should seek legal counsel with regard to how long records need to be kept.

Risk Management: An Important Management Function

Fitness professionals often are employed in management positions within a facility. In these positions, they perform numerous management functions in areas such as human resource management, financial management, facility management, marketing and promotion, strategic planning, customer service, scheduling of programs and services, and information technology. However, risk management is one of the most important management functions because it focuses on participant safety. Developing and implementing the risk management strategies described in this chapter that help ensure the safety of participants should be the number one priority of all fitness professionals. These risk management strategies also reflect the many legal duties fitness professionals have toward their participants. In addition to minimizing injuries and subsequent litigation, risk management has other benefits such as enhancing operational efficiency and improving the quality of services (23).

Risk Management Pyramid

This chapter has focused on negligence, a major legal issue facing fitness professionals. The risk management pyramid in figure 27.5 depicts seven lines of defense that can help minimize negligence claims and lawsuits for fitness professionals and facilities. Each line of defense is briefly described, summarizing the key concepts presented within this chapter:

- First line of defense: Risk managers and liability insurance company executives and underwriters have known for many years that a genuinely friendly, caring,

Record-Keeping Tips

Keeping records can help provide evidence that legal duties were properly carried out. Examples include the following:

- Credentials of staff members (e.g., degrees, current certifications)
- Criminal background checks of personnel
- Staff trainings (e.g., dates, staff members attending, content covered)
- Preactivity screening forms (e.g., screening device, physician clearance)
- Waivers and informed consents
- Medical release forms
- Written scope-of-practice guidelines for staff members
- Participant facility orientations (e.g., dates, participants attending, content covered)
- Job performance evaluations of staff members
- Facility and equipment inspections
- Facility and equipment maintenance records
- Written EAP
- Completed incident report forms and related evidence
- Written exposure control plan (OSHA's BBP Standard)

and professional environment will minimize not only the occurrence of incidents, which can lead to claims and suits, but the actual assertion of claims and suits as well! As a starting point such an environment should be created – not just for liability reasons but for business and professional reasons as well.

• Second line of defense: Sadly, it appears that a significant number of health/fitness professionals do not know, understand, appreciate, or adhere to the law and published standards of practice. Health/fitness facilities must adhere to the law and should comply with published standards of practice. These standards are the established benchmarks of expected behavior for the profession and will be used to evaluate and judge the care that is provided in the event an incident may occur, which results in claim and suit. Familiarity with such standards is clearly the starting point for compliance with the standard of care.

• Third line of defense: Because all programs and services in any health/fitness facility are provided through personnel, the basic core for any facility's service delivery system will always be evaluated through those persons. Only qualified and competent personnel – be they employees or independent contractors should be permitted to deliver service. Education, training, and certification and/or "national board" testing should serve as the basic starting point for all facility personnel.

• Fourth line of defense: Based upon the law and published standards of practice, all health/fitness facilities should adopt written policies and procedures dealing with pre-activity health screening, health/fitness assessment and prescription, and instruction and supervision provided to participants as well as a variety of issues related to exercise equipment and the fitness facility. Compliance to these policies and procedures not only helps to prevent medical emergencies in the first place but also can help to successfully defend against any negligence claim/lawsuit by being able to demonstrate that no legal duties were breached.

• Fifth line of defense: If a medical emergency does occur, it is important that a written Emergency Action Plan (EAP) be in place to be properly carried out by staff members in order to meet the standard of care. Follow-up procedures such as completing an incident report also are important. To help make sure that these steps are properly carried out, staff members should practice all aspects of the EAP periodically throughout the year and possess current certifications related to the process (e.g., CPR/AED and first-aid). Written and practiced EAPs can help mitigate a medical emergency and minimize any subsequent liability that may occur.

• Sixth line of defense: If a court rules that a participant's personal injury or wrongful death was caused by

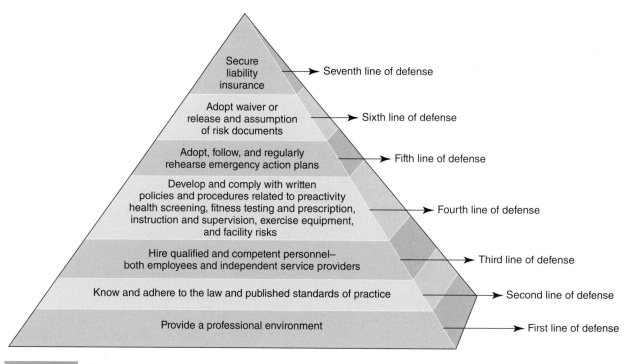

FIGURE 27.5 The risk management pyramid.

Reprinted, by permission, from J. Eickhoff-Shemek, D. Herbert, and D. Connaughton, 2009, *Risk management for health/fitness professionals: Legal issues and strategies* (Lippincott Williams & Wilkins, Baltimore, Maryland).

the negligence of a health/fitness facility or its personnel, a properly written and administered release/waiver can protect the health/fitness facility from any liability for "ordinary" negligence in most states. If it is determined that a participant's untoward event was due to the inherent risks of the activity (not based upon negligence or in those jurisdictions where releases/waivers are barred or not recognized), an assumption of risk document (e.g., express assumption of risk, agreement to participate, informed consent) can help strengthen the assumption of

risk defense for a health/fitness facility, which also helps to protect the facility from any liability.

• Seventh line of defense: If a claim is filed, applicable liability insurance will provide a defense to the claim. In addition, if a facility is found liable for negligence, liability insurance will pay for the resultant damages up to the amount of coverage allowed in the policy, thus protecting the financial assets of the facility. Both general and professional liability insurance should be considered to provide this protection.

STUDY QUESTIONS

1. Describe the types of injuries that can occur while participating in physical activity.
2. Describe the three primary sources of law and give an example of each.
3. Define the following legal terms: *stare decisis*, *respondeat superior*, *compensatory damages*, *punitive damages*, and *exculpatory clause*.
4. Define the following risk management terms: *loss-prevention strategies*, *loss-reduction strategies*, *contractual transfer of risks*, *general liability insurance*, and *professional liability insurance*.
5. Describe the type of conduct that would be considered ordinary negligence and gross negligence.
6. Explain why the primary assumption of risk was not an effective defense in the *Corrigan* and *Santana* cases. Also, describe how the courts in these cases distinguished sport and physical activity with regard to this defense.
7. Describe why fitness professionals should have a waiver reviewed and edited by a competent lawyer before having participants signing it.
8. Describe how the professional standard of care can be determined in negligence cases.
9. Explain how a fitness professional could be qualified but not competent. Then describe why it is essential from a legal perspective that fitness professionals be competent.
10. List the names of the negligence cases described in this chapter where the defendant (fitness professional) was likely practicing outside the scope of practice.

CASE STUDIES

You can check your answers by referring to appendix A.

World's Best Fitness Center (WBFC) is located in Virginia. Upon joining the fitness center, John Smith signed a membership contract that included an exculpatory clause (waiver). Mr. Smith was not offered any type of orientation or instruction on how to use the equipment and the facility. One day while at the club, he decided to perform some exercises with an exercise ball. He had never used an exercise ball before but had observed other members using them. No fitness staff members were around that day instructing or supervising in the fitness area, so he went ahead and tried these new exercises on his own.

While performing these exercises, the ball exploded and he fell hard and fast to the floor. The fall caused extreme pain to his lower back and he could not move. A staff member, who had just entered the fitness area, immediately went to his aid and called EMS. All emergency procedures were carried out properly by the staff members according to ACSM standards and guidelines. At the hospital, Mr. Smith was diagnosed with a severe spinal injury that will require spinal fusion surgery. His lawyer has filed a personal injury lawsuit against WBFC seeking damages for Mr. Smith's injury.

WBFC never assigned or trained a staff member to inspect the exercise balls to detect any signs of wear or proper inflation. In addition, a week before Mr. Smith's injury, another member was seriously injured from an exploding exercise ball.

1. What negligence claims will Mr. Smith and his lawyer likely file against WBFC?
   a. How will the court determine the duties owed to the plaintiff in this case?
   b. What type of damages will Mr. Smith seek?

2. What defenses will WBFC likely use in this case?

    a. Will these defenses be effective in protecting WBFC from any liability?

    b. Why or why not?

3. What risk management strategies should WBFC have implemented that might have prevented Mr. Smith's injury?

4. As a risk management strategy, WBFC provided general liability insurance coverage for their employees. If WBFC is found liable for negligence, will the insurance company pay out the damages in this case? Why or why not?

REFERENCES

1. Abbott, A.A. 2009. Fitness professionals: Certified, qualified, and justified. *The Exercise Standards and Malpractice Reporter* 23(2): 17, 20-22.

2. ADA Title III Part 36: Nondiscrimination on the basis of disability by public accommodation and commercial facilities. 2010. Available at www.ada.gov/reg3a.html. Accessed December 5, 2010.

3. *Americans with Disabilities Act (ADA).* 2004. 42 U.S.C. 12181(7) (L) and 12182.

4. *Alack v. Vic Tanny International of Missouri, Inc.* 923 S.W.2d 330 (Mo., 1996).

5. Blair, S.A. 2003. Implementing HIPAA. *ACSM's Health & Fitness Journal* 7(5): 25-27.

6. *Bloodborne pathogens.* 2009. 29 C.F.R. § 1910.1030. New York: Thomson Reuters.

7. Brathwaite, A., D. Davidson, and J.M. Eickhoff-Shemek. 2006. Recruiting, training, and retaining qualified group exercise leaders: Part I. *ACSM's Health & Fitness Journal* 10(2): 14-18.

8. Brathwaite, A., and J.M. Eickhoff-Shemek. 2007. Preparing quality personal trainers: A successful pilot program. *The Exercise Standards and Malpractice Reporter* 21(2): 25-31.

9. *Capati v. Crunch Fitness International, Inc., et al.* Analyzed in: Herbert, D.L. 1999. $320 million lawsuit filed against health club. *The Exercise Standards and Malpractice Reporter* 13(3): 33, 36.

10. *Capati v. Crunch Fitness International, Inc., et al.* Analyzed in: Herbert, D.L. 2006. Wrongful death case of Anne Marie Capati settled for in excess of $4 million. *The Exercise Standards and Malpractice Reporter* 20(3): 36.

11. Carper, D.L., N.J. Mietus, and B.W. West BW. 2000. *Understanding the law.* 3rd ed. Cincinnati, OH: West Legal Studies in Business/Thomson Corporation.

12. *Chai v. Sports & Fitness Clubs of America, Inc.* Analyzed in: Failure to defibrillate results in new litigation. 1999. *The Exercise Standards and Malpractice Reporter* 13(4): 55-56.

13. Clarkson, K.W., R.L. Miller, G.A. Jentz, and F.B.Cross. 2001. *West's business law.* 8th ed. St. Paul, MN: West.

14. *Corrigan v. Musclemakers, Inc.*, 258 A.D.2d 861 (N.Y. App. Div., 1999).

15. Cotten, D.J., and M.B. Cotten. 2010. *Waivers and releases of liability.* 7th ed. Statesboro, GA: Sport Risk Consulting.

16. Craig, A., and J.M. Eickhoff-Shemek. 2009. Educating and training the personal fitness trainer: A pedagogical approach. *ACSM's Health & Fitness Journal* 13(2): 8-15.

17. Davidson, D., A. Brathwaite, and J.M. Eickhoff-Shemek. 2006. Recruiting, training, and retaining qualified group exercise leaders: Part II. *ACSM's Health & Fitness Journal* 10(3): 22-26.

18. Dobbs, D.B. 2000. *The law of torts.* St. Paul, MN: West.

19. *Duncan v. World Wide Health Studios*, 232 S.2d 835 (La. Ct. App. 1970).

20. Eickhoff-Shemek, J.M., and D.L. Herbert. 2007. Is licensure in your future? Issues to consider—part 1. *ACSM's Health & Fitness Journal* 11(5): 35-37.

21. Eickhoff-Shemek, J.M., and D.L Herbert. 2008. Is licensure in your future? Issues to consider—part 2. *ACSM's Health & Fitness Journal* 12(1): 36-38.

22. Eickhoff-Shemek, J.M. and D.L. Herbert. 2008. Is licensure in your future? Issues to consider—part 3. *ACSM's Health & Fitness Journal* 12(3): 36-38.

23. Eickhoff-Shemek, J.M., D.L. Herbert, and D.P. Connaughton. 2009. *Risk management for health/fitness professionals: Legal issues and strategies.* Baltimore: Lippincott Williams & Wilkins.

24. Eickhoff-Shemek, J.M, and N.P. Pronk. 2009. Applying the HIPAA nondiscrimination rules into employer-sponsored wellness programs. *ACSM's Health & Fitness Journal* 13(5): 35-39.

25. *Elledge v. Richland/Lexington School District Five*, LEXIS 108 (S.C. Ct. App. 2000).

26. *Goynias v. Spa Health Clubs, Inc.*, 148 N.C.App. 554 (N.C. Ct. App., 2002).

27. *Guthrie v. Crouser.* Analyzed in: Herbert, D.L. 2008. Qualifications/certifications of personal trainers again in the news. *The Exercise Standards and Malpractice Reporter* 22(3): 33, 36-38, and in: Jury verdict in favor of personal trainer client. 2011. *The Exercise Standards and Malpractice Reporter* 25(1): 11.

28. Head, G.L., and S. Horn. 1997. *Essentials of risk management: Vol. I.* 3rd ed. Malvern, PA: Insurance Institute of America.

29. Herbert, D.L. 2010. New Jersey reintroduces personal trainer legislation. *The Exercise Standards and Malpractice Reporter* 24(3): 37-41.

30. Herbert, D.L., and W.G. Herbert. 2002. *Legal aspects of preventive, rehabilitative and recreational exercise programs.* 4th ed. Canton, OH: PRC.

31. *Hicks v. Bally Total Fitness Corp.* Analyzed in: Herbert, D.L. 2009. New AED case filed. *The Exercise Standards and Malpractice Reporter* 23(1): 1, 4-7.

32. *Makris v. Scandinavian Health Spa, Inc.*, Ohio App. LEXIS 4416 (Ct. of Appeals, 7th Dist., 1999).

33. Moorman, A.M., and J.M. Eickhoff-Shemek. 2007. Risk management strategies for avoiding and responding to sexual assault complaints. *ACSM's Health & Fitness Journal* 11(3): 35-37.

34. *Nondiscrimination and wellness programs in health coverage in the group market: Final rules.* 2006. 71 Fed. Reg. 75,013. (26 C.F.R. pt. 54, 29 C.F.R. pt. 2590, 45 C.F.R. pt. 146). Available at: www.dol.gov/ebsa/Regs/fedreg/final/2006009557.pdf.

35. *Ohio Board of Dietetics, Bulletin #8, General Non-Medical Nutrition Information.* 2009. Available at: www.dietetics.ohio.gov/bulletins/bulletin8.pdf.

36. *Ohio Board of Dietetics v. Brown*, 83 Ohio App. 3rd 242 (Ohio App. LEXIS 88, 1993).

37. *Randas v. YMCA of Metropolitan Los Angeles*, 17 Cal. App.4th 158 (Cal. App. 2 Dist., 1993).

38. *Restatement of the law third. Restatement of the law—torts.* 2006. Philadelphia: American Law Institute.

39. *Restatement of the law third. Restatement of the law torts: Liability for physical harm.* 2005. Proposed Final Draft No. 1, § 12. Knowledge and skills. Philadelphia: American Law Institute.

40. *Rostai v. Neste Enterprises*, 41 Cal. Reptr.3rd 411 (Cal. Ct. App., 4th Dist. 2006).

41. *Rutnik v. Colonie Center Court Club, Inc.*, 672 N.Y.S 2d 451 (1998 N.Y. App. Div. LEXIS 4845).

42. *Sanford v. Vision Quest Sport and Fitness.* Analyzed in: Herbert, D.L. 2009. Personal trainer sued in Washington. *The Exercise Standards and Malpractice Reporter* 23(1): 8-10.

43. *Santana v. Women's Workout and Weight Loss Centers, Inc.* (2001 Cal. App. LEXIS 1186).

44. Sass, C., J.M. Eickhoff-Shemek, M.M. Manore, and L.J. Kruskall. 2007. Crossing the line: Understanding the scope of practice between registered dietitians and health/fitness professionals. *ACSM's Health & Fitness Journal* 11(3): 12-19.

45. *Seigneur v. National Fitness Institute, Inc.*, 132 Md. App. 271 (Md. Ct. Spec. App., 2000).

46. Springer, J., J.M. Eickhoff-Shemek, and E. Zuberbuehler. 2009. An investigation of preactivity cardiovascular screening procedures in health/fitness facilities, part I: Is adherence with national standards decreasing? *Preventive Cardiology* 12(3): 155-162.

47. Springer, J., J.M. Eickhoff-Shemek, and E. Zuberbuehler. 2009. An investigation of preactivity cardiovascular screening procedures in health/fitness facilities, part II: Rationale for low adherence with national standards. *Preventive Cardiology* 12(4): 176-183.

48. Tharrett, S.J. and J.A. Peterson, eds. 2012. *ACSM's health/fitness facility standards and guidelines.* 4th ed. Champaign, IL: Human Kinetics.

49. *Thomas v. Sport City, Inc.* 738 So. 2d 1153 (La. Ct. App. 2 Cir., 1999).

50. Thompson, W.R., ed. 2010. *ACSM's guidelines for exercise testing and prescription.* 8th ed. Philadelphia: Lippincott Williams & Wilkins.

51. van der Smissen, B. 2007. Elements of negligence. In *Law for recreation and sport managers*, 4th ed. Ed. D.J. Cotton and J.T. Wolohan. Dubuque, IA: Kendall/Hunt.

52. van der Smissen B. 1990. *Legal liability and risk management for public and private entities: Vol. 2.* Cincinnati, OH: Anderson.

53. *Xu v. Gay*, 668 N.W.2d 166 (Mich. App., 2003).

54. *York Insurance Company v. Houston Wellness Center, Inc.*, 261 Ga. App. 854 (Ga. Ct. App., 2003).

APPENDIX A
Case Study Answers

Chapter 1

1. You might state that the physical activity recommendations in the government report were aimed at people who are currently sedentary and not those who are habitually active and involved in strenuous exercise. In addition, you might indicate that participation in more strenuous exercise is associated with other health-related benefits (increases in CRF, or $\dot{V}O_2max$) that are more difficult to achieve with moderate-intensity exercise.

2. You might respond by admitting that there are risks related to exercise, with 1 death occurring each year for every 15,000 to 18,000 exercisers. However, more people die while sleeping or after eating and yet few people advocate the cessation of those activities. In addition, deterioration of the cardiovascular system through sedentary living causes a much higher risk of major health problems compared with being active. Finally, exercise-related risks can be minimized by starting slowly and gradually increasing the amount and intensity of work done during exercise.

3. You might begin by telling him that the health-related benefits of physical activity occur in all people, independent of body weight or body fatness. Further, it is important to establish a pattern of physical activity as one of the new behaviors needed to help maintain the weight loss once the goal is achieved.

Chapter 2

1. Ask Barbara to confirm that she has not been diagnosed with high BP and is not taking a prescribed medication to control it. If she does take BP medication, make certain she has taken it within the last 24 hr. Next, inquire if she has eaten, consumed caffeine, smoked, or performed physical activity within the last hour. If she answers these questions to your satisfaction, it is likely her elevated HR and BP may be attributed to anxiety regarding the fitness assessment. You may want to review the procedures for the fitness tests, reassure her of their safety, and remind her that she can stop any test at any time if she desires to do so. You may also want to discuss activities she enjoys for a couple of minutes in order to help her relax. Next, reassess her HR and BP. If they are within normal values, continue with the fitness tests. Be certain to reassure her throughout each test. If HR and BP remain high, then you may ask her to make a second appointment when it is convenient for her.

2. Although she is 65 yr old, she did not indicate any risk factors on her PAR-Q, has had a recent physician-administered exam, and participates regularly in moderate-intensity exercise. Thus, she is classified as moderate risk and does not need physician consent before participation in moderate-intensity physical activities. She should be instructed to alert the instructor if she experiences any abnormal responses to exercise (e.g., unusual shortness of breath, dizziness), to begin with light weights such as 3 to 5 lb (1.4-2.3 kg) dumbbells, and to expect some mild soreness for 1 to 2 days after class participation.

3a. Tom's primary risk factors for CHD include age (>45 yr), hypertension (taking medication for the condition), high cholesterol (taking medication for the condition and LDL ≥130 mg · dl^{-1}), and physical inactivity (does not accumulate 30 min of moderate intensity at least 3 days · wk^{-1}). Thus, he has four risk factors and would be classified as moderate risk.

3b. According to the AHA and ACSM guidelines for physician consent, the fitness professional should contact Tom's physician to obtain medical clearance because he was classified as moderate risk and wants to pursue high-intensity (i.e., vigorous) exercise. Although Tom has seen his physician recently, it was not necessarily to inquire if he should begin exercising regularly. Contacting the physician ensures that she is aware of Tom's plans to pursue regular physical activity and provides the fitness professional with consent from a medical authority.

Chapter 3

1. Explain to the exerciser that the hip and knee extensors that are used to push against the weights are also working to control the descent. The press requires concentric contraction; the return requires eccentric contraction. Both kinds of contractions lead to increases in strength.

2. When she's doing the wrist curls with her palms down (radioulnar pronated position), the wrist extensors are the contracting muscles; when her palms are up (supinated position), the wrist flexors are the working muscles. The wrist flexors are usually stronger than the wrist extensors.

The explanation is different for the pull-ups. The elbow flexor muscles are working regardless of the position of the radioulnar joint. However, when the palms are facing away (pronation), the distal tendon of the biceps brachii is wrapped around the radius bone and therefore this muscle cannot exert as much force as when the palms are facing toward the body (supinated position).

3. He should make a conscious effort to maintain a backward pelvic tilt. He should also keep his arms in front of his head instead of by his ears and his knees slightly flexed to help maintain the backward tilt.

Chapter 4

1. The lactate threshold is the point during a GXT when the blood lactic acid concentration suddenly increases. The lactate threshold has been used to indicate performance because the speed at which it occurs closely relates to the speed that can be maintained in distance runs (10K or marathon). As she improves her training, the lactate threshold occurs later in the GXT, indicating that she can maintain a faster pace in distance runs.

2. You need to confirm your client's feeling that the heart is stronger after training and, as a result, can pump more blood out per beat (increased SV). As a result, the heart does not have to beat as many times to deliver the same amount of oxygen to the tissues. This is a more efficient way for the heart to pump blood, and the heart does not have to work as hard at this lower heart rate.

3. You might begin by briefly stating that running speed in distance races relates to the amount of oxygen the runner can deliver to the muscles. When more oxygen can be delivered, the running speed is faster. The elite female distance runner differs from the elite male distance runner in three ways that have a bearing on this issue: Her heart size is smaller and she cannot pump as much oxygen-rich blood to the muscles per minute, the oxygen content of her blood is lower due to the lower hemoglobin concentration, and she is also carrying relatively more body fat, which negatively affects sustained running speed even at the same level of fitness.

Chapter 5

1. This athlete weighs 86.4 kg. The ACSM, ADA, and Dietitians of Canada position statement (4) suggests that such an athlete may benefit from ingesting 1.2 to 1.4 g of protein for each kilogram of body weight. This athlete is consuming approximately 525 kcal of protein each day (3,500 kcal ·

0.15 = 525 kcal). This amount roughly equals 131 g of protein (525 kcal ÷ 4 kcal · g^{-1} = 131.25 g), or approximately 1.5 g · kg^{-1} (131.25 g ÷ 86.4 kg = 1.52 g · kg^{-1}). Additional protein intake appears unwarranted. If the athlete is unable to maintain weight, endurance, or strength with his current eating habits, a registered dietitian or sports dietitian should be consulted.

2. Mr. Flanagan is asking important questions about his overall wellness and, as a fitness professional, you are positioned to help him in several ways. First, point out to Mr. Flanagan the general recommendations contained in the Dietary Guidelines for Americans, which outline healthy eating practices that Americans should incorporate into their daily lives. The information contained in table 5.4 is a summary of some of these recommendations. Second, encourage Mr. Flanagan to begin tracking his dietary habits (see form 5.1). Tell him about the MyPlate website and encourage him to examine how his food intake matches recommended levels. Third, share with Mr. Flanagan recipes for healthy and easy to cook meals.

3. Because Mrs. Ortez has a metabolic disease, type 2 diabetes, it is important that she seek out advice from a number of medical professionals, including her physician and a registered dietitian. However, as a fitness professional, you are a critical member of her overall wellness team. Here are things that you should do: (1) Encourage Mrs. Ortez to carefully follow the instructions of her physician regarding medications, weight loss, and any exercise limitations; (2) encourage Mrs. Ortez to consult a registered dietitian about her dietary habits (if necessary, point her to registered dietitians in your area); (3) provide general recommendations from the Dietary Guidelines for Americans about healthy eating habits; (4) provide examples of easy, low-calorie recipes; and (5) help her track her progress with exercise goals and weight loss and monitor her response to exercise for any unhealthy signs.

Chapter 6

1. $3.5 \text{ mi} \cdot \text{hr}^{-1} \cdot 26.8 \text{m} \cdot \text{min}^{-1} = 93.8 \text{m} \cdot \text{min}^{-1}$

$93.8 \text{m} \cdot \text{min}^{-1} \left(\dfrac{0.1 \text{ml} \cdot \text{kg}^{-1} \cdot \text{min}^{-1}}{\text{m} \cdot \text{min}^{-1}} \right) +$

$3.5 \text{ml} \cdot \text{kg}^{-1} \cdot \text{min}^{-1} = 12.9 \text{ml} \cdot \text{kg}^{-1} \cdot \text{min}^{-1}$

$12.9 \text{ml} \cdot \text{kg}^{-1} \cdot \text{min}^{-1} \cdot 75 \text{kg} =$

$968 \text{ml} \cdot \text{min}^{-1}, \text{ or } 0.97 \text{L} \cdot \text{min}^{-1}$

$0.97 \text{L} \cdot \text{min}^{-1} \cdot 5 \text{kcal} \cdot \text{L}^{-1} = 4.85 \text{kcal} \cdot \text{min}^{-1}$

$4.85 \text{kcal} \cdot \text{min}^{-1} \cdot 30 \text{min} = 146 \text{kcal}$

2. $$100 \text{ W} = 600 \text{ kpm} \cdot \text{min}^{-1}$$

$$\dot{V}O_2 = \frac{(600 \text{ kpm} \cdot \text{min}^{-1} \cdot 1.8 \text{ ml O}_2 \cdot \text{min}^{-1})}{60 \text{ kg} + 7 \text{ ml} \cdot \text{kg}^{-1} \cdot \text{min}^{-1}}$$

$$25 \text{ ml} \cdot \text{kg}^{-1} \cdot \text{min}^{-1} =$$

$$18 \text{ ml} \cdot \text{kg}^{-1} \cdot \text{min}^{-1} + 7 \text{ ml} \cdot \text{kg}^{-1} \cdot \text{min}^{-1}$$

3. $3 \text{ mi} \cdot 1,610 \text{ m} \cdot \text{mi}^{-1} = 4,830 \text{ m} \div 24 \text{ min} = 201 \text{ m} \cdot \text{min}^{-1}$

$$201 \text{ m} \cdot \text{min}^{-1} \left(\frac{0.2 \text{ ml} \cdot \text{kg}^{-1} \cdot \text{min}^{-1}}{\text{m} \cdot \text{min}^{-1}} \right) +$$

$$3.5 \text{ ml} \cdot \text{kg}^{-1} \cdot \text{min}^{-1} = 43.7 \text{ ml} \cdot \text{kg}^{-1} \cdot \text{min}^{-1}$$

$$43.7 \text{ ml} \cdot \text{kg}^{-1} \cdot \text{min}^{-1} \cdot 70 \text{ kg} =$$

$$3,059 \text{ ml} \cdot \text{min}^{-1}, \text{ or } 3.06 \text{ L} \cdot \text{min}^{-1}$$

$$3.06 \text{ L} \cdot \text{min}^{-1} \cdot 5 \text{ kcal} \cdot \text{L}^{-1} =$$

$$15.3 \text{ kcal} \cdot \text{min}^{-1} \cdot 24 \text{ min} = 367 \text{ kcal}$$

4. $$12 \text{ METs} = 12 \text{ kcal} \cdot \text{kg}^{-1} \cdot \text{hr}^{-1} \cdot 70\% =$$

$$8.4 \text{ kcal} \cdot \text{kg}^{-1} \cdot \text{hr}^{-1}$$

5. You might indicate that the cost of jogging 1 m · min^{-1} (0.2 ml · kg^{-1} · min^{-1}) is about twice that for walking (0.1 ml · kg^{-1} · min^{-1}) due to the extra energy needed to propel the body off the ground and absorb the force of impact on each step. You might provide a summary table he can use describing the caloric cost of walking and running 1 mi (1.6 km).

Chapter 7

1. Requiring sedentary middle-aged participants to take a maximal, unmonitored test at the beginning of their fitness program is inappropriate. You might suggest the club replace the 1.5 mi (2.4 km) run with the 1 mi (1.6 km) walk test, which should be used after the participants have demonstrated that they can comfortably walk 1 mi.

2. His estimated $\dot{V}O_2$max = 37.8 ml · kg^{-1} · min^{-1}. His level of CRF is adequate for most activities and just short of being good for his age group.

3. The HR response of 100 beats · min^{-1} at the work rate of 300 kgm · min^{-1} should be ignored. The HR values are extrapolated to 170 beats · min^{-1}, and the vertical line dropped from that point indicates a work rate of about 1,050 kgm · min^{-1},

$$\dot{V}O_2 = \frac{(1050 \text{ kpm} \cdot \text{min}^{-1} \cdot 1.8 \text{ ml O}_2 \cdot \text{kpm}^{-1})}{81.7 \text{ kg} + 7 \text{ ml} \cdot \text{kg}^{-1} \cdot \text{min}^{-1}}$$

$$= \frac{30.1 \text{ ml} \cdot \text{kg}^{-1} \cdot \text{min}^{-1}}{3.5 \text{ ml} \cdot \text{kg}^{-1} \cdot \text{min}^{-1}} = 8.6 \text{ METs}$$

4. The graph should ignore the HR value of 96 beats · min^{-1}. The line is extrapolated to 190 beats · min^{-1}, and the vertical line dropped from that point indicates a value of about 16.75% grade, which

equals a $\dot{V}O_2$ of about 35.6 ml · kg · min^{-1}. This is 10.2 METs, or 1.94 L · min^{-1}.

5. The reference point for the scale is the zero point established when the free-swinging pendulum stops (with the cycle on a flat surface). All scale values are relative to this zero, and if the zero is off, all scale readings are off. If the pendulum does not rest at zero when no weight is attached, the entire scale is off by the amount the zero value is off by. For example, if the scale reads 0.25 kg when no weight is attached, each scale value shifts 0.25 kg upward when known weights are attached.

Chapter 8

1. Height, weight, BMI, %BF, and waist and hip circumference

2. BMI = 97.7 kg ÷ (1.778 m · 1.778 m) = 30.9 kg · m^{-2}, which is in the obese range.

WHR = 41 in. ÷ 39 in. = 1.05, which is considered high risk.

To calculate %BF, first calculate body density using the three-site formula:

D_b = 1.10938 − 0.0008267 (sum of skinfolds) + 0.0000016 (sum of skinfolds)^2 − 0.0002574 (age)

= 1.10938 − 0.0008267 (104) + 0.0000016 (104)^2 − 0.0002574 (48)

= 1.0283.

Next, use the Siri equation to convert the density into %BF:

%BF = (495 ÷ D_b) − 450 = (495 ÷ 1.0283) − 495 = 31.4%, which is in the obese range.

3. First calculate fat mass and fat-free mass:

FM = weight · %BF = 215 · 31.4% = 67.5 lb (30.6 kg).

FFM = total weight − FM = 215 − 67.5 = 147.5 lb (66.9 kg).

Now calculate target weight:

Target weight = FFM ÷ (1 − desired %BF) = 147.5 ÷ (1 − 0.28) = 205 lb (93.0 kg).

Chapter 9

1a. Please see pages 186-187 for a summary of the push-up test.

1b. Please see pages 186-187 for a summary of the curl-up test.

1c. Please see page 185 for a summary of the 1RM test.

Chapter 10

1. The sacral angle should be at least 80° (a book or board on edge placed against the sacrum would be snug if the angle were 90°). Next examine the curvature of the spine; it should be smooth with no evident flatness or hypermobility in any one particular area. Arm–leg length discrepancy might also be a factor (e.g., long arms in relation to legs).

2. Most false positives in the Thomas test result when the person being tested brings the thigh too close to the chest. This can result in excessive posterior rotation of the pelvis, which can make it appear that the hip flexors are tight.

3. As with most conditions, a scoliosis may be minor and not necessitate any special consideration. In some cases a client's scoliosis might seem to be a problem that might benefit from a few specific exercise routines; however, even though this might be true in some cases, because the cause of a scoliosis can be quite complex, it would be inappropriate for an exercise leader to prescribe exercises involving spinal movement in an attempt to correct a scoliosis without discussing this with the client and obtaining proper consultation. Has the client been under the care of an orthopedist, physiatrist, chiropractor, or other medical personnel for the condition? Have any specific exercises or activities been recommended for the scoliosis? Are there any contraindicated exercises or activities?

Chapter 11

1. If a person has a normal response to a GXT, HR and SBP increase with each stage of the test, whereas the DBP remains the same or decreases slightly. In addition, the ECG shows no significant ST segment depression or elevation and no significant arrhythmias. In these cases it can be assumed that the last load achieved on the test represents the true functional capacity (max METs). The GXT presented in this case study is representative of such a test.

Paul has normal resting BP and a negative family history for CHD. Risk factors include a relatively high percentage of body fat, a sedentary lifestyle, and a poor blood lipid profile. Based on these findings, a THR range of 158 to 177 beats $\cdot$ min^{-1} was calculated (60%-80% $\dot{V}O_2$max as measured during the maximal GXT); this HR range corresponds to work rates equal to 6.3 to 8.4 METs. Initially, he will work at or below the lower end of the calculated THR range, with the emphasis on the duration of activity. As he becomes more active he will be able to work within the THR range, depending, of course, on his interests. He was referred for nutritional counseling to improve his blood lipid profile.

Paul has an estimated HRmax of 174 beats $\cdot$ min^{-1}; his measured HR was 24 beats $\cdot$ min^{-1} higher. Given the inherent biological variation in the estimated HRmax, use the measured values when they are available.

2. Mary's maximal work rate was estimated to be 750 kpm $\cdot$ min^{-1} by extrapolating the relationship between HR and work rate to the predicted maximal HR (see chapter 5). This is equivalent to a $\dot{V}O_2$max of 29 ml $\cdot$ kg^{-1} $\cdot$ min^{-1}, or 8.3 METs.

Her blood chemistry values and BP are normal. Her family history is negative for CHD. Her HR response to the test is normal and indicates poor CRF. The low maximal aerobic power is related to the sedentary lifestyle, the cigarette smoking (carbon monoxide), and the 30% body fat. She was encouraged to participate in a smoking-cessation program and was given the names of two local professional groups.

The recommended exercise program emphasized the low end of the THR zone (70% HRmax: 127 beats $\cdot$ min^{-1}) with long duration. She preferred a walking program because of the freedom it gave her schedule. She was given the walking program in chapter 14 and was asked to record her HR response to each of the exercise sessions.

A body-fat goal of 22% resulted in a target body weight of 121 lb (55 kg). She did not feel the need for dietary counseling at this time, but she agreed to record her food intake for 10 days to determine the patterns of eating behavior that would be beneficial to change (see chapters 5, 12, and 19). She made an appointment with the fitness professional in 2 wk to discuss the progress with her program.

3. You might begin by talking about the importance of regular physical activity in reducing the risk of numerous chronic diseases. In addition, you could indicate that the risk associated with regular participation in moderate-intensity physical activity is very low. Then, give them a copy of the PAR-Q to read over and help them make a determination about whether or not they should see their physician before beginning a physical activity program. Next, you might recommend a walking program that begins with short (e.g., 10 min) bouts of activity done at a comfortable pace each day. Encourage them to gradually increase the number of 10 min bouts done per day until they could do a single 30 min walk each day. On the other hand, if some wanted to continue to do 10 min bouts because it fit their schedules, that would be fine. Finally, you might suggest that their weekly goal be at least 150 min of walking, but more is better relative to health benefits derived.

Chapter 12

1. EER = 354 − 6.91(age) + PA[9.36(weight) + 726(height)],

   EER = 354 − 6.91(55) + 1.12[9.36(72.7) + 726(1.65)],

   $$EER = 2,078 \text{ kcal} \cdot \text{day}^{-1}.$$

2. $1,578 \text{ kcal} \cdot \text{day}^{-1}$ (deficit of $500 \text{ kcal} \cdot \text{day}^{-1}$) should be recommended.

3. Approximately $4.5 \text{ kcal} \cdot \text{min}^{-1} \cdot 30 \cdot \text{min day}^{-1} = 135 \text{ kcal} \cdot \text{day}^{-1}$.

   If Ms. Kim engages in this activity 5 days $\cdot$ wk^{-1}, that will add up to 675 kcal $\cdot$ wk^{-1}, which will add an extra pound (0.5 kg) of weight loss every 5 wk.

Chapter 13

1. Since it is not possible to improve at the same rate over long-term training, it is important to vary the resistance training program over time to limit training plateaus and optimize adaptations. By periodically varying the program variables (e.g., choice of exercise, sets, and repetitions), long-term performance gains will be optimized and exercise adherence will be improved. One option for this member is to follow an undulating or nonlinear training program, which is characterized by daily fluctuations in volume and intensity. For example, over time he could progress to 2 or 3 sets of 8 to 10 repetitions with a moderate load on Monday, 3 or 4 sets of 6 repetitions with a heavy load on Wednesday, and 1 or 2 sets of 12 to 15 repetitions with a light load on Friday. In addition, he should seek advice from a fitness professional and learn how to safely incorporate free-weight exercises and other training systems (e.g., preexhaustion and assisted training) into his program.

2. Although this client should be encouraged to continue swimming, resistance training can offer additional benefits in terms of musculoskeletal strength. A fitness professional should discuss the potential health and fitness benefits of regular weight-bearing physical activity with the client and should dispel any preconceived concerns regarding resistance training. In short, females will not develop bulky muscles if they participate in a resistance training program, but they will improve their musculoskeletal strength and reduce their risk of developing osteoporosis later in life. Since this client does not have any resistance training experience, she should begin with a single set of 8 to 12 repetitions on a variety of single and multijoint exercises to improve her confidence and exercise compliance. Over time, she should progress to a multiple-set system using various combinations of sets and repetitions to optimize gains in musculoskeletal strength.

3. Regular resistance training can offer observable health and fitness benefits to older adults; however, the health status of seniors should be assessed before resistance training begins in order to identify any preexisting medical conditions. Also, fitness professionals who have experience working with older populations should be available to provide instruction and assistance as needed. General program design considerations that should be discussed with the director of this assisted living center include the following: (1) Resistance training should begin with minimal resistance during the first few weeks so participants can learn proper exercise technique and have time for musculoskeletal adaptation; (2) the resistance, repetitions, or number of sets should be gradually increased to maximize gains in muscular fitness; and (3) over time, exercises that reduce the base of support, stress postural muscle groups, and reduce sensory input should be sensibly incorporated into the resistance training program to enhance balance, agility, and proprioception. Further, the importance of exercising in a group setting should not be underemphasized since social support can enhance exercise adherence in older populations.

Chapter 14

1. Although it is possible that this exercise might be appropriate for some people with well-developed abdominal musculature, it is not appropriate for the masses since the quality of the movement is so critical. A person with extremely well-developed abdominal muscles may be able to perform this exercise and keep her low back in contact with the exercise surface throughout its execution; however, someone with weaker abdominal muscles or tight hip flexors will invariably anteriorly tilt the pelvis, and the resulting lumbar lordosis places the lumbar vertebrae in a potentially compromising position. Undoubtedly the physical therapists who use this activity use it only as a test on a one-to-one basis, which enables them to immediately stop the activity if they believe it is compromising to the individual.

2. It is good that the exercise leader emphasizes the importance of not doing ballistic stretches even from the sitting position; however, there are other factors that she should also consider. This maneuver is a fair exercise for improving hamstring extensibility. However, if the participant has extremely tight hamstrings (i.e., if the sacrum should be less than 80° to 90° with the exercise surface in the sit-and-reach), the forward stretching from this position could potentially stretch the tissues of the

low back instead of the hamstrings. Therefore, the sit-and-reach exercise may be contraindicated for people with fairly tight hamstrings, and the standing toe touch could be worse because of the effect of gravity on the moment arm of force.

3. Although isometric exercises have become less popular for strength development in most applications (joint injury would be an exception), they can be used most appropriately for strengthening trunk musculature, assuming the exerciser does not have high BP. The oblique curl could be particularly advantageous since the internal and external oblique muscles play an important role in stabilizing the spine. This factor may decrease the likelihood of having low-back problems; for the individual who is symptomatic, developing these muscles in this way may enable him to better maintain a neutral spine and avoid postures that exacerbate his condition.

Chapter 15

1. Refer the parent to the recommendations for resistance training in children, explaining that the emphasis should be on proper form, supervision, and endurance at this age. After puberty, he can include resistance training with fewer repetitions.

2. Acknowledge that reading and math are important. The school needs to provide a good foundation in these areas, but it cannot possibly do it all—some reading and math work will need to be done at home and in the community. Including physical activity (through physical education and recess) is essential for the health of the children. Basic health is a prerequisite for other learning. In the same way that the school cannot provide all the necessary math and reading, the school cannot provide all the recommended physical activity, but it can provide a foundation that can be supplemented in the home and community.

3. You might provide a summary of the psychological and social benefits that can be realized through participation in sport. These benefits are considerable and include the following:

   ○ Psychological assets

     a. Self-determined motivation toward physical activity

     b. Positive values toward physical activity

     c. Feelings of self-determination, autonomy, and choice

     d. Positive identity, body image, and self-esteem

     e. Perceived physical competence and self-efficacy

     f. Positive affect and stress relief

     g. Moral identity, empathy, and social perspective-taking

     h. Cognitive functioning and intellectual health

     i. Hope and optimism about the future

   ○ Social assets

     a. Support from significant adults and peers

     b. Feelings of social acceptance

     c. Close friendship and friendship quality

     d. Leadership, teamwork, and cooperation

     e. Respect, responsibility, courtesy, and integrity

     f. Sense of civic engagement and contribution to community

     g. Resistance to peer pressure to engage in risky behaviors

Chapter 16

1. You should begin by finding out when he had his last physical and what his physician told him about his arthritis. A submaximal cycle ergometer test should be carried out to obtain some baseline measures (HR, RPE) to use as reference points for subsequent follow-ups. Establish a THR zone for him (50%-70% of HRR), and verify that this elicits an RPE of about 10 to 13. Have him begin his exercise program at 50% HRR, performing work–relief intervals (5 min on, 1 min off) to determine if he can do a series of these intervals with little or no joint discomfort. The goal is 30 min of continuous activity as long as the discomfort is little or nothing. Increase the work interval to 10 min in the second week. If joint discomfort is a problem, stay with intervals within his tolerance. Intensity can be increased after he has achieved 30 min of total exercise time. Introduce him to a variety of weight-supported exercise modes (cycle, rower, water aerobics) that he should be able to use with less joint discomfort than what he experienced with jogging. Workouts should be done 3 to 4 times each week and include regular warm-up and flexibility activities.

2. This 55-yr-old woman is clearly fit, but she needs to add other types of activities to her regular routine to improve bone health. You might recommend that she add a resistance training program that will not only improve bone strength but also her swimming performance. In addition, you might suggest that she add regular walking to her weekly activities to provide some downward loading to the bone that she is not experiencing in her swim workouts.

3. You might begin by using the SFT (Senior Fitness Test) to obtain some baseline values for the various fitness components. Based on those test results, you should develop a program of activities that include walking (graduated in a manner that encourages multiple short walks with plenty of rest) and muscle-strengthening activities using either very light dumbbells or low-tension elastic bands (again, with only a few reps in the beginning).

Chapter 17

1. This client will benefit from both weight-bearing aerobic activity and resistance training. To increase her aerobic fitness, protect her against chronic disease, and load her bones, a walking program is appropriate. She should gradually progress to a 30 min brisk walk on most, preferably all, days of the week. Additionally, she should engage in resistance training 2 to 3 days · wk^{-1}. The program should include upper- and lower-body exercises and focus on areas at high risk for osteoporotic fractures (hip, spine, wrist). Three sets of approximately 70% of 1RM (8-12 reps) are appropriate. Suggested exercises include the standing toe raise, leg press, leg extension, leg curl, back extension (use care to avoid hyperextension), bench press, shoulder press, biceps curl, triceps extension, and wrist curl. Additionally, the client should consume adequate amounts of calcium and vitamin D (see chapter 5).

2. Given that Janice's physician cleared her to continue running, there is no medical reason to stop running at this point in her pregnancy. However, it is understandable that both Janice and her mother-in-law have concerns. The first step is to alleviate fears through education. Give Janice background information on the health benefits of remaining active during pregnancy. Also, provide her with the warning signs that she should seek medical help (e.g., vaginal bleeding, dyspnea before exertion). Then encourage her to remain as active as she feels comfortable with during her pregnancy. Talk with her about using HR and RPE as a guide to her exercise intensity. Also, acknowledge that the types and intensity of exercise will likely need to change as she gets closer to term. Discuss with her the types of exercise that should be avoided (e.g., supine exercise).

3. This is a potentially difficult and dangerous situation. At the very least, Samantha is exhibiting signs of poor physical and emotional health. Begin a dialogue with Samantha addressing your concerns. Gently ask questions about her weight and eating habits (e.g., "Have you been doing anything different with your eating or exercise?"). Encourage her to take her health seriously. Explain to her how important it is to eat a healthy diet in order to optimize performance as well as remain healthy. Encourage her to discuss with her health care providers the recurrent stress fractures that she is experiencing. She is still a minor, so if you have a relationship with her parents, you may also want to engage them in a conversation. But before you engage either Samantha or her parents in conversation about your concerns, you need to seek out a support system for assistance. Find out the names of nutritionists, physicians, and mental health professionals in your area who specialize in eating disorders, particularly with athletes. Given that Samantha is already exhibiting diminished health and signs associated with disordered eating, she is likely going to require the assistance of a multidisciplinary team.

Chapter 18

1. Since John is a 46-yr-old male with typical effort-induced angina and an elevated total cholesterol–HDL ratio over 5.0 (signifying increase risk), he has a high likelihood of CHD. A reasonable next step would be to refer him for a GXT in the presence of a physician to see if signs or symptoms of CHD occur. If they do, a more definitive diagnostic test such as coronary angiography might be recommended.

2. Jane's GXT results indicated that her maximal aerobic capacity was 7 METs; therefore, prescribing exercise at about 60% of this value, or around 4 METs, would be appropriate. Suitable exercises would include treadmill walking, stationary cycling, and arm cranking. Realize that her maximal HR is low because she is taking a beta-blocker. Thus, exercise could be prescribed on the basis of RPE (e.g., a target rating of *somewhat hard* on the Borg RPE scale). Light resistance exercises using dumbbells and elastic bands, as tolerated, would also be acceptable. The resistance should be selected so as to allow her to perform 12 to 15 repetitions with good form.

3. Because Ralph has had a chest incision and heart surgery, he must proceed cautiously. A resistance training program consisting of light, seated exercises using 1 to 2 lb (.5-.9 kg) dumbbells and light-weight elastic bands is appropriate in the beginning. He could perform 12 to 15 repetitions of several exercises while maintaining good form and proper breathing. The goal should be to slightly overload the muscles and maintain ROM. He should stop if he feels pain or movement in the area of the incision. Also, he should be instructed to avoid holding his breath or straining while lifting. Over time, the weights can be gradually increased.

Chapter 19

1a. Because Marsha is hypertensive, has extreme (class III) obesity, is inactive, has a strong family history of CVD and diabetes, and has not undergone a medical examination in several years, medical clearance before beginning an exercise program is recommended. The medical examination should be used to reveal any underlying medical conditions that would make it unsafe for Marsha to engage in moderate or vigorous exercise.

1b. In addition to height and weight, measurement of waist and hip circumference is recommended. In addition to BMI calculations and examination of abdominal adiposity, an estimate of body-fat percentage could be useful, but only if methods are chosen that are both reliable and accurate for obese individuals (see chapter 8). CRF could be assessed with either a treadmill or a cycle ergometer protocol. Standard flexibility and strength tests could be used.

1c. A conversation with Marsha is crucial to determine her goals and interests. To increase adherence, close attention should be paid to her willingness to engage in a variety of activities. Attempts should be made to increase lifestyle activity and structured exercise. Assuming that Marsha is willing to invest an hour a day, 3 days $\cdot$ wk^{-1}, in structured exercise and is willing to exercise on her own on other days, the following program would target a weight loss of 2 lb $\cdot$ wk^{-1} (0.9 kg $\cdot$ wk^{-1}).

  o Exercise 6 days $\cdot$ wk^{-1} and try to expend 300 kcal of energy on each of these days. The structured exercise should focus on improving CRF, strength, and flexibility. On 3 days $\cdot$ wk^{-1} Marsha could walk on her own (preferably with an exercise partner) for 1 hr (could be divided into shorter sessions). This increase in activity will increase her caloric expenditure by approximately 1,800 kcal $\cdot$ wk^{-1}. Given that Marsha is very inactive now, a progressive program must be included in order to build up to this level of exercise.

  o She should target an energy intake that is approximately 745 kcal below her estimated calorie need. Using the formula in chapter 12, Marsha's daily energy need is approximately 2,480 kcal. Targeting a daily caloric intake of approximately 1,735 kcal $\cdot$ day^{-1} will result in a caloric deficit of 5,200 kcal $\cdot$ wk^{-1} from caloric restriction.

  o The combination of caloric restriction (5,200 kcal $\cdot$ wk^{-1}) and energy expenditure (1,800 kcal $\cdot$ wk^{-1}) will result in a weight loss of approximately 2 lb (0.9 kg) each week. Weekly weigh-ins and consultation with the fitness professional are recommended in order to adjust the program as needed.

2. Exercise goals—develop a plan that will allow Kevin to accumulate 300 min $\cdot$ wk^{-1} in moderate-intensity exercise. Better yet, given that Kevin is healthy and young, encourage him to spend at least some of his exercise time in vigorous exercise. Determine Kevin's exercise preferences and develop a program that meets aerobic recommendations and also addresses muscular fitness needs (resistance training 2 days $\cdot$ wk^{-1} and flexibility training during cool-downs from all workouts).

Lifestyle goals—encourage Kevin to eat a well-rounded diet as described in chapter 5. He is at a fairly healthy BMI, so making weight loss a major consideration is unnecessary. However, for a person like Kevin, weight-loss maintenance can be a struggle. Therefore the following can be useful: (1) Encourage him to weigh himself each morning, (2) encourage him to keep a journal of his food intake and exercise, and (3) encourage him to seek out a support system. As his fitness trainer, you will be a primary part of his support system, but encourage him to seek out friends who can provide additional support and encouragement for his healthy eating and exercise habits.

3. Shala has a long way to go to become an active person, but the fact that she has undergone bariatric surgery and that she is following her doctor's advice to become more active suggests that she is serious about improving her health. It is imperative that you begin the process of encouraging her to take small steps toward her fitness. Given the fact that she has never been active, it is unlikely that she has ever found enjoyment with exercise. Additionally, ADLs (e.g., walking in from her car) leave her breathless. This means you must start with small steps and build up.

During the first week, encourage her to walk at a pace that feels comfortable for 10 min each day. Also, encourage her to decrease her TV viewing time. Ask her to keep a journal of her daily exercise and how she feels during and following the exercise bouts. Reassess and modify goals the following week based on any symptoms or difficulties she experiences. Use this process to gradually build up her exercise time. Encourage her to try a variety of exercise modes. In addition to aerobic activity, devise a resistance training and flexibility program, again with a focus on slow progression. Encourage her to get additional support through either personal training or a facility with a focus on helping people with extreme obesity. She will need to develop a supportive network if she is to evolve into an active person. Because she has undergone bariatric surgery, she should follow her doctor's orders regarding her nutritional needs.

Chapter 20

1. Recommend aerobic and resistance training for Mr. Conner.

   Month 1: Begin with 5 days · wk^{-1} of supervised sessions (3 days of aerobic exercise and 2 days of aerobic exercise and resistance training). Although this may seem like a lot of supervised sessions, it is designed to assist with compliance and to help him make the significant lifestyle adjustment. His history indicates he is not likely to exercise without support. Additionally, because he is new to the medication regiment, he needs supervision in case of a hypoglycemic event.

   ○ Aerobic component—begin with 2 bouts of walking, 10 min each in duration, separated by 5 min of stretching. Use RPE (target 12 on 2-20 scale). If joint pain is an issue, use walking for one bout and select another mode of aerobic activity for the other bout. After the second week, move to 12 min bouts.

   ○ Resistance component—select 8 multijoint exercises with upper- and lower-body exercises as a part of the workout. Have Mr. Conner complete 1 set of 8 to 12 repetitions during the first month. Do these exercises following his walking bouts on 2 days · wk^{-1}.

   Month 2: Continue with 5 days of supervised exercise, but also encourage him to build activity into his daily life and on his unsupervised days. Focus on building activity into his routine (e.g., parking farther from his office door, taking stairs). Encourage him to buy a pedometer and track his steps during the day. On his unsupervised days, encourage him to engage in active leisure activities (e.g., trips to the park, walking at the mall, visiting local outdoor markets).

   ○ Aerobic component—gradually build up to 2 bouts of 20 min each, separated by 5 min of stretching. Use RPE (target 13-14 on the 6-20 scale).

   ○ Resistance component—continue with same exercises, but add a second set.

   Month 3: Continue with 5 supervised sessions per week. If Mr. Conner is doing well (no hypoglycemic events and he appears motivated), you might consider dropping off to 3 supervised sessions per week. On his days off, set specific exercise goals and have him report his activity.

   ○ Aerobic component—gradually convert his walking to a 30 min bout followed by a 15 min bout, separated by 5 min of stretching. Use RPE (target 12-16 on the 6-20 scale).

   ○ Resistance component—same as month 2.

2. Weight-loss goals: Mr. Conner should restrict calories and increase exercise to achieve a weekly weight loss of 1 to 2 lb (0.5-0.9 kg). Use strategies outlined in chapter 12 to calculate caloric intake goals at approximately 500 kcal · day^{-1} below energy needs. Focus on low-fat food options. He has likely been given eating recommendations by his physician; incorporate those recommendations into his plan.

3. Mr. Conner will benefit from building a supportive network. Help him identify friends, family members, coworkers, and so on who will encourage his healthy lifestyle. Encourage him to keep a journal of his eating and exercise. Help him develop strategies to deal with challenges (e.g., travel, time management). Encourage him to monitor his weight, and check in with his physician regularly. It will be important to monitor his CVD risk factors. If he makes the changes you suggest and he follows the medication regimen prescribed by his physician, his risk-factor profile should improve.

Chapter 21

1. Find out if she has worked with her physician and is currently experiencing any problems with her medication. In addition, ask if she carries a bronchodilator with her to class, and determine that she knows how to use it at when she has shortness of breath. Lastly, pay special attention to her during the early phases of the class.

2. The patient likely has emphysema and possibly bronchitis, two forms of COPD that commonly result from cigarette smoking. This is shown by his reduced ability to exhale air quickly (decreased FEV$_1$). The logical course of treatment is a program to help him stop smoking, followed by a pulmonary rehabilitation program to help him regain his ability to exercise so that he can carry out ADLs.

3. The patient has a limited ability to exercise, but intermittent treadmill walking (with treadmill level), cycle ergometry, and rowing would be suitable. Arm exercises with very light weights or stretch cords for upper-body conditioning are also appropriate. During physical training his oxygen saturation, ECG, and symptoms of dyspnea should be closely monitored. Supplemental oxygen will help increase his oxygen saturation, maintaining it above 90%.

Chapter 22

1. Topics to address include
   - paying attention to signs and symptoms that indicate problems, with instructions to act on them with a visit to the physician;
   - choosing proper shoes;
   - choosing appropriate clothing for the season and locations for exercise (e.g., safety, surface, lighting);
   - using a buddy system to encourage participation, and
   - identifying an alternative walking location for poor weather (e.g., shopping mall).

2. You should encourage her to continue her walking program, reinforcing the fact that she is gaining a wide variety of health-related benefits by doing so. However, you might also inquire whether she would like to simply try a Zumba class to see if she likes it. If she does, she could add an occasional class to her exercise routine to have some variety. If she doesn't, she has her walking program to keep her active.

3. You should use the graduated jogging program outlined in this chapter to help her make the transition from walking to walk–jog intervals and then to steady jogging. You will need to educate her to check her HR more often and to not rush toward her goal. If she is not ready by the date she has picked, there will be plenty of fun runs to come.

4. The fact that the client has been regularly active at a high intensity allows you to recommend a wide range of activities that will reduce the loading on the knees. At the top of the list are cycle ergometers (including spinning classes) and rowing machines. Both should take a load off the knee (you should verify that this is the case) and can accommodate a wide variety of intensity levels. Encourage the client to make a gradual transition to these new activities by beginning at lower intensities and working up to the desired intensity over several sessions.

Chapter 23

1. Dana is in the preparation stage and has low exercise self-efficacy. She has had a bad experience with exercise in the past, so you want to educate her about what to expect at the beginning of an exercise program and make sure the prescription is appropriate for her fitness level. Use the fitness evaluation to give her a realistic idea of her current fitness level and how much progress she can expect based on a sensible prescription. In setting goals with her, find out what *she* wants to achieve and activities she might enjoy. Brainstorm about her barriers to exercise and how to counter them. Identify supports and ways she could reward herself during the program. Target her low exercise self-efficacy with a beginners' exercise class where she would have social support. Make sure she gets individual attention and encouragement, especially during the first few weeks. A behavioral contract with Mike doing something she wants him to do when she meets short-term goals could provide incentives and support that she will need to keep her program going.

2. Jack is in the action stage and is especially susceptible to relapse. You could make a point of walking with Jack the next time he comes in to provide support and education about relapse prevention. Extra work at the end of the term is a high-risk situation for him; he is discouraged and at risk of relapse. Talk with him about setting short-term goals that can be readjusted during exams. Help him to make the goals realistic and reachable. He might want to take walk breaks for 10 to 15 min during the days he can't get to the facility. Point out that these breaks will help him stay on track and give him a way to manage stress at work. Praise him for how far he has come and for continuing even though he is very busy. Help him see that the high-risk situation is time limited, and brainstorm ways he can reward himself for the walking he can do. Recruit veteran walkers to provide support and encouragement.

3. Marty is in the maintenance stage, but his motivation has shifted from intrinsic to extrinsic by focusing on beating his brother Jim in the Thanksgiving race. His relationship with Jim is beyond your role, but you can help him train most effectively for this race. Ask if he has an exercise log you could review together to learn more about his training, or get him to log his miles, speed, and physical and psychological responses over the next week. Find out his experiences with resistance training and stretching to discover why he skips these activities. He might not know their benefits or he might not enjoy lifting weights and stretching. Invite Marty to a resistance class that has several runners who have benefited from lifting weights. Introduce him to a fast runner who has a balanced training program and can show Marty stretching routines that have helped his running performance.

Chapter 24

1. You could refer him to an experienced and certified Alexander teacher for 2 to 4 sessions. The Alexander teacher will observe the subject running, perhaps sprinting, and will observe posture,

movement mechanics, and breathing pattern. She will particularly stress a more efficient alignment of the runner's head, neck, shoulders, and spine. The Alexander teacher will help the runner relearn more efficient alignment, movement, and breathing patterns, which will be especially useful during the more stressful segments of a race.

2. In addition to a low- to moderate-intensity aerobic exercise program 3 to 5 days · wk^{-1}, such as variable terrain walking, you find a yoga therapist who specializes in restorative yoga and low-back pain. She introduces this gentleman to a series of therapeutic restorative yoga asanas that incorporates a variety of props and bolsters to support his back while allowing him to progressively stretch his low-back and hamstring muscles. Some of the key restorative yoga asanas incorporated in his program are supported cobra, child's, and modified bridge poses. After 8 wk, the magnitude and frequency of low-back pain has decreased and his hamstring muscles are more flexible.

3. One appropriate option is to start them on an 8 wk series of tai chi chih exercises, which are very simple and with a graduated increased focus on whole-body balance. All tai chi forms entrain balance, but tai chi chih exercises are relatively easy and safe for seniors and are graduated throughout the 20 choreographed movements. Throughout the series of sessions you can ascertain how these sessions are affecting their daily functional activities as well as their balance and fear of falling.

Chapter 25

1a. HR = 1500 ÷ 12 = 125 beats · min^{-1}.

PR interval duration = 0.12 sec.

QRS complex duration = 0.08 sec.

QT interval duration = 0.32 sec.

1b. She has sinus tachycardia, a fast HR over 100 beats · min^{-1}.

1c. Common causes of sinus tachycardia are anxiety, nervousness, caffeine, or low fitness.

2a. He has atrial fibrillation—jagged baseline with irregularly spaced PVCs.

2b. Ventricular rate = 6 cardiac cycles in a 6 sec strip · 10 = 60 beats · min^{-1}.

3a. Trigeminy—every third heartbeat is a PVC.

3b. Gradually decrease treadmill speed and grade, and notify the physician.

4. Because the person was on Inderal (a nonselective beta-blocker) at the time of his exercise test, HR would have been suppressed. Now that he is no longer taking the medication, his previously calcu-

lated THR will be too low. The exercise intensity should be adjusted upward.

5. Isordil contains nitroglycerin and is used to reduce the chance of having an angina attack. The drug relaxes vascular smooth muscle and might cause pooling of blood in the extremities. This pooling could decrease BP and result in symptoms of dizziness.

Chapter 26

1a. Suspect insulin shock.

1b. Ask the following questions:

a. What happened?

b. Are you a diabetic?

c. Have you taken your insulin today?

d. Have you eaten?

1c. Check the medical-alert tag. If insulin shock is still suspected, administer sugar (orange juice, candy, sugar granules). If unconscious or recovery is slow (greater than 1-2 min), refer to a physician.

2a. Suspect heatstroke.

2b. Implement EMS (call 911). This is a medical emergency.

a. Cool quickly, starting at the head and working down.

b. Expose as much skin surface as possible.

c. Monitor vital signs

d. Treat cramps by stretching and by applying ice, direct pressure, and gentle massage.

e. Treat for shock.

f. Wrap in cold, wet sheets for transport.

2c. Emergency plans and materials should include the following:

○ Access to cooling agents, such as water, ice, ice towels, and a cool environment

○ Access to a phone and EMS and emergency phone numbers

○ Knowledge of roles in emergency: person in charge, person who assists person in charge, person responsible for making emergency phone call, person who meets and directs the emergency vehicle to the injured

○ Knowledge of rules to move a person, if necessary.

3a. Suspect hyperventilation.

3b. Rule out the following:

a. Heart condition

b. Heat illness

c. Shock

3c. Procedures and treatment:

- Reassure and calm participant.
- Encourage deep, slow breathing.
- Cup hands or use paper bag to cover nose and mouth to help restore CO_2 levels.
- Monitor vital signs, if indicated.
- Treat for shock and implement EMS if indicated.

4a. Suspect that pollution is affecting breathing or that the participant is experiencing exercise-induced asthma.

4b. Take action:

a. Slow down or stop activity.

b. Check HR and allow normal breathing pattern to return.

c. Ask if there is any history of breathing problems, asthma, or allergies.

d. Monitor other vital signs.

e. When recovered, use judgment as to whether to stop, continue walking or running while staying within THR, or resume with an indoor activity.

5a. Suspect shin splints.

b. Rule out stress fracture, metabolic or vascular disorder, compartment syndrome, and muscular strain.

c. Symptoms:

- A dull ache in the lower leg after workouts
- Decreased performance and output because of pain
- Soft-tissue pain
- Mild swelling along area of inflammation
- Slight temperature elevation at the site of inflammation
- Pain when moving the foot up and down

Chapter 27

1. Mr. Smith and his lawyer will likely file the following negligence and gross negligence claims:

- Negligence (ordinary) claims

1) WBFC failed to provide Mr. Smith with any orientation or instruction on how to use the exercise equipment or facility.

2) WBFC failed to provide any instruction or supervision of members while exercising in the fitness area.

3) WBFC failed to assign and train a staff member to carry out regular inspections of their exercise balls based on the manufacturer's specifications.

- Gross negligence

1) WBFC's conduct was reckless because they knew of a danger or risk (exploding exercise ball that caused an injury prior to Mr. Smith's injury) and did nothing to prevent a future injury from happening. (The plaintiff also may file a separate product liability claim against the manufacturer of the exercise ball, alleging some type of defect.)

1a. There are several ways the court can determine duty in this case. For example, the court will likely classify the relationship that was formed between WBFC and Mr. Smith as an inherent relationship. In this type of relationship, the defendant has a legal duty to provide reasonably safe programs and services, which requires taking steps to prevent foreseeable injury risks, such as providing instruction and inspecting for dangers and risks. In addition, according to van der Smissen, there is an inherent duty to instruct and supervise program participants (52).

It is likely that an expert witness will introduce standards of practice published by professional organizations as evidence of the duty owed to the plaintiff (i.e., standards and guidelines that require or recommend that participants receive instruction and supervision). Also, specifications published by the manufacturer of the exercise ball regarding its proper inspection and maintenance may be introduced by an expert witness as evidence of a duty owed to the plaintiff.

The court also will likely classify Mr. Smith as an invitee—the duty owed to an invitee is reasonable inspection and correction or warning of any risks or dangers. In addition, the court will use precedent (opinions from similar case law) to help determine the duty owed to the plaintiff (see the court's ruling in *Thomas* regarding instruction).

1b. He will seek compensatory damages for the negligence claims and punitive damages for the gross negligence claim.

2. The defendant will likely use the waiver defenses and primary assumption of risk.

2a. No.

2b. Though Mr. Smith signed a waiver (included in the membership agreement), waivers are against public policy in Virginia for personal injury and, therefore, unenforceable. It is unlikely that primary assumption of risk will protect the defendant because this defense is effective for inherent injuries only, not negligence, which likely occurred in this case. Also, the primary assumption of risk requires that the plaintiff knows, understands, and appreciates the inherent risks and voluntarily assumes them. Because Mr. Smith did not receive any instruction on how to use the exercise ball, it is unlikely he fully understood and appreciated all the risks.

3. Risk strategies should have included the following:

   o Provide new members with an orientation and instruction on how to use the equipment and facility.

   o Provide staff supervision of the fitness area at all times.

   o Assign and train a staff member to inspect the equipment and facility on a regular basis for any dangers or risks. If any dangers are found, correct them, remove them, or provide warning signage.

   o Follow manufacturer's specifications for inspection and maintenance of exercise equipment and document that such inspection and maintenance has been completed.

4. If the defendant is found liable for any of the ordinary negligence claims, the general liability insurance carrier will likely pay out compensatory damages up to the limits of the policy, but it will not pay out punitive damages if the defendant is found liable for the gross negligence claim.

Calculation of Oxygen Uptake and Carbon Dioxide Production

Calculation of Oxygen Consumption ($\dot{V}O_2$)

The air we breathe is composed of 20.93% oxygen (O_2), 0.03% carbon dioxide (CO_2), and the balance, 79.04%, nitrogen (N_2). When we exhale, the fraction of the air represented by O_2 is decreased and the fraction represented by CO_2 is increased. To calculate the volume of O_2 used by the body ($\dot{V}O_2$), we simply subtract the number of liters of O_2 exhaled from the number of liters of O_2 inhaled. Equation 1 summarizes these words.

1. Oxygen consumption =
(volume of O_2 inhaled) − (volume of O_2 exhaled)

Now, using $\dot{V}O_2$ to mean volume of oxygen used, V_I to mean volume of air inhaled, V_E to mean volume of air exhaled, F_{IO_2} to mean fraction of oxygen in inhaled air, and F_{EO_2} to mean fraction of oxygen in exhaled air, equation 2 can be written.

2. $\dot{V}O_2 = (V_I \cdot F_{IO_2}) - (V_E \cdot F_{EO_2})$

You know that $F_{IO_2} = 0.2093$, and F_{EO_2} will be determined on an oxygen analyzer. Consequently, you are left with only two unknowns: the volume of air (liters) inhaled (V_I) and the volume of air (liters) exhaled (V_E). It appears that you must measure both volumes, but fortunately, this is not necessary. It was determined years ago that N_2 is neither used nor produced by the body. Consequently, the number of liters of N_2 inhaled must equal the number of liters of N_2 exhaled. Equation 3 states this equality using the symbols mentioned earlier.

3. $V_I \cdot F_{IN_2} = V_E \cdot F_{EN_2}$

This is an important relationship because it permits you to calculate V_E when V_I is known or vice versa. Using equation 3, here are two formulas, one giving V_E when V_I is known and one giving V_I when V_E is known.

$$V_I = \frac{V_E \cdot F_{EN_2}}{F_{IN_2}}, \quad V_E = \frac{V_I \cdot F_{IN_2}}{F_{EN_2}}$$

Now that you know how to do this, you need only one other piece of the puzzle to calculate $\dot{V}O_2$. The value for F_{IN_2} is constant (0.7904), so we must determine F_{EN_2}. When the expired gas sample is analyzed, you will obtain a value for F_{EO_2} and F_{ECO_2} but not F_{EN_2}. However, since all the gas fractions must add up to 1.0000, you can calculate F_{EN_2} in the same way we calculated F_{IN_2}: 1.0000 − 0.0003 (CO_2) − 0.2093 (O_2) = 0.7904.

Problem: Calculate F_{EN_2} when $F_{EO_2} = 0.1600$ and $F_{ECO_2} = 0.0450$

Answer: $F_{EN_2} = 1.0000 - 0.1600 - 0.0450 = 0.7950$

The following problem shows how these equations are used. Given that V_I equals 100 L, $F_{EO_2} = 0.1600$, and $F_{ECO_2} = 0.0450$, calculate V_E.

$$V_E \cdot F_{EN_2} = V_I \cdot F_{IN_2}, \text{ so } V_E = \frac{V_I \cdot F_{IN_2}}{F_{EN_2}}$$

$F_{IN_2} = 0.7904$ and

$F_{EN_2} = 1.0000 - 0.1600 - 0.0450 = 0.7950$.

$$V_E = 100 \text{ L} \cdot \frac{0.7904}{0.7950} = 99.4 \text{ L}$$

At this point, the equation for $\dot{V}O_2$ can be rewritten using V_I, V_E, F_{IO_2}, and F_{EO_2}.

$$\dot{V}O_2 = V_I \cdot F_{IO_2} - V_E \cdot F_{EO_2}$$

Assuming that you measure only V_I, this formula is rewritten:

$$\dot{V}O_2 = V_I \cdot F_{IO_2} - \frac{V_I \cdot F_{IN_2}}{F_{EN_2}} \cdot F_{EO_2}$$

V_I can be factored out of this equation, so

$$\dot{V}O_2 = V_I \left[F_{IO_2} - \frac{F_{IN_2}}{F_{EN_2}} \cdot F_{EO_2} \right]$$

We will repeat the last two steps assuming that V_E is the volume that is measured and then factor out V_E.

$$\dot{V}O_2 = \frac{V_E \cdot F_{EN_2}}{F_{IN_2}} \cdot F_{IO_2} - V_E \cdot F_{EO_2}$$

$$= V_E \left[\frac{F_{EN_2}}{F_{IN_2}} \cdot F_{IO_2} - F_{EO_2} \right]$$

At this point you know how to calculate $\dot{V}O_2$. If you ever get stuck, always go back to the formula: $\dot{V}O_2 = V_I \cdot F_{IO_2} - V_E \cdot F_{EO_2}$. Simply substitute for V_E or V_I depending on what was measured.

Some comments:

1. You must always match the volume measurement with the F_{EO_2} and F_{ECO_2} values measured in that expired volume. If you measure V_I for 2 min, you must have a single 2 min bag of expired gas to get F_{EO_2} and F_{ECO_2} values. If you measure a 30 sec volume, your expired bag must be collected over those 30 sec.

2. $\dot{V}O_2$ and $\dot{V}CO_2$ are usually expressed in liters per minute: the *rate* at which O_2 is used or CO_2 is produced per minute. To signify this rate, we write $\dot{V}O_2$ (read *vee dot*). You would convert 30 sec or 2 min volumes to 1 min values before calculating $\dot{V}O_2$.

Sample problem:

$\dot{V}_I = 100 \text{ L} \cdot \text{min}^{-1}$, $F_{EO_2} = .1600$, and $F_{ECO_2} = .0450$

Calculate $\dot{V}O_2$.

$$\dot{V}O_2 = V_I \cdot F_{IO_2} - \dot{V}_E \cdot F_{EO_2}, \text{ and}$$

$$\dot{V}_E = \frac{\dot{V}_I \cdot F_{IN_2}}{F_{EN_2}}$$

$$\dot{V}O_2 = \dot{V}_I \cdot F_{IO_2} - \frac{\dot{V}_I \cdot F_{IN_2}}{F_{EN_2}} \cdot F_{EO_2}$$

$$= \dot{V}_I \left[F_{IO_2} - \frac{F_{IN_2}}{F_{EN_2}} \cdot F_{EO_2} \right]$$

$$F_{EN_2} = 1,0000 - 0.1600 - 0.0450 = 0.7950$$

$$\dot{V}O_2 = 100 \text{ L} \cdot \text{min}^{-1} \left[0.2093 - \frac{0.7904}{0.7950} \cdot 0.1600 \right]$$

$$= 5.02 \text{ L} \cdot \text{min}^{-1}$$

The volume (let's assume that $\dot{V}_E$ was measured) used in the previous equations was measured at room temperature (23 °C) and at the barometric pressure of that moment (740 mmHg). The environmental conditions under which the volume was measured are called *ambient conditions*. If this volume of gas were transported to 10,000 ft (3,050 m) above sea level, where the barometric pressure is lower, the volume would increase because of the reduced pressure. The volume of a gas varies inversely with pressure (at a constant temperature). Another factor influencing the volume of a gas is the temperature. If that volume, measured at 23 °C, were placed in a refrigerator at 0 °C, the volume of gas would decrease. The volume of gas varies directly with the temperature (at constant pressure).

Since the volume ($\dot{V}_E$) is influenced by both pressure and temperature, the value measured as O_2 used ($\dot{V}O_2$) might reflect changes in pressure or temperature rather than a change in workload, training, and so on.

Consequently, it would be convenient to express $\dot{V}_E$ in such a way as to make measurements comparable when they are obtained under different environmental conditions. This is done by standardizing the temperature, barometric pressure, and water vapor pressure at which the volume is expressed. By convention, volumes are expressed at standard temperature and pressure, dry (STPD): 273 K (equals 0 °C), 760 mmHg pressure (sea level), and with no water vapor pressure. When $\dot{V}O_2$ is expressed at STPD, you can calculate the number of molecules of oxygen actually used by the body because at STPD, 1 mole of oxygen equals 22.4 L.

Let's make the correction to STPD one step at a time. Let's assume that a volume ($\dot{V}_E$) was measured at 740 mmHg and 23 °C and equaled 100 L · min⁻¹. This expired volume is *always* saturated with water vapor.

To correct for temperature, use 273 K as the standard (0 °C).

$$\text{Volume} \cdot \frac{273 \text{ K}}{273 \text{ K} + °C} = \frac{273 \text{ K}}{273 + 23}$$

$$100 \text{ L} \cdot \text{min}^{-1} \cdot \frac{273 \text{ K}}{296 \text{ K}} = 92.23 \text{ L} \cdot \text{min}^{-1}$$

When we correct for pressure, we must remove the effect of water vapor pressure because the gas volume is adjusted on the basis of the standard pressure (760 mmHg), which is a dry pressure.

To correct the volume to the standard 760 mmHg pressure (dry), use this:

$$\text{Volume} \cdot \frac{\text{barometric pressure} - \text{water vapor pressure}}{760 \text{ mmHg (dry)}}$$

Water vapor pressure is dependent on two things: the temperature and the relative humidity. In expired gas, the gas volume is saturated (100% relative humidity). Consequently, you can obtain a value for water vapor pressure directly from the following table.

Going back to our pressure correction:

$$92.23 \text{ L} \cdot \text{min}^{-1} \cdot \frac{740 - 21.1}{760} = 87.24 \text{ L} \cdot \text{min}^{-1} \text{(STPD)}.$$

To combine the temperature and pressure correction:

$$100 \text{ L} \cdot \text{min}^{-1} \cdot \frac{273 \text{ K}}{273 \text{ K} + 23} \cdot \frac{740 - 21.1}{760} =$$
$$87.24 \text{ L} \cdot \text{min}^{-1} \text{(STPD)}$$

Temperature (°C)	Saturation water vapor pressure (mmHg)
18	15.5
19	16.5
20	17.5
21	18.7
22	19.8
23	21.1
24	22.4
25	23.8
26	25.2
27	26.7

A special note must be made here. If you are using an inspired (inhaled) volume ($\dot{V}_I$), you are rarely dealing with a gas saturated with water vapor. Consequently, when you correct for pressure you must find how much water vapor is in the inspired air. You do this by finding the relative humidity of the air. You then multiply this value by the water vapor pressure value for saturated air at whatever the temperature is. To clarify, if your volume in the previous example was $\dot{V}_I$ and had a relative humidity of 50%, the pressure correction would have been as follows:

$$volume \cdot \frac{740 - (.50 \cdot 21.1 \text{ mmHg})}{760 \text{ mmHg}}$$

This may seem like a minor point, but it is critical to the accurate measurement of $\dot{V}O_2$ that the proper water vapor correction be used. When calculating $\dot{V}O_2$, you usually find the STPD factor first since you will be multiplying this factor by each volume measured.

Problem: Given $\dot{V}_I = 100$ L · min^{-1}, $FEO_2 = 0.1700$, and $FECO_2 = 0.0385$. Temperature = 20 °C, barometric pressure = 740 mmHg, and relative humidity = 30%.

Answer:

$$STPD \text{ factor} = \frac{740 \text{ mmHg} - (.30)\ 17.5 \text{ mmHg}}{760}$$

$$\cdot \frac{273 \text{ K}}{273 \text{ K} + 20 \text{ °C}} = .900$$

$$100 \text{ L} \cdot \text{min}^{-1} \cdot 0.900 = 90 \text{ L} \cdot \text{min}^{-1} \text{ STPD}$$

$$\dot{V}O_2 = \dot{V}_{I_{STPD}} \left[F_{IO_2} - \frac{F_{IN_2}}{F_{EN_2}} \cdot F_{EO_2} \right]$$

$$\dot{V}O_2 = 90 \text{ L} \cdot \text{min}^{-1} \left[0.2093 - \frac{0.7904}{0.7915} \cdot 0.1700 \right]$$

$$\dot{V}O_2 = 3.56 \text{ L} \cdot \text{min}^{-1}$$

Carbon Dioxide Production ($\dot{V}CO_2$)

When O_2 is used, CO_2 is produced. The ratio of CO_2 production ($\dot{V}CO_2$) to O_2 consumption ($\dot{V}O_2$) is an important measurement in metabolism. This ratio ($\dot{V}CO_2 \div \dot{V}O_2$) is called the *respiratory exchange ratio* and is abbreviated as *R*.

How do we measure $\dot{V}CO_2$? We start at the same step as for $\dot{V}O_2$:

$$\dot{V}CO_2 = \text{liters of } CO_2 \text{ expired} - \text{liters of } CO_2 \text{ inspired}$$

$$= \dot{V}_E \cdot F_{ECO_2} - \dot{V}_I \cdot F_{ICO_2}$$

The steps to follow are the same as those for measuring $\dot{V}O_2$. Always use an STPD volume in your calculations. The following is the equation to use when $\dot{V}_I$ is measured:

$$\dot{V}CO_2 = \dot{V}_{I_{STPD}} \left[\frac{F_{IN_2}}{F_{EN_2}} \cdot F_{ECO_2} - \dot{V}_I \cdot F_{ICO_2} \right]$$

The following steps summarize the calculations for $\dot{V}CO_2$ and *R* for the previous problem.

$$\dot{V}CO_2 = 90 \cdot \text{L} \cdot \text{min}^{-1} \left[\frac{0.7904}{0.7915} \cdot 0.0385 - 0.0003 \right]$$

$$= 3.43 \text{ L} \cdot \text{min}^{-1}$$

$$R = \dot{V}CO_2 \div \dot{V}O_2 = 3.43 \text{ L} \cdot \text{min}^{-1} \div 3.56 \text{ L} \cdot \text{min}^{-1}$$

$$R = 0.96$$

Compendium of Physical Activities

The Compendium of Physical Activities was developed to support the use of physical activity questionnaires to help track the physical activity patterns of various populations and quantify how much energy was expended as a result of the physical activity. In this way, investigators could link the energy expenditure of physical activity to various health outcomes and determine, for example, the relationship of physical activity to the risk of type 2 diabetes.

Dr. Bill Haskell of Stanford University conceptualized the idea of the Compendium and developed a prototype that was used in studies examining physical activity, exercise, and fitness patterns in populations. In 1993, the first complete version of the Compendium was published, followed by an update in 2000 (see following references). Both articles had a long list of activities that included specific codes to identify the activity and energy cost values expressed in METs, where 1 MET is equal to $3.5\ \text{ml} \cdot \text{kg}^{-1} \cdot \text{min}^{-1}$ or $1\ \text{kcal} \cdot \text{kg}^{-1} \cdot \text{hr}^{-1}$. In 2011, an update of the Compendium was published, but this time the list of activities, their codes, and MET values were published on a website that will be updated regularly, rather than the seven to 10 years between previous updates (http://sites.google.com/site/compendiumofphysicalactivities/home).

The following examples are provided to show how to use the information on the website to estimate the energy cost of activities your clients are doing. Please keep in mind that the energy cost values in the Compendium are measured or estimated values of a group; large interindividual variation in energy cost may exist for some activities.

Example 1: Your client, who weighs 60 kg, bicycles to and from work each day (1 hour round trip) and wants to know how much energy she is using each day.

1. On the home page of the website choose Activity Categories in the top menu bar.

2. Select bicycling and scroll down to "bicycling to and from work, self-selected pace." The MET value is 6.8.

3. $6.8\ \text{kcal} \cdot \text{kg}^{-1} \cdot \text{hr}^{-1} \cdot 1\ \text{hr} \cdot \text{day}^{-1} \cdot 60\ \text{kg} = 408\ \text{kcal} \cdot \text{day}^{-1}$.

Example 2: Your client, who weighs 80 kg, does a 30-minute brisk walk 5 days a week and wants to know how much energy he is using per week with this activity.

1. On the home page of the website choose Activity Categories in the top menu bar.

2. Select walking and scroll down to "walking, 3.5 mph, level, brisk, firm surface, walking for exercise" The MET value is 4.3.

3. $4.3\ \text{kcal} \cdot \text{kg}^{-1} \cdot \text{hr}^{-1} \cdot 2.5\ \text{hr} \cdot \text{wk}^{-1} \cdot 80\ \text{kg} = 860\ \text{kcal} \cdot \text{wk}^{-1}$.

Past Compendium references

1993 Compendium Ainsworth BE, Haskell WL, Leon AS, Jacobs DR Jr, Montoye HJ, Sallis JF, Paffenbarger RS Jr. Compendium of physical activities: Classification of energy costs of human physical activities. *Medicine and Science in Sports and Exercise*, 1993;25:71-80.

2000 Compendium Ainsworth BE, Haskell WL, Whitt MC, Irwin ML, Swartz AM, Strath SJ, O'Brien WL, Bassett DR Jr, Schmitz KH, Emplaincourt PO, Jacobs DR Jr, Leon AS. Compendium of Physical Activities: An update of activity codes and MET intensities. *Medicine and Science in Sports and Exercise*, 2000;32 (Suppl):S498-S516.

Suggested citation for Current Compendium and website:

Manuscript: Ainsworth BE, Haskell WL, Herrmann SD, Meckes N, Bassett Jr DR, Tudor-Locke C, Greer JL, Vezina J, Whitt, Glover MC, Leon AS. 2011 Compendium of Physical Activities: a second update of codes and MET values. *Medicine and Science in Sports and Exercise*, 2011;43(8):1575-1581.

Website: Ainsworth BE, Haskell WL, Herrmann SD, Meckes N, Bassett Jr DR, Tudor-Locke C, Greer JL, Vezina J, Whitt-Glover MC, Leon AS. The Compendium of Physical Activities Tracking Guide. Healthy Lifestyles Research Center, College of Nursing & Health Innovation, Arizona State University. Retrieved [date] from the World Wide Web. https://sites.google.com/site/compendiumofphysicalactivities/

APPENDIX D
Common Medications

β-Blockers

Use or condition: Hypertension, angina, arrhythmias including supraventricular tachycardia, increasing AV block to slow ventricular response in atrial fibrillation, acute myocardial infarction, migraine headache, anxiety; mandatory as part of therapy for HF due to systolic dysfunction

Drug name	Brand name†
Acebutolol**	Sectral**
Atenolol	Tenormin
Betaxolol	Kerlone
Bisoprolol	Zebeta
Esmolol	Brevibloc
Metoprolol	Lopressor SR, Toprol XL
Nadolol	Corgard
Penbutolol**	Levatol**
Pindolol**	Visken**
Propranolol	Inderal
Sotalol	Betapace
Timolol	Blocadren

**β-Blockers with intrinsic sympathomimetic activity.

β-Blockers in Combination With Diuretics

Use or condition: Hypertension, diuretic, glaucoma

Drug name	Brand name†
Atenolol, chlorthalidone	Tenoretic
Bendroflumethiazide, nadolol	Corzide
Bisoprolol, hydrochlorothiazide	Ziac
Metoprolol, hydrochlorothiazide	Lopressor HCT
Propranolol, hydrochlorothiazide	Inderide
Timolol, hydrochlorothiazide	Timolide

α- and β-Adrenergic Blocking Agents

Use or condition: Hypertension, chronic heart failure, angina

Drug name	Brand name†
Carvedilol	Coreg
Labetalol	Normodyne, Trandate

α1-Adrenergic Blocking Agents

Use or condition: Hypertension, enlarged prostate

Drug name	Brand name†
Doxazosin	Cardura
Tamsulosin	Flomax
Prazosin	Minipress
Hytrin	Terazosin

Central α2-Agonists and Other Centrally Acting Drugs

Use or condition: Hypertension

Drug name	Brand name†
Clonidine	Catapres, Catapres-TTS patch
Guanfacine	Tenex
Methyldopa	Aldomet
Reserpine	Serpasil

Central α2-Agonists in Combination With Diuretics

Use or condition: Hypertension

Drug name	Brand name†
Methyldopa + hydrochlorothiazide	Aldoril
Reserpine + chlorothiazide	Diupres
Reserpine + hydrochlorothiazide	Hydropres

Nitrates and Nitroglycerin

Use or condition: Angina, vasodilator in chronic HF

Drug name	Brand name†
Amyl nitrite	Amyl Nitrite
Isosorbide mononitrate	Ismo, Imdur, Monoket
Isosorbide dinitrate	Dilatrate, Isordil, Sorbitrate
Nitroglycerin, sublingual	Nitrostat, NitroQuick
Nitroglycerin, translingual	Nitrolingual
Nitroglycerin, transmucosal	Nitrogard
Nitroglycerin, sustained release	Nitrong, Nitrocine, Nitroglyn, Nitro-Bid
Nitroglycerin, transdermal	Minitran, Nitro-Dur, Transderm-Nitro, Deponit, Nitrodisc, Nitro-Derm
Nitroglycerin, topical	Nitro-Bid, Nitrol

Calcium Channel Blockers (Nondihydropyridines)

Use or condition: Angina, hypertension, increasing AV block to slow ventricular response in atrial fibrillation, paroxysmal supraventricular tachycardia, headache

Drug name	Brand name†
Diltiazem extended release	Cardizem CD, Cardizem LA, Dilacor XR, Tiazac
Verapamil immediate release	Calan, Isoptin
Verapamil long acting	Calan SR, Isoptin SR
Verapamil COER-24	Covera HS, Verelan PM

Calcium Channel Blockers (Dihydropyridines)

Use or condition: Hypertension, angina, neurological deficits after subarachnoid hemorrhage

Drug name	Brand name†
Amlodipine	Norvasc
Felodipine	Plendil
Isradipine	DynaCirc CR
Nicardipine sustained release	Cardene SR
Nifedipine long acting	Adalat, Procardia XL
Nimodipine	Nimotop
Nisoldipine	Sular

Cardiac Glycosides

Use or condition: Chronic heart failure in the setting of dilated cardiomyopathy, increasing AV block to slow ventricular response with atrial fibrillation

Drug name	Brand name†
Digoxin	Lanoxin

Direct Peripheral Vasodilators

Use or condition: Hypertension, hair loss, vasodilation for heart failure

Drug name	Brand name†
Hydralazine	Apresoline
Minoxidil	Loniten

Angiotensin-Converting Enzyme (ACE) Inhibitors

Use or condition: Hypertension, coronary artery disease, chronic heart failure due to systolic dysfunction, diabetes, chronic kidney disease, heart attack, scleroderma, migraine

Drug name	Brand name†
Benazepril	Lotensin
Captopril	Capoten
Cilazapril*	Inhibace
Enalapril	Vasotec
Fosinopril	Monopril
Lisinopril	Zestril, Prinivil
Moexipril	Univasc
Perindopril	Aceon
Quinapril	Accupril
Ramipril	Altace
Trandolapril	Mavik

*Available only in Canada.

ACE Inhibitors in Combination With Diuretics

Use or condition: Hypertension, chronic heart failure

Drug name	Brand name†
Benazepril + hydrocholorthiazide	Lotensin
Captopril + hydrocholorthiazide	Capozide
Enalapril + hydrocholorthiazide	Vaseretic
Lisinopril + hydrocholorthiazide	Prinzide, Zestoretic
Moexipril + hydrocholorthiazide	Uniretic
Quinapril + hydrocholorthiazide	Accuretic

ACE Inhibitors in Combination With Calcium Channel Blockers

Use or condition: Hypertension, chronic heart failure, angina

Drug name	Brand name†
Benazepril + amlodipine	Lotrel
Enalapril + felodipine	Lexxel
Trandolapril + verapamil	Tarka

Angiotensin II Receptor Antagonists

Use or condition: Hypertension

Drug name	Brand name†
Candesartan	Atacand
Eprosartan	Tevetan
Irbesartan	Avapro
Losartan	Cozaar
Olmesartan	Benicar
Telmisartan	Micardis
Valsartan	Diovan

Angiotensin II Receptor Antagonists in Combination With Diuretics

Use or condition: Hypertension, chronic heart failure, angina

Drug name	Brand name†
Candesartan + hydrochlorothiazide	Atacand HCT
Eprosartan + hydrochlorothiazide	Teveten HCT
Irbesartan + hydrochlorothiazide	Avalide
Losartan + hydrochlorothiazide	Hyzaar
Telmisartan + hydrochlorothiazide	Micardis HCT
Valsartan + hydrochlorothiazide	Diovan HCT

Diuretics

Use or condition: Edema, chronic heart failure, polycystic ovary syndrome, certain kidney disorders (i.e., kidney stones, diabetes insipidus, female hirsutism, osteoporosis) Thiazides

Drug name	Brand name†
Chlorothiazide	Diuril
Hydrochlorothiazide (HCTZ)	Microzide, Hydrodiuril, Oretic
Indapamide	Lozol
Metolazone	Mykron, Zaroxolyn
Polythiazide	Renese

"Loop" Diuretics

Drug name	Brand name†
Bumetanide	Bumex
Ethacrynic acid	Edecrin
Furosemide	Lasix
Torsemide	Demadex

Potassium-Sparing Diuretics

Drug name	Brand name†
Amiloride	Midamor
Triamterene	Dyrenium

Aldosterone Receptor Blockers

Drug name	Brand name†
Eplerenone	Inspra
Spironolactone	Aldactone

Diuretic Combined With Diuretic

Drug name	Brand name†
Amiloride + hydrochlorothiazide	Moduretic
Triamterene + hydrochlorothiazide	Dyazide, Maxzide

Antiarrhythmic Agents

Use or condition: Specific for drug but include suppression of atrial fibrillation and maintenance of NSR, serious ventricular arrhythmias in certain clinical settings, increase in AV nodal block to slow ventricular response in atrial fibrillation

Drug name	Brand name†
CLASS IA	
Disopyramide	Norpace
Moricizine	Ethmozine
Procainamide	Pronestyl, Procan SR
Quinidine	Quinora, Quinidex, Quinaglute, Quinalan, Cardioquin
CLASS IB	
Lidocaine	Xylocaine, Xylocard
Mexiletine	Mexitil
Phenytoin	Dilantin
Tocainide	Tonocard
CLASS IC	
Flecainide	Tambocor
Propafenone	Rythmol

(continued)

(continued)

Drug name	Brand name†
CLASS II	
β-Blockers	Refer to previous tables in appendix a
CLASS III	
Amiodarone	Cordarone, Pacerone
Bretylium	Bretylol
Sotalol	Betapace
Dofetilide	Tikosyn
CLASS IV	
Calcium channel blockers	Refer to previous tables in appendix a

Antilipemic Agents

Use or condition: Elevated blood cholesterol, low-density lipoproteins, triglycerides, low high-density lipoproteins, and metabolic syndrome

Category	Drug name	Brand name†
A	Cholestyramine	Questran, Cholybar, Prevalite
A	Colesevelam	Welchol
A	Colestipol	Colestid
B	Clofibrate	Atromid
B	Fenofibrate	Tricor, Lofibra
B	Gemfibrozil	Lopid
C	Atorvastatin	Lipitor
C	Fluvastatin	Lescol
C	Lovastatin	Mevacor
C	Lovastatin + niacin	Advicor
C	Pravastatin	Pravachol
C	Rosuvastatin	Crestor
C	Simvastatin	Zocor
D	Atorvastatin + amlodipine	Caduet
E	Niacin	Niaspan, Nicobid, Slo-Niacin
F	Ezetimibe	Zetia
F	Ezetimibe + simvasatin	Vytorin

A = bile acid sequestrants; B = fibric acid sequestrants; C = HMG-CoA reductase inhibitors; D = HMG-CoA reductase inhibitors + calcium channel blocker; E = nicotinic acid, F = cholesterol absorption inhibitor.

Blood Modifiers (Anticoagulant or Antiplatelet)

Use or condition: To prevent blood clots, heart attack, stroke, intermittent claudication, or vascular death in patients with established peripheral arterial disease (PAD) or acute ST-segment elevation myocardial infarction; also used to reduce aching, tiredness, and cramps in hands and feet. Plavix is critical to maintain for one year after PCI for DES patency.

Drug name	Brand name†
Cilostazol	Pletal
Clopidogrel	Plavix
Dipyridamole	Persantine
Pentoxifylline	Trental
Ticlopidine	Ticlid
Warfarin	Coumadin

Respiratory Agents

Main drug classes for respiratory conditions include steroidal anti-inflammatory agents and bronchodilators.

Steroidal Anti-Inflammatory Agents

Use or condition: Allergy symptoms including sneezing, itching, and runny or stuffed nose; shrinking nasal polyps; various skin disorders; asthma

Drug name	Brand name†
Beclomethasone	Beclovent, QVAR
Budesonide	Pulmicort
Flunisolide	AeroBid
Fluticasone	Flovent
Fluticasone and salmeterol (β2 receptor agonist)	Advair Diskus
Triamcinolone	Azmacort

Bronchodilators

Use or condition: Dilate the bronchi and bronchioles to decrease airway resistance and facilitate airflow. Bronchodilators include anticholinergics (acetylcholine receptor antagonists and anticholinergics with sympathomimetics), sympathomimetics (β2-Receptor Agonists), xanthine derivatives, leukotriene antagonists and formation inhibitors, and mast cell stabilizers.

Anticholinergics (Acetylcholine Receptor Antagonists)

Use or condition: To prevent wheezing, shortness of breath, and troubled breathing caused by asthma, chronic bronchitis, emphysema, and other lung diseases

Drug name	Brand name†
Ipratropium	Atrovent

Anticholinergics With Sympathomimetics (β2-Receptor Agonists)

Use or condition: Chronic obstructive pulmonary lung disease (COPD)

Drug name	Brand name†
Ipratropium and albuterol	Combivent

Sympathomimetics (β2-Receptor Agonists)

Use or condition: To prevent wheezing, shortness of breath, and troubled breathing caused by asthma, chronic bronchitis, emphysema, and other lung diseases

Drug name	Brand name†
Albuterol	Proventil, Ventolin
Metaproterenol	Alupent
Pirbuterol	Maxair
Salmeterol	Serevent
Salmeterol and fluticasone (steroid)	Advair
Terbutaline	Brethine

Xanthine Derivatives

Use or condition: To prevent wheezing, shortness of breath, and troubled breathing caused by asthma, chronic bronchitis, emphysema, and other lung diseases

Drug name	Brand name†
Theophylline	Theo-Dur, Uniphyl

Leukotriene Antagonists and Formation Inhibitors

Use or condition: To prevent wheezing, shortness of breath, and troubled breathing caused by asthma, chronic bronchitis, emphysema, and other lung diseases

Drug name	Brand name†
Montelukast	Singulair
Zafirlukast	Accolate
Zileuton	Zyflo

Mast Cell Stabilizers

Use or condition: To prevent wheezing, shortness of breath, and troubled breathing caused by asthma, chronic bronchitis, emphysema, and other lung diseases

Drug name	Brand name†
Cromolyn inhaled	Intal
Nedocromil	Tilade
Omalizumab	Xolair

Antidiabetic Agents

Use or condition: To control glucose levels. Antidiabetic agents include biguanides, glucosidase inhibitors, insulins, meglitinides, sulfonylureas, thiazolidinediones, and incretin mimetics.

Biguanides (Decrease Hepatic Glucose Production and Intestinal Glucose Absorption)

Use or condition: Type 2 or adult-onset diabetes

Drug name	Brand name†
Metformin	Glucophage, Riomet
Metformin and glyburide	Glucovance

Glucosidase Inhibitors (Inhibit Intestinal Glucose Absorption)

Use or condition: Type 2 or adult-onset diabetes

Drug name	Brand name†
Miglitol	Glyset

Insulins

Use or condition: Type 1, or sometimes type 2 or adult-onset diabetes

Rapid acting	Intermediate acting	Intermediate- and rapid- acting combination	Long acting
Humalog	Humulin L	Humalog Mix	Humulin U
Humulin R	Humulin N	Humalog 50/50	Lantus injection
Novolin R	Iletin II Lente	Humalog 70/30	Levemir
Iletin II R	Iletin II NPH	Novolin 70/30	
	Novolin L		
	Nivalin N		
Humalog	Humulin L	Humalog Mix	Humulin U

557

Meglitinides (Stimulate Pancreatic Islet Beta Cells)

Use or condition: Type 2 or adult-onset diabetes

Drug name	Brand name†
Nateglinide	Starlix
Repaglinide	Prandin, Gluconorm

Sulfonylureas (Stimulate Pancreatic Islet Beta Cells)

Use or condition: Type 2 or adult-onset diabetes

Drug name	Brand name†
Chlorpropamide*	Diabinese
Gliclazide	Diamicron
Glimepiride*	Amaryl
Glipizide*	Glucotrol
Glyburide	DiaBeta, Glynase, Micronase
Tolazamide*	Tolinase
Tolbutamide*	Orinase

*These drugs have been associated with increased cardiovascular mortality.

Thiazolidinediones (Increase Insulin Sensitivity)

Use or condition: Type 2 or adult-onset diabetes

Drug name	Brand name†
Pioglitazone	Actos
Rosiglitazone	Avandia

Incretin mimetics (Increase Insulin and Decrease Glucagon Secretion)

Use or condition: Type 2 diabetes

Drug name	Brand name†
Glucagon-like peptide 1	Byetta

Obesity Management

Main drug classes include appetite suppressants and lipase inhibitors.

Appetite Suppressants

Use or condition: Morbid obesity and metabolic syndrome

Drug name	Brand name†
Phentermine Adipex-P	Termene
Diethylpropion Durad	Tenuate
Phendimetrazine Adipost	Bontril PDM

Lipase Inhibitors

Use or condition: Morbid obesity and metabolic syndrome

Drug name	Brand name†
Orlistat Alli	Xenical

†Represent selected brands; these are not necessarily all-inclusive.

Adapted, by permission, from ACSM, 2009, *ACSM's exercise management for persons with chronic diseases and disabilities,* 3rd ed. (Champaign, IL: Human Kinetics), 97-406; Adapted from *ACSM's guidelines for exercise testing and prescription,* 7th ed. (Philadelphia, PA: Lippincott, Williams, and Wilkins).

TABLE D-1 Effects of Medications on Heart Rate, Blood Pressure, the Electrocardiogram (ECG), and Exercise Capacity

Medications	Heart rate	Blood pressure	ECG	Exercise capacity
I. β-Blockers (including carvedilol and labetalol)	↓* (R and E)	↓ (R and E)	↓ HR* (R) ↓ ischemia† (E)	↑ in patients with angina; ↓ or ↔ in patients without angina
II. Nitrates	↑ (R) ↑ or ↔ (E)	↓ (R) ↓ or ↔ (E)	↑ HR (R) ↑ or ↔ HR (E) ↓ ischemia† (E)	↑ in patients with angina ↔ in patients without angina; ↑ or ↔ in patients with chronic heart failure (CHF)
III. Calcium channel blockers Amlodipine Felodipine Isradipine Nicardipine Nifedipine Nimodipine Nisoldipine	↑ or ↔ (R and E)	↓ (R and E)	↑ or ↔ HR (R and E) ↓ ischemia† (E)	↑ in patients with angina; ↔ in patients without angina
Diltiazem Verapamil	↓ (R and E)		↓ HR (R and E) ↓ ischemia† (E)	
IV. Digitalis	↓ in patients with atrial fibrillation and possibly CHF Not significantly altered in patients with sinus rhythm	↔ (R and E)	May produce non-specific ST-T–wave changes (R) May produce ST-segment depression (E)	Improved only in patients with atrial fibrillation or in patients with CHF
V. Diuretics	↔ (R and E)	↔ or ↓ (R and E)	↔ or PVCs (R) May cause PVCs and "false positive" test results if hypokalemia occurs May cause PVCs if hypomagnesemia occurs (E)	↔, except possibly in patients with CHF
VI. Vasodilators, nonadrenergic	↑ or ↔ (R and E)	↓ (R and E)	↑ or ↔ HR (R and E)	↔, except ↑ or ↔ in patients with CHF
ACE inhibitors, and angiotensin II receptor blockers	↔ (R and E)	↓ (R and E)	↔ (R and E)	↔, except ↑ or ↔ in patients with CHF
α-Adrenergic blockers	↔ (R and E)	↓ (R and E)	↔ (R and E)	↔
Antiadrenergic agents without selective blockade	↓ or ↔ (R and E)	↓ (R and E)	↓ or ↔ HR (R and E)	↔

(continued)

TABLE D-1 *(continued)*

Medications	Heart rate	Blood pressure	ECG	Exercise capacity
VII. Antiarrhythmic agents (all antiarrhythmic agents may cause new or worsened arrhythmias [proarrhythmic effect])				↔
Class I Quinidine Disopyramide	↑ or ↔ (R and E)	↓ or ↔ (R) ↔ (E)	↑ or ↔ HR (R) May prolong QRS and QT intervals (R) Quinidine may result in "false negative" test results (E)	↔
Procainamide	↔ (R and E)	↔ (R and E)	May prolong QRS and QT intervals (R) May result in "false positive" test results (E)	↔
Phenytoin	↔ (R and E)	↔ (R and E)	↔ (R and E)	↔
Tocainide Mexiletine				
Moricizine	↔ (R and E)		May prolong QRS and QT intervals (R) ↔ (E)	↔
Propafenone	↓ (R) ↓ or ↔ (E)	↔ (R and E) ↔ (R and E)	↓ HR (R) ↓ or ↔ HR (E)	
Class II β-Blockers (see I)				
Class III Amiodarone Sotalol	↓ (R and E)	↔ (R and E)	↓ HR (R) ↔ (E)	↔
Class IV Calcium channel blockers (see III)				
VIII. Bronchodilators	↔ (R and E)	↔ (R and E)	↔ (R and E)	Bronchodilators ↑ exercise capacity in patients limited by bronchospasm
Anticholinergic agents	↑ or ↔ (R and E)	↔	↑ or ↔ HR	
Xanthine derivatives			May produce PVCs (R and E)	
Sympathomimetic agents	↑ or ↔ (R and E)	↑, ↔, or ↓ (R and E)	↑ or ↔ HR (R and E)	↔
Cromolyn sodium	↔ (R and E)	↔ (R and E)	↔ (R and E)	↔
Steroidal anti-inflammatory agents	↔ (R and E)	↔ (R and E)	↔ (R and E)	↔

Medications	Heart rate	Blood pressure	ECG	Exercise capacity
IX. Antilipemic agents	Clofibrate may provoke arrhythmias, angina in patients with prior myocardial infarction Nicotinic acid may ↓ BP All other hyperlipidemic agents have no effect on HR, BP, and ECG			↔
X. Psychotropic medications Minor tranquilizers	May ↓ HR and BP by controlling anxiety; no other effects			
Antidepressants	↑ or ↔ (R and E)	↓ or ↔ (R and E)	Variable (R)	
Major tranquilizers	↑ or ↔ (R and E)	↓ or ↔ (R and E)	Variable (R)	
Lithium	↔ (R and E)	↔ (R and E)	May result in T-wave changes and arrhythmias (R and E)	
XI. Nicotine	↑ or ↔ (R and E)	↑ (R and E)	↑ or ↔ HR May provoke ischemia, arrhythmias (R and E)	↔, except ↓ or ↔ in patients with angina
XII. Antihistamines	↔ (R and E)	↔ (R and E)	↔ (R and E)	↔
XIII. Cold medications with sympathomimetic agents	Effects similar to those described for sympathomimetic agents, although magnitude of effects is usually smaller			↔
XIV. Thyroid medications Only levothyroxine	↑ (R and E)	↑ (R and E)	↑ HR May provoke arrhythmias ↑ ischemia (R and E)	↔, unless angina worsened
XV. Alcohol	↔ (R and E)	Chronic use may have role in ↑ BP (R and E)	May provoke arrhythmias (R and E)	↔
XVI. Hypoglycemic agents Insulin and oral agents	↔ (R and E)	↔ (R and E)	↔ (R and E)	↔
XVII. Blood modifiers (anticoagulants and antiplatelets)	↔ (R and E)	↔ (R and E)	↔ (R and E)	↔ ↑ or ↔ in patients limited by intermittent claudication (for cilostazol only)
XVIII. Pentoxifylline	↔ (R and E)	↔ (R and E)	↔ (R and E)	↔ in patients limited by intermittent claudication
XIX. Anti-gout medications	↔ (R and E)	↔ (R and E)	↔ (R and E)	↔

(continued)

TABLE D-1 *(continued)*

Medications	Heart rate	Blood pressure	ECG	Exercise capacity
XX. Caffeine	Variable effects depending on previous use Variable effects on exercise capacity May provoke arrhythmias			
XXI. Anorexiants/diet pills	↑ or ↔ (R and E)	↑ or ↔ (R and E)	↑ or ↔ HR (R and E)	Increased HR and BP common with norepinephrine reuptake inhibitors (e.g., sibutramine)

*β-Blockers with intrinsic sympathomimetic activity lower resting HR only slightly.

†May prevent or delay myocardial ischemia (see text).

Abbreviations: PVCs = premature ventricular contractions; ↑ = increase; ↔ = no effect; ↓ = decrease; R = rest; E = exercise; HR = heart rate.

APPENDIX E
Fitness Assessment

This appendix provides a foundation for the areas of fitness assessment covered in part III, allowing you to better explain what fitness test scores mean. In part III, we examined the assessment of cardiorespiratory fitness (CRF), body composition and nutrition, muscular strength and endurance, and flexibility and low-back function.

The first step in fitness testing is choosing your fitness tests wisely. You must consider the following factors in your selection:

- **Reliability:** Can I get consistent results with this test?

- **Objectivity:** Do different test administrators get the same results on this test?

- **Validity:** Does the test measure the characteristic I'm interested in evaluating?

Although a test can be reliable and objective and still not be valid, tests that are unreliable or lack objectivity cannot be valid. Once the consistency of the test is ensured, there are ways to determine whether the test measures what it is supposed to measure. For example, do experts agree that the test is valid? Does the test compare favorably with an established test (a standard) in the same area?

The fitness tests recommended in this book have been shown to be reliable and objective when carefully administered by trained professionals. There also is evidence that the tests in this book are valid (experts recommend them or the tests compare favorably with valid tests).

Fitness professionals can do several things to maximize accuracy (i.e., minimize error) in testing:

- Properly prepare the person being tested.
- Organize the testing session.
- Attend to details.

Fitness testing has many uses in a fitness setting, from prescribing exercise to refining programs. Fitness professionals must know how to interpret test scores and provide feedback to all program participants.

You can help participants evaluate their fitness test scores by doing the following (3, 4):

- Emphasize health status rather than comparison with others.

- For those needing improvement, emphasize change rather than current status.

- Provide specific recommendations based on the test data and your understanding of the participant.

One common approach to evaluating test scores is to compare the fitness participant with people of the same gender and similar age (i.e., use percentiles). Much of the way the individual compares with others is based on heredity and early experience. There are limits to how much people can change even with great effort. It is unfortunate that many people in fitness programs try to use the performance model of being number one. The emphasis should not be on who can run the fastest or who has the lowest cholesterol but on helping all people understand, obtain, and maintain CRF, healthy body composition, and low-back function.

The current edition of *ACSM's Guidelines for Exercise Testing and Prescription* (1) uses percentiles for evaluation of fitness tests. Much more research is needed before health criteria can be finalized; however, we think that attempting to set health criteria is better, even with its limitations, than relying on percentiles. For example, a person could weigh significantly more now than in 1980 and be at the same percentile because the whole population gained weight. In addition, a person could gain fat and lose muscle with age and stay at the same percentile.

The table provides fitness standards based on what is needed for good health. Although performance decreases with age, the minimal fitness standards listed in the table are the same for adults of all ages. This is similar to a serum cholesterol value ≥ 200 mg $\cdot$ dl^{-1} or SBP ≥ 140 mmHg being the same cutoff values used for risk-factor assessment in adults, independent of age. More research is needed so that we can refine these fitness standards; as we find out more about the relationship between test scores and positive health, some of these standards may need to be modified.

The most important question for a fitness participant is not what her health status is at this moment in life, but what it will be 6 mo, 2 yr, or 20 yr from now. In this way, the person is encouraged to deal with her current status (compared with health standards) so that she can set reasonable, desirable, and achievable goals for the next testing time.

Test results can also help people work toward and eventually achieve specific goals. It may be that the fitness standards are not appropriate or reasonable for an individual. For example, the standards for running the mile cannot be used for people who swim for their fitness workouts or for people who use wheelchairs. However, individual goals for covering a certain distance in the water or in a wheelchair can be established. Or, the fitness professional may want to set intermediary goals for a person who is very unfit. For example, a person who can only walk a quarter of a mile without stopping would be discouraged by discussing

FITNESS TEST Standards for Ages 6 Through 70

Test item		6-9 yr	10-12 yr	13-15 yr	16-30 yr	31-50 yr	51-70 yr
1 mi (1.6 km) run in min							
Males	Good	14	12	11	10	10	10
	Borderline	16	14	13	12	12	12
	Needs work	≥18	≥16	≥15	≥14	≥14	≥14
Females	Good	14	12	13	12	12	12
	Borderline	16	14	15	14	14	14
	Needs work	≥18	≥16	≥17	≥16	≥16	≥16
Percent body fat (%)							
Males	Good	7-18	7-18	7-18	7-18	7-18	7-18
	Borderline	22	22	22	22	22	22
	Needs work	>25	>25	>25	>25	>25	>25
Females	Good	7-18	7-18	16-25	16-25	16-25	16-25
	Borderline	22	22	27	27	27	27
	Needs work	>25	>25	>30	>30	>30	>30
Curl-ups (#)							
	Good	≥20	≥25	≥30	≥35	≥35	≥35
	Borderline	12	10	22	25	25	25
	Needs work	≤5	≤10	≤13	≤15	≤15	≤15
Sit-and-reach (in./cm)[a]							
	Good	12/30.5	12/30.5	12/30.5	12/30.5	12/30.5	12/30.5
	Borderline	8/20.3	8/20.3	8/20.3	8/20.3	8/20.3	8/20.3
	Needs work	≤6/15.2	≤6/15.2	≤6/15.2	≤6/15.2	≤6/15.2	≤6/15.2
Modified pull-ups (#)							
	Good	≥10	≥12	≥15	≥15	≥15	≥15
	Borderline	6	8	10	10	10	10
	Needs work	≤2	≤4	≤5	≤5	≤5	≤5

[a]The feet touch the base of the box at 9 in. (22.9 cm). A score of 9 (22.9) indicates the person can touch her feet.

People over 70 yr should be encouraged to do the walk test (see chapter 5) and strive to monitor the other fitness components.

Adapted from Corbin and Lindsey 2002; Cooper Institute for Aerobics Research 1992; President's Council on Physical Fitness and Sports 2001; Franks 1989.

the standards for running 1 mi (1.6 km). The initial goal for that person may be to work up to being able to walk 1 mi without stopping. As indicated in chapter 23, it is important to set goals and subgoals to help people begin and continue healthy behaviors.

Fitness and lifestyle behaviors (e.g., getting adequate exercise, nutrition, and rest; avoiding substance abuse; coping with stress) and fitness test scores are interrelated. The fitness professional should emphasize fitness *behaviors*. It is more important for people to begin and continue regular physical activity than to reach a certain level on a graded exercise test (GXT). Likewise, it is more important for people to develop healthy eating habits than to have a certain percentage of body fat. By emphasizing healthy behaviors, fitness professionals can recognize people for their effort, and in the long run, living a consistent, healthy lifestyle is the best way for a client to improve fitness test scores and overall health.

Overemphasizing test scores can discourage some participants. Two good examples of programs that recognize fitness behaviors are the Canadian *Active Living Challenge*

(2) and the President's Council on Fitness, Sports and Nutrition's Presidential Active Lifestyle Award (*PALA*) programs (7). Both programs award people who do various physical activities for a certain number of hours, thus rewarding the behavior rather than the test result.

Many people have one or more disabilities resulting in mild to severe limitations regarding physical activity and assessment. It is beyond the scope of this book to recommend specific activities and tests to deal with each possible condition (8). The fitness professional can, however, apply the following general principles:

- Almost all people with disabilities can benefit from regular physical activity.

- Most of these individuals can participate in a variety of activities with simple adaptations.

- People with disabilities can gain motivation from periodic assessment.

- The same types of fitness tests can be used with simple adaptations.

- Adaptations of activities and assessments are often simply commonsense adjustments made by the fitness professional and the participant.
- Experts in adapted physical education, therapeutic recreation, and special education can provide additional assistance.

Fitness professionals are challenged with determining whether programming is meeting clients' needs. For example, "Is my spin class improving the fitness of my attendees?" Analyzing test scores from various fitness classes can help the fitness professional decide what revisions need to be made in the overall fitness program. How many people drop out of various classes? What kind of changes in CRF, body fatness, and low-back function are being made? How many injuries relate to the various classes? The answers to such questions help you evaluate, revise, and improve your fitness programs. You might consider your programs to be improving steadily rather than having reached perfection. This improvement can result from program evaluation.

Another use of test scores is to educate the public and to get positive attention for your program. What percentage of the participants stay with the program long enough to make important fitness gains? What is the total amount of fat lost by participants over a year? How many miles have the participants run during the year? Careful testing, record keeping, and analysis can provide helpful information about your program to the public.

REFERENCES

1. American College of Sports Medicine (ACSM). 2010. *ACSM's guidelines for exercise testing and prescription.* 8th ed. Philadelphia: Lippincott Williams & Wilkins.

2. Canadian Association for Health, Physical Education, Recreation and Dance. 1994. *The Canadian Active Living Challenge.* Gloucester, ON: Author.

3. Cooper Institute for Aerobics Research. 1992. *Prudential Fitnessgram test administration manual.* Dallas: Author.

4. Corbin, C.B., and R. Lindsey. 2002. *Fitness for life.* 4th ed. Champaign, IL: Human Kinetics.

5. Franks, B.D. 1989. *YMCA youth fitness test.* Champaign, IL: Human Kinetics.

6. President's Council on Physical Fitness and Sports (PCPFS). 2001. *President's challenge physical activity and fitness award program.* Washington, DC: Author.

7. President's Council on Fitness, Sports and Nutrition. 2011. *Presidential Active Lifestyle Award.* www.fitness.gov/presidents-challenge/presidential-active-lifestyle-award/index.html.

8. Seaman, J.A. 1999. Physical activity and fitness for persons with disabilities. *PCPFS Research Digest* 3(5).

GLOSSARY

1-repetition maximum (1RM)—The heaviest weight that can be lifted only once using good form.

A band—Portion of the sarcomere composed of myosin and actin; the length of the A band remains constant during muscle shortening.

abduction—Movement of a bone laterally away from the anatomical position.

absolute intensity—Can be expressed in a number of ways: kilocalories (kcal) of energy produced per min (kcal · min⁻¹), milliliters of oxygen consumed per kilogram of body weight per minute (ml · kg⁻¹ · min⁻¹), or METs, where one MET is taken as RMR and is equal to 3.5 ml · kg⁻¹ · min⁻¹.

acceptable macronutrient distribution range (AMDR)—The percentages of calories from carbohydrate, fat, and protein that are thought to promote good health.

actin—The thin contractile filament of the sarcomere to which myosin binds to release the energy in the activated crossbridges, leading to sarcomere shortening.

adduction—The return to the anatomical position from the abducted position.

adequate intake (AI)—The amount of a nutrient considered adequate although insufficient data exist to establish an RDA.

adipose tissue—Tissue composed of fat cells.

administrative law—A primary source of law (from the executive branch of the government) that is formed by numerous administrative agencies that exist at both the federal and state levels.

aerobic energy—When oxygen is used to help supply energy (ATP) to a person who is working.

agility—Ability to start, stop, and move the body quickly in different directions.

agonist—A muscle that is very effective in causing a certain joint movement; also called the *prime mover.*

air displacement plethysmography—Method of assessing body composition that estimates body density from body volume and body weight.

airway obstruction—Blockage of the airway that can be caused by a foreign object. Swelling is secondary to direct trauma or allergic reaction.

alcohol—Ethanol; a depressant that may affect the response to an exercise test.

amenorrhea—Absence of menses.

amino acids—Nitrogen-containing building blocks for proteins that can be used for energy.

amortization phase—Time between the eccentric and concentric phases of a muscle action.

amphiarthrodial joint—A joint that allows only slight movement in all directions; also called the *cartilaginous joint.*

anaerobic energy—Energy (ATP) supplied without oxygen. Creatine phosphate and glycolysis supply ATP without using oxygen.

android-type obesity—Obesity in which there is a disproportionate amount of fat in the trunk and abdomen.

aneurysm—A spindle-shaped or saclike bulging of the wall of a blood-filled vein, artery, or ventricle.

angina pectoris—Severe cardiac pain that may radiate to the jaw, arms, or legs. Angina is caused by myocardial ischemia, which can be induced by exercise in susceptible people.

angular momentum—The quantity of rotation. Angular momentum is the product of rotational inertia and angular velocity.

anorexia nervosa—An eating disorder in which a preoccupation with body weight leads to self-starvation.

antagonist—A muscle that causes movement at a joint in a direction opposite to that of the joint's agonist (prime mover).

antiarrhythmics—Drugs that reduce the number of arrhythmias.

anticoagulants—Drugs that delay blood clotting.

antihistamines—Drugs that relieve allergy symptoms, thus making it easier to breathe.

antihypertensives—Drugs that lower BP.

antioxidant vitamins—Substances that attach to free radicals and diminish their effects. Antioxidants are touted as effective in decreasing the risk of CVD and cancer.

aortic valve—Heart valve located between the aorta and the left ventricle.

apnea—Temporary cessation of breathing; often caused by an excess amount of oxygen or too little carbon dioxide in the brain.

aponeuroses—Broad, flat, tendinous sheaths attaching muscles to one another.

arterioles—Blood vessels between the artery and the capillary that are involved in the regulation of blood flow and BP.

arteriovenous oxygen difference—Volume of oxygen extraction; calculated by subtracting the oxygen content of mixed venous blood (as it returns to the heart) from the oxygen content of the arterial blood.

arthritis—Inflammation of a joint.

articular capsule—A ligamentous structure that encloses a diarthrodial joint.

articular cartilage—Cartilage covering bone surfaces that articulate (meet or come into contact) with other bone surfaces.

atherosclerosis—A form of arteriosclerosis in which fatty substances are deposited in the inner walls of the arteries.

atrial fibrillation—The atrial rate is 400 to 700 beats · min^{-1}, whereas the ventricular rate is 60 to 160 beats · min^{-1}; P waves cannot be seen on the ECG.

atrial flutter—The atrial rate is 200 to 350 beats · min^{-1}, whereas the ventricular rate is 60 to 160 beats · min^{-1}; ECG shows a sawtooth pattern between QRS complexes.

atrioventricular (AV) node—The origin of the bundle of His in the right atrium of the heart. Normal electrical activity of the heart passes through the AV node before depolarization of the ventricles.

atrophy—A reduction in muscle fiber size.

avascular—Without a blood supply.

balance—Ability to maintain a certain posture or to move without falling.

ballistic movement—A rapid movement with three phases: an initial concentric action by agonist muscles to begin movement, a coasting phase, and a deceleration by the eccentric action of the antagonist muscles.

bariatric surgery—A surgical procedure designed to help with weight loss. These surgeries alter the gastrointestinal system to restrict food intake and nutrient uptake.

baroreceptors—Receptors that monitor arterial BP.

behavioral contracts—Written, signed, public agreements to engage in specific goal-directed activities. Contracts include a designated time frame and clear consequences of meeting and not meeting the agreed-upon objectives.

bench stepping—A GXT that can be used for both submaximal and maximal testing to evaluate CRF. The height of the bench and the number of steps per minute determine the intensity of the effort. Bench stepping is also a popular conditioning exercise.

beta-adrenergic blocking medications (beta-blockers)—Drugs that block receptors that respond to catecholamines (epinephrine and norepinephrine); they slow HR.

beta-adrenergic receptors—Receptors in the heart and lungs that respond to catecholamines (epinephrine and norepinephrine).

beta-carotene—A precursor of vitamin A and an important antioxidant.

binge-eating disorder—An eating disorder characterized by consuming large amounts of food in a short time.

bioelectrical impedance analysis (BIA)—Method of body composition assessment based on the electrical conductivity of various tissues in the body.

black-globe temperature (T_g)—A measure of radiant heat energy; a measurement taken in the sunlight to evaluate the potential to gain or lose heat by radiation.

body composition—Description of the tissues that make up the body; typically refers to the relative percentages of fat and nonfat tissues in the body.

body fat distribution (fat patterning)—Pattern of fat accumulation that often is inherited.

body mass index (BMI)—Measure of the relationship between height and weight; calculated by dividing weight in kilograms by height in meters squared.

bodybuilding—A competitive sport in which the primary goal is to enhance muscular size, symmetry, and definition.

bone mineral density (BMD)—Amount of bone mineral per unit area. Typically measured with DXA and used for clinical diagnosis of osteoporosis.

bradycardia—Slow HR, below 60 beats · min^{-1} at rest. Bradycardia is healthy if it is the result of physical conditioning.

bronchodilators—Drugs that dilate the bronchioles, providing relief from an asthma attack.

bulimia nervosa—An eating disorder characterized by consuming large amounts of food followed by food purging.

bundle branch—Bundle of nerve fibers between both ventricles of the heart; conducts impulses.

bundle of His—Conduction pathway that connects the AV node with bundle branches in the ventricles.

bursae—Fibrous sacs lined with synovial membrane that contain a small quantity of synovial fluid. Bursae are found between tendon and bone, between skin and bone, and between muscle and muscle. Their function is to facilitate movement without friction between these surfaces.

calcium channel blockers—Medications that act by blocking the entry of calcium into the cell; used to treat angina, arrhythmias, and hypertension.

caloric equivalent of oxygen—Approximately 5 kcal of energy is produced per liter of oxygen consumed (5 kcal · L^{-1}).

carbohydrate—An essential nutrient composed of carbon, hydrogen, and oxygen that is an energy source for the body.

carbohydrate loading—Increasing carbohydrate intake and decreasing activity in the days preceding competition.

carbon monoxide (CO)—A pollutant derived from the incomplete combustion of fossil fuels; binds to hemoglobin to reduce oxygen transport and thus reduce maximal aerobic power.

cardiac output (Q)—The volume of blood pumped by the heart per minute; calculated by multiplying HR (beats · min⁻¹) by SV (ml · beat⁻¹).

cardiopulmonary resuscitation (CPR)—Established procedures to restore breathing and blood circulation.

cardiorespiratory fitness (CRF)—The ability of the circulatory and respiratory systems to supply oxygen to muscles during dynamic exercise involving a large muscle mass.

case law—A primary source of law (from the judicial branch of government) that is derived from written court opinions at both the federal and state levels.

cholesterol—A fatty substance in which carbon, hydrogen, and oxygen atoms are arranged in rings; may be deposited in the arterial walls, contributing to atherosclerosis.

chronic obstructive pulmonary diseases (COPDs)—Diseases that obstruct the flow of air in the airways of the lung.

claudication—Interference with the blood supply to the legs, often resulting in limping.

closed-circuit spirometry—The subject breathes 100% oxygen from a spirometer while carbon dioxide is absorbed; the decrease in the volume of oxygen in the spirometer is proportional to the oxygen consumption.

communication—Interaction, often verbal, to share information and emotions.

compartment syndrome—Increased pressure within a muscular compartment that compromises blood flow and nerve supply.

complex carbohydrate—Polysaccharides formed by combining three or more sugar molecules. Polysaccharides include starches and fiber and are found in high numbers in rice, pasta, and whole-grain breads.

concentric action—A shortening of the muscle; causes movement at the joint.

concreteness—Being specific about events and ideas; not abstract.

conduction—Heat-exchange mechanism in which heat is lost from warmer to cooler objects in direct contact with each other.

confrontation—Pointing out incongruities or inconsistencies between what a person says and does that are observable facts.

convection—Special case of conduction related to heat loss. Heat is transferred to air or water in direct contact with the skin; warm air or water is less dense and rises, carrying heat away from the body.

coordination—Ability to perform a task that integrates movements of the body and various parts of the body.

coronary angiography—A diagnostic procedure where a flexible guide wire is inserted into a coronary artery, and a catheter is then passed over it. A radiographic contrast dye is then injected into the artery to reveal any potential blockages.

coronary arteries—Blood vessels that supply the heart muscle.

coronary artery bypass graft (CABG)—Procedure in which arteries or veins are sutured above and below a blocked coronary artery to restore adequate blood flow to that portion of the myocardium.

coronary heart disease (CHD)—Atherosclerosis of the coronary arteries. Also called *coronary artery disease (CAD)*.

creeping obesity—Slow accumulation of adipose tissue with aging.

criterion method—Method used as the gold standard, or the method against which other methods are compared.

crossbridge—Part of myosin filament that binds to actin, releasing energy that results in shortening of the sarcomere.

cycle ergometer—A one-wheeled stationary cycle with adjustable resistance used as a work task for exercise testing or conditioning.

daily caloric need—Number of calories needed to maintain current body weight. This number is composed of RMR, calories for activity, and the thermic effect of food.

daily values (DVs)—Indicate the percentage of daily recommended levels of nutrients that are contained in a food. DVs are based on a calorie intake of 2,000 kcal · day⁻¹.

DASH diet—The DASH (Dietary Approaches to Stop Hypertension) diet was originally designed to help people control their BP. This diet is characterized by sodium restriction; an emphasis on vegetables, fruits, low-fat milk products, whole grains, and lean meats; and elimination or minimization of added sugars and processed meats. Several studies have shown that this dietary approach can be helpful in reducing BP and weight.

decongestants—Drugs that reduce nasal and bronchial congestion and dry out the airways.

defendant—The individual or entity whom the plaintiff (injured party) is suing in a civil law case, such as in a negligence lawsuit, or the individual or entity who is accused of committing a crime (violating a statute) in a criminal law case.

diabetes mellitus—Group of metabolic diseases characterized by high blood glucose concentrations.

diaphysis—The shaft of a long bone.

diarthrodial joint—A freely moving joint characterized by its synovial membrane and capsular ligament; also called a *synovial joint*.

diastolic blood pressure (DBP)—The pressure blood exerted on the vessel walls during the resting portion of the cardiac cycle, measured in millimeters of mercury by a sphygmomanometer.

dietary fiber—Substances found in plants that cannot be broken down by the human digestive system.

dietary reference intake (DRI)—Set of values used to evaluate dietary intake.

digitalis—A drug that augments the contraction of the heart muscle and slows the rate of conduction of cardiac impulses through the AV node.

direct calorimetry—A method of measuring the metabolic rate using a closed chamber in which a subject's heat loss is picked up by water flowing through the walls of a chamber; the gain in temperature of the water plus that lost in evaporation determines the metabolic rate.

disc—Located between vertebrae; acts as a shock absorber and frequently is involved in low-back pain.

disordered eating—Unhealthy eating pattern that can in some cases be a precursor to eating disorders.

diuretics—Drugs that increase urine production, thereby ridding the body of excess fluid.

dose—The quantity (intensity, frequency, and duration) of exercise needed to bring about a response (e.g., lower resting BP).

double product—See *rate–pressure product*.

dry-bulb temperature (T_{db})—The temperature of the air measured in the shade by an ordinary thermometer.

duration—The length of time for a fitness workout or a bout of physical activity.

dynamic testing—Strength assessment that involves movement of the body (e.g., push-up) or an external load (e.g., bench press).

dyspnea—Difficult or labored breathing beyond what is expected for the intensity of work. The exercise test or activity should be stopped.

dyspnea rating scale—An instrument used to rate the severity of a patient's symptoms of shortness of breath.

eating disorders—Clinical eating patterns that result in severe negative health consequences.

eccentric action—Lengthening of the muscle during its action; controls speed of movement caused by another force.

ectopic focus—An irritated portion of the myocardium or electrical conducting system; gives rise to extra heartbeats that do not originate from the SA node.

effect—The desired response resulting from exercise training (e.g., lower resting BP).

ejection fraction—The fraction of the EDV ejected per beat (SV divided by EDV).

elasticity—Ability of ligaments and tendons to lengthen passively and return to their resting length.

electrocardiogram (ECG)—Graphic recording of the electrical activity of the heart. The ECG is obtained with the electrocardiograph.

electrolytes—Particles in solution that convey an electrical charge. Most electrolyte drinks are diluted solutions of glucose, salt, other minerals, and artificial flavoring. Other than sodium, the minerals provided by an electrolyte solution do not provide much benefit.

embolism—Sudden obstruction of a blood vessel by a solid body such as a clot carried in the bloodstream.

emergency medical system (EMS)—A system designed to handle medical emergencies; 911 or other community emergency numbers.

emergency procedure—Plan of action to follow in emergency situations.

empathy—Identification with the thoughts or feelings of another person and the effective communication that the other person's feelings are understood.

end-diastolic volume (EDV)—The volume of blood in the heart just before ventricular contraction; a measure of the stretch of the ventricle.

endothelial cells—Cells that form the interior lining of the blood vessels, heart, and lymphatic vessels.

end-ROM—Point at which further movement may stretch ligaments or other soft-tissue structures such as discs.

epimysium—The connective-tissue sheath surrounding a muscle.

epiphyseal plates—The sites of ossification in long bones.

epiphyses—The ends of long bones.

ergogenic aids—Substances taken in hopes of improving athletic performance.

essential amino acids—The eight amino acids that the body cannot synthesize and therefore must be ingested.

essential fat—The minimum amount of body fat needed for good health.

evaporation—Conversion of water from liquid to gas by means of heat, as in evaporation of sweat; results in the loss of 580 kcal for each liter of sweat evaporated.

excess postexercise oxygen consumption (EPOC)—The amount of oxygen used during recovery from work that exceeds the amount needed for rest. Also called *oxygen debt* and *oxygen repayment*.

exculpatory clause—A clause within a waiver (prospective release) that can absolve (protect) defendants from their ordinary negligence.

exercise—A subset of physical activity that is planned, structured, and repetitive and is meant to improve or maintain physical fitness.

exercise-induced asthma—A reactive airway disease in which exercise tends to cause the bronchioles to constrict.

exercise tests—A series of tests that evaluate prospective exercise participants' current level of fitness and commonly include CRF, muscular strength and endurance, body composition, and flexibility.

exertional heat stroke (EHS)—most severe form of heat-related injury with body temperature above 41.1° C (106° F); treat as medical emergency.

extension—Increasing the angle at a joint, such as straightening the elbow.

external rotation—Movement of a bone around its longitudinal axis away from the midline of the body in the anatomical position.

facet joint—Junction of the superior and inferior articular processes of the vertebrae.

fascicles—Bundles of muscle fibers surrounded by perimysium.

fast glycolytic fiber—See *type IIx fiber.*

fast oxidative glycolytic fiber—See *type IIa fiber.*

fat—Non-water-soluble substance composed of hydrogen, oxygen, and carbon that serves a variety of functions in the body, including energy production.

fat mass (FM)—The mass of the fat tissues in the body.

fat-free mass (FFM)—Weight of the nonfat tissues of the body.

fat patterning—See *body-fat distribution.*

female athlete triad—A condition sometimes observed in female athletes that is characterized by disordered eating, amenorrhea, and osteoporosis.

first-degree AV block—The delayed transmission of impulses from atria to ventricles (in excess of 0.20 sec).

flexibility—The ability to move a joint through its full ROM without discomfort or pain.

flexion—Anterior or posterior movement that brings two bones together.

force arm (*FA*)—Perpendicular distance from the axis of rotation to the direction of the application of the force-causing movement.

forced expiratory volume in 1 sec (FEV₁)—The maximal amount of air that can be forcibly exhaled in 1 sec, as measured by spirometry; this variable is used to diagnose COPD. A person who can expel less than 75% of her VC in 1 sec should be referred to a physician.

free radicals—Molecules or fragments of molecules formed during metabolic processes that are highly reactive and can damage cellular components.

frequency—Refers to the number of days per week that physical activity is done.

functional capacity—Maximal oxygen uptake, expressed in milliliters of oxygen per kilogram of body weight per minute, or in METs.

functional curve—Spinal curve (e.g., lordotic curve) that can be removed by assuming different postures.

genuineness—Being authentic and sincere in a relationship with another person.

glucose—A simple sugar that is a vital energy source in the human body.

glycemic index—A rating system used to indicate how rapidly a food causes blood glucose to rise.

glycogen—The storage form of carbohydrate in the human body.

glycolysis—The metabolic pathway producing ATP from the anaerobic breakdown of glucose. This short-term source of ATP is important in all-out activities lasting less than 2 min.

goal setting—Goals are desired tasks to accomplish in a specific amount of time; they provide direction and foster persistence in the search for task strategies. Effective goal setting includes establishing objectives that can be measured, concretely defined, and practically achieved.

good nutrition—A diet in which foods are eaten in the proper quantities and with the needed distribution of nutrients to maintain good health in the present and in the future.

graded exercise test (GXT)—A multistage test that determines a person's physiological responses to various intensities of exercise and the person's maximal aerobic power.

gynoid-type obesity—Obesity in which there is a disproportionate amount of fat in the hips and thighs.

H zone—The middle area of the sarcomere that contains only myosin.

health—Being alive with no major health problem. Also called *apparently healthy.*

health-related fitness—Refers to muscular strength and endurance, CRF, flexibility, and body composition.

heart rate (HR)—The number of heartbeats per minute.

Heimlich maneuver—Procedure used to dislodge material caught in the respiratory passage that is blocking the airway.

hemorrhage—The escape of a large amount of blood from a vessel.

hepatitis B (HBV)—A type of hepatitis (viral infection of the liver) that is transmitted by sexual or blood-to-blood contact.

high-density lipoprotein cholesterol (HDLC)—This form of cholesterol protects against the development of CHD by transporting cholesterol to the liver, where it is eliminated. Thus, low levels of HDL-C are related to a high risk of CHD.

high-risk situation—An event, thought, or interaction that challenges a person's perceived ability to maintain a desired behavioral change.

human immunodeficiency virus (HIV)—A virus that destroys the body's ability to fight infection; causes AIDS.

hydrostatic weighing—Method of assessing body composition based on Archimedes' principle; also called *underwater weighing*. Hydrostatic weighing is often used as the criterion method for assessing %BF.

hyperglycemia—Blood glucose concentrations above normal (fasting plasma glucose of 110 mg · dl^{-1}).

hypertension—High BP. Normally SBP exceeds 140 mmHg or DBP exceeds 90 mmHg in someone who has hypertension.

hyperthermia—An elevation of the core temperature; if unchecked, it can lead to heat exhaustion or heatstroke and death.

hypertrophy—An enlargement in muscle fiber size.

hyperventilation—A level of ventilation beyond that needed to maintain the arterial carbon dioxide level; can be initiated by a sudden increase in the hydrogen ion concentration attributable to lactic acid production during a progressive exercise test.

hypotension—Low BP.

hypothermia—Below-normal body temperature.

hypoxemia—Abnormally low oxygen content in the arterial blood but not total anoxia.

I band—An area of the sarcomere that is bisected by the Z line and is composed of actin; the I band decreases during muscle shortening as the actin slides over the myosin.

impaired fasting glucose—A fasting blood glucose level between 100 and 125 mg · dl^{-1}; commonly considered a precursor to the development of diabetes.

impaired glucose tolerance (IGT)—A condition in which the body does not normally process glucose; often an intermediate step before development of type 2 diabetes.

indirect calorimetry—Estimating energy production on the basis of oxygen consumption.

informed consent—A procedure used to obtain a person's voluntary permission to participate in a program. Informed consent requires a description of the procedures to be used as well as the potential benefits and risks and written consent of the participant.

inherent risks—Injury risks that exist during participation in sport or physical activity that are no one's fault; they just happen and are inseparable from the activity.

insulin resistance—A condition in which the body's insulin receptors no longer respond normally to insulin.

intensity—Describes the rate of work (e.g., how much energy is being expended per minute) or the degree of effort required to carry out the task (percent of maximal HR).

intercalated discs—Junctions between adjacent cardiac muscle cells that allow electrical impulses to pass from cell to cell into both ventricles (see *bundle of His*).

internal rotation—Movement of a bone around its longitudinal axis toward the midline of the body in the anatomical position.

intracoronary stent—A device placed within the lumen of the artery to keep the artery open.

iron-deficiency anemia—A condition characterized by a decreased amount of hemoglobin in red blood cells and a resultant decrease in the ability of the blood to transport oxygen.

isokinetic testing—The assessment of maximal muscle tension throughout a range of joint motion at a constant angular velocity (e.g., 60° · sec^{-1}).

isometric action—A muscle action in which the muscle length is unchanged; the muscle exerts a force that counteracts an opposing force. Isometric action is also called *static action*.

J point—On an ECG, the point at which the S wave ends and the ST segment begins.

joint cavity—The space between bones enclosed by the synovial membrane and articular cartilage.

kyphotic—Describes the condition of kyphosis, a convex curvature of the spine (e.g., the thoracic curve).

lactate threshold—The point during a GXT at which the blood lactate concentration suddenly increases; a good indicator of the highest sustainable work rate. Also called the *anaerobic threshold*.

lean body mass—Term often used synonymously with *fat-free mass*.

liability—Legal responsibility.

ligament—The connective tissue that attaches bone to bone.

lipoproteins—Large molecules responsible for transporting fat in the blood.

local muscular endurance—The ability of a muscle or muscle group to perform repeated contractions against a submaximal resistance.

lordotic curve—Describes the condition of lordosis; a forward, concave curve of the lumbar spine when the spine is viewed from the side.

low-back problems—Strong discomfort in the low-back area, often caused by lack of muscular endurance and flexibility in the midtrunk region or improper posture or lifting.

low-density lipoprotein cholesterol (LDLC)—The form of cholesterol that is responsible for the buildup of plaque in the inner walls of the arteries (atherosclerosis). Thus, high levels of LDL-C are related to a high risk of CHD.

lumbosacral area—Area encompassing the lumbar vertebrae and the sacrum.

lumen—The open space inside a structure such as an artery or intestine.

macrocycle—A phase of training that lasts about 1 yr.

malnutrition—A diet in which there is underconsumption, overconsumption, or unbalanced consumption of nutrients that leads to disease or increased susceptibility to disease.

maximal aerobic power or **maximal oxygen uptake ($\dot{V}O_2$max)**—The maximal rate at which oxygen can be used by the body during maximal work; related directly to the maximal capacity of the heart to deliver blood to the muscles. Expressed in $L \cdot min^{-1}$ or $ml \cdot kg^{-1} \cdot min^{-1}$.

maximum voluntary contraction (MVC)—Maximum amount of force that can be elicited during a single repetition.

medical release—A document that is signed by a person that grants permission to release that person's private medical information to a third party. For example, a medical release form can be signed by a client so the client's personal fitness trainer can obtain medical information from the client's physician such as stress test results, cholesterol, and so on.

Mediterranean diet patterns—Mediterranean diet patterns have become popular in recent years. These patterns vary somewhat based on region but generally emphasize grains (particularly whole grains), fruits, vegetables, olive oil, and nuts. More monounsaturated fatty acids than saturated fatty acids are consumed in this pattern. Wine consumption along with meals is also common. This eating pattern has been linked with a lower prevalence of CVD.

menisci—Partial, semilunar-shaped discs between the femur and the tibia at the knee.

mesocycle—A phase of training that lasts for several months.

microcycle—A phase of training that lasts about 1 wk.

mindful exercise—Low to moderate physical activity performed with a meditative, proprioceptive, or sensory-awareness component.

minerals—Inorganic atoms or ions that serve a variety of functions in the human body.

mitochondria—Cellular organelles responsible for generating energy (ATP) through aerobic metabolism.

mitral valve—Heart valve located between the left atrium and left ventricle.

Mobitz type I AV block—On an ECG, the PR interval progressively increases until the P wave is not followed by a QRS complex. The site of the block is within the AV node.

Mobitz type II AV block—On an ECG, a constant PR interval with some but not all P waves followed by QRS. The site of the block is the bundle of His.

moderate intensity—Refers to an absolute intensity of 3 to 5.9 METs and a relative intensity of 40% to 59% $\dot{V}O_2$max.

monounsaturated fatty acids—Fat that has a single double bond between carbon atoms in the fatty acid chain. Examples are olive and canola oil.

motion segment—Fundamental unit of the lumbar spine; made up of two vertebrae and their intervening disc.

motor unit—The functional unit of muscular action that includes a motor nerve and the muscle fibers that its branches innervate.

muscle fiber—Muscle cell. Contains myofibrils that are composed of sarcomeres; uses chemical energy of ATP to generate tension, which, when greater than the resistance, results in movement.

muscle group—A group of specific muscles that are responsible for the same action at the same joint.

muscular endurance—The ability of the muscle to perform repetitive contractions over a prolonged time.

muscular fitness—Describes the integrated status of muscular strength and muscular endurance.

muscular strength—The ability of muscle to generate the maximum amount of force.

myocardial infarction (MI)—Death of a section of heart tissue in which the blood supply has been cut off; commonly called a *heart attack.*

myocardial ischemia—A lack of blood flow to the heart tissue.

myocardium—The middle layer of the heart wall; involuntary, striated muscle innervated by autonomic nerves.

myofibril—Component inside muscle fibers that is composed of a long string of sarcomeres.

myosin—The thick contractile filament in sarcomeres that can bind actin and split ATP to generate crossbridge movement and develop tension.

MyPlate—The USDA's individualized recommendations for food intake based on age, sex, and current activity patterns. The plan contains recommendations for five food groups: grains, fruits, vegetables, dairy, and protein. MyPlate corresponds with the Dietary Guidelines for Americans and aims to help Americans eat a healthy diet and maintain a healthy weight.

negative caloric balance—When less energy is consumed than is expended, which decreases body weight.

negative health—Negative health is associated with morbidity (incidence of disease) and premature mortality.

negligence—The failure to do something that a reasonable, prudent professional would do or doing something that a reasonable, prudent professional would not have done under the same or similar circumstances.

nicotine gum—Gum containing nicotine that is used for smoking cessation. Nicotine is absorbed through the oral mucosa, providing sufficient plasma nicotine concentrations to curb the craving to smoke.

nitrates—A class of medications used to treat angina pectoris, or chest pain.

nutrient density—The amount of essential nutrients in a food compared with the calories it contains.

nutrient—A substance that the body requires for the maintenance, growth, and repair of tissues.

obesity—Condition in which a person has an excessive accumulation of fat tissue; also may be classified by the relationship between weight and height.

oligomenorrhea—Irregular menses.

open-circuit spirometry—Measuring oxygen consumption by inhaling room air while collecting and analyzing the expired air.

oral antiglycemic agents—Medications used to treat non-insulin-dependent diabetes mellitus; they stimulate the pancreas to secrete more insulin.

ossification—The replacement of cartilage by bone.

osteoarthritis—Most common form of arthritis (90%-95% of all cases); affects joints whose articular cartilage is damaged or injured.

osteopenia—When bone has been lost but has not yet reached osteoporotic levels.

osteoporosis—A disease characterized by a decrease in the total amount of bone mineral and a decrease in the strength of the remaining bone.

overload—To place greater than usual demands on some part of the body (e.g., picking up more weight than usual overloads the muscle involved). Chronic overloading leads to increased function.

overweight—Condition in which a person is above the recommended weight-to-height range but is below obesity levels.

oxygen consumption ($\dot{V}O_2$)—The rate at which oxygen is used during a specific intensity of an activity; oxygen uptake.

oxygen deficit—The difference between the steady-state oxygen requirement of a physical activity and the measured oxygen uptake during the first minutes of work.

ozone—An active form of oxygen formed in reaction to UV light and as an emission from internal combustion engines; exposure can decrease lung function.

P wave—On an ECG, a small positive deflection preceding a QRS complex, indicating atrial depolarization. The P wave is normally less than 0.12 sec in duration, with an amplitude of 0.25 mV or less.

pars interarticularis—The part of the vertebra between its upper elements (superior articular process and transverse process) and its lower elements (inferior articular process and spinous process).

percent body fat (%BF)—Percentage of the total weight composed of fat tissue; calculated by dividing fat mass by total weight and multiplying by 100.

percentage of HRR (%HRR)—The HR reserve (HRR) is calculated by subtracting resting HR from maximal HR. The %HRR is a percentage of the difference between resting and maximal HR and is calculated by subtracting resting HR from exercise HR, dividing by HRR, and multiplying by 100%.

percentage of maximal HR (%HRmax)—HR expressed as a simple percentage of the maximal HR.

percentage of maximal oxygen uptake (%$\dot{V}O_2$max)—Ratio of submaximal oxygen uptake to maximal oxygen uptake, multiplied by 100%.

percentage of oxygen uptake reserve (%$\dot{V}O_2$R)—$\dot{V}O_2$R is calculated by subtracting 1 MET ($3.5 \text{ ml} \cdot \text{kg}^{-1} \cdot \text{min}^{-1}$) from the subject's $\dot{V}O_2$max. The %$\dot{V}O_2$R is a percentage of the difference between resting $\dot{V}O_2$ and $\dot{V}O_2$max and is calculated by subtracting 1 MET from the measured oxygen uptake, dividing by the subject's $\dot{V}O_2$R, and multiplying by 100%.

percutaneous transluminal coronary angioplasty (PTCA)—A surgical procedure in which a flexible guide wire is inserted into a partially blocked coronary artery, and then a catheter with an inflatable balloon near the tip is passed over the guide wire. The balloon is inflated and then deflated and removed in order to open the coronary artery.

performance—The ability to perform a task or sport at a desired level. Also called *motor fitness* or *skill-related fitness*.

perimysium—The connective tissue surrounding fasciculi within a muscle.

periodization—A process of varying the training stimulus to promote long-term fitness gains and to avoid overtraining.

periosteum—The connective tissue surrounding all bone surfaces except the articulating surfaces.

phosphocreatine (PC)—A high-energy phosphate compound that represents the primary immediate anaerobic source of ATP at the onset of exercise. PC is important in all-out activities lasting a few seconds.

phospholipids—Fatty compounds that are essential constituents of cell membranes.

physical activity—Any bodily movement produced by skeletal muscle that results in energy expenditure; associated with occupation, leisure time, household chores, sport, and so on.

physical fitness—A set of health- or skill-related attributes that people have or achieve relating to their ability to perform physical activity.

plaintiff—The injured party who is seeking damages to recover from a personal injury (or property loss) caused by the conduct of the defendant in a civil law case, such as negligence.

polyunsaturated fatty acid—Fat that has two or more double bonds between carbon atoms in the fatty acid chain. Examples are fish, corn, soybean, and peanut oils.

positive caloric balance—When more calories are consumed than are expended, resulting in weight gain.

positive health—Optimal quality of life, including social, mental, spiritual, and physical fitness components; capacity to enjoy life and withstand challenges, not just the avoidance of disease.

positron emission tomography (PET)—A scanning technique that involves infusing the blood with radionuclides. The photons emitted by destruction of positrons are used to generate color images that correspond to blood flow and uptake of substances in various tissues, such as the heart.

power—Ability to exert muscular strength quickly.

powerlifting—A competitive sport in which athletes attempt to lift maximal amounts of weight in the squat, deadlift, and bench press.

PR interval—The time interval between the beginning of the P wave and the QRS complex. The upper normal limit is 0.2 sec. This segment is normally used as the isoelectric baseline.

PR segment—Forms the isoelectric line, or baseline, from which ST segment deviations are measured.

prediabetes—A condition in which a person has impaired fasting glucose or impaired glucose tolerance. Without treatment, prediabetes typically evolves into type 2 diabetes.

premature atrial contraction—On an ECG, the rhythm is irregular and the R-R interval is short; the origin of the beat is somewhere other than the SA node.

premature junctional contraction (PJC)—On an ECG, the ectopic pacemaker in the AV junctional area causes a QRS complex; frequently seen with inverted P waves.

premature ventricular contraction (PVC)—Wide, bizarrely shaped QRS complex originating from an ectopic focus in the His-Purkinje system. The QRS interval lasts longer than 0.12 sec, and the T wave is usually in the opposite direction.

prepubescent—Describes children who have not yet reached puberty.

pressure points—The points where to apply pressure over major arteries to control bleeding.

prevalence—The percentage of a population that has a particular characteristic. For example, obesity prevalence is calculated by dividing the number of people classified as obese by the total number of people.

PRICE—The suggested treatment for minor sprains and strains: protection, rest, ice, compression, and elevation.

primary amenorrhea—The absence of menarche (i.e., first menses) in girls aged 16 or older.

primary assumption of risk—A legal theory in which a plaintiff is generally not allowed to seek damages for an injury that was due to inherent risks as long as the plaintiff knew, understood, and appreciated the inherent risks and voluntarily assumed them.

principle of reversibility—A corollary to the principle of overload; loss of a training effect with disuse.

product liability—A type of liability imposed upon a manufacturer for a defect (design, manufacturing, or marketing) in a product that is considered unreasonably dangerous to the user.

protein—Nutrients composed of amino acids that serve a variety of functions in the human body.

pubescent—Describes the transition from child to adult.

pulmonary function testing—Procedures used to test the capacity of the respiratory system to move air into or out of the lungs.

pulmonary valve—A set of three crescent-shaped flaps at the opening of the pulmonary artery; also called the *semilunar valves*.

pulmonary ventilation—The number of liters of air inhaled or exhaled per minute.

pulse oximeter—Device used to measure the percent saturation of hemoglobin in the arterial blood.

Purkinje fibers—The fibers found beneath the endocardium of the heart; the impulse-conducting network of the heart.

Q wave—The initial negative deflection of the QRS complex on an ECG.

QRS complex—The largest complex on an ECG, indicating a depolarization of the left ventricle and normally lasting less than 0.1 sec.

QT interval—The time interval from the beginning of the QRS complex to the end of the T wave. The QT interval reflects the electrical systole of the cardiac cycle.

R wave—The positive deflection of the QRS complex in the ECG.

radiation—The process of heat exchange from the surface of one object to another that depends on a temperature gradient but does not require direct contact between objects, for example, heat loss from the sun to the earth.

rate–pressure product—The product of HR and SBP; indicative of the oxygen requirement of the heart during exercise. Training lowers the rate–pressure product at rest and during submaximal work. Also called the *double product*.

rating of perceived exertion (RPE)—Borg's scale used to quantify the subjective feeling of physical effort. The original scale was from 6 to 20; the revised scale is from 0 to 10.

recommended dietary allowance (RDA)—The amount of a nutrient found to be adequate for approximately 97% of the population.

recruitment—Stimulation of additional motor units to increase the strength of a muscle action.

reinforcement—Positive reinforcement involves adding something positive to increase the frequency of the target behavior. Negative reinforcement also increases the frequency of the desired behavior, but it is the removal of something negative, such as losing weight because of a regular walking program. Reinforcement can be administered by oneself (self-reinforcement) or by other people (social reinforcement).

relapse prevention—Way to identify and successfully deal with high-risk situations by educating the client about the relapse process and using a variety of strategies to foster an effective coping response.

relative humidity—A measure of the relative wetness of the air; the ratio of the amount of water vapor in the air to the maximum the air can hold at that temperature times 100%. High relative humidity in a warm environment helps determine the potential for losing heat by evaporation.

relative intensity—Describes the degree of effort required to expend energy and is influenced by the person's maximal aerobic capacity or CRF ($\dot{V}O_2max$). Relative intensity can be expressed as a percentage of $\dot{V}O_2max$ or a percentage of maximal HR (HRmax).

relative leanness—The relative amounts of body weight that are fat and nonfat. Also called *body composition*.

repetition—One complete movement of an exercise, which typically consists of a concentric (lifting) and eccentric (lowering) phase.

repetition maximum (RM)—The maximum amount of weight that can be lifted for a predetermined number of repetitions with proper exercise technique. For example, 5RM is the most weight that can be lifted five but not six times.

rescue breathing—Artificial respiration; used to promote oxygenation of blood in an unconscious person who is not breathing.

resistance arm (RA)—Perpendicular distance from the axis of rotation to the direction of the application of the force resisting movement.

resistance force (R)—The opposing force that is resisting another force.

resistance training—A method of exercise designed to enhance musculoskeletal strength, power, and local muscular endurance. Resistance training encompasses a wide range of training modalities, including weight machines, free weights, medicine balls, elastic cords, and body weight.

respect—Objective, nonjudgmental regard for another person's values, beliefs, rights, and property.

respiratory quotient (RQ) or **respiratory exchange ratio (R)**—The ratio of the volume of carbon dioxide produced to the volume of oxygen used during a given time ($\dot{V}CO_2 \div \dot{V}O_2$).

respiratory shock—A condition in which the lungs are unable to supply enough oxygen to the circulating blood.

respondeat superior—A legal doctrine that imposes vicarious liability (a form of strict liability) upon an employer for the negligent acts of its employees while performing their job responsibilities.

resting metabolic rate (RMR)—Number of calories needed to sustain the body under normal resting conditions.

restrictive lung diseases—Diseases that restrict a person's ability to expand the lungs.

rheumatoid arthritis—Debilitating arthritis of unknown cause that can affect a few joints (pauciarticular) or many joints (polyarticular).

risk factor—A characteristic, sign, symptom, or test score that is associated with increased probability of developing a health problem. For example, people with hypertension have increased risk of developing CHD.

risk management—A proactive administrative process that involves four steps: (1) assessment of legal liability exposures, (2) development of risk management strategies, (3) implementation of the risk management plan, and (4) evaluation of the risk management plan. The major goal of risk management is to minimize injuries and subsequent litigation.

rotational inertia—Reluctance to rotate; proportional to the mass and distribution of the mass around the axis.

R-R interval—The time interval from the peak of the QRS of one cardiac cycle to the peak of the QRS of the next cycle.

S wave—The first negative wave (preceded by Q or R waves) of the QRS complex in the ECG.

salt tablets—Supplements that generally are not recommended as a means to increase salt in the diet; if used, they must be taken with large amounts of water.

sarcomeres—The basic units of muscle contraction. They contain actin and myosin; tension develops as the myosin crossbridges pull the actin toward the center of the sarcomere.

sarcoplasmic reticulum (SR)—The network of membranes that surround the myofibril; stores calcium needed for muscle contraction.

saturation pressure—Water vapor pressure that exists at a particular temperature when the air is saturated with water.

sciatic nerve—Nerve originating in the sacral area; it is involved in low-back problems that can result in loss of feeling and control in the legs.

scoliosis—An abnormal lateral curvature of the spine.

scope of practice—Activities performed by fitness professionals while carrying out their responsibilities that are within the limitations (or boundaries) of their education, training, certifications, and experiences.

secondary amenorrhea—A lack of menses for 3 or more consecutive months occurring in females after menarche.

secondary prevention—Steps taken to prevent the recurrence of a heart attack.

second-degree AV block—On an ECG, some but not all P waves precede the QRS complex and result in ventricular depolarization.

set—A group of repetitions performed without stopping.

simple sugars—Monosaccharides and disaccharides, such as glucose, fructose, and sucrose. These forms of carbohydrate provide the majority of calories in candy, soft drinks, and fruit drinks.

sinoatrial (SA) node—A mass of tissue in the right atrium of the heart, near the vena cava, that initiates the heartbeat.

sinus arrhythmia—A normal variant in sinus rhythm in which the R-R interval varies by more than 10% per beat.

sinus bradycardia—Normal heart rhythm and sequence, with a slow HR (below 60 beats · min^{-1} at rest). Sinus bradycardia may indicate a high level of fitness or a mental illness such as depression.

sinus rhythm—The normal timing and sequence of the cardiac events, with the sinus node as a pacemaker; resting rate is between 60 and 100 beats · min^{-1}.

sinus tachycardia—The normal heart rhythm and sequence, with a fast HR (above 100 beats · min^{-1} at rest). Sinus tachycardia may indicate illness or stress.

skill-related (performance-related) fitness—Refers to agility, balance, coordination, speed, power, and reaction time that are linked to games, sport, dance, and so on.

sliding-filament theory—The theory that muscular tension is generated when the actin in the sarcomere slides over the myosin because of the action of the myosin crossbridges.

slow oxidative fiber—See *type I fiber.*

specificity—The principle that states that training effects derived from an exercise program are specific to the exercise done (endurance versus strength training) and the types of muscle fibers involved.

speed—The ability to move the whole body quickly.

sphygmomanometer—A BP measurement system.

spondylolisthesis—Condition in which the vertebral body and transverse processes slip anteriorly (forward) on the vertebral body below; it is common for L5 to slip over L4.

spondylolysis—A stress fracture in the pars interarticularis.

spot reduction—The myth that exercise emphasizing a particular body part will cause that area to lose fat faster than the rest of the body loses it.

ST segment—The part of the ECG between the end of the QRS complex and the beginning of the T wave. Depression below (or elevation above) the isoelectric line indicates ischemia.

ST segment depression—When the ST segment of the ECG is depressed below the baseline; may signify myocardial ischemia.

ST segment elevation—When the ST segment of the ECG is elevated above the baseline; may signify the early (acute) stages of an MI.

stability—The ease with which balance is maintained.

stage 1 hypertension—An SBP of 140 to 159 mmHg or a DBP of 90 to 99 mmHg.

stage 2 hypertension—An SBP of 160 to 179 mmHg or DBP of 100 to 109 mmHg; typically controlled through medication.

stage 3 hypertension—A persistent elevation in BP (SBP >180 mmHg or DBP >110 mmHg) with target-organ damage.

standard deviation (SD)—A measure of the deviation from the mean (average) value generalized to the population. One SD above and below the mean includes about 68% of the population, 2 SD includes about 95%, and 3 SD includes about 99% of the population. For example, if the mean $\dot{V}O_2$max = 25 ml · kg^{-1} · min^{-1} and SD = 3 ml · kg^{-1} · min^{-1}, then you would expect 68% of the population to have $\dot{V}O_2$max values between 22 (25 − 3) and 28 (25 + 3) ml · kg^{-1} · min^{-1}, 95% of the population to be between 19 and 31 ml · kg^{-1} · min^{-1}, and almost all of the population to be between 16 and 34 ml · kg^{-1} · min^{-1}. The *standard error of estimate (SEE)* is used to indicate the standard deviation of any estimate derived for a prediction formula.

statutory law—A primary source of law (from the legislative branch of government) that is enacted through the legislative process at both the federal and state levels.

steady-state oxygen requirement—When the oxygen uptake levels off during submaximal work so that the oxygen uptake value represents the steady-state oxygen (ATP) requirement for the activity.

strength—The maximal force a muscle or muscle group can generate at a specified velocity.

strength training—See *resistance training*.

stroke—A vascular accident (embolism, hemorrhage, or thrombosis) in the brain, often resulting in sudden loss of body function.

structural curve—Curve that cannot be removed in normal movement because of chronically shortened musculotendinous units or ligaments.

submaximal—Less than maximal (e.g., an exercise that can be performed with less than maximal effort).

sulfur dioxide (SO$_2$)—A pollutant that can cause bronchoconstriction in people with asthma.

summation—The additive effect of force generated during higher rates of stimulation when the muscle fiber does not completely relax between stimuli.

sweating—The process of moisture coming through the pores of the skin from the sweat glands, usually as a result of heat, exertion, or emotion.

synarthrodial joint—Immovable joint.

synovial membrane—The inner lining of the joint capsule; secretes synovial fluid into the joint cavity.

systolic blood pressure (SBP)—The pressure exerted on the vessel walls during ventricular contraction, measured in millimeters of mercury by a sphygmomanometer.

T wave—On an ECG, the wave that follows the QRS complex and represents ventricular repolarization.

tachycardia—HR greater than 100 beats · min^{-1} at rest. Tachycardia may be seen in deconditioned people or people who are apprehensive about a situation (e.g., an exercise test).

tachypnea—Excessively rapid breathing that may be a sign of overexertion, shock, or hyperventilation.

talocrural joint—Ankle joint.

target heart rate (THR)—The HR recommended for fitness workouts.

tendon—A band of tough, inelastic, fibrous connective tissue that attaches muscle to bone.

tetanus—Increase in skeletal muscle tension in response to high-stimulation frequencies. The resulting contractions fuse together into a smooth, sustained, high-tension contraction.

thermic effect of food—The energy needed to digest, absorb, transport, and store the food that is eaten.

third-degree AV block—On an ECG, the QRS appears independently, the PR interval varies with no regular pattern, and HR is less than 45 beats · min^{-1}.

threshold—The minimum level needed for a desired effect; often used to refer to the minimum level of exercise intensity needed for improving CRF.

tolerable upper intake level (UL)—The highest intake of a nutrient believed to pose no health risk.

torque (*T*)—The effect produced by a force causing rotation; the product of the force and length of the force arm.

total cholesterol—The sum of all forms of cholesterol in the bloodstream. Because LDL-C is usually the primary factor in the total amount, a high level of total cholesterol is also a risk factor for CHD.

total work—The amount of work accomplished during a workout.

tranquilizers—Medications that bring tranquility by calming, soothing, quieting, or pacifying.

trans fat (trans-fatty acid)—Hydrogenated fat created to be solid at room temperature and to be used in cooking. Consuming this type of fat lowers HDL-C and raises LDL-C.

transfer of angular momentum—Angular momentum can be transferred from one body segment to another by stabilizing the initial moving part at a joint.

transtheoretical model—A general model of intentional behavior change in which behavior change is seen as a dynamic process that occurs through a series of interrelated stages. Basic concepts emphasize the person's motivational readiness to change, the cognitive and behavioral strategies for changing behavior, self-efficacy, and the evaluation of the pros and cons of the new behavior.

transverse tubule—Connects the sarcolemma (muscle membrane) to the sarcoplasmic reticulum; action potentials move down the transverse tubule to cause the sarcoplasmic reticulum to release calcium to initiate muscle contraction.

treadmill—A machine with a moving belt that can be adjusted for speed and grade, allowing a person to walk or run in place. Treadmills are used extensively for exercise testing and training.

tricuspid valve—A valve located between the right atrium and right ventricle of the heart.

triglycerides—The primary storage form of fat in the human body.

tropomyosin—A protein (part of the thin filament) that regulates muscle contraction; works with troponin.

troponin—A protein (part of the thin filament) that can bind the calcium released from the sarcoplasmic reticulum; works with tropomyosin to allow the myosin crossbridge to interact with actin and initiate crossbridge movement.

two-compartment model—Model that divides the body into fat and fat-free components.

type 1 diabetes—Type of diabetes mellitus in which insulin is not produced. It is caused by damage to the beta cells of the pancreas.

type 2 diabetes—Type of diabetes mellitus in which the insulin receptors lose their sensitivity to insulin.

type I (slow oxidative) fiber—A muscle fiber that contracts slowly and generates a small amount of tension, with most of the energy coming from aerobic processes; active in light to moderate activities and possesses great endurance.

type IIa (fast oxidative glycolytic) fiber—A muscle fiber that contracts quickly, can produce energy aerobically, and generates great tension; adds to the tension of type I fibers tension as exercise intensity increases.

type IIx (fast glycolytic) fiber—A muscle fiber that contracts quickly and generates great tension; produces energy by anaerobic metabolism and fatigues quickly.

universal precautions—Safety measures taken to prevent exposure to blood or other body fluids.

USDA Food Patterns—The USDA Food Patterns suggest daily amounts that people should consume from five major food groups (vegetables, fruits, grains, dairy products, and proteins). Suggested limits on intake for certain products (e.g., solid fats) are also included. This plan is based on the established DRIs for nutrients and the Dietary Guidelines for Americans. This approach allows a great deal of flexibility in choosing foods and is adaptable to a vegetarian lifestyle.

ventilatory threshold—The intensity of work at which the rate of ventilation increases sharply during a GXT.

ventricular fibrillation—The heart contracts in an unorganized, quivering manner, with no discernible P waves or QRS complexes on the ECG; requires immediate emergency attention.

ventricular tachycardia—An extremely dangerous condition in which three or more consecutive PVCs occur. Ventricular tachycardia may degenerate into ventricular fibrillation.

vigorous intensity—Refers to an absolute intensity of 6 or more METs and a relative intensity of 60% to 84% $\dot{V}O_2$max.

vital capacity (VC)—The greatest amount of air that can be exhaled after a maximal inspiration. A person whose VC is less than 75% of the value predicted for her age, sex, and height should be referred to a physician for further testing.

vitamins—Organic substances essential to the normal functioning of the human body. They may be subdivided into fat soluble and water soluble.

volume—Refers to the total amount of energy expended or work accomplished in an aerobic activity; equals the product of the absolute intensity, frequency, and time. In resistance training it is the product of the sets, reps, and weight lifted.

waist-to-hip ratio (WHR)—Waist circumference divided by hip circumference; often used as an indicator of android-type obesity.

waiver—A protective legal document, also referred to as a *prospective release*, that contains an exculpatory clause and is signed by a participant before participation in sport or physical activity.

water vapor pressure gradient—The gradient between the water vapor pressure on the skin and the water vapor pressure in the air.

weightlifting—A competitive sport in which athletes attempt to lift maximal amounts of weight in the snatch and the clean and jerk.

wet-bulb globe temperature (WBGT)—Heat stress index that considers dry-bulb, wet-bulb, and black-globe temperatures.

wet-bulb temperature (T_{wb})—Air temperature measured with a thermometer whose bulb is surrounded by a wet wick; an indication of the ability to evaporate moisture from the skin.

windchill index—The temperature equivalent, under calm air conditions, attributable to a combination of temperature and wind velocity.

Z line—Connective-tissue elements that mark the beginning and end of the sarcomere.

INDEX

Note: The italicized *f* and *t* following page numbers refer to figures and tables, respectively.

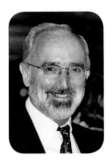

Edward T. Howley, PhD, FACSM, FNAK, earned his bachelor's degree from Manhattan College and his master's and doctorate degrees from the University of Wisconsin at Madison. He then completed a one-year postdoctoral appointment at Penn State University and was hired in 1970 as a faculty member at the University of Tennessee at Knoxville. Howley taught a variety of courses, including an undergraduate course in fitness testing and prescription and undergraduate and graduate courses in exercise physiology. He retired in 2007 and holds the rank of professor emeritus.

In addition to the previous editions of this book, Dr. Howley has authored three books, four book chapters, and 61 research articles dealing with exercise physiology, fitness testing, and prescription. He is a fellow in the National Academy of Kinesiology and served as chair of the Science Board of the President's Council on Physical Fitness and Sports in 2006-2007. In 2007-08 he served on the Physical Activity Guidelines Advisory Committee that evaluated the science related to physical activity and health and generated a report for use by the U.S. Department of Health and Human Services to write the *2008 Physical Activity Guidelines for Americans*.

Most of Dr. Howley's volunteer efforts have been with the American College of Sports Medicine (ACSM). He was involved in the development of certification programs and served as president in 2002-03. He served as editor in chief of *ACSM's Health & Fitness Journal* for seven years and as chair of the program planning committee for the annual ACSM Health and Fitness Summit meeting. In 2007, Howley was recognized for his professional contributions with the ACSM Citation Award. In his leisure time, he likes to golf, ride his bike, travel, and play with his grandchildren.

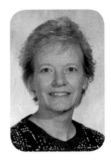

Dixie L. Thompson, PhD, FACSM, FNAK, is a professor and head of the department of kinesiology, recreation, and sport studies at the University of Tennessee at Knoxville. She is also the director of the Center for Physical Activity and Health at the university. She graduated from the 2008 class of the Higher Education Resource Services (HERS) Bryn Mawr Summer Institute, held at Bryn Mawr College. The Summer Institute is a professional development program dedicated to the advancement of female leaders in administration of higher education. She also participated in the 2009-2010 Academic Leadership Development Program sponsored by the Southeastern Conference Academic Consortium.

Dr. Thompson focuses her research on the health benefits of exercise for women and techniques used for body composition assessment. She is the author of over 60 peer-reviewed publications and articles for fitness professionals and general audiences. She is a former associate editor in chief for *ACSM's Health & Fitness Journal* and is currently the editor in chief for *ACSM's Fit Society Page Newsletter*.

Dr. Thompson is a fellow of the American College of Sports Medicine (ACSM) and a fellow of the National Academy of Kinesiology. She is active in professional societies and is a past president of the Southeast Chapter of ACSM. She is also a former chair of the Physical Fitness Council for the American Alliance for Health, Physical Education, Recreation and Dance.

Dr. Thompson received her BA in physical education and MA in exercise physiology from the University of North Carolina at Chapel Hill. She earned her PhD from the University of Virginia.

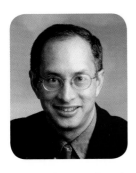

David R. Bassett Jr. is a professor in the department of kinesiology, recreation, and sport studies at the University of Tennessee in Knoxville. He is a fellow of the American College of Sports Medicine and a certified exercise specialist. He is also a frequent reviewer for several scientific journals. Dr. Bassett teaches courses in exercise physiology, clinical exercise physiology, and fitness testing and exercise prescription. His primary research focus is on objective methods of measuring physical activity, including pedometers, accelerometers, and heart rate monitors. He also studies the role of the built environment as a determinant of physical activity and health, at the community level. In his spare time he enjoys hiking, bicycling, and swimming.

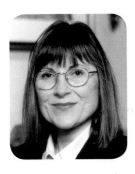

Janet Buckworth, PhD, FACSM, is an associate professor of exercise science at The Ohio State University and part of the Health and Exercise Behavior Research Group. Her research areas are exercise adherence and the psychobiology of exercise, mental health, and obesity. Dr. Buckworth coordinates the undergraduate program in exercise science and works with various campus groups on exercise and weight management. She directed a campus wellness program before earning her PhD in exercise psychology at the University of Georgia. She is the coauthor of *Exercise Psychology* with Dr. Rod Dishman and a fellow of the American College of Sports Medicine.

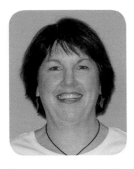

Sue Carver, ATC, MPT, CMT, is currently co-owner and practicing clinician at A World of Difference Therapy Services, an outpatient physical therapy clinic in Little Rock, Arkansas. She has been a licensed physical therapist since 1987 and has been practicing in Little Rock since 1989. She received her National Athletic Trainers certification in 1978. She served as the women's athletic trainer at the University of Tennessee at Knoxville from 1978 to 1982. In 1984 Ms. Carver was a volunteer athletic trainer at the U.S. Olympic Training Center in Colorado Springs. She was selected to work at the National Sports Festival VI in Baton Rouge in 1985 and the U.S. Olympic Track and Field Trials in Indianapolis in 1988. She was a volunteer trainer for track and field at the 1996 Summer Olympic Games in Atlanta.

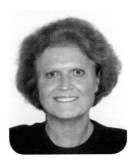

JoAnn M. Eickhoff-Shemek, PhD, FACSM, FAWHP, is a professor and the coordinator of the undergraduate exercise science program at the University of South Florida in Tampa. At her former institution, the University of Nebraska at Omaha, she developed and coordinated a master's degree program in health and fitness management and received the College of Education's Outstanding Teaching Award. Dr. Eickhoff-Shemek is the lead author of a groundbreaking, comprehensive textbook titled *Risk Management for Health/Fitness Professionals: Legal Issues and Strategies*. Published by Lippincott Williams & Wilkins, this is the first textbook to address the law, legal liability, and risk management principles designed specifically for exercise science and health/fitness students and professionals. For 10 years (2001-2011), Dr. Eickhoff-Shemek served as an associate editor and the legal columnist for *ACSM's Health & Fitness Journal*. Prior to becoming a full-time academician in 1994, she worked as a health/fitness manager in various settings for nearly 20 years. Dr. Eickhoff-Shemek is an active member of professional organizations having served in numerous elected and appointed leadership positions. She is an ACSM certified health/fitness director, exercise test technologist, and health fitness specialist and is a fellow of the ACSM and the former AWHP. She received her PhD at the University of Nebraska-Lincoln in 1995.

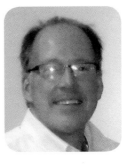

Avery D. Faigenbaum, EdD, CSCS, FACSM, is a full professor in the department of health and exercise science at the College of New Jersey at Ewing, New Jersey. He is a fellow of the American College of Sports Medicine and lectures nationally and internationally to health and fitness organizations. He is the author of over 150 scholarly publications, 30 book chapters, and eight books including *Youth Strength Training*. As an active researcher and practitioner in the field of pediatric exercise science, he continues to develop successful strength and conditioning programs for children and adolescents.

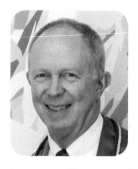

Ralph La Forge, MS, is a clinical lipid specialist and managing director of the Duke lipid disorder and disease management training program at Duke University Medical Center, Division of Endocrinology, Metabolism and Nutrition. He has worked for 29 years in clinical cardiology and endocrinology and as an instructor of exercise physiology and psychobiology at the University of California at San Diego. He is currently a faculty member of the Center for Complementary Medicine and Alternative Therapies at the University of North Carolina at Chapel Hill.

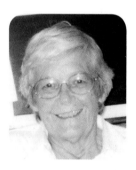

Jean Lewis received her doctorate in education (physical education with an emphasis in exercise physiology) from the University of Tennessee at Knoxville, where she is now a professor emeritus. She was involved in the establishment of undergraduate major concentrations in physical fitness and exercise physiology and has also developed courses in applied anatomy, applied kinesiology, and weight control, fitness, and exercise. Dr. Lewis was known for innovative teaching methods, which helped physical education majors understand how to apply kinesiological concepts. Recently retired, she misses the students and teaching, but is enjoying working in her garden and workshop.

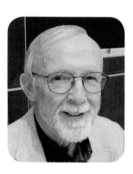

Wendell Liemohn received his BA from Wartburg College in Waverly, Iowa, and his MA from the University of Iowa at Iowa City. After coaching and teaching on the collegiate level, he returned to the University of Iowa and completed his PhD. He was on the faculty of Indiana University for 7 years, where his research centered on psychomotor functioning in special populations. In 1978 he accepted a position as professor at the University of Tennessee. At Tennessee he started the graduate specialization in biomechanics and sports medicine. He is a former president of the Research Consortium for AAHPERD and is a fellow of ACSM and in the American Academy of Kinesiology and Physical Education. His research in sports medicine relates to flexibility and low-back functioning, and he authored the book *Exercise Prescription and the Back* (McGraw-Hill Medical Publishing, 2000). He retired from teaching in January 2005; however, he is still doing research on core stability.

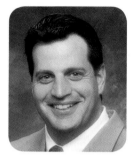

Kyle J. McInnis, ScD, is professor and chair in the department of exercise and health sciences at the University of Massachusetts in Boston. Dr. McInnis is an experienced researcher and practitioner in the area of health/fitness and chronic disease prevention. He is a Fellow of the American College of Sports Medicine (ACSM) and a senior coeditor of the *ACSM's Health and Fitness Facilities Standards and Guidelines, Fourth Edition.* He resides in New Hampshire with his wife, Susan, and their three children, Brendan, Riley, and Shane.

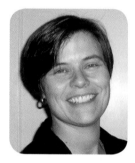

Clare E. Milner, PhD, FACSM, is an associate professor in the department of kinesiology, recreation, and sport studies at the University of Tennessee Knoxville. Her research interests are in the biomechanics of lower-extremity injury, injury prevention, and rehabilitation. She focuses on overuse injuries in runners, knee injuries in recreationally active women, and walking after knee replacement. Dr. Milner teaches undergraduate and graduate classes in applied anatomy and biomechanics. She is a fellow of the American College of Sports Medicine.

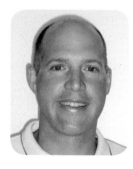

Michael Shipe, PhD, RCEP, is an assistant professor of exercise science and the department chair in the health, physical education, and sport science department at Carson Newman College in Jefferson City, Tennessee. He attained his registered clinical exercise physiologist certification in 1999. Mr. Shipe served as the fitness director for the Blount Memorial Wellness Center from 1997 to 2001. He was director of the medical fitness and cardiac rehabilitation programs at Blount Memorial Hospital from 2002 to 2004.